SCIENCE AND MEDICINE
IN SPORT

DEDICATION

To Noelene, Robyn and Val, who have
continued to support us very strongly,
both personally and professionally.

SCIENCE AND MEDICINE IN SPORT

EDITOR-IN-CHIEF

John Bloomfield

Professor, Department of Human Movement
University of Western Australia

EDITOR

Peter A. Fricker

Director of Medical Services, Department of Sports Medicine
Australian Institute of Sport

EDITOR

Kenneth D. Fitch

Medical Consultant, Department of Human Movement
University of Western Australia
Visiting Fellow
Australian Institute of Sport

SECOND EDITION

b

**Blackwell
Science**

© 1992, 1995 by
Blackwell Science Pty Ltd
Editorial Offices:
54 University Street, Carlton
  Victoria 3053, Australia
Osney Mead, Oxford OX2 0EL
25 John Street, London WC1N 2BL
23 Ainslie Place, Edinburgh EH3 6AJ
238 Main Street, Cambridge
  Massachusetts 02142, USA

Other Editorial Offices:
Arnette Blackwell SA
  1, rue de Lille, 75007 Paris
  France

Blackwell Wissenschafts-Verlag GmbH
  Kurfürstendamm 57
  10707 Berlin, Germany

  Feldgasse 13, A-1238 Wien
  Austria

First published 1992
Reprinted with corrections 1992
Second edition published 1995

Typeset by Solo Typesetting, Adelaide
Printed in Singapore

DISTRIBUTORS
Blackwell Science Pty Ltd
54 University Street
Carlton, Victoria 3053, Australia
(*Orders*: Tel: 03 9347 0300
          Fax: 03 9349 3016)

North America
  Blackwell Science, Inc.
  238 Main Street
  Cambridge, MA 02142
  (*Orders*: Tel: 800 215-1000
                  617 876-7000
          Fax: 617 492-5263)

United Kingdom
  Marston Book Services Ltd
  PO Box 87
  Oxford OX2 0DT
  (*Orders*: Tel: 01865 791155
          Fax: 01865 791927
          Telex: 837515)

Cataloguing-in-Publication Data

Science and medicine in sport.

  2nd ed.
  Bibliography.
  Includes index.
  ISBN 0 86793 321 6.

  1. Sports medicine. 2. Sports sciences.
  I. Bloomfield, John, 1932– .
  II. Fricker, Peter, 1950– .
  III. Fitch, K. D. (Kenneth D.), 1932– .
  IV. Title: Textbook of science and medicine
  in sport.

CONTENTS

SECTION 5

SPECIAL CONSIDERATIONS IN SPORTS MEDICINE 477

EDITORS

PROFESSOR JOHN BLOOMFIELD AM MSc PhD DipPE FACHPER FASMF CBiol FIBiol FAIBiol, is a former national champion sportsman, a former high-level coach and currently an academic at the University of Western Australia. He has been Chairman of the Australian Institute of Sport, the Australian Sports Science Council and the Australian Sports Medicine Federation, and has written two government reports and numerous papers in the field of sport and sports science. Professor Bloomfield is also the author of one book and co-author of two others.

ADJUNCT PROFESSOR PETER FRICKER OAM MB BS FASMF FACSM FACSP, is currently Director of Medical Services at the Australian Institute of Sport and has been a medical officer of the Commonwealth and Olympic Games teams in 1986, 1988, 1990, 1992 and 1994. He is first a practising sports physician but is also an active researcher, having published widely in the field of sports medicine.

ADJUNCT PROFESSOR KEN FITCH AM MB BS MD FRACGP FACRM FASMF FACSP, is a practising sports physician with appointments at various institutions throughout Australia. He is currently Chairman of the Medical Commission of the Australian Olympic Committee and the Oceania National Olympic Committees, as well as being a member of the Medical Commission of the International Olympic Committee. He has also been the Senior Medical Director of the Australian Olympic Games teams in 1976, 1980 and 1984 and has published widely in the field of sports medicine.

LIST OF AUTHORS

T. R. Ackland MPE PhD   Senior Lecturer, Department of Human Movement, The University of Western Australia.

I. F. Anderson MB BS FRACR   Radiologist, Sports X-ray, North Sydney Orthopaedic and Sports Medicine Centre.

J. Bloomfield AM MSc PhD DipPE FACHPER FASMF CBiol FIBiol FAIBiol   Professor, Department of Human Movement, The University of Western Australia.

J. W. Bond BEd MA DipPE TSTC, Dip Clin Hyp   Head, Department of Sport Psychology, Australian Institute of Sport.

J. A. Booth MB BS FRACP DDU   Physician, Nuclear Medicine and Diagnostic Ultrasound, John James Memorial Hospital, Canberra.

J. R. Brotherhood MB BS   Research Medical Officer, National Institute of Occupational Health and Safety and Senior Lecturer, Department of Occupational Medicine, University of Sydney.

L. Burke BSc GradDipDiet PhD   Head of Sports Nutrition Program, Australian Institute of Sport.

R. J. Carbon MB BS DipSptMed FACSP   Sports Physician, Royal London Hospital, and British Olympic Medical Centre, Northwick Park Hospital.

D. J. Chisholm MB BS FRACP   Professor of Endocrinology, University of New South Wales and Head, Metabolic Division, Garvan Institute of Medical Research, St Vincents Hospital, Sydney.

B. Cooper DRM DCRT   Massage and Acupuncture Therapist, Department of Sports Medicine, Australian Institute of Sport.

K. J. Crichton MB BS Grad DipSptSc FACSP FASMF   Sports Physician, North Sydney Orthopaedic and Sports Medicine Centre, Crows Nest and Sydney Sports Medicine Centre, Olympic Park, Homebush Bay.

V. Deakin BSc DipT GradDipNutrandDiet MDAA   Sports Dietitian, ACT Academy of Sport, Canberra, Lecturer, University of Canberra.

B. C. Elliott MEd PhD DipPE FACHPER FAIBiol FASMF   Professor, Department of Human Movement, The University of Western Australia.

K. E. Fallon MB BS MEx&SpSc FRACGP FACSP   Sports Physician, Department of Sports Medicine, Australian Institute of Sport, and Senior Lecturer in Sports Medicine, University of Canberra.

K. D. Fitch AM MB BS MD FRACGP FACRM FACSM FASMF   Adjunct Professor, Department of Human Movement, University of Western Australia and Physician and Head, Sports Injuries Clinic, Royal Perth Rehabilitation Hospital.

J. P. Fricker BDS MDSc GradDipAdultEd FRACDS   Senior Clinical Associate, Westmead Dental School, Visiting Lecturer, University of Canberra and Consultant, Australian Institute of Sport.

P. A. Fricker OAM MB BS FASMF FACSM FACSP   Director of Medical Services, Department of Sports Medicine, Australian Institute of Sport and Adjunct Professor of Sports Medicine, University of Canberra.

A. P. Garnham MB BS Dip RACOG FACSP   Sports Physician, Alphington Sports Medicine Clinic, Northcote, Victoria.

P. N. Gilchrist MB BS FRANZCP DipPsychother   Clinical Director, Weight Disorder Unit, Flinders Medical Centre, Adelaide.

A. M. D. Gordon MA MEd PhD DipPE DipEd   Senior Lecturer, Department of Human Movement, The University of Western Australia.

A. B. Gray Dip Ed Dip T BSc PhD   Lecturer, Faculty of Nursing and Health Sciences, Griffith University, Queensland.

J. R. Grove MA PhD Senior Lecturer, Department of Human Movement, The University of Western Australia.

A. G. Hahn BPE PhD DipPE HDipTch Senior Physiologist, Department of Physiology and Applied Nutrition, Australian Institute of Sport.

S. P. Haynes FILMS Chief Executive, Australian Sports Drug Agency, Canberra.

B. E. F. Hockings MB BS MD FRACP Consultant Cardiologist, Royal Perth Hospital.

G. Hoy MB BS FRACS FASMF FACSP Orthopaedic Surgeon, Melbourne Orthopaedic Group, Melbourne.

W. Johnson MB BS FRACS FACS FRCS Consultant Surgeon, Alfred Hospital, Melbourne.

J. J. Kellett MB BS BHMS DipSptMed FACSP Sports Physician, Canberra.

R. N. Marshall MSc PhD Senior Lecturer, Department of Human Movement, The University of Western Australia.

K. F. Maguire MB BS BMedSc FRACP FASMF FACSP Sports Physician, Perth Orthopaedic and Sports Medicine Centre.

W. A. McDonald BSc MB BS FACSP Sports Physician, Department of Sports Medicine, Australian Institute of Sport.

B. P. Miller BEd MA Consultant Sports Psychologist, British Olympic Association, London.

A. R. Morton MSc EdD DipPE FACSM FASMF FACHPER CBiol FIBiol FAIBiol Professor, Department of Human Movement, The University of Western Australia.

B. W. Oakes MB BS MD FASMF Senior Lecturer, Department of Anatomy, Monash University and Director, Sports Medicine Centres of Victoria.

M. L. O'Neill BDS Consultant Dental Surgeon, Department of Sports Medicine, Australian Institute of Sport.

C. R. Purdam DipPhty GradDipSptPhysio FASMF Head Physiotherapist, Department of Sports Medicine, Australian Institute of Sport.

F. S. Pyke MEd PhD DipPE FACHPER Executive Director, Victorian Institute of Sport.

D. B. Pyne MApp Sc PhD Sports Physiologist, Department of Physiology and Applied Nutrition, Australian Institute of Sport.

R. A. Reid MB BS FACSP FASMF DipSptMed Sports Physician, Canberra.

B. G. Sando OAM MB BS FRACGP FASMF Sports Physician, Sportscare, Adelaide.

J. R. Sutton MB BS DSc FRACP FACSP Professor and Head, Department of Biological Sciences, Cumberland College, University of Sydney.

A. S. Watson MB BS FASMF GradDipSptSc FACSP Director, Narrabeen Sports Medicine Centre, Sydney.

G. A. Wood MSc PhD DipEd DipPE Associate Professor, Department of Human Movement, The University of Western Australia.

SPECIAL CONTRIBUTORS

Dr J. A. Atha, Loughborough University of Technology, UK.

Dr G. Bower, Nuclear Physician, WA.

Dr P. D. Brukner, Sports Physician, Olympic Park Sports Medicine Centre, Vic.

Dr A. B. Corrigan, (Retired), Dee Why, NSW.

Dr C. Danta, Royal Canberra Hospital, ACT.

Mr B. C. Edwards, Mount Hospital Medical Centre, WA.

Prof. K. B. Fields, Moses Centre Memorial Hospital, Greensboro, USA.

Dr J. H. Green, University of Leeds, UK.

Dr P. T. Keenan, Mount Hospital Medical Centre, WA.

Ms K. King, Mount Hospital Medical Centre, WA.

Mr S. R. Lawrence, Western Australian Institute of Sport, WA.

Dr L. Mackinnon, University of Queensland, Qld.

Prof. C. A. Michaels AM, University of Western Australia, WA.

Dr J. Orchard, Sports Physician, NSW.

Dr R. L. Prince, University of Western Australia, WA.

Dr P. T. Pullen, Mount Hospital Medical Centre, WA.

Dr N. Roydhouse, St Michaels Clinic, Auckland, N.Z.

Dr R. Smith, Australian Institute of Sport, ACT.

Dr P. F. Soh, Private Practitioner, WA.

Prof. J. E. Taunton, Alan McGavin Sports Medicine Centre, UBC, Canada.

Mr D. McA. Tumilty, Physiologist, Australian Institute of Sport, ACT.

Dr T. A. Welborn, Sir Charles Gairdner Hospital, WA.

Dr S. White, Olympic Park Sports Medicine Centre, Vic.

Prof. C. Williams, Loughborough University of Technology, UK.

Dr J. G. P. Williams, Bon Secours Hospital, Beaconsfield, UK.

Prof. J. H. Wilmore, University of Texas, USA.

Dr G. J. Wilson, New England University, NSW.

PREFACE TO FIRST EDITION

The fields of sports science and sports medicine are relatively new developments in biological science and medicine and during the past two decades a large body of scientific knowledge has been gathered to cater for the increasing number of people who are taking part in competitive sport. In fact it has been recently estimated that Westernized countries have between 25 and 30% of their populations actively competing in a wide variety of sports. The age range of the competitors has also been greatly extended, so that we now have very young as well as older athletes in regular training and competition.

Because many humans are competitive and strive for excellence, the amateur training methods used in the past are no longer adequate for them, so they seek scientific information from the various professionals involved in sport to help them improve their performance. This has led to the rapid development of a new group of professionals whose expertise is widely sought in the fields of coaching, sports science and sports medicine.

This book has been developed because of demands for more applied information from coaches, sports scientists, medical doctors and other allied health professionals in the above areas. As well as serving this purpose, it has also been designed as a textbook for a 1 year course for various professionals specializing in sports science and sports medicine.

Science and Medicine in Sport has been divided into five sections, the first three of which are specifically related to sports science. They incorporate functional anatomy and biomechanics, the physiology of training and applied nutrition, as well as sports psychology and performance enhancement. The fourth section, by far the largest in the book, comprises the area of sports medicine. Rather than dealing only with injuries, it consists of a detailed coverage of the mechanisms of injury, repair and healing, principles of treatment and imagery in sports medicine and then covers in detail various sports injuries to all regions of the body. The fifth and final section deals with areas which need to be given special consideration in sports medicine. These include children in sport, the female athlete, the disabled athlete, aquatic sports, doping and the problems of the asthmatic, epileptic and diabetic athlete.

In the past there has not been a close relationship in the application of science and medicine to sport, despite the fact that they are inextricably linked. It has therefore been a definite policy of ours to integrate the two areas as much as possible and readers will notice that there is frequent cross-referencing in many places in the text.

Because the medical profession is now becoming more aware of the relatively new area of prevention, the authors have suggested various preventive measures wherever possible. Where it is not possible to fully rehabilitate patients with certain serious injuries or medical conditions, the alleviation of their problems using various aids and devices has also been discussed, so that these athletes will at least be able to continue in sport at one level or another.

The book has been written by 39 highly-qualified

Australian authors who are all intimately connected with professional or high-level amateur athletes as well as average performers. They have each been chosen because of their special expertise in the various areas of sports science and medicine. The authors have also been supported by 22 additional contributors who have added some very specialized information to various chapters and we would like to formally thank them for their assistance.

All the chapters were sent out for peer review and over 30 highly-qualified specialists have vetted the contributions. The most pleasing feature of this process has been the reviewers' endorsement of the material in the text, as only minor modifications have been necessary.

We would like to sincerely thank all the authors who contributed to this work. They were under the constraints of space for both text and illustrative material and also had to conform to rigid editorial guide-lines. They did this with good grace and in a very co-operative fashion.

Finally, there are several people who have been extremely helpful in the preparation of this book. Mark Robertson, the Managing Director of Blackwell Scientific Publications (Australia) Pty Ltd has been of great assistance since the project commenced, while Aileen Boyd-Squires and Penny Bowers have been most helpful. At the Australian Institute of Sport, Dr Ross Smith and Mrs Shirley Steer have given great support, while Joan Williams at The University of Western Australia has been a tower of strength with the typing and organization of the vast majority of the manuscript. We are also grateful to Noelene Bloomfield for her constructively critical reading of the manuscript during the final stages of the preparation of the book.

John Bloomfield
Peter A. Fricker
Kenneth D. Fitch
Editors

PREFACE TO SECOND EDITION

After the international success of *Science and Medicine in Sport* during its first 2 years of sales, a decision was made to update all chapters of the book and expand 20 of them, to include significant new research. Two new chapters were added to the sports medicine section, providing a comprehensive coverage of the field both in breadth and in depth.

Five new authors have contributed to this edition, and all the expanded and new chapters have been peer reviewed. Therefore a total of 43 authors and 28 special contributors have been responsible for the content.

We would like to thank all the authors, the special contributors and reviewers who have assisted in making this second edition a highly specialized and authoritative work. Again they were constrained by space for both text and illustrative material, as well as having to conform to strict editorial guidelines.

Finally, there are many people who helped to prepare this edition and it is only fitting that we thank them for their contribution. Aileen Boyd-Squires, the Publishing Director of Blackwell Science has been of enormous assistance since the project commenced, and Penny Bowers, Marnie Hannagan and Alice King have also contributed greatly. More recently at the Australian Institute of Sport, Mrs Shirley Steer has again given great support. From the Department of Human Movement of The University of Western Australia, Paul Ricketts and Roger Dickinson have been of assistance with the artwork, while Kerry Langton and Pat Stevenson were most helpful with various aspects of the preparation of the manuscript. A special note of thanks must go to Dianne Newton who so capably typed and organized the entire manuscript. We are again grateful to Noelene Bloomfield for her constructive reading of various parts of the manuscript.

John Bloomfield
Peter A. Fricker
Kenneth D. Fitch
Editors

ACKNOWLEDGEMENTS

The support of the Australian Sports Commission with the first edition of this book is gratefully acknowledged; it was their grant which enabled the illustrations to be of such high quality from the beginning. In the second edition, the Developmental Unit for Instructional Technology of The University of Western Australia significantly improved several key figures and photographs in the text, while the secretarial services of the Department of Human Movement of The University of Western Australia have been invaluable in the completion of this edition.

SECTION 1

THE ANATOMY AND BIOMECHANICS
OF SPORT PERFORMANCE

CHAPTER 1

APPLIED ANATOMY

T. R. Ackland and J. Bloomfield

Human anatomy does not represent the end product of a perfectly designed structure but rather, continues to be characterized by changes in response to various environmental stresses. Many structural changes have been required for an essentially ape-like creature with a quadrupedal form of locomotion to develop the anatomy and bipedal gait of the modern human. The most important evolutionary changes which have affected locomotion have been as follows:

- An upward shift in the centre of gravity to a less stable position
- A shortening and broadening of the pelvis to permit the centre of gravity to remain within the base of support
- Elongation of the legs as the major propulsive limbs
- A change in foot function from semi-support and grasping to one of specialized weight-bearing and resilience
- An S-shaped vertebral column instead of the ape-like C-shaped curve
- A transference of the foramen magnum towards the base of the skull more directly above the vertebral column, thereby reducing the torque about the neck region

It should be noted that although humans stand on two legs, their skeleton was originally designed for four and that incomplete evolution has left several weaknesses with which we must contend. An ana-

tomical structure best described as a compromise system produces areas of weakness, particularly within the feet, knee joints, abdominal wall, lumbar vertebrae and neck regions, which are often affected by stress-related activities.

These weaknesses are far outweighed by the positive results of evolution, as the human body has successfully developed the capability to perform a wide variety of motor tasks. None of these skills individually can compete with the specialized expertise exhibited by various animals in speed, agility or strength, but humans are capable of successfully coping with the physical environment because of their versatility.

Clearly, the strong relationship between structure and function has been demonstrated throughout human evolution. Until recently, however, documentation of the anatomical variability among the human species and the subsequent modification of human physical capacities to improve sports performance has received little systematic scientific scrutiny. The aim of this chapter is to review the body of knowledge in the field of applied anatomy and to demonstrate how its application can improve human performance in sport. It should be further noted that some physical capacities such as body proportions may not be altered; however, others such as body composition and strength may be modified easily over a short period of time. Furthermore, human physical capacities are often closely related and therefore physicians, coaches and sports scientists should be aware that modification of one parameter will invariably affect others. For example, body shape and composition are closely related, as are strength, power and speed.

BODY SHAPE

There have been many attempts by biological scientists in the last 100 years to place humans into various body types. Sheldon (1954) used a sample of 46 000 males to identify three basic builds: the endomorph or obese individual; the mesomorph or muscular type; and the ectomorph, who is characterized by a high degree of linearity. Each of these components was rated on a seven-point scale, which indicated the degree of dominance of the above characteristics. To describe each body type, three numbers were given in order to denote the rating in endomorphy, mesomorphy and ectomorphy, respectively (Fig. 1.1). For example, a somatotype rating of 6–1–1 or 7–2–1 indicates dominance in the endomorphic component, so that such individuals would be classified as endomorphs. Similarly, a rating of 2–7–1 would denote primary mesomorphy, while 1–2–7 would rate the subject as a primary ectomorph. Most people, however,

demonstrate a combination of two physique types rather than a single dominance.

In all, Sheldon (1954) isolated 88 body types which can be used for comparative purposes. Heath and Carter (Carter 1975) have refined the Sheldon system by giving it a high degree of objectivity and by extending the original seven-point scale to nine in ectomorphy and mesomorphy, and to 12 in endomorphy. Rather than assessing only photographs of the subject, the following direct anthropometric measurements are now made: standing height, body mass, four skinfolds, two limb girths and two bone widths. These measurements are taken and then placed on a rating chart to determine the somatotype of each subject. Photographs can also be taken to further refine the technique.

Significance of Body Shape for Athletic Performance

Body shape plays an important role in the self-selection of individuals for competitive sport. There

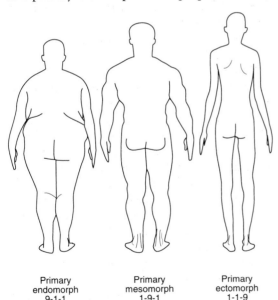

Fig. 1.1 The three basic physique types (Bloomfield *et al.* 1994).

Primary endomorph 9-1-1   Primary mesomorph 1-9-1   Primary ectomorph 1-1-9

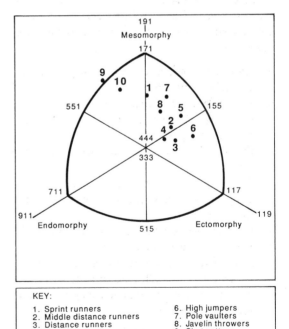

KEY:
1. Sprint runners
2. Middle distance runners
3. Distance runners
4. Marathon runners
5. Long jumpers
6. High jumpers
7. Pole vaulters
8. Javelin throwers
9. Shot putters
10. Discus throwers

Fig. 1.2 A somatotype distribution of Olympic track and field athletes.

is also a considerable body of information in the sports science literature on the suitability of various types not only to particular sports, but also to specific events or positions within those sports. Because many factors are involved in the physical make-up of a champion sportsman or woman, there is not going to be one perfect body shape for a particular sport or event within that sport. However, there will be a small range of shapes which cluster around the mean of each group. Figure 1.2 illustrates the distribution on the somatochart of Olympic track and field athletes, with the specific numbers on the chart showing the mean somatotype of the various specialists within that sport.

Exceptions to the Standard Body Shapes

It is not uncommon to find athletes at the state or national level and occasionally at the international level, whose physiques do not appear to be suited to a sport or a specialized event within a sport. One must decide when not to interfere with an individual's body build, and Peter Snell from New Zealand provides a good example of this phenomenon. Snell was an outstanding middle distance runner, winning gold medals at Tokyo in 1964 for the 800 and 1500 m events despite the fact that his muscular physique appeared more suited to the 200 m distance. However, with a $\dot{V}_{O_2max}$ of 5.502 L·min^{-1} (73.3 mL·min^{-1}·kg^{-1}) Snell possessed the circulatory capacity to successfully endure the middle distance events (Pyke & Watson 1978) even though he was carrying more body mass than his fellow competitors (Fig. 1.3).

More recently, the marathon performances of Robert De Castella from Australia have interested sports scientists. Between 1981 and 1986 De Castella won six international marathons including the World championship in 1983, despite being approximately 5 cm taller than other elite runners and 10–12 kg greater in body mass (R. D. Telford personal communication). However, with a $\dot{V}_{O_2max}$ of 83 mL·min^{-1}·kg^{-1} he possessed the endurance capacity needed for the marathon event.

When one carefully examines participants in every sport, it is possible to find 'exceptions to the rule'

because of the many factors which make up a championship performance.

It is important to know the sports for which certain body shapes are best suited. Expert guidance on diet and intensive exercise can assist athletes to partially modify their somatotype within the limits of his or her genetic make-up. If the individual is within a standard deviation of the mean for a particular group, little modification is needed, whereas those athletes outside it need a special programme to assist them to move closer to the mean of their group. Previous research has shown that somatotypes tend to change very little throughout life and, as a result, adult somatotypes can

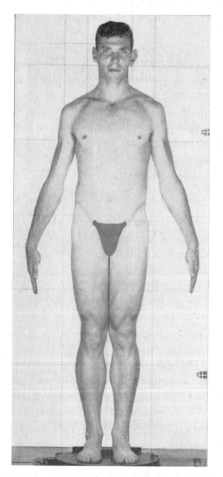

Fig. 1.3 An exception to the standard body type of a world champion 1500 m runner (courtesy of Tanner 1964).

4

be predicted with some accuracy during pre-adolescence.

BODY COMPOSITION

It is obvious that human body shape and composition are very closely related. The relative proportions of bone, muscle and fat determine the shape and composition of each individual, fat being the variable which can be modified most easily. A methodology which very accurately monitors changes in human body composition, yet remains economically viable, has not yet been developed.

Body Composition Assessment

WEIGHT/HEIGHT INDICES

In previous epidemiological studies a significant correlation between weight/height indices and body composition standards has been reported. This does not imply, however, that they can be used on an individual basis to predict body composition. Unfortunately, the widespread adoption of measures such as the Body Mass Index and Ponderal Index has often been based on practical and economic criteria without regard to test validity.

DENSITOMETRY

In anatomical terms, and for practical purposes, the body can be divided into a simple two-compartment system. The first compartment is the fat-free mass or lean body mass (LBM) which includes bone, muscle, connective tissue and organs, while the second component is fat mass (FM). The relative amounts of each of these compartments may be estimated by weighing the individual in water to determine the density of the body. Densitometry is thus used as an indirect method for estimating per cent fat by assuming that the FM has a uniform density of 0.90 g·mL^{-1} and LBM a density of 1.10 g·mL^{-1}. It is important to understand that body-weight itself provides no real indication of tissue composition as is illustrated in the following example.

Subject A in Fig. 1.4 is composed of a high proportion of LBM with a total body mass of 90 kg and a density of 1.082 g·mL^{-1}. The LBM is com-

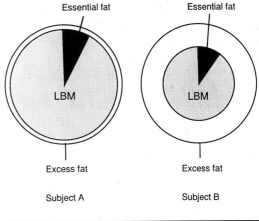

LBM	86 kg	LBM	63 kg
FM		FM	
Essential fat	2 kg	Essential fat	2 kg
Excess fat	2 kg	Excess fat	25 kg
Total Body Mass	90 kg	Total Body Mass	90 kg
Density 1.082 g·mL^{-1}		Density 1.035 g·mL^{-1}	

Fig. 1.4 Tissue composition for two individuals of similar body mass.

prised of bone, muscle, connective tissue and organs, but a certain proportion of fat is necessary to support normal function and is thus included in the inner circle. In subject B the inner circle encompasses tissue similar to A in density and composition but differs in mass by 23 kg. The outer circle circumscribes an accumulation of 25 kg of excess fat. The density of this 90 kg individual is 1.035 g·mL^{-1}.

In the past, coaches and sports scientists have considered body composition in terms of the percentage of body fat, on the assumptions that:

- The constituent tissues of LBM are in fixed proportions and that each has a constant density
- The density of fat is constant

However, research from the Brussels Cadaver Study (Martin *et al*. 1986) does not support these assumptions. It is now generally believed that the accurate measurement of body density should be used for monitoring change in the composition of an individual, rather than attempting to predict the proportion of body fat.

SKINFOLDS

The width of a compressed, double fold of skin plus the subcutaneous adipose tissue underneath it may be measured using a skinfold caliper at various standard sites on the body; however, measurement errors due to tester inaccuracy and poor site location sometimes lead to inaccurate results. In addition, five assumptions have traditionally been made when measuring skinfolds:

- That the skinfold is constantly compressible
- That skin thickness is a constant proportion of the skinfold
- That interindividual fat patterning is constant
- That fat represents a constant proportion of adipose tissue
- That the proportion of subcutaneous fat to internal fat is constant

The validity of these assumptions has been partially refuted by Martin *et al.* (1984) using data derived from the Brussels Cadaver Study.

Data from skinfold measurements have been used in a variety of ways to estimate body composition. It has been common for skinfold values to be included as independent variables in formulae which attempt to predict body mass proportions. These prediction strategies often used criteria derived from densitometry. Thus, the failings of both densitometry and skinfold methodologies are incorporated in these regression equations. These body composition prediction strategies are therefore of little scientific value and it is now commonly believed that the skinfold measures should be used directly for comparison without modification. Values from at least eight sites (two from the upper limb, four from the trunk and two from the lower limb) provide an adequately representative sample of the fat distribution and the logarithmic sum of these values may be compared across populations.

The O-Scale system (Ross & Ward 1984) provides a method of comparing individual skinfold results with a normative data base from more than 20 000 observations, categorized by age and gender. Individual adiposity ratings are determined from nine standard intervals (stanines), which provide divisions at the percentile equivalents of P4, 11, 23, 40, 60, 77, 89 and 96.

OTHER METHODS

As well as these methods of estimating FM and LBM, many other accurate chemical and electrical techniques have been developed to determine the relative amounts of lean and fat tissue, but they require costly and sophisticated equipment. Potassium 40 counting, helium dilution, isotope dilution, radiographic analysis, photon absorptiometry, ultrasound, computerized tomography and magnetic resonance imaging devices are beyond the scope of most laboratory budgets, but may in the future be employed to provide more accurate estimates of body composition.

Body Composition Requirements for Athletic Performance

A glut of information has become available on the body compositional requirements for various sports as it is often assumed that success not only demands a particular physique but also a certain ratio of LBM to FM. However, caution is required before there is wholesale adoption of this information, because of the manner in which the data were collected and treated. A lack of standardization of techniques within the field in the past, together with the use of a variety of data treatment strategies, has meant that the pooling of some of the results for profiling and comparative purposes cannot be done with accuracy. Bloomfield *et al.* (1994) have summarized the related literature and report values for the sum of skinfolds of various sport participants. However, without providing specific values for body composition components, the following examples illustrate the current understanding of the relationship between LBM/FM requirements and athletic performance.

- In contact football, backs generally possess a low proportion of FM (density = $1.072\,\mathrm{g \cdot mL^{-1}}$) while forwards may require a higher proportion of FM to increase their inertia and assist in the protection of skeletal structures from repeated impacts
- Class weight-lifters and wrestlers have almost no excess body fat, while the heavyweight performers require a high proportion of FM to

increase their inertia and provide greater stability while lifting

- Field games competitors in agility events such as jumping have minimal excess fat, whereas those who throw heavy implements possess the most

Body composition can be altered by diet, exercise or a combination of both, which will affect the relative proportions of bone, muscle and fat in the individual. These concepts are discussed in more detail in Chapter 5. The exercise programme emphasis towards either endurance or strength training will determine which of these components is altered most. Increased knowledge of the degree of modification which can be safely made will ultimately assist the coach to improve the performance of athletes.

PROPORTIONALITY

Even the casual observer will have noted that human body proportions vary greatly from person to person. These variations play an important part in the self-selection process for various sports and events, and it is obvious that there is little that can be done to alter many body proportions, especially extremity lengths. It is possible in many sports, however, for the coach to modify techniques successfully to suit individuals whose proportions are less advantageous from a mechanical viewpoint than those of their opponents.

Kinanthropometric Assessment

Human size and proportions are assessed by the use of anthropometry. The most common anthropometric measures are those which assess the lengths, widths, girths and volumes of body segments based on conventional landmarks which employ precision instruments as described in detail by Cameron (1978). Anthropometric variables are often expressed as indices to allow a more meaningful description of physique to be made. The relationship of the length of the lower leg to the thigh, or the crural index, can be calculated in the following way:

$$\text{crural index} = \frac{\text{foreleg length} \times 100}{\text{thigh length}}$$

Similarly, the brachial index, which demonstrates the length of the forearm with respect to the arm, may be calculated:

$$\text{brachial index} = \frac{\text{forearm length} \times 100}{\text{arm length}}$$

When various anthropometric measures have been taken and the indices computed, it is possible for individuals to be compared with elite competitors in the same sports or events. This could help them in their selection of a sport or event, which they may pursue seriously in the future.

Proportionality Applied to Sport Performance

The basic laws of physics as they relate to leverage, play an important part in sport. The length of bones and insertion points of muscles can either be an advantage or a disadvantage depending on the physical demands of the sport in which the individual competes.

Bone lengths are absolute when the individual has reached full maturity and cannot be altered by training. Similarly, the tendinous insertion of muscles and the distance from the joint axis determine the mechanical advantage of the lever system. These aspects of proportionality, together with the muscle fibre composition, combine to determine an athlete's propensity for power, strength or endurance events.

Proportionality Characteristics of Athletes

When comparing proportions of athletes it is important to be aware of the basic differences which exist between the various races. Africans and African Americans generally have longer extremities and shorter trunks than Europeans, while Asians have shorter legs and longer trunks. This does not mean that some Europeans might not have similar leg–trunk proportions to either of these groups, but it is only towards the ends of the range that they are similar. It is for this reason that certain sports are dominated by particular racial groups. For example, Europeans seem particularly well suited to swimming; Africans, especially the Nilotic people originally from north-eastern Africa, seem to be dominant in the game of basketball and excel in long distance running; while Asians appear to have an advantage in such sports as gymnastics, diving, weight-lifting and some martial arts because of their body proportions. It should be noted, however, that although they are important factors there are still a large number of physiological and psychological variables to be taken into consideration. See Chapters 4 and 7–9 for further details.

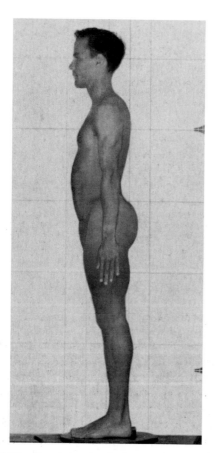

Fig. 1.5 This sprinter is of medium height with short legs. He also displays an anterior pelvic tilt and protruding buttocks (courtesy of Tanner 1964).

There are also large differences not only between sportsmen and women and the average person in the community, but also between individuals within the same sports. For example, a proportionality examination of sprint runners reveals that they are mostly of medium height with comparatively short muscular legs (Fig. 1.5). Their trunks are of normal length with an average crural index (Fig. 1.6). Dintiman (1974) found that high-level sprinters can execute 4.5–5.0 strides per second and that such rapid leg movements provide greater ground contact, allowing more propulsive force to be generated, and this is aided by the sprinter's short lower limb lever length. A shorter lever has a lower moment of inertia or resistance to movement than a longer lever and this concept is explained more fully in the kinetics section of Chapter 2.

Jumpers are another special group whose proportions play an important part in their performance. They are the tallest subgroup of all the track and field athletes with long legs and relatively short trunks for their height. They have a high crural index, suggesting that long forelegs in relation to thighs are a definite advantage in jumping. High-level open class wrestlers also have special proportions which greatly assist them in a combative sport. They have thick muscular bodies and short solid legs in comparison with their trunk lengths and a low crural index. This leg structure ensures a low centre of gravity, which is essential if one is to have a stable base of support while competing (Bloomfield 1979).

Another specialized group comprises high-level swimmers, who are heavier, taller and have longer trunks, shorter legs and larger hands and feet than lower level competitors. Even among top level swimmers there are special characteristics which differentiate them from one stroke to another. If a comparison is made between sprint swimmers and middle-distance swimmers, the differences are quite marked. For example, sprint swimmers have a higher brachial index than middle-distance swimmers because of their longer forearms and shorter upper arms. Sprinters have high crural indices which tend to give them a mechanical advantage for crawl-stroke kicking over middle-distance swimmers (Bloomfield & Sigerseth 1965).

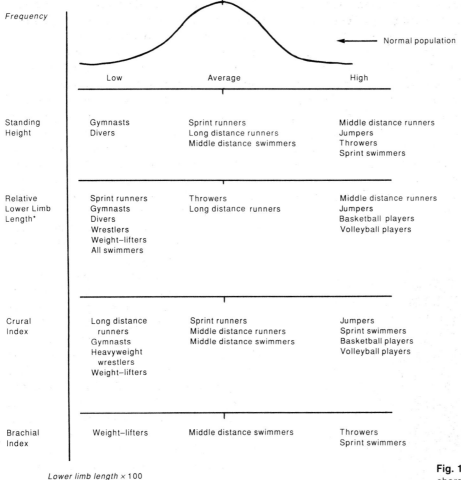

Fig. 1.6 Proportionality characteristics of Olympic athletes.

$$^*RLLL = \frac{Lower\ limb\ length \times 100}{standing\ height}$$

Individual Comparisons

One possible limitation of using raw anthropometric data for comparative purposes, whether on the same individual over time, or between groups, is being able to appreciate the magnitude of a linear or circumferential measure with respect to body size. A number of strategies have been proposed to overcome this limitation including the somatogram (Behnke & Wilmore 1974) and the Phantom (Ross et al. 1988), both of which are discussed in Bloomfield et al. (1994).

Body Modification

Except under extenuating circumstances, human proportions cannot be modified using a simple intervention programme, because the mature athlete's bone lengths are absolute and cannot be changed. As a matter of interest, some bodies have been modified either accidentally or by design. However, on both moral and ethical grounds, deliberate changes are not recommended under any circumstances.

Bloomfield et al. (1994) provide examples of

enforced growth plate compaction through heavy weight-bearing exercise by children. This has the effect of producing short, thick bones in the extremities and advantages the athlete in weight-lifting events. A further example is given whereby an athlete became stronger following the reinsertion of a ruptured tendon more distal to its original attachment point.

Technique Modification

The specific proportionality requirements for various athletic events clearly demonstrate the important role of this capacity in high-level performance. Human proportions cannot be modified in the same manner as other capacities and so remain a significant parameter in the process of self-selection into various sports and events. The coach or educator, however, may be able to modify the lever system via technique changes in order to minimize any adverse mechanical effect caused by an individual's body proportions. Such a strategy may be identified in the following examples and relates to the discussion on lever systems in Chapter 2.

- Swimmers with long extremities and relatively weak propulsive musculature may, in addition to increasing their strength, shorten the propulsive lever by flexing the forearm more than is normally recommended (Fig. 1.7)
- Tennis players of tall stature with long extremities and relatively weak musculature may be able to produce more powerful volleys by flexing the forearm during the stroke. Similarly, the player may adopt a double-handed technique for ground strokes which not only shortens the striking lever, but may also facilitate greater stability, an increased racquet velocity at impact and better technique to hit a top spin shot (Fig. 1.7)

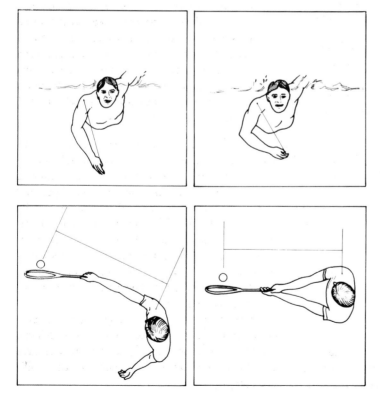

Fig. 1.7 Shortening the effective lever in the crawl-stroke and using a two-handed backhand in tennis.

- A golfer with long lower limbs should set up to the ball with a wider stance than a shorter limbed player, in order to prevent swaying laterally 'past the ball', which causes the club face to be slightly open at impact and can result in a push-slice being made

Proportionality is a self-selector for various sports and events and some athletes are born with proportions which are highly suited to some sports but not at all suited to others. If an athlete has many of the physical characteristics which are suitable for a particular sport, but lacks the leverage capacity to do this, then the intelligent coach can modify his or her technique to partially overcome this physical disadvantage.

POSTURE

Static posture may be defined as the relative arrangement of body segments and this arrangement indicates a state of muscular and skeletal balance within the body. 'Good posture' therefore, is a balanced state in which the supporting structures (bone, ligaments, muscle and other connective tissues) are protected against progressive deformity. It should be noted that a balanced state may be achieved with any arrangement of body segments; however, that which requires the least muscular effort or ligament strain is more efficient. A faulty relationship of body segments which increases the stress on supporting structures may then be termed 'poor posture'. We often think of good and poor standing postures but these principles also apply to other positions such as sitting and lying.

Furthermore, the coach and sports physician are also interested in this relative arrangement of body segments while the body is in motion or when performing a skill. This is known as dynamic posture, and a high correlation usually exists between good static and dynamic posture.

Postural Defects

At the beginning of this chapter several skeletal adaptations to bipedal locomotion were observed and resulting areas of anatomical weakness noted.

These anatomical compromises provide the potential for the development of poor posture, while the following factors actually cause postural defects. Several of these factors may be passed to successive generations through heredity and are as follows:

- *Injury* — when a bone, ligament or muscle is injured it is apt to weaken the support normally provided to the total framework. Therefore, as long as the condition is present, good posture may not be attainable
- *Disease* — diseases often weaken bones and muscles or cause joints to lose their strength thus upsetting posture. Examples of such diseases include arthritis and osteoporosis
- *Habit* — postural habits are acquired by repeating a body alignment on many occasions, such as leaning over a desk or slouching in a chair. Body segments held out of alignment for extended periods cause the surrounding musculature to rest in a lengthened or shortened position
- *Skeletal imbalance* — the most familiar imbalance of skeletal lengths is seen in the lower limbs and in extreme cases causes a lateral pelvic tilt and may result in the development of scoliosis. However, more subtle skeletal differences such as the location of the acetabulum and length of the clavicle provide equal potential for defective posture

Of further interest is the relationship between static postural defects and musculoskeletal injuries. Lorenzton (1988) reported in a study of injured runners, that 40% of them had a variety of postural defects, muscle weakness and imbalance, or decreased flexibility. Malalignment problems identified in this study included pronated or flat feet, poor leg–foot alignment, eversion of the calcaneus, high arches (pes cavas), knock knees (genu valgum), bow legs (genu varum) and leg length discrepancies accompanied by pelvic tilt.

These injuries can be partially eliminated with early screening and treatment of these defects. Astute observation and early action can often save an athlete from developing a chronic and debilitating injury.

Posture Assessment

Static posture is usually assessed subjectively in the standing position using a rating chart as a guide for the observers (Bloomfield *et al.* 1994), while more objective tests involving the use of medical imaging techniques may be employed to focus on a particular postural deformity. Instrumentation and methodologies for measuring dynamic posture are not generally available; however, these may eventually be developed in association with the biomechanical techniques of cinematography and electrogoniometry, which are fully discussed in Chapter 3.

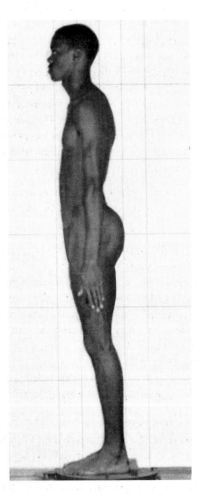

Fig. 1.8 This jumper has a similar hip and buttock posture to sprinters (courtesy of Tanner 1964).

Desirable Postures for Sports Performance

There are various postural types that are well suited to different sports and events, because the alignment of the bones and the muscles covering them give a mechanical advantage, with speed, power or balance (Bloomfield 1979). For example, people with inverted feet, or a 'pigeon-toed' gait, have excellent dynamic balance and possess above average agility. This characteristic is of great advantage to players in agility sports, such as tennis, squash, football (in specialized positions) and basketball. Individuals with lordosis or a 'sway back' and protruding buttocks, where anterior pelvic tilt (APT) is present, appear to have an advantage in sprint running, as this characteristic appears to assist them in the extension phase of the running stride (Fig. 1.5). This type of posture is also found in top level jumpers (Fig. 1.8) and many gymnasts.

Swimmers are another group who exhibit various postures which inherently assist them. Many good breast-stroke swimmers for example, have everted feet or 'duck feet', which give them a natural kicking advantage, while those with inverted feet have a definite advantage in backstroke, crawl-stroke and butterfly kicking.

Modification of Posture and Technique to Improve Performance

As discussed in the previous section, there are several postures which may be advantageous to top athletic performance. Therefore, there should be no attempt to modify these characteristics in any way, even though at first glance they may appear to be partially defective. Other postures, however, may be detrimental to performance, so that a strategy should be worked out to modify them.

A decision therefore must be made by the coach as to whether the athlete should undergo a modification programme or not. The following actions can be taken:

- The first approach should be to modify any *static* defects that may need correction, using a series of exercises which will stretch tight muscles and strengthen those which have become slack. This corrective programme should be undertaken if at all possible in pre- or early adolescence. In post-adolescence it will take longer, but reasonable results can still be obtained at this time if the programme is intensive enough

- The second action is to accentuate those postures which are known to be advantageous for various sports. This is particularly important for individuals who appear to have almost all of the other necessary physical capacities for optimal performance, but who lack the postural characteristics needed for highly specialized events. Bloomfield *et al.* (1994) provide examples in this regard to increase APT for sprint runners and to increase tibial torsion (inverted feet) for agility athletes. It should be stressed again that posture modification will only occur with an intense intervention programme taking place, often over several years

- *Dynamic* posture can also be changed with good skills coaching, and this has been done by enlightened coaches for the last half century in technique-oriented sports, such as track and field and swimming. These coaches know how to incorporate various postural positions into their athletes' techniques, such as tilting the pelvis, rounding the back, tucking in the chin, squaring the shoulders, everting the feet and so on. However, less attention has been paid to dynamic posture in individual and team sports where agility is an important factor in the game and more specialization in various positions is becoming necessary. Bloomfield *et al.* (1994) suggest that round-shouldered players have a natural advantage over square-shouldered players in collision sports. The latter are more prone to injury when running into rucks, mauls and packs; or for closed field running, where tacklers are able to hit the ball carrier with little notice

MUSCULAR STRENGTH AND POWER

Training to improve strength and power is now considered important for successful performance in many sports, not just for those in which muscular strength is the principal factor. These capacities are very important in agility sports, such as basketball, netball, football and gymnastics, but are equally important where the athlete has to propel an object or missile in sports, such as baseball or cricket and in various field events. This change in attitude has led to a proliferation of methods and equipment in an attempt to achieve maximum gains in these capacities. Muscular strength and power are two parameters which are easily modified and have a directly observable benefit on sports performance. A considerable proportion of this chapter, therefore, is devoted to the discussion of the factors which determine the status and trainability of these capacities.

With increased interest in strength and power training has also come a profusion of popular jargon, which has served to mystify and confuse many participants. For clarity in the following discussion, strength is defined as the amount of force a muscle can exert against a resistance in one maximal effort while muscular power is dependent on two interrelated factors, namely strength and contraction velocity, that is

$$power = force\ (strength) \times velocity$$
$$= \frac{force\ (strength) \times distance}{time}$$

Thus, muscular power may be developed by increasing the athlete's strength or speed of movement or both. Further, power training in either strength or speed should be specific to the skill and where possible, carried out in a similar posture to the event itself. In order to present this topic in a balanced way a brief review of muscle structure and function is warranted.

Muscle Structure and Function

There are three types of muscle within the body: smooth, cardiac and skeletal. Each has an individual and specific role in the maintenance of homeostasis and production of human movement. However, as strength and power generation are caused by skeletal muscle activity, the remainder of this section will focus on its structure and function alone.

With over 400 individual skeletal muscles comprising 40–50% of the total body mass, only 75 pairs are involved in controlling posture and producing gross movement. Each muscle is surrounded by a fascia of connective tissue called the epimysium, beneath which bundles of muscle fibres or fasciculi are surrounded by a second layer of connective tissue, the perimysium (Fig. 1.9). The fasciculus contains a number of muscle fibres, which are elongated cells with many nucleii. Surrounding the fibre is another layer of connective tissue, the endomysium as well as the cell membrane or sarcolemma. Inside each muscle fibre are numerous myofibrils, which resemble individual fine wires in an electrical cable. The myofibril appears striated or striped due to the repetitive pattern formed by the sarcomeres, which are joined in series and represent the contractile units of the skeletal muscle tissue.

An individual sarcomere, as shown in Fig. 1.9, is composed of many myofilaments, which are the contractile proteins actin and myosin. Actin proteins are the thinner filaments and are situated between the thicker myosin filaments. The alignment of filaments is presumed to be responsible for the alternative dark and light bands, which characterize skeletal muscle appearance. Each sarcomere

is delineated by a Z-line situated in the centre of the light I-band, which contains only actin filaments. The A-band is darker in appearance and consists of both actin and myosin filaments. A distinctly lighter band within the A-band, called the H-zone, represents an area of myosin filaments only. The H-zone will disappear when the muscle contracts, as the actin filaments slide into this region with muscle shortening.

The precise mechanism used to shorten the sarcomere is not fully understood; however, it is believed that when activated, the actin and myosin filaments slide past one another due to the action of cross-bridges extending from myosin to the actin proteins (causing the Z-lines to converge). Wilmore and Costill (1994) provide a description of the physiology of muscular contraction, which is beyond the scope of this chapter.

MUSCLE FIBRE TYPES

While the muscle fibre is seen as the basic structural unit of the system, the smallest functional unit is termed the motor unit. A motor unit consists of the motor nerve or α motor neuron plus all of the muscle fibres it innervates. A single α motor neuron may innervate as few as three muscle fibres in

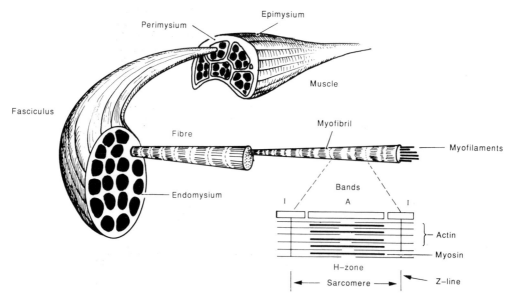

Fig. 1.9 The structure of human skeletal muscle. (Wilmore & Costill 1988; used with permission.)

regions where fine movement control is required, for example in muscles controlling eye movement, or as many as 800 muscle fibres in the larger muscles producing gross movements of the body. These nerves controlling the activation of muscle fibres also determine their physiological and endurance properties. Increases in muscular force production are neurally controlled by first increasing the firing rate of motor units, and second in the recruitment of additional units.

Two discrete categories of muscle fibre types have been identified based on their histochemical staining qualities as well as their physiological characteristics. The slow twitch (ST or Type I) type accounts for approximately 50% of normal human skeletal muscle fibres, which are characterized as possessing an aerobic endurance quality. The fast twitch (FT or Type II) fibre may be further divided into three categories based on their stained appearance as well as their propensity for recruitment. FT type 'a' (FTa or Type IIa) constitute about half of the FT muscle fibres, with the remainder predominantly apportioned to the FT 'b' (FTb or Type IIb). Only a very small number of FT 'c' (FTc

or Type IIc) have been identified. The FT fibres produce more force than ST fibres; however, they fatigue more rapidly. For this reason, ST fibres are preferentially recruited during low-intensity activities and as the muscle tension requirements increase, more motor units controlling FT fibres are activated (Wilmore & Costill 1994).

Endowment of the various muscle fibre types within skeletal muscle would presumably affect the performance capabilities of an athlete. At present the scientific evidence regarding the dominance of genetic versus training influences on muscle fibre composition is equivocal. Komi (1988) provides a summary of the relevant arguments and proposes that at the time of peak performance, the muscle fibre composition of an athlete is dependent upon both influences. Using needle biopsy and histochemical staining techniques, several studies have reported data for the fibre composition of various athletic groups, examples of which are shown in Fig. 1.10. Long distance runners, cyclists, rowers, orienteers and cross-country skiers possess a greater proportion of ST fibres compared with the normal population, whereas power athletes such as throwers,

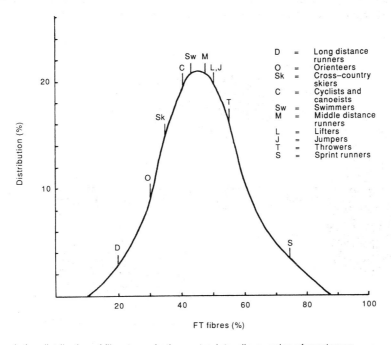

Fig. 1.10 The relative distribution of fibre types in the vastus lateralis muscles of sportsmen.

sprinters and jumpers have proportionally more FT fibres.

FORCE PRODUCTION

The arrangement of fibres with respect to the tendon is a very important consideration in calculating force production capability. Two categories of skeletal muscle have been described based on the gross arrangement of muscle fibres.

- *Fusiform (strap-like)*. These muscle fibres are arranged longitudinally with respect to the tendon, for example in the gracilis m. These muscles produce low force but are capable of shortening over a large range. There are few muscles of fusiform structure and they are mostly located in the extremities of the body (Fig. 1.11)
- *Penniform*. These muscle fibres are arranged at an angle with respect to the tendon. They produce large forces, while the tendons shorten over a relatively small range. Three-quarters of the skeletal muscles are of the penniform variety, of which the three following subcategories exist:

— unipennate muscle fibres to one side of the tendon, for example, semimembranosis m
— bipennate muscle fibres to both sides of a central tendon, for example rectus femoris m
— multipennate muscle fibres to both sides of a number of tendons, giving a herring-bone appearance, for example, deltoid m

Given that most lever systems in the human body are of the third class category (see Chapter 2), it is necessary for most of the musculature to possess the force production and degree of shortening capabilities of the penniform types.

A muscle can develop a maximum force of approximately $50 \, \text{N} \cdot \text{cm}^{-2}$ of muscle cross-section. Thus, a reasonable estimation of muscle strength can be gained by measuring the physiological cross-sectional area of the muscle contractile tissue; however, other factors also play an important role. These neuromuscular factors are presented in more detail in Chapter 2 and include the type of muscular action, muscle length, speed of contraction, fibre composition, neural innervation pattern and muscle compliance.

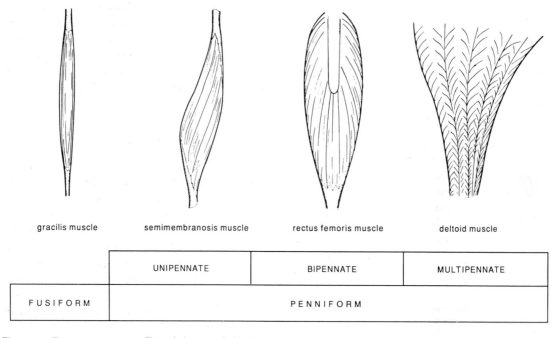

| | gracilis muscle | semimembranosis muscle | rectus femoris muscle | deltoid muscle |

	UNIPENNATE	BIPENNATE	MULTIPENNATE
FUSIFORM	PENNIFORM		

Fig. 1.11 The arrangement of fibres in human skeletal muscle.

RATE OF FORCE PRODUCTION

The rate at which force is developed, which is only one component of muscle power, depends upon the internal characteristics of the skeletal muscle as outlined below.

The number of sarcomeres in series

This depends primarily on the muscle fibre composition. The myofibrils of the ST fibres have long sarcomeres (approximately 6.0 μm) and thus comparatively fewer will fit in series over the fibre length. As a result their rate of shortening is slow. The FT fibres, however, have many sarcomeres in series as the sarcomere length is only approximately 2.4 μm. Thus, they are capable of rapid force development.

The rate at which individual cross-bridges work

Once again this is dependent upon fibre composition. The ST fibres contain myofilaments where the cross-bridges work at a slow rate and thus are useful in more sustained contractions. Crossbridge action of the FT fibres is more rapid and thus the rate of shortening is increased.

AGGREGATE MUSCLE ACTIONS

Skeletal muscles rarely work individually, but more often as part of a team to create movement. In order to appreciate this it is necessary to understand the modes in which a muscle may contract. The following aggregate muscle actions may be identified.

- *Concentric contraction* — when the tension developed is greater than the force necessary to overcome resistance, then the muscle shortens
- *Eccentric contraction* — when the tension developed is less than the force necessary to overcome resistance, then the muscle lengthens
- *Isometric contraction* — when the tension developed equals the resistance, then muscle length remains unchanged[1]

---

[1] When limb movement is prevented mechanically, muscle is still able to shorten due to stretching of the series elastic components (see Chapter 2), thus the isometric state is not achieved until shortening is complete.

All skeletal muscles are capable of performing under each mode of contraction as they assist in producing movement. Further comment related to these modes of contraction may be found in Chapter 2.

When a muscle or group of muscles is contracting (concentric) on one side of a body segment, it is usual that another group is lengthening on the opposite side. The two terms used here are:

- *Agonists or 'prime movers'* — cause movement due to their concentric contraction
- *Antagonists or 'prime stoppers'* — are located on the opposite side of the joint and act to slow or partially resist the original movement by contracting eccentrically

In addition, the musculature surrounding one attachment of the agonist or antagonist must also contract (isometrically) to stabilize that bone in order to permit tension development. These muscles, termed fixators or stabilizers play an important but often neglected role in the production of movement and they must be trained in conjunction with the agonists and antagonists to minimize any strength imbalance. The final aggregate muscle action is that of muscle synergy whereupon muscles act cooperatively to produce a desired movement. These muscles may generally oppose one another but, by their combined actions, allow a particular movement to occur. For example, the contraction of wrist extensor muscles and finger flexor muscles facilitates effective grasping movements of the hand.

Strength Assessment

Traditionally, muscular strength has been assessed using an isotonic (concentric), or an isometric mode of contraction. By setting a specific weight on a barbell for example, it was incorrectly presumed that a constant load or isotonic stress was placed on the active muscle group. However, variations in strength due to the muscle length, angle of tendon insertion, changes in movement velocity and proportionality characteristics of the subject rendered this method of assessment invalid. Attempts to standardize strength measurement then led to isometric protocols whereby the limb segment was placed in a standard position and force production recorded by a strain gauge or other form of dynamometer. These isometric tests are of limited use as they only measure force at one point in the range of motion and are also affected by body proportionality, that is, the lever length of the subject.

More recent methods for the assessment of the dynamic characteristics of muscle strength have required the use of an 'isokinetic' dynamometer which, as discussed in Chapter 3, is more correctly described as an isokinematic dynamometer. These machines attempt to accommodate to the torque being applied by the subject by offering a commensurate resistance throughout the range of motion, thus permitting movement of the body segment at a set angular velocity. The maximum torque output throughout this range may then be assessed. Both concentric and eccentric activity, as well as reciprocal activity, may be assessed by these machines.

Power Assessment

Power is a difficult component of performance to quantify and its assessment has generally been limited to a number of field tests. The Margaria-Kalamen test for example, measures the power output required to raise the bodyweight vertically in a short period of time as the subject ascends a flight of stairs. Other tests which have more tenuous links with this capacity as defined previously, include the vertical jump, 40 m sprint and standing long jump tests.

One laboratory test of power which has received widespread adoption is the Wingate Anaerobic Test. This 30 s bicycle test involves the subject pedalling maximally at a constant resistance based on his or her bodyweight. Power output is calculated for each 5 s period throughout the test.

Furthermore, the isokinetic dynamometers may be used to assess muscle power, which is computed as the product of torque and angular velocity. Bloomfield *et al.* (1994) provide an expanded discussion on the various methods used to measure muscular strength and power, which includes the recently developed Plyometric Power System. Developed at Southern Cross University, this system allows dynamically loaded activities, such as squat

jumps and bench press throws to be performed, with the option of engaging an electronically controlled brake to reduce potentially hazardous impact forces. The system permits the safe performance of these and many other standard resistance training movements. A rotary encoder, fixed to the shaft of the machine, records the direction and distance of bar movements and relays this information to a computer to enable the calculation of the distance moved, work done, average power output and peak velocity.

The Development of Strength and Power

TRAINING PRINCIPLES

Several principles underlie the development of strength and power, whether it be to improve sport performance or to rehabilitate sports injuries. If they are adhered to they will facilitate maximum gains in these parameters. Further information related to training principles may also be found in Chapter 4.

Variation principle

The principle of variation recognizes that when a training stimulus is consistently presented to the body in exactly the same way, its effectiveness will diminish and training gains will be reduced.

The training year should be divided into phases in which the emphasis on time, volume, intensity or type of exercise may vary considerably to achieve a desired outcome. These phases permit variety in training so that boredom and fatigue may be minimized, adequate fitness established within the early part of the season and peak performance levels reached at critical times during the competition period. For example, preparation of the musculoskeletal system for power training may be more effectively or safely achieved by a preceding phase of strength work using slower, controlled speed repetitions of greater load. Thus the hypertrophied muscle, connective tissues and bone may be better able to respond to the high stresses imposed in a power training phase.

Smaller units of time or microcycles within these phases require that consideration be given to resting the body and thereby avoiding overtraining, which may lead to fatigue and possibly injury. Periodic rest should occur during the training week to permit recovery from the exercise and allow physiological adaptation to occur.

Progressive overload principle

For gains in strength and power to be achieved, it is necessary to undertake a training load in excess of that to which the body is normally accustomed. As the body adapts to this new level of force it will be necessary to readjust the training stimulus in order that added stress be placed on the musculoskeletal system. This accepted principle has been referred to in the scientific literature for over 100 years and, with later refinements, may be demonstrated in Fig. 1.12. The body adapts to an overload by increasing the strength threshold and so, for further improvements to occur, the training level must again increase. If the body is underloaded for a period of time due to illness, bed-rest or lack of training, strength will be lost as the threshold level decreases. It is important, however, that the overload be sufficient to stimulate adaptation, but not so great as to cause injury.

Once strength levels have been increased due to training they may be maintained by the performance of one maximal contraction per week for each muscle group. Data from Berger (1962) showed strength levels marginally improved over a 6 week period using this maintenance programme, whereas strength levels diminished when training ceased altogether.

Specificity principle

Similarity should exist between the training conditions and those required in the actual athletic performance. Strength and power training should therefore involve the muscle groups which cause the desired movement and in addition, those antagonist and stabilizer muscle groups which assist in the production of the movement should be trained. This will permit a balanced strength increase, protecting the body from potential injury. Furthermore, strength and power training should be undertaken in a posture which resembles that used in the performance for maximal benefit. An example of this can be seen with the 'power driver' developed by Nautilus (Fig. 1.13).

Specificity also relates to the type of training

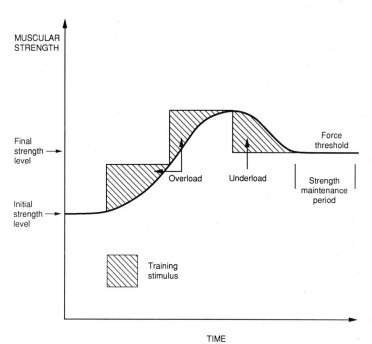

Fig. 1.12 Muscular strength variation under various conditions of the training stimulus.

19

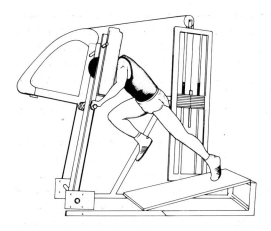

Fig. 1.13 Strength training in a sprinting posture using the 'Power Driver' (adapted from Nautilus 1975).

emphasis followed to achieve increases in muscle hypertrophy, strength or power. Komi (1988) refers to this as the force–velocity principle and proposes that the training mode model in Fig. 1.14 reflects this principle. If the training loads are selected from the high force part of the curve (low velocity) then the training effect is primarily reflected in that

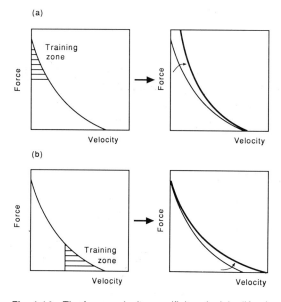

Fig. 1.14 The force–velocity specificity principle. (Komi 1988; used with permission.)

part of the force–velocity curve (see Chapter 2). Conversely, exercising with lower loads at high velocities will affect the force–velocity curve in the manner shown in Fig. 1.14b.

Depending upon the current training state of the individual, however, these responses may not be so rigid. An untrained person for example, will initially experience global improvements in the force–velocity curve despite the type of training undertaken. This specificity concept is supported by Wilmore and Costill (1994) who suggest that training at a slow pace with low loads will emphasize the use of only the ST fibres, inducing little training effect on the FTa or FTb fibres. Long, slow bouts of training do not prepare muscles for the demands of competition in which a greater reliance on the FT fibres is required.

Recovery principle

Muscle growth and adaptation occur between training sessions and therefore, an adequate recovery is essential. According to Bloomfield *et al.* (1994), a recovery period of approximately 48–72 h should be interposed between intensive resistance training sessions of the same muscle group. Too little recovery time will result in reduced performance and may also lead to injury.

STRENGTH TRAINING METHODS

Isometric training (static)

Gaining great popularity in the mid-1950s with the promise of unprecedented strength gains, isometric training has since been largely overlooked by coaches and athletes, especially with the subsequent inability of research to substantiate these claims. Nevertheless, strength improvements do occur when muscle groups are contracted against a fixed, immovable resistance. Isometrics therefore may be a valuable training method for sports such as gymnastics, where positions must be held for several seconds, or as a strength maintenance regimen when limbs are immobilized. It is also used extensively in the rehabilitation of sports injuries. Little research has been devoted to this form of training for sport; however, it is commonly believed that the best results are obtained by performing a maximal, or near-maximal contraction for 6 s and repeating the efforts five or six times, on four or five occasions per week. Strength gains are thought to be specific to the joint angle (muscle length) at which training occurs and thus it is suggested that isometric exercises be performed at various joint angles if possible.

Isotonic training (concentric/eccentric)

Isotonic training methods have traditionally used resistances in the form of dumb-bells and barbells, or more recently pinloaded weight machines and pulley weights. Research during the past half century has attempted to determine the optimum combination of weights and repetitions to maximize strength gains. Early contributions by DeLorme and Watkins (1948) have been slightly modified in recent years to suggest that isotonic training be performed at five to seven repetitions maximum (RM), with three sets being accomplished per exercise at one session. The frequency of training should be approximately three or four sessions per week. The RM concept of DeLorme and Watkins repre-

sented the maximum number of repetitions which could be continuously performed at a given resistance, thus 6 RM referred to the resistance for which only six repetitions could be achieved. This system provided a suitable method of incorporating the overload principle, as persons were able to exercise at their individual loads yet still conform to the RM concept.

Several limitations exist for this type of training and there has been a proliferation of machines which claim to improve on the isotonic training mode. When using a barbell as in Fig. 1.15, the weight of the bar does not change throughout the movement, but the effective resistance, determined statically by the torque about the axis of rotation located at the elbow joint, varies considerably. This torque is minimal at position A and maximal at position D. However, under dynamic conditions the bar may be accelerated from position A so that the momentum generated through the remainder of the curl causes a reduction in the experienced load, compared with the static load at subsequent

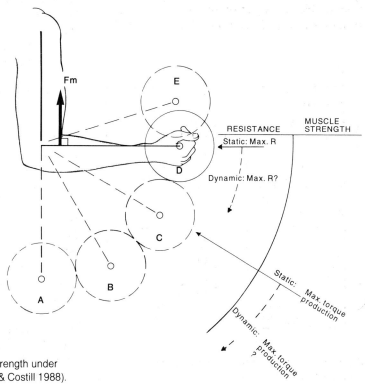

Fig. 1.15   Variation in resistance and strength under isotonic loading (adapted from Wilmore & Costill 1988).

positions. This is especially so during fast repetitions (power training), but not so critical when slow movements are performed.

Furthermore, the ability to perform the curl also varies with the location of the bar. Statically, the torque produced by the forearm flexors is maximal when the optimal combination of tendon insertion angle and muscle length is reached. Given that the optimum tendon insertion angle of 90° would occur approximately at position D, but that maximum contractile capability at the resting length of the muscle occurs between points A and D, then the position of maximum torque production would lie at approximately 120° of extension (position C). The greatest muscular force could be developed isometrically at each position, but under dynamic conditions where the bar is elevated with some velocity, force production throughout the range of motion would be less than maximal. Under dynamic conditions therefore, many of these variables will be altered, yet the muscle group is not permitted to train maximally throughout the entire range of motion. Isotonic exercise loads are limited to the resistance which may be overcome at the 'sticking point' of the movement. If maximum muscular torque is experienced before or after the 'sticking

point', then the muscle will not be maximally stressed at these times. In other words a lift would be maximal only at the weakest point in the range of motion.

In an effort to overcome this limitation, free weight trainers perform forced repetitions, using spotters or assistants to help them through the sticking region. In this way repetitions can be performed, which enable the production of maximal effort throughout a greater range of motion and over a number of repetitions.

Variable resistance training

Several machines have been produced in recent years, which attempt to overcome some of the shortcomings of the traditional isotonic mode. These variable resistance machines enable a load to be altered during the range of motion so that the effective resistance matches the torque-producing capability of the muscle group. Special cams have been designed to change the moment arm by which a weight stack exerts its resistance or pneumatic cylinders have been developed to carry out a similar function. Although often claimed to produce iso-kinetic motion, these variable resistance machines do not fully restrict the body segment to constant

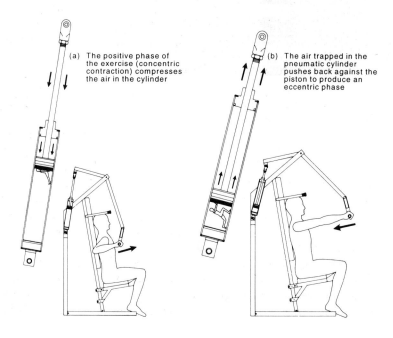

Fig. 1.16 A seated chest press using a Keiser Air-powered exercise machine. (Keiser 1989; used with permission.)

(a) The positive phase of the exercise (concentric contraction) compresses the air in the cylinder

(b) The air trapped in the pneumatic cylinder pushes back against the piston to produce an eccentric phase

velocity motion. Examples of these include the Nautilus, Polaris, Eagle Pulstar and Keiser (Fig. 1.16) systems.

Accommodating resistance training

These devices attempt to control the speed of contraction through various mechanisms including electronic servo-motor control systems (Fig. 1.17), and hydraulic chambers. They are described as accommodating resistance machines, as they attempt to exactly match the variation in torque produced throughout a movement with an appropriate resistance. Thus the limb moves with a constant angular velocity and the muscle group is trained maximally through the range of motion. Examples of these machines include the Cybex, Kincom, Biodex and Orthotron systems.

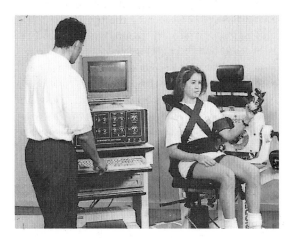

Fig. 1.17 Accommodating resistance training using the Biodex system (courtesy of Bloomfield *et al.* 1994)

POWER TRAINING METHODS

The use of heavy loads will improve power to a greater extent than training with relatively light loads (Schmidtbleicher & Buehrle 1987). According to the size theory of motor unit recruitment, the large FT motor units will only be recruited if relatively large forces are involved in the exercise. Consequently, heavy loads must be used in training to develop dynamic athletic performance, provided the athlete attempts to lift these loads explosively.

Plyometric training

Traditional plyometric training uses the acceleration and deceleration of bodyweight as the overload in dynamic activities such as depth jumps and bounds. Coaches and athletes maintain that plyometric training represents the bridge between strength and power and perceive it as a method of training that will directly enhance competitive performance. They often see strength training as a means of increasing general strength and plyometrics as a way to apply this strength to improve performance. Such a perception appears well supported in the literature, with many studies reporting that the combination of plyometric and strength training resulted in superior performance gains when compared with plyometric or strength training alone.

Bloomfield *et al.* (1994) describe a number of advantages of plyometric over traditional heavy weight training including:

- Plyometric exercise tends to be performed in a more explosive manner than traditional strength training
- Plyometric exercises do not involve a large deceleration phase during concentric movement
- Plyometric exercises are performed at higher velocities than those achieved using traditional strength training
- Plyometric exercises involve a dynamic stretch–shorten cycle movement similar to that adopted in most sporting activities

Despite these advantages, this training modality has a number of limitations associated with its use, which are as follows:

- High impact forces can occur when landing from depth jumps or bounds
- Plyometric training has typically been limited to the use of the athlete's body mass providing the load stimulus, although some coaches report that the use of weight vests, belts or anklets can increase this load
- A limited number of exercises can be performed plyometrically
- Plyometric exercises are generally performed with very limited or no feedback
- Due to the high velocities achieved when perform-

ing plyometric exercises, the forces produced tend to be lower than those achieved in traditional strength training

Bloomfield *et al.* (1994) provide further discussion on this topic, with particular reference to training prerequisites, training principles and training 'tips'. This last topic includes recommendations for optimal drop height, ground contact time, recovery periods and feedback.

Maximal power training

Maximal explosive power training involves the performance of dynamic weight training at the load which maximizes mechanical power output. This training strategy involves lifting relatively light loads (~30–45% of maximum) at high speed and results in the production of the highest mechanical power output (Fig. 1.18). Berger (1963) reported

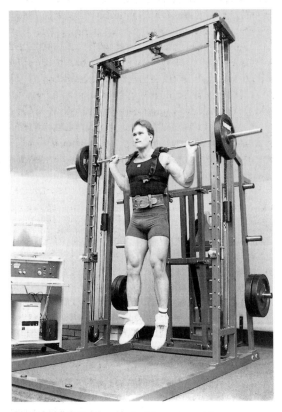

Fig. 1.18 Maximal power training: plyometric squats performed at a load which maximizes power output (courtesy of Bloomfield *et al.* 1994).

that the performance of squat jumps at a load of approximately 30% of maximum resulted in greater increases in vertical jump height (2.8 cm) than those achieved in traditional weight training (2.3 cm), isometric training (0.8 cm) or unweighted vertical jumps (−1.0 cm).

One important point to consider in the application of maximal power training is that standard weight training exercises such as bench press or squats, where the bar must achieve zero velocity at the end of the movement range, cannot be used. In such instances maximal power training is relatively ineffective, because of the large deceleration phase. This means that high-force levels are achieved only through a very small range of the movement and suboptimal training gains result (Schmidtbleicher & Buehrle 1987). This is also the reason why this form of training is not popular at present with athletes or coaches.

Bloomfield *et al.* (1994) reviewed a number of studies which had compared power training methods. The consensus among researchers was that athletes should train using a load that maximizes the mechanical power output of the lift (~30–45% of maximum force) to optimally enhance athletic performance. Furthermore, a number of practical applications of this strategy are discussed by Bloomfield *et al.* together with some new directions for this training modality, such as the development of the Plyometric Power System which is demonstrated in Fig. 1.18.

Adaptations to Resistance Training

A number of adaptations occur within the body as a result of resistance training, in response to an increased load to protect structures from injury, or in order to promote a strength or power improvement. Furthermore, significant benefits may be gained during rehabilitation from injury as described in Chapter 13. Wilmore and Costill (1994) discuss these issues at length and refer to the following adaptations in particular.

MUSCLE SIZE ADAPTATIONS

Once believed to be the sole factor responsible for improvements in strength, increases in muscle size still contribute significantly to individual strength levels, although other mechanisms have now been shown to play an equally important role. Chronic hypertrophy refers to the increase in muscle size resulting from resistance training and is distinguished from transient hypertrophy or 'pumping-up' of a muscle which occurs during a single exercise session as a result of fluid accumulation or muscle oedema. Research findings which attempt to explain the exact mechanism for muscle hypertrophy are equivocal, with the bulk of evidence supporting an increase in the size of existing fibres rather than an increase in fibre number (hyperplasia). It is interesting to note that the majority of muscle hypertrophy that occurs in response to high-intensity resistance training, tends to be in the FT muscle fibres.

NEUROLOGICAL ADAPTATIONS

Evidence for the role of a neural adaptation to resistance training may be found in many situations, including the fact that strength gains achieved early in a training programme often occur in the absence of muscle hypertrophy. This is especially so for women for whom strength levels have reportedly doubled without any appreciable change in the size of the muscle. Evidence exists that each α motor neuron is affected by both excitatory and inhibitory influences. These inhibitory influences may result from sensory feedback from kinesthetic receptors located within joints, muscles and tendons (autogenic inhibition), or from some higher level centre within the brain. It is proposed that these inhibitory influences may be overcome or counteracted with training, thus permitting greater levels of force to be developed. Gains in strength may well be the result of an increase in the ability to recruit additional motor units and to better synchronize their firing pattern.

OTHER ADAPTATIONS

Many other adaptations as a result of resistance training also occur within bone and connective tissue in response to an increase in load. Furthermore, changes affecting the endocrine and cardiovascular systems have also been reported, but more specific discussion in this regard is beyond the scope of this chapter.

Modification strategies aimed at improving muscular strength and power will elicit changes more easily and will be of greater magnitude than any other physical capacity. It is therefore not surprising that many coaches incorporate strength and power programmes as part of the training regimen for a variety of sports. Because muscular strength responds so dynamically to training and its effect on performance is almost immediately observed, a continual assessment of technique as well as of muscular strength and power should be performed. This is especially so during the late and post-adolescent period for males when the rate of strength development is maximal.

FLEXIBILITY

Suppleness or flexibility has been traditionally defined as the range of motion in a joint and is usually specific to a joint or combination of them. Thus the coach cannot say that an individual is generally flexible, as some areas of the body may have an extensive range of movement while others may only be of average or below average flexibility. The limiting factors which affect this capacity are muscle bulk, the surrounding connective tissue, the structure of the bony articulations and skin suppleness. It is also one of the capacities, together with body composition and strength, which is able to be modified easily.

Levels of flexibility are normally tested in the static position; however, several sports scientists have proposed other types of flexibility assessment. For example, the term dynamic flexibility has been used to describe an ability to move body segments rapidly or to make quick, repeated movements. Functional flexibility, however, has been used to describe the range of joint motion displayed by an athlete while performing a particular skill. For example, golfers display functional flexibility during the back-swing phase of a full golf shot because an increased back-swing, if made with body control, allows more time and distance for clubhead speed to be developed during the down-swing phase. For the remainder of this section the discussion will be limited to static and functional flexibility parameters.

Flexibility is influenced by a number of factors including the level of normal activity and range of motion normally required of a joint, as well as others such as gender, age, body type, temperature and psychological stress. The influence of these factors on joint mobility has been reviewed by Holland (1968).

Specific Benefits of Stretching

Many coaches and sports scientists now believe that flexibility exercises are of more value than was previously thought. In the past they have been used as part of the warm-up programme for various sports, but their value in technique and increasing the explosive power in a movement has only recently been realized. It is for these reasons that stretching has become an integral part of the modern training programme in a similar way to that of strength and power, speed and mental skills training.

Bloomfield et al. (1994) provide an expanded discussion related to the specific benefits of stretching. These benefits may be summarized as follows:

- Improved performance — with respect to improving the aesthetic appearance, range of motion and force development capability
- Prevention of injury — not only do stretching exercises decrease the incidence, intensity and duration of musculotendinous and joint injury but, as a result of an increased range of motion, may act to help avoid these injuries
- Relief of muscle soreness — a brief period of static stretching (10 min) performed after exercise can alleviate soreness
- Muscle relaxation — static stretching is of great value to alleviate muscular tension

Flexibility Measurement

As static flexibility is a joint-specific, rather than a general athletic capacity, gross movement tests such as the sit and reach provide only limited information. The most simple device which will provide accurate measures of joint mobility is the goniometer, which is used to measure the angle between two body segments at the extreme ends of their range of motion. An electrogoniometer or 'elgon' is a more advanced form of the goniometer, incorporating a potentiometer at the axis of the two measurement arms. Changes in joint angle are recorded as voltage fluctuations thus providing a real-time, analogue display of joint motion. This device may therefore be used to provide measurements of static as well as functional flexibility (see Chapter 3).

Rather than measure the angle between two segments, the Leighton flexometer, a device containing two rotating and weighted dials, may be used to record the motion of a single, isolated segment with respect to the perpendicular plane. With this instrument it is of paramount importance that other body segments be held rigid so that only movements of the isolated segment be recorded. A full discussion related to flexibility testing may be found in Bloomfield et al. (1994).

Flexibility and Sports Performance

It is well known that high levels of flexibility are necessary for top performance in many sports. It is essential for example, that the hurdler has a high degree of trunk flexion, thigh abduction in the trail leg and thigh flexion in the lead leg to 'stride over' each hurdle rather than jump it. In several other sports such as swimming, diving and gymnastics, it is necessary to have very high levels of flexibility in specific joints within the body. Even in throwing and striking sports such as baseball, golf and the racquet sports, it is an advantage to have above average flexibility levels of the trunk and shoulder region.

It should be noted that high levels of flexibility are not always advantageous for sport performance, and in several regions of the body it is a disadvantage for the athlete to possess an extreme range of motion. Persons competing in body contact sports and in those which require evading manoeuvres would be disadvantaged by excessive mobility of the knee and ankle joints, as the extra mobility predisposes the joint to injury during body contact. Generally, however, a high degree of joint mobility in certain regions of the body is not only important to attain the correct technique but also for the prevention of musculoskeletal injuries. Lorenzton (1988) cites muscle tightness, as well as weakness and strength imbalance, as significant contributors to muscle rupture and tendinitis.

Stretching is frequently used in the rehabilitation of muscle tissue. The muscle must be very slowly returned to its original length with gentle stretching exercises, which will encourage it to re-form in its long state, thus reducing cross-adhesions. At the same time as the above process is occurring, proprioception and tension will be returning.

Methods Used to Increase Flexibility

From the previous discussion it is clear that no generalized programme of flexibility should be adopted across all sports. As the movement requirements of each event are analysed, a specific flexibility programme, concentrating on the appropriate joint movements, needs to be devised.

The first and oldest system of flexibility training is *ballistic stretching* (de Vries 1986) where the athlete uses rhythmical actions to cause the muscle group to undergo a series of elongations as the limbs or trunk are forced to the end of their range of motion. De Vries (1986), however, did not favour this method because of the high incidence of soft-tissue injury and muscle soreness, which was observed in athletes who performed ballistic stretching.

Some coaches still support ballistic stretching because they maintain that many movements in sport are ballistic in nature. Its supporters suggest that it is specific to sport and provided it is done with caution and the athlete does not overstretch, it can be an effective way to increase flexibility. However, it is of great importance that the musculature be thoroughly warmed prior to performing ballistic stretching.

A more recent method, called *static stretching*, involves holding a static position for a period of time after the limb has already been stretched and has become very popular during the past decade, because it is both effective and relatively safe. Simply put, it involves a slow stretch (to inhibit the firing of the stretch reflex) almost to the point of resistance, where it is then held for 20–30 s or even up to 60 s if necessary. During this time the tension

partially diminishes (due to the inverse stretch reflex) and the athlete slowly moves into a deeper stretch and repeats the above once or several times (Bloomfield *et al.* 1994).

A third system is *proprioceptive neuromuscular facilitation* (PNF) or sometimes called 3-S or *Scientific Stretching for Sport*. This technique has been developed by Holt (1974) specifically for sport and offers an alternative stretching method to both the traditional static and ballistic regimens. It is based on Herman Kabat's therapeutic principles, whereby it is hypothesized that increased range of motion is promoted through the principles of successive induction, autogenic inhibition and active mobilization of connective tissues (Holt 1974). Specifically, it is suggested that greater muscle relaxation occurs after a significant contraction of the muscle. This may occur as a result of a reduced afferent discharge from the muscle spindle or a reflex inhibition of the muscle due to increased Golgi tendon organ discharge. In each exercise the muscle is initially placed in a lengthened position, then isometrically contracted against the immovable resistance of a partner for a period of 6 s. This is followed by a *very brief* period of relaxation, after which the athlete contracts the opposite muscle group, which is aided by a partner who applies light pressure for 6–10 s enabling greater range of movement (ROM) to be achieved (Fig. 1.19). The exercise is then repeated three or four times. Improvements in joint mobility using each method of flexibility training have been shown in the literature; however, no clear conclusion as to the best technique has yet been reached.

Finally, for athletes in sports which need an extreme range of flexibility in certain joints, the *passive stretching* system is of great value. When using this technique the athlete stays relaxed and makes no active contribution to the stretch, which should be done slowly and with care. An external force is usually applied by a partner (Fig. 1.20). More detail on the above techniques and additional ones, can be found in Bloomfield *et al.* (1994).

Achieving optimal levels of flexibility has become a very important goal for high-performance athletes. For example, in sports where the performance is judged, competitors are required to achieve certain

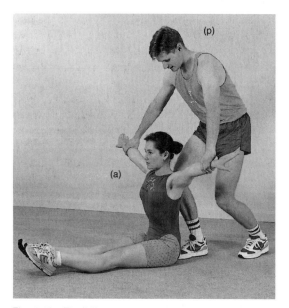
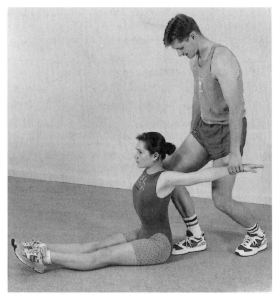

Fig. 1.19 Flexibility training using the principles of proprioceptive neuromuscular facilitation to stretch the pectoral muscle group. (a) Athlete; (p) partner (courtesy of Bloomfield *et al.* 1994).

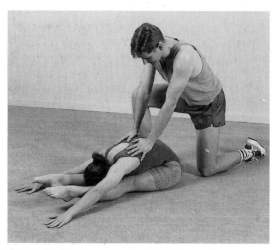

Fig. 1.20 An elite gymnast undergoing passive stretching (courtesy of Bloomfield *et al.* 1994).

set positions in order to score high artistic marks. Furthermore, the potential for an athlete to develop more force or velocity becomes possible when the range of motion of the body segment is increased. This is an important factor in hitting, throwing and kicking sports.

SPEED

Movement speed is an essential physical capacity in the majority of sports and results from the ability to perform fast motor actions in a short period of time. While speed has many connotations, in this chapter it refers to the maximum possible speed, which is achieved in single or repeated maximal efforts of short duration. Thus it refers not only to running velocity, but also to arm movements in swimming strokes or in a throwing action, a leg action in a kick, or the development of impact velocity of a club, bat or racquet. Speed is another capacity which may be modified with appropriate training.

It should also be noted that speed is a specific capacity which relates to a particular movement pattern, rather than a general quality. Thorstensson (1988) provides an overview of the biomechanical, muscular, neural and general factors which influence this capacity. These factors may enhance or counteract movement speed and therefore the coach or sports scientist is obliged not only to promote the positive factors, but also to limit those which hinder the production of movement speed.

Basic Determinants of Speed

There are several major factors which, when integrated, go to make up a speedy movement. At this point in the development of sports science, it has not been possible to rate them in order of importance; however, the following list attempts to classify them from the research and anecdotal information that is currently available (Bloomfield *et al*. 1994):

- Muscle fibre type — the relative proportions of FT and ST fibres
- Skill — neuromuscular co-ordination
- Muscle insertion point — affects the mechanical advantage of the lever system
- Lever length — an optimal lever length needs to be developed in order for a fast movement to occur
- Posture — the alignment of muscles as they cross various joints to give a mechanical advantage
- Elastic energy — adopting techniques to take advantage of the storage of elastic energy in the musculotendinous unit

The Development of Speed

The aim of speed training is to condition the athlete to move at high velocity, employing maximal power when needed. In order to do this the neuromuscular system must be conditioned to very fast movements and training needs to be very specific (especially to cadence, posture and skill), with a very high anaerobic component.

As a prerequisite to specific speed training, high levels of both cardiovascular and musculoskeletal fitness are necessary. If these are neglected, then there is a strong possibility that an injury will be sustained. Therefore, a solid foundation provided by a strength training programme as well as flexibility and power training and aerobic conditioning should be created.

SPEED-RESISTED TRAINING

This type of training involves the performance of a skill with an increased load or resistance and is usually confined to the pre-season or early season period. Examples of this regimen are as follows:

- Running up gradual hills, specially built ramps (4–5° inclines), and stairs; using a power trainer, pulling a specially weighted sled or tyre; running with a small parachute behind; or using weighted shoes
- Cycling in high gear at as fast a cadence as possible, or pulling a sled or tyre behind the cycle
- The use of weight bands or weighted vests, weighted boots or weighted equipment in mobile field games
- Swimming with hand paddles; using pull buoys; towing a sea anchor; or using a speed trainer (e.g. the Sparta Speed Trainer)
- Rowing, canoeing or kayaking using large oars or paddle blades. Heavy boats, canoes or kayaks are also of assistance in this form of training
- Competing against heavier opponents in the combative sports
- Using very light dumb-bells for boxers (shadow sparring) or for other athletes who use their arms to strike, hit or pump, as in running

SPEED-ASSISTED TRAINING

In order to condition the neurological system to perform very fast movements it has been proposed that skills be performed with reduced loads. Examples of this regimen, which should be confined to the early to mid-season period, include the following:

- Running on a speeded-up treadmill, down a 2° ramp, or behind a vehicle or motor bike holding on to an extension of it; using surgical tubing to pull the athlete, towing with the Sprint Master (Bloomfield *et al*. 1994)
- Agility training drills for players in mobile field sports using very rapid sprint and directional changes. To do this sharp commands and shrill whistles should be used
- Cycling in low gear at a fast cadence, on rollers, or riding in the slip-stream behind a motor bike while on the cycling track
- Swimming using a sprint towing device or modified flippers
- Rowing, canoeing or kayaking using a *slightly* smaller oar or paddle blade, or with several small holes bored in the blade

SKILL TRAINING

No speed-resisted or speed-assisted training should take place beyond the mid-season period. Beyond that time, specific skill or technique training should be encouraged at a maximal speed. Skill is the most important single factor in the attainment of movement speed and this must not be overshadowed by any of the others.

If the athlete is to reach full potential in a sport and if speed of movement is a necessary component in it, the speed and velocity demands of that sport must be carefully analysed. Several examples of sport-specific speed training are discussed by Bloomfield et al. (1994).

MODIFYING HUMAN PHYSICAL CAPACITIES AND TECHNIQUE TO IMPROVE PERFORMANCE

The modification of human physical capacities and technique to improve sports performance, as proposed by Bloomfield (1979), has received little systematic attention from sports coaches. Coaches in the past have tended to teach standard techniques, especially those which have been used by World or Olympic champions, whether they suit their own athletes or not. Many of them have not yet realized that improved athletic performances can be achieved when the athlete's physical capacities are modified to suit a particular technique, or when a technique has been modified to suit the individual athlete.

There are certain biomechanical principles which are determined by the laws of motion and must be adhered to in all skilled performances for the optimal result to be obtained. Because there is such great variability in human morphology, the way in which coaches apply these principles can vary considerably. Too often, however, they attempt to modify technique with little or no consideration of the athlete's physical capacity to adapt to a new skill. Certain physical characteristics will be very advantageous for a particular sport, whereas others will be a distinct handicap. This is known as the principle of self-selection for various sports and events.

When applying the above concept, the coach must first develop the physical capacities of the individual to an optimal level and this is done after a profile (see Chapter 11) has been developed which will point out the strengths and weaknesses of the athlete. When this has been achieved a set of technique preferences can be applied by the coach which will best utilize the inherent physical strengths of the athlete. At this point trade-offs must be made in order to obtain the best result. The following example will illustrate this point.

In the right-handed golf swing, one must decide whether the player should transfer more weight to the right side in the back-swing, thus enabling a little more lateral motion to be applied in the down-swing, which in turn will give more velocity at contact and greater hitting distance for the player, or whether they should develop a more compact swing with only a minor weight shift to the right side and not gain quite as much distance with the shot. The latter ultimately gives less distance but greater accuracy and such a decision relates mainly to body build, proportions and the power of the golfer. A smaller, shorter-levered and less powerful player may prefer to take the risks which are inherent in a swing which has a slightly higher degree of lateral shift, in order to gain a longer distance with each shot, whereas the taller, long-levered and more powerful player may not.

Similar modifications may be made in other sports. For example, if a butterfly swimmer's flexibility level has not improved to the point where the style is economical and mechanically effective, despite an intensive stretching programme for the shoulder joints, then the coach should teach that competitor the side-breathing technique. Also contact sports players with long legs tend to stride out during on-field running, and this lowers their level of dynamic balance. In order to improve it, they should bend their legs a little more and consciously take short, very fast steps, especially when near or contacting opponents. By adopting such a technique, they keep their base of support under their body, thereby improving their dynamic balance.

Many coaches have thought little about this aspect of coaching, but knowing the physical capacities of the athlete and selecting the preferences which suit that individual is the very essence of a scientific approach. However, in such a selection, a great deal of assessment and reassessment needs to be done while always adhering to the basic mechanical principles.

As a general tenet it is believed that the coach should strive to modify the physical capacities which provide an advantage for the particular sport initially, then seek to modify technique as discussed in Chapters 2 and 3. Finally, success will be achieved through constant monitoring and modification of both the athlete's physical capacities and his or her technique.

REFERENCES

Behnke A. R. & Wilmore J. H. (1974) *Evaluation and Regulation of Body Build and Composition.* Prentice-Hall, New Jersey.

Berger R. (1962) Optimum repetitions for the development of strength. *The Research Quarterly* **33**, 334–338.

Berger R. (1963) Effect of dynamic and static training on vertical jumping. *The Research Quarterly* **34**, 419–424.

Bloomfield J. (1979) Modifying human physical capacities and technique to improve performance. *Sports Coach* **3**, 19–25.

Bloomfield J. & Sigerseth P. O. (1965) Anatomical and physiological differences between sprint and middle distance swimmers at the University level. *The Journal of Sports Medicine and Physical Fitness* **5**, 76–81.

Bloomfield J., Ackland T. R. & Elliott B. C. (1994) *Applied Anatomy and Biomechanics in Sport*, pp. 47, 62, 73–75, 91, 104, 106, 108, 144–152, 195, 209–210, 218–220, 252–258, 315–318, 325–329, 332–349. Blackwell Scientific Publications, Melbourne.

Cameron N. (1978) The methods of auxological anthropometry. In Faulkner F. & Tanner J. M. (eds) *Human Growth*, Vol. 2, *Postnatal Growth*. Plenum Press, New York.

Carter J. E. L. (1975) *The Heath-Carter Somatotype Method.* San Diego State University, CA.

DeLorme T. L. & Watkins A. L. (1948) Techniques of progressive resistance exercise. *Archives of Physical Medicine* **29**, 263–273.

de Vries H. A. (1986) *Physiology of Exercise — For Physical Education and Athletics*, p. 467. Wm C. Brown, Dubuque, IA.

Dintiman G. B. (1974) *What Research Tells the Coach about Sprinting.* AAHPER Press, Washington DC.

Holland G. L. (1968) The physiology of flexibility: A review of literature. *Kinesiology Reviews* **1**, 49.

Holt L. E. (1974) *Scientific Stretching for Sport (3-S)*, pp. 1–8. Sport Research Ltd, Nova Scotia.

Komi P. V. (1988) The musculoskeletal system. In Dirix A., Knuttgen H. G. & Tittel K. (eds) *The Olympic Book of Sports Medicine I*, pp. 23–27. Blackwell Scientific Publications, Oxford.

Lorenzton R. (1988) Causes of injuries: Intrinsic factors. In Dirix A., Knuttgen H. G. & Tittel K. (eds) *The Olympic Book of Sports Medicine I*, pp. 376–390. Blackwell Scientific Publications, Oxford.

Martin A. D., Ross W. D., Drinkwater D. T. & Clarys J. P. (1984) Prediction of body fat by skinfold calipers: Assumptions and cadaver evidence. *International Journal of Obesity* **7**, 17–25.

Martin A. D., Drinkwater D. T., Clarys J. P. & Ross W. D. (1986) The inconsistency of the fat-free mass: A reappraisal with implications for densitometry. In Reilly T., Wilson J. & Borms J. (eds) *Kinanthropometry III*. Spon, London.

Pyke F. & Watson G. (1978) *Focus on Running*, pp. 47–48. Pelham Books, London.

Ross W. D. & Ward R. (1984) *The O-Scale System.* Rosscraft, Vancouver.

Ross W. D., DeRose E. H. & Ward R. (1988) Anthropometry applied to sports medicine. In Dirix A., Knuttgen H. G. & Tittle K. (eds) *The Olympic Book of Sports Medicine I*, pp. 233–265. Blackwell Scientific Publications, Oxford.

Schmidtbleicher D. & Buehrle M. (1987) Neuronal adaptations and increase of cross-sectional area studying different strength training methods. In Johnson G. (ed.) *Biomechanics X-B*, Vol. 6-B, pp. 615–620. Human Kinetics Publishers, Champaign, IL.

Sheldon W. H. (1954) *Atlas of Men.* Gramercy Publishing, New York.

Thorstensson A. (1988) Speed and acceleration. In Dirix A., Knuttgen H. G. & Tittle K. (eds) *The Olympic Book of Sports Medicine I*, pp. 218–329. Blackwell Scientific Publications, Oxford.

Wilmore J. H. & Costill D. L. (1988) *Training for Sport and Activity*, 3rd edn, pp. 6–16. Wm C. Brown, Dubuque, IA.

Wilmore J. H. & Costill D. L. (1994) *Physiology of Sport and Exercise*, pp. 26–41, 68–86. Human Kinetics Publishers, Champaign, IL.

CHAPTER 2

BIOMECHANICAL PRINCIPLES

B. C. Elliott and G. A. Wood

Academic and professional interest in sport biomechanics may be related to a wide range of factors important in sport performance or in the prevention of injury. Biomechanically based questions of interest might include:

- What technique(s) should a player use for optimal performance?
- What technique(s) should a player use to reduce the possibility of injury?
- What effect does a change in equipment design have on the performance of an athlete during training and competition?
- How often can a particular activity be repeated before 'overuse injuries' become a major consideration of both the athlete and the coach?

As the term suggests, biomechanics involves a study of the structure and function of the human body using mechanics. The biomechanics of human movement, therefore deals with the mechanical basis of movements, such as running, hitting a tennis ball, performing a somersault in gymnastics or a pirouette in dance. The criterion measure of human performance, that is, the successful achievement of a task in an injury-free environment, makes it imperative that medical and paramedical personnel interested in movement have an understanding of biomechanics.

A critical variable in the aetiology of pain, injuries and performance in general, is load (Nigg *et al.* 1984). A schematic diagram of the factors in-

fluencing load in sporting movement is included as Fig. 2.1. This chapter discusses the mechanics of movement, a major factor in the determination of load on the body in general or a segment or joint in particular. Sections outlining the neuromuscular factors that influence muscle force production and the effect of external conditions such as the equipment used for a particular activity are also included. The biomechanical enhancement of sport performance and measurement techniques in biomechanics are discussed in Chapter 3.

MECHANICS AND MOVEMENT

The study of biomechanics involves an understanding of both statics and dynamics. Statics deals with the equilibrium state of bodies at rest or the special state of constant velocity, whereas dynamics deals with the general case of bodies in motion as a result of the action of forces.

Statics

FORCES

Forces are pushes or pulls, and while these actions are necessary to produce movement, there are many instances in biomechanics where the forces acting are balanced in a way that no motion is produced. The most practical way in which to measure a force is to counter it with another force of known magnitude, as is done when we weigh ourselves on a set

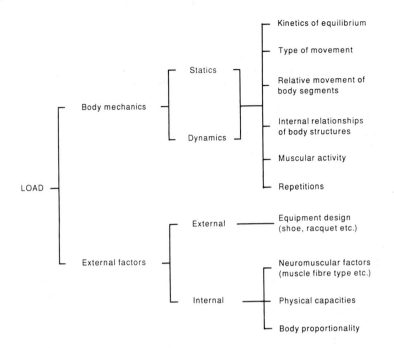

Fig. 2.1 The factors which influence load in sports performance. (modified from Nigg *et al.* 1984.)

of bathroom scales. In this instance the force being measured is the pull of gravity acting on our body, a force we call bodyweight (BW; although the number on the scales is often taken as a measure of body mass) and is counterbalanced by a force exerted by the scale's spring mechanism whose deformation characteristics are known. These two forces act in equal but opposite ways on the body, and in so doing provide the state of rest necessary to obtain

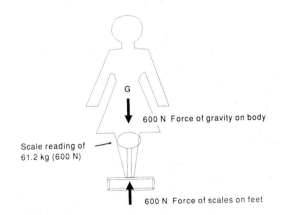

Fig. 2.2 The free-body diagram of a static force system (upright stance).

an accurate reading. This static force situation is shown in Fig. 2.2: a diagrammatic representation of a force system that is referred to as a free-body diagram. Here all external effects acting on the body are represented as force vectors whose magnitude (600 N), line (vertical), point of application (at feet and centre of body mass) and sense (up or down, as indicated by the arrowhead) are detailed, and the body is thereby effectively isolated from its environs and readily amenable to analysis. Vector quantities indicate both magnitude and direction (line plus sense), whereas scalar quantities (e.g. mass, length, time, temperature) indicate only magnitude. Throughout this chapter standard symbols representing vector quantities are printed in boldface (e.g. **F**).

A free-body diagram of a sprinter poised in a crouch starting position awaiting the starter's gun is shown in Fig. 2.3. Here too the human body is stationary, and as all external influences, that is supportive forces (e.g. buoyancy), pushes (e.g. R_1, R_2 and R_3), pulls, wind resistance, gravitational force (BW), and magnetism have been accounted for where necessary, then the force system that is depicted must be in static equilibrium. In both

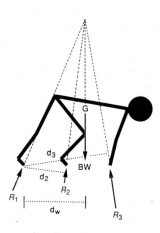

Fig. 2.3 The free-body diagram of a sprinter 'set' in a crouch start position.

Table 2.1 Moments of force about the sprinter's rear foot

Force	Perpendicular distance	Moment
R_1 250 N	d_1 0.0 m (unseen)	0 N m
R_2 175 N	d_2 0.6 m	105 N m
BW 650 N	d_w 0.9 m	− 585 N m
R_3 400 N	d_3 1.2 m	480 N m
Sum of moments		0 N m

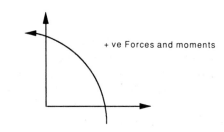

Sign convention for motion, forces and moments of force

cases, therefore, the algebraic sum (Σ) of all the forces and their respective turning effects or moments of force, about any common axis must be equal to zero. That is:

$$\Sigma \, \mathbf{F} = 0 \text{ and } \Sigma \, \mathbf{M} = 0.$$

In the coplanar, or two-dimensional, example given in Fig. 2.3 the forces shown can be resolved into perpendicular components representing the separate horizontal (x) and vertical (y) effects of each force. The algebraic sum of each directional set of force components is still zero, but the solution of unknown forces is sometimes simplified by such an approach. This procedure is adopted later in this chapter for the analysis of musculoskeletal forces (Fig. 2.5).

In Fig. 2.2 all forces acting on the body are collinear, that is they acted in the same plane about any point on the body. However, in Fig. 2.3 the forces acting are neither collinear nor parallel, and rotation would occur were it not for the fact that the net turning effect of all forces acting in combination is still zero. The turning potential of a force about a point is called its moment, a quantity which is also a vector and is measured by the product of the force and the perpendicular distance of its line of action from that point, that is, its moment arm. The moments of each force about the rear foot shown in Fig. 2.3 are given in Table 2.1, based on the sign convention shown (+ or −), and are seen to sum to zero. It can also be seen that the lines of action of all forces in Fig. 2.3 meet at one point, that is the forces are concurrent. This situation is also an indicator that there is no net turning effect present (i.e. the athlete is in equilibrium), a condition that the starter must ensure before firing the gun.

The forces acting at the hands and feet of the sprint runner depicted in Fig. 2.3 arise as a result of the body's contacts with the track surface. These forces are reaction forces and are equal in magnitude but opposite in direction to the force actions generated by the sprinter against the ground. The reciprocity of these contact forces was first recognized by Sir Isaac Newton in the seventeenth century and formalized at that time as the third of his three laws of motion. This law is commonly stated today as: 'For every action there is an equal and opposite reaction'. It is the reaction forces from the ground that will cause the sprinter to move forward and upward in response to the starter's gun, but movement will only occur if the net (resultant) force acting on the body is non-zero, and the type of motion produced (i.e. linear or angular) will depend on the action line of this resultant force with respect to the mass centre of the sprinter. The size of these ground reaction forces at footstrike, however, is one of the primary causes of impact and overuse injuries. This concept will be fully discussed in the section on external forces on the body.

BALANCE AND STABILITY

Equilibrium, often referred to as balance, describes the state of a body that is not being accelerated. Some sporting activities such as archery, gymnastics, shooting or certain holds in judo demand static balance, where the body is kept at rest, while others require dynamic balance, which occurs when the body is moving with a constant velocity. The location of the centre of mass distribution of the body relative to its base of support is a critical factor in both static and dynamic balance.

GRAVITATIONAL FORCES AND THE CENTRE OF GRAVITY

The law of gravitation, another of Newton's laws, states that:

Between every two particles in the Universe there is a force of gravitational attraction which is proportional to the product of the masses of the two particles and inversely proportional to the square of the distance between them.

This force, which acts along a line joining the two particles, is given by:

$$\mathbf{F}_G = G \cdot \frac{m_1 \cdot m_2}{d^2}$$

Where: $\mathbf{F}_G$ = the force of gravitational attraction

G = the universal gravitational constant (6.67×10^{-11} N m$^2 \cdot$ kg^{-2})

m_1, m_2 = the masses of the two particles or objects, and

d = the distance between their centres of mass.

By far the greatest gravitational force that our bodies encounter is that between the earth and ourselves, because of the earth's size relative to any other object. Every particle of our body experiences an attractional force with the earth and the resultant of all these attractional forces is our bodyweight. The weight of a person or object such as a shot will vary if the force of gravitational attraction varies. Owing to the fact that the radius of the earth at the equator is greater than the radius at the poles, the force of gravity is marginally greater at the poles than at the equator. This not only affects body-weight but also the time in flight of projectiles thrown at different locations on the earth's surface. That is, if all other variables are held constant then an object thrown near the equator will travel further than an object thrown near the earth's poles.

The resultant force of gravitational attraction on the body (bodyweight) is considered to act in a vertically downward direction towards the centre of the earth and through a point at the centre of the body's mass distribution. This point is referred to as the centre of gravity of the body.

STABILITY

Stability describes the resistance of a body to losing its static or dynamic balance. A body can be considered to have some degree of stability when at rest, such as in pistol shooting; when moving in a straight line, such as in water skiing or a 'tug-o'-war'; or when resisting rotary motion, such as in arm wrestling. The stability of a body in equilibrium depends primarily on four factors, namely:

- The weight of the body
- The vertical line of the centre of gravity with reference to the base of support
- The height of the centre of gravity with reference to the base of support
- Friction

The weight of the body

The greater the weight of the body the greater will be its stability. The weight of Sumo wrestlers, linemen in American football or front row forwards in rugby, where stability is an essential feature for success, together with the use of weight classifications in wrestling and judo, bear testimony to the importance of weight as a factor in stability.

The vertical line of the centre of gravity with reference to the base of support

Stability is increased if the line of the centre of gravity is central to the base of support, which is created by a wide (yet comfortable) positioning of the feet. Sports that require a stable platform from which to project an object, for example in archery, or where continued stability is required following the application of an external force, such as in wrestling, usually depict this posture with the centre of gravity centrally located. If the direction of an external force is known, an athlete might displace his or her centre of gravity closer to the edge of the base of support nearest to the external force in order to enhance stability.

The sprinter using the crouch start in Fig. 2.4 has moved his centre of gravity forward of the front foot on the command 'set' to decrease stability in the forward direction. In this situation equilibrium can only be maintained if the counter-clockwise moment created by the weight of the body is balanced by the clockwise moment of the reaction force at the hands. The system would become immediately unstable if the line of the centre of gravity moved forward of the hand support. Likewise, when the hands of the crouched sprinter shown in Fig. 2.4 are lifted on 'go' his stability is immediately upset, allowing for a quicker start than would occur if the sprinter's centre of

gravity was more centrally located over the feet as is the case with the upright stance in Fig. 2.4. Performers who are required to move quickly from one location to another, such as a tennis player, often 'remain on the toes' to displace their centre of gravity forward towards the front of the base of support so that only a small force is necessary to initiate movement toward the ball.

The height of the centre of gravity with reference to the base of support

Stability is generally increased by lowering the centre of gravity. A higher centre of gravity increases the moment arm, and hence the turning effect, of an external force applied through this location with reference to the axis of rotation (the feet). Lowering the centre of gravity decreases this moment arm and makes the body more stable, particularly when the body must maintain stability in the presence of external forces, such as those encountered in body contact sports. In pistol shooting this lowering is not required unless a very strong wind has to be countered as no external force, other than the reaction to the shot, is apparent.

Friction

Friction is a force which opposes motion or impending motion. It is a force that must be exceeded to create motion and there is always a resistance to

Fig. 2.4 The location of the body's centre of gravity as a factor in stability.

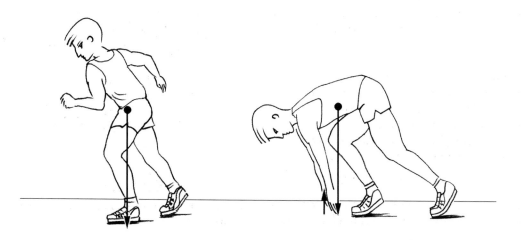

motion present when a body moves over a surface or through a fluid. In many sporting activities this frictional force is undesirable and equipment and technique modifications are often designed to reduce its effect on movement. In ice skating the blades are quite narrow to help reduce the force of friction in opposing motion. Friction may, however, be of advantage in sporting activities. Cleats in football boots and rubber-soled shoes in court games increase the frictional force between the foot and playing surface and thus enable the athlete to maintain a stable position during activities which require sudden changes of direction.

The discussion of static mechanics to this point has focused on force systems that are external to the human body as a whole, but a full appreciation of the biomechanics of human movement is only realized by an understanding of the musculoskeletal forces generated within the body, and of the interactions between body parts. If, for example, one was interested in the forces acting about the ankle joint during the 'set' position of the sprinter depicted earlier in Fig. 2.3, then a free-body diagram could be constructed of the foot independent of all other body parts. Again, all forces that impinge on the foot as a result of the influences of other external structures are shown, together with the pull of gravity on the foot which is negligible in comparison with the other forces present. The completed free-body diagram is shown in Fig. 2.5 and includes some detail of the geometry of the foot which could be readily obtained from external examination or a photographic record, together with an indication of the magnitude and direction of the ground reaction force, which would need to have been obtained from a force-measuring device such as a force platform.

On the basis of the information detailed in Fig. 2.5 it is possible to calculate the magnitude of the net muscular force acting about the ankle (F_M) as well as the magnitude and direction of the joint reaction force (F_J). Equilibrium equations which apply to a system of forces that is static, are:

$$\Sigma\,F = 0 \text{ and } \Sigma\,M = 0.$$

As more is known about the lines of action of the forces than their respective magnitudes, moments about the ankle joint are summed in order to calculate the unknown magnitude of the ankle extensor force (F_M) using the sign convention introduced in Fig. 2.3.

Taking moments about the ankle joint:

$$(F_R \cdot 10) + (-F_G \cdot 3 \cdot \cos 45) + (F_J \cdot 0) + (F_M \cdot 4 \cdot \cos 20) = 0.$$

That is:

$$(F_R \cdot 10.0) + (-F_G \cdot 2.12) + (F_M \cdot 3.76) = 0.$$

And, substituting for known force values:

$$F_M = (8\,N \cdot 2.12 - 250\,N \cdot 10.0)/3.76 = (-)\,660.38\,N.$$

The negative sign simply indicates that the muscular force is tending to rotate the foot in a negative (clockwise) direction with respect to the ankle joint.

Now that the ankle plantar flexor force is known, the other equilibrium equation can be used to calculate the joint reaction force, being the downward and backward push of the shank (leg) on the foot arising from the weight of the structures above, combined with the reaction to the muscular pull at the ankle.

As: $$\Sigma\,F = 0$$

and therefore:

$$\Sigma\,F^X = 0 \text{ and } \Sigma\,F^Y = 0$$

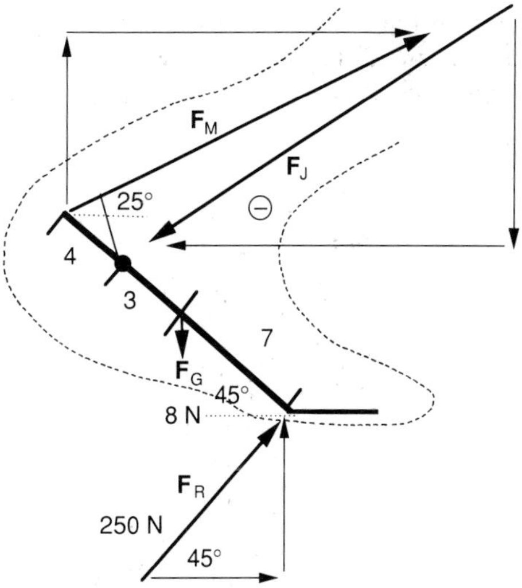

Fig. 2.5 A free-body diagram of a sprinter's rear foot system.

Then:
$$\mathbf{F}_M^X + \mathbf{F}_J^X + \mathbf{F}_R^X = 0$$

and
$$\mathbf{F}_M^Y + \mathbf{F}_J^Y + \mathbf{F}_G + \mathbf{F}_R^Y = 0.$$

That is:
$$(\mathbf{F}_M \cdot \cos 25) + \mathbf{F}_J^X + (\mathbf{F}_R \cdot \cos 45) = 0$$

and therefore
$$\mathbf{F}_J^X = (-598.5) + (-176.8)$$
$$= -775.3 \text{ N.}$$

And:
$$(\mathbf{F}_M \cdot \sin 25) + \mathbf{F}_J^Y + \mathbf{F}_G + (\mathbf{F}_R \cdot \sin 45) = 0$$

and therefore
$$\mathbf{F}_J^Y = (-279.1) + 8 + (-176.8)$$
$$= -447.9 \text{ N.}$$

The composition of these two perpendicular components of the joint reaction force is then undertaken using the Pythagorean theorem, thus:

$$\mathbf{F}_J = \sqrt{(-775.3)^2 + (-447.9)^2}$$
$$= 895.4 \text{ N}$$

and the direction of this resultant force is found by taking the inverse tangent of the ratio of the two perpendicular components:

$$\theta = \tan^{-1}[-447.9 / -775.3]$$
$$= 30°$$

which, in terms of the normal reference system, where all measures are given with respect to a right-hand horizontal, would be 210°.

The magnitude of these musculoskeletal forces is surprisingly large in comparison with the external forces that are generated and reflect the rather inefficient leverage systems that have evolved in the human body. This is the reason why health professionals must be very careful when increasing weights which may be attached to body segments (e.g. the foot) during rehabilitation exercises (e.g. leg extension at the knee joint), as a small increase in external load requires a large increase in muscle force for movement to occur and proportionately greater joint forces.

Dynamics

Dynamics is that part of biomechanics which deals with bodies in motion. It is comprised of: kine-matics, which is a description of the geometry of motion; and kinetics, which is concerned with the causes of motion. A key area in the study of kinematics is the precise description of how the centre of gravity of the human body, or in fact individual segments of the body, move in a straight line (linear motion) and/or in a circular path (rotary or angular motion).

LINEAR KINEMATICS

The change in position of a particle or body segment landmark (e.g. hip, shoulder, centre of gravity, or greater trochanter of the femur) in a straight line, is referred to as the linear displacement ($\Delta \mathbf{r}$) of that point provided direction is taken into consideration. During his airborne phase the runner in Fig. 2.6 has a linear displacement $\Delta \mathbf{r}$ for the hip (often used to represent the centre of gravity of the body) of 0.8 m, being the change from an initial position at toe-off, $\mathbf{r}_i$, to the final position at footstrike, $\mathbf{r}_f$ (i.e. $\Delta \mathbf{r} = \mathbf{r}_f - \mathbf{r}_i$).

The linear velocity, $\mathbf{v}$ of the centre of gravity of this runner is the time rate of change of the position vector $\mathbf{r}$.

$$\mathbf{v} = \frac{\Delta \mathbf{r}}{\Delta t} \text{ or } \frac{d\mathbf{r}}{dt}$$

A coach, keen to reduce the horizontal retarding effect of footstrike on forward movement, may be interested in the instantaneous linear velocity of

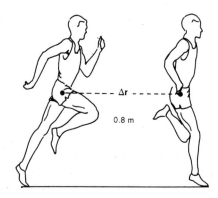

Fig. 2.6 The linear displacement of a runner's hip during the flight phase in running.

the hip at footstrike rather than the average velocity for the race. An instantaneous velocity at footstrike can be calculated by considering the time taken for a very small change in the linear position of the hip at footstrike. If the displacement was 0.1 m and the time taken was 0.015 s, then:

$$v_{instantaneous} = \frac{\Delta r}{\Delta t} = \frac{0.1}{0.015}$$
$$= 6.7 \text{ m·s}^{-1}.$$

Certainly, the velocity fluctuations during a breast-stroke cycle or a leg extension exercise for example, would be extremely important to the coach interested in developing an efficient stroke, or to the health professional interested in the rehabilitation of the quadriceps muscle group.

The linear acceleration, a, for the centre of gravity of this runner is the time rate of change of the velocity vector:

$$a = \frac{\Delta v}{\Delta t} = \frac{dv}{dt}$$

If the runner's hip velocity in Fig. 2.6 decreased from an initial value (v_i) of 6.7 m·s^{-1} at footstrike to a value (v_f) of 5.7 m·s^{-1} by mid-support in 0.05 s then the average linear (de)acceleration of the hip is:

$$a_{average} = \frac{v_f - v_i}{\Delta t} = \frac{5.7 - 6.7}{0.05}$$
$$= -20.0 \text{ m·s}^{-2}.$$

Although difficult to completely avoid, this retarding affect has important implications for the sprinter attempting to attain a high velocity or for the distance runner trying to maintain efficiency.

ANGULAR KINEMATICS

When a body segment rotates from one angular position to another, the angular displacement ($\Delta\theta$) of this segment is given by the angle between the start and finishing positions. For example, the angular displacement between the leg's flexed and extended positions in Fig. 2.7 is 100°. Direction again must be considered and the 100° change in this instance is in a counter-clockwise or positive direction. Angular displacement can be measured

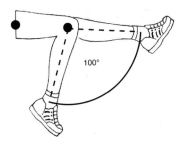

Fig. 2.7 An angular displacement of the lower leg during knee extension.

in a variety of units; however, degrees or radians are the most common units.

The angular velocity (ω) is the time rate of change of angular displacement.

$$\omega = \frac{\Delta\theta}{\Delta t} \text{ deg·s}^{-1} \text{ or rad·s}^{-1}$$

The average angular velocity for the movement of the leg in Fig. 2.7 during 0.2 s is:

$$\omega_{average}(\text{deg}) = \frac{\Delta\theta}{\Delta t} = \frac{100}{0.2}$$
$$= 500 \text{ deg·s}^{-1}.$$

or

$$\omega_{average}(\text{rad}) = \frac{\Delta\theta}{\Delta t} = \frac{100}{0.2 \cdot 57.3}$$
$$= 8.7 \text{ rad·s}^{-1}.$$

The instantaneous angular velocity of the leg at any point during the running cycle in Fig. 2.6 can therefore be calculated in a similar manner to the calculation of instantaneous linear velocity, by reducing the time interval and thus the angular displacement.

The angular acceleration of a segment (α) is the time rate of change of angular velocity, that is:

$$\alpha = \frac{\Delta\omega}{\Delta t} \text{ , or } \frac{\omega_f - \omega_i}{\Delta t}$$

Like its linear equivalent a, α is a variable that must be considered in the understanding of movement because of its link to moment of force ($M_0 = I_G\alpha$) discussed later in this chapter.

THE INTERACTION OF LINEAR AND ANGULAR MOTION

In the majority of sporting or general body movements the angular motion of a body segment is used to increase the linear velocity of the end-point of that segment. In throwing, the angular velocity of the upper limb combined with the forward movement of the body (manifested as the linear velocity of the shoulder) produces a high linear velocity of the hand at release. In hitting sports such as tennis, the angular velocity of an extended upper limb and striking implement produces a high linear velocity of the point of impact with the ball.

Two factors influence the linear velocity of a segment end-point or the point of impact of an implement during rotary motion. The linear velocity of the impact position on the racquet head in tennis or hand in throwing, tangential to the path of the racquet or hand, respectively (v_T), is equal to the angular velocity of the rotating segment (ω; measured in rad·s^{-1}) multiplied by the distance from the axis of rotation to the end-point, or impact point, of the rotating segment (l), that is:

$$v_T = \omega \cdot l.$$

When a segment or implement is rotating about an axis that is itself moving with some linear velocity, for example in softball pitching as depicted in Fig. 2.8, then the linear velocity of the shoulder at

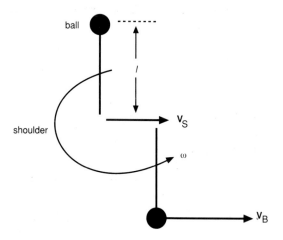

Fig. 2.8 The angular motion of the pitching arm of a softball pitcher.

release (v_S) is added to the angular velocity of the upper limb at release (ω) multiplied by the length of the upper limb (l) to produce the linear velocity of the hand and ball at release (v_B).

$$v_B = v_S + \omega \cdot l$$

(*Note.* No consideration is given here to the role of hand movement during the pitching action.)

A discus thrower in endeavouring to increase the linear velocity of the discus at release could, therefore:

- Increase the linear velocity of the body in the movement across the circle; and/or
- Increase the angular velocity of the upper limb at release of the discus; and/or
- Increase the distance from the axis of rotation (the central axis of the body) to the discus

Projectile motion

In a movement where the body leaves the ground the centre of gravity follows the curvilinear path of a projectile similar to that of a ball or any other object. The equations for uniformly accelerating motion (Hay 1985) can be used to describe this motion for situations where the release and landing heights are at the same level, provided the effects of air resistance on the path of the projectile are ignored. Those interested in the effects of air resistance on various forms of human movement in sport are referred to Daish (1972) and Kyle (1979). A general treatment of projectile motion is also presented by Hay (1985).

FORCE, MASS AND ACCELERATION

The essence of biomechanics is embodied in the relationships between the kinematic measures defined above and the kinetic factors which bring about change in these quantities. The most fundamental of these relationships is that between an applied force and the resulting motion of a body, first formulated by Sir Isaac Newton: 'The rate of change of momentum of a body is proportional to the resultant applied force, and takes place in the direction in which that force acts'. The term momentum is used to describe the quantity of motion a body possesses and is defined as the product of its mass (m) and velocity (**v**). Therefore the rate of change in momentum ($\Delta \mathbf{p}$) to which Newton referred is mathematically equivalent to mass $\times$ velocity/time, where time (Δt) is the period during which the change in velocity occurred (assuming mass remains constant). Thus force (**F**) is proportional to:

$$\text{rate of change in momentum } \frac{\Delta \mathbf{p}}{\Delta t} = m \cdot \frac{\Delta \mathbf{v}}{\Delta t}$$

and as the entity $\Delta \mathbf{v} \div \Delta t$ is equivalent to acceleration (**a**), this relationship is usually simplified to:

$$\mathbf{F} = m \cdot \mathbf{a}.$$

A force with which we are all very familiar is bodyweight and it so happens that this force would cause our bodies to accelerate toward the centre of the earth at approximately 9.8 m·s^{-2} (the rate of gravitational acceleration) if no resistance was offered. The acceleration due to gravity is usually symbolized as g, and from the above formulation it therefore follows that:

$$\text{Weight} = m \cdot g,$$

where weight is measured in newtons and mass in kilograms.

IMPULSE–MOMENTUM RELATIONSHIP

Relationships between the application of forces and resulting motion are sometimes more easily appreciated by considering Newton's second law as originally expressed in terms of changes in momentum. From the equations presented above it will be remembered that:

$$\mathbf{F} = m \cdot \mathbf{a} = m \cdot \frac{\Delta \mathbf{v}}{\Delta t}$$

and therefore

$$\mathbf{F} \cdot \Delta t = m \cdot \Delta \mathbf{v}.$$

The entity $\mathbf{F} \cdot \Delta t$ is called the impulse of a force and this equation, which expresses the relationship between the duration of application of a force and the change in momentum that would occur, is known as the impulse–momentum relationship. The force–time record for a runner during one

episode of contact with the ground is graphically portrayed in Fig. 2.9. The time courses of both the horizontal component and the vertical component of the ground reaction force are shown, and the area under each force curve represents the impulse of that force component. While the largest vertical forces are observed immediately following foot-strike, little change to the runner's vertical motion arises at this time due to the brevity of this phase of force application. Rather, the arrest of the downward momentum acquired during the latter part of the preceding flight phase, together with the generation of sufficient upward momentum to become airborne again is achieved during the production of the second force peak, which is of a much longer duration. The effect of this peak and the time of its application will be discussed in the section on external factors and load on the body.

While the magnitude of the horizontal forces is much less, the reversal of direction of force application here gives an important indicator to the effectiveness of the runner's propulsion. The initial negative force–time phase indicates a period of retardation or 'braking' during which the runner's forward momentum is decreased. For efficient running it is necessary to reduce this effect to a minimum so that performance can be enhanced and the chance of injury reduced. Later the application of a positive horizontal force generates new forward momentum, and if the area under this region of the force–time curve is greater than that of the earlier

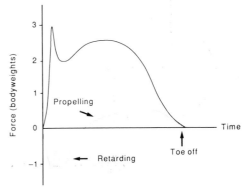

Fig. 2.9 A force–time record of ground reaction forces during running. Vertical (——); fore-aft (.....).

retardation phase, that is, if the net impulse is positive, then the runner's forward velocity will increase.

KINETIC ANALYSES

The impulse–momentum relationship is often used to calculate movement arising from the application of known forces, or, alternatively, to identify the average magnitude of forces applied when only the resulting change in motion is known. When, however, the forces acting at an instant in time are required then the relationship between force, mass and acceleration must be used. For example, if one wished to calculate the muscular forces acting on the leg just prior to footstrike in running, then that question could be answered in the following way:

- First, an accurate record of the instantaneous linear and angular accelerations of the leg must be obtained, using the appropriate procedures outlined in Chapter 3
- Second, the leg's mass and location of mass centre, together with its mass moment of inertia must be obtained
- Third, a free-body diagram is constructed which identifies all forces and moments of force acting on the body segment; the known characteristics of this system are expressed through equations based on Newton's second law of motion (Fig. 2.10)

The force system depicted on the far left in Fig. 2.10 is not immediately amenable to solution in that there are more unknown variables than there are equations defining known relationships between these variables. In order to simplify this force system, the rotary effects of the knee flexors ($\mathbf{F_F}$) and extensors ($\mathbf{F_E}$) can be combined into a single resultant muscle moment of force ($\mathbf{M_M}$) acting on the segment. The non-rotary components of the muscular forces (components whose lines of action pass directly through the joint) are then combined with the joint reaction force ($\mathbf{F_J}$) to produce a resultant joint–muscle force ($\mathbf{F_R}$) acting at the joint centre. These simplifications are shown in the central diagram, with the known dynamic state illustrated on the right. As there are now only two unknowns indicated ($\mathbf{M_M}$ and $\mathbf{F_R}$), values for these can be found using the linear form of Newton's second law, together with its angular equivalent which states the relationship between moments of force ($\mathbf{M}$), angular acceleration (α) and the moment of inertia (I_G), of the body part. That is:

$$\Sigma\,\mathbf{F} = m \cdot \mathbf{a}$$

or $\qquad \Sigma\,\mathbf{F}^X = m \cdot \mathbf{a}^X$ and $\Sigma\,\mathbf{F}^Y = m \cdot \mathbf{a}^Y$

and $\qquad\qquad \Sigma\,\mathbf{M} = I_G \cdot \alpha$

where $\mathbf{a}^X$ and $\mathbf{a}^Y$ are the horizontal and vertical components, respectively, of the linear acceleration

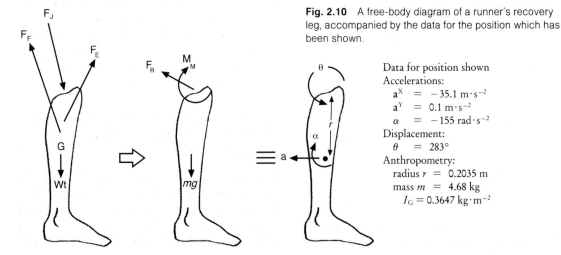

Fig. 2.10 A free-body diagram of a runner's recovery leg, accompanied by the data for the position which has been shown.

Data for position shown
Accelerations:
$\quad a^X \;=\; -35.1 \; \mathrm{m \cdot s^{-2}}$
$\quad a^Y \;=\; 0.1 \; \mathrm{m \cdot s^{-2}}$
$\quad \alpha \;\;=\; -155 \; \mathrm{rad \cdot s^{-2}}$
Displacement:
$\quad \theta \;\;=\; 283°$
Anthropometry:
$\quad$ radius $r \;=\; 0.2035 \; \mathrm{m}$
$\quad$ mass $m \;=\; 4.68 \; \mathrm{kg}$
$\qquad I_G = 0.3647 \; \mathrm{kg \cdot m^{-2}}$

of the segment's mass centre, and I_G the moment of inertia of the leg about the centre of mass of the segment. These equations can then be solved in a similar manner to the static example included earlier in this chapter.

A more extensive portrayal of the dynamics of the runner's recovery leg actions is presented in Fig. 2.11. Here it can be seen that a period of moderate knee extensor effort is followed by larger knee flexor moments. The action of the quadriceps muscle group is needed to swing the leg through and the hamstring muscle group then acts to retard the forward rotation of the leg thus preparing it for footstrike. Muscle power is also shown in this figure and is a measure of the rate at which work is done or energy is expended. As work is the product of force (or moment of force) and distance moved as a result of that force, it follows that:

$$\text{Power } (P) = \frac{\mathbf{F} \cdot \mathbf{d}}{\Delta t}$$
$$= \mathbf{F} \cdot \mathbf{v}$$

or, in this case of muscular actions:

$$\text{muscle power } (P_M) = \mathbf{M}_M \cdot \omega_j.$$

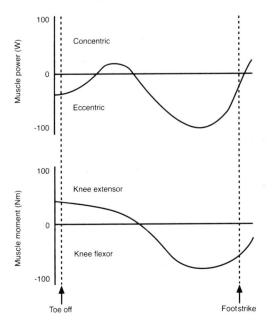

Fig. 2.11 Knee joint moments of force and muscle power during leg recovery in running.

When muscle power is positive, muscles are said to be producing energy, or doing work on a body segment; when negative, energy from the segment is being absorbed by muscles. These alternative muscular actions are often referred to as concentric (producing) and eccentric (absorbing) work. That is, a negative muscle power measure indicates that the resultant muscle action is in the opposite direction to which the segment is rotating, and therefore the muscles concerned are acting eccentrically.

It can be seen from Fig. 2.11 that most of the muscular action about the knee joint during the recovery phase in running is eccentric in nature (negative power). To a large extent the impetus for the forward swing of the lower limb is initiated by the hip flexors, and the knee extensors act initially to prevent the leg from folding up too much as the thigh is pulled forward. During mid-recovery there is a brief period of power production of the knee extensors (a concentric action), but then the knee flexors dominate and provide a vigorous eccentric effort to control an otherwise excessive whip-like action, absorbing the energy acquired by the leg and slowing it down in preparation for footstrike. Kinetic analysis has also shown that the hip extensors are dominant during the same time period, which clearly points to the prominent role that the two-joint hamstring muscles play in leg recovery. Indeed it is during this phase that a runner is most susceptible to hamstring muscle strain, and the predominance of power-absorbing muscle activity at the knee clearly points to the need for eccentric muscle conditioning, particularly for sprint runners. It has also been shown that the eccentric force capacity of this muscle group is the major factor limiting a sprinter's performance.

NEUROMUSCULAR FACTORS THAT INFLUENCE MUSCULAR FORCE PRODUCTION

Although muscle involvement can be predicted from kinetic analyses based on force–mass–acceleration relationships, whereby the cause (muscle force) is inferred from the effect (kinematic behaviour), there are many factors which can influence the effective force that a muscle or muscle group can produce, which are not revealed by these analyses. In most instances of kinetic analysis only a net muscle moment of force can be predicted, and then only for a group of muscles with some commonality of action. Experimental studies of muscle function have, however, identified a number of neuromuscular factors which play an important role in the internal behaviour of muscles. Listed below are some of these factors, with brief illustrations of their influence on muscle force production. More details of the structures involved are discussed in Chapter 1.

Type of Muscular Action

The generation of active force within a muscle is achieved through the attachment of cross-bridges between actin and myosin filaments, which brings about a tendency for these filaments to slide past one another making new attachments (the sliding filament theory). However, the expected shortening in muscle length will only occur if the total force generated by the cross-bridge attachments exceeds the external and internal resistances that are encountered. In many instances the external load applied to a musculotendinous unit is greater than the internally generated force, and so the muscle fibres lengthen during their active state. This effect is referred to as an *eccentric* muscle action, whereas a muscle shortening effect is called a *concentric* action. When there is a complete balance between force generation and external resistance the action is referred to as *isometric*. For reasons that are still not fully understood, there are differences in the force capability of muscle when it is acting under each of these three conditions. Maximal activity under eccentric loading will produce more force than is possible during a maximal concentric action, while a muscle acting maximally in an isometric state will generate an intermediate amount of force. The predominance of eccentric muscle action during the leg recovery phase in sprint running shown in Fig. 2.11 is obviously related to the high incidence of hamstring muscle strain commonly encountered in this activity, and indicates the wisdom of eccentric muscle conditioning for these athletes.

Muscle Length

The overall length of muscle fibres in an active state determines the number of effective cross-bridge linkages between actin and myosin filaments, and thereby the contractile force that can be generated. As the length of a muscle approaches either its shortest or longest extents, there is a reduction in the number of cross-bridge attachments possible, and the maximal level of muscular force capability diminishes. However, if a muscle is stretched beyond its normal resting length, even in an inactive state, some additional tension is produced as a result of the elasticity of passive structures (e.g. connective tissue) that are in parallel with the contractile elements. The combined effects of these two factors can be seen in Fig. 2.12, which depicts the classical length–tension curve of isolated skeletal muscle. The eccentric actions of the hamstring muscle group identified above take place when that muscle group is slightly stretched beyond its normal resting length and suggests that more elastic (compliant) muscle may be beneficial in preventing muscle tears. Recent research has shown that muscle elasticity can be increased by following a programme of flexibility exercises. It has also been shown that ageing increases musculature stiffness and therefore increases the potential for muscle and associated tissue injury. This trend is reduced for those elderly persons that follow an exercise programme.

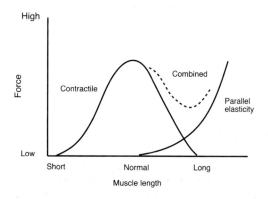

Fig. 2.12 The length–tension curve for an isolated skeletal muscle.

Rate of Change in Length of Muscle

The speed with which muscle fibres shorten or lengthen during an active state governs the effectiveness of the cross-bridge bindings between actin and myosin filaments, and therefore the amount of tension that can be generated. With an increasing rate of change in the length of a muscle, eccentric actions have some capacity for greater force production whereas concentric actions become weaker. These effects, together with the influence of type of muscular action, can be seen in Fig. 2.13. Ideally muscle conditioning should be undertaken in a manner that is specific both to the type of muscle action and the rate of change in length encountered in the activity; that is a tennis player should follow a muscle conditioning programme that is not only specific with reference to the muscles exercised, but at least some of the activities in the programme must be performed at a rate similar to that of the segment movements in tennis.

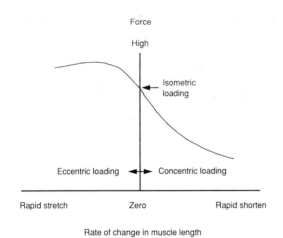

Fig. 2.13 The force–velocity relationship for skeletal muscle.

Muscle Architecture

The arrangement of fibres within a muscle can vary in several ways and these design features will govern the amount of force that can be generated by a whole muscle, as well as its speed of shortening. The sliding filaments mentioned above lie within functional units called sarcomeres. The number of end-to-end connections of these sarcomeres within a muscle fibre determines the extent and rate of shortening of each muscle fibre and therefore the whole muscle, while the number of sarcomeres arranged side-to-side dictates the inherent force capability of a muscle. The ankle plantar flexors for example have approximately 15 sarcomeres per fibre length, whereas the dorsiflexors have twice that number. However, the ankle plantar flexors have a much greater number of sarcomeres lying side by side, and therefore can exert a much greater overall force, a capacity in keeping with the functional role that each muscle must play during movement. However, if the fibres themselves are oriented at some angle to the overall line of pull of a muscle (an angle of pinnation greater than zero, as is the case with the ankle plantar flexors) then there will be a reduction in the ability of each fibre to contribute to both the overall strength and shortening capacity of the whole muscle.

Fibre Composition of Muscle

Muscle fibres together with the spinal neuron from which they receive their innervation (collectively called a motor unit) vary in type, some producing slow muscular actions, others much faster. The faster acting units are also able to generate more force, and these functional differences are largely due to the number of fibres per neuron (the innervation ratio), together with the diameter of each fibre (number of sarcomeres in parallel). Thus, the force capability of a particular muscle will depend on the percentage of each motor unit type it contains. It is therefore not unexpected that sprint runners have a high percentage of fast twitch muscle fibres in their lower limb muscles, whereas marathon runners have a predominance of slow twitch fibres.

Neural Innervation Pattern

Muscle force can be regulated by the nervous system in several different ways. The number of motor units recruited as well as their type would affect the amount and rate of tension capability of a muscle. However, despite the obvious benefits to be gained in some instances by a selective innervation of fast-acting high-force fibres, recruitment normally proceeds in an orderly fashion: first, the slow-acting, low-force-producing units followed by the faster acting units as the tension level rises. Nevertheless, by the time approximately 50% of maximal force is reached all muscle fibres are usually activated, and thereafter it is the pattern of neural stimulus that largely governs the level of force generated. As the rate of discharge of action potentials from the neuron increases, so does the level of muscle fibre force output. Furthermore, it has been shown that a more forceful muscular action will arise when neurons tend to discharge synchronously (i.e. at similar intervals in time). These neural factors that govern the force output of a muscle are respectively referred to as motor unit recruitment and rate coding effects. For example, it has been found that workers accustomed to heavy manual work display a more synchronous pattern of motor unit firing than their clerical counterparts, and that weight-training will promote more synchronous firing.

Muscle Compliance

Active muscle, together with its tendinous insertions and connective tissue, is quite elastic in nature, and when stretched is able to store energy. Some of this energy is subsequently dissipated as heat, but if the stretching eccentric phase is followed closely by a concentric action, then a significant portion of the stored energy can be recovered in the form of useful work. The dissipation of elastic energy with an increased pause time between the eccentric and concentric phases of a bench press can be represented by a negative exponential equation with a 0.85 s half-life of decay (Fig. 2.14). After a delay of approximately 1 s 55% of the stored energy is lost, after 2 s 80% of the stored energy is lost and after a 4 s delay almost all the stored energy is lost (Wilson *et al.* 1991). This elastic behaviour of muscle is advantageous in that it increases the effectiveness and efficiency of muscular work which involves a stretch–shorten cycle of muscle action (e.g. in jumping, running and throwing), and also, it prevents damage occurring to structural elements during strong eccentric actions. This spring-like

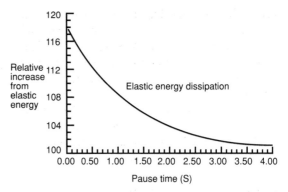

Fig. 2.14 Dissipation of elastic energy with increased pause time.

capacity of a musculotendinous unit can be measured in terms of the amount of elongation produced per unit of applied force, a mechanical measure called compliance.

It has been calculated that the Achilles tendon stretches approximately 18 mm on ground contact during running at moderate speed and that 42 J of energy are stored (Alexander & Bennet-Clark 1977). The stored energy is then recovered during the push-off phase, thereby increasing the efficiency of the runner's action, in that additional work is accomplished by the plantar flexors without a corresponding increase in muscle metabolism. This recovery of strain energy, which represents a significant proportion of the total energy required for running at moderate speed, also benefits the runner in that a greater force or speed of shortening of the

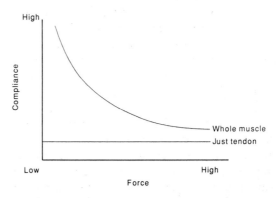

Fig. 2.15 The compliance–force relationship for a musculotendinous structure.

plantar flexors is possible: that is the force–velocity curve illustrated above is moved toward the right (Bosco & Komi 1979). A muscle's compliance decreases with an increase in force generation (more motor units recruited), but eventually it plateaus at a level commensurate with the compliance of the elastic structures which are in series (i.e. end-to-end) with the contractile elements, principally its tendon. These relationships are illustrated in Fig. 2.15.

EXTERNAL FACTORS AND LOAD ON THE BODY

All human movements are the result of internal and/or external forces which act on the body. The previous section outlined how muscles, ligaments, tendons and associated tissues are subjected to internal forces, the intensity of which largely depends on the type of activity being performed. Movements in sport certainly are characterized by loads that produce biological responses ranging from structural and functional adaptations, to overuse injuries or the destruction of tissues.

The link between load and injury is difficult to establish. While it seems that mechanical overload is often the cause of injury, an actual quantification of this relationship is very difficult to achieve. While the measurement of external forces can be accomplished using current instrumentation, the direct measurement of internal forces is considerably more complex. Komi (1990) recorded *in vivo* forces by surgically attaching a 'buckle-type' transducer to the Achilles tendon. This procedure, which was performed under local anaesthesia, allowed measurements to be taken for 3 h before the transducer was removed. Hennig and Lafortune (1989) used a triaxial accelerometer fastened to a Steinmann traction pin, which was inserted into the lateral condyle of the tibia to internally measure the acceleration of the tibia. This procedure enabled the internal influence of impact forces to be determined. Resultant joint reaction forces and muscle moments of force can, however, be estimated from data derived from high-speed motion analysis and internal load can sometimes be inferred from electromyographic activity, but both techniques

have their limitations, which are discussed in Chapter 3. Consequently, the majority of scientific studies on load have focused on external parameters, particularly ground reaction forces, and their influence on the body.

External Forces on the Body

The forces produced in many sports are larger than those experienced during normal gait. However, these loads cannot be classified as healthy or unhealthy, as the body reacts to load as a living organism and therefore the reaction of the body to load may be biopositive or bionegative (Nigg *et al.* 1981). Bionegative effects may be the result of no force or too little force. For example, space travel or convalescence often cause muscle atrophy, excessive force can cause a bone fracture, or repeated submaximal forces can lead to a stress fracture. An optimum exists where, for a given level and frequency of repetitive stress, the effect is biopositive (e.g. strengthening of bone with training). The following sections briefly outline the magnitude of forces associated with selected sporting activities.

LOADING IN SPORTING ACTIVITIES AND GAIT

Walking is a popular fitness activity, particularly for the elderly, as the peak ground reaction forces (GRF) recorded are of the magnitude of 1.2 BW vertically, while peak anteroposterior levels of −0.2 BW are generally recorded. Research has shown that these GRF are velocity related in that vertical GRF for running are approximately 2.5 BW while for sprinting they approach 3.6 BW. Similarly, anteroposterior levels of −0.5 BW (running) increase to −0.8 BW for sprinting. While these forces recorded during running are relatively low, it must be stressed that internal forces are considerably higher. Komi (1990) demonstrated that loading of the Achilles tendon in some cases during running reached values corresponding to 12.5 BW. In an attempt to reduce the injury level of aerobic exercise classes, instructors have replaced high-impact, high-energy activities (jogging) with activities where the GRF are minimized and yet the energy expenditure is kept high (power walking).

Ramey (1970), in a study of the long jump take-off, recorded peak vertical GRF of almost 7 BW for jumps of approximately 4.2 m. These GRF increased to levels between 7 and 12 BW in the triple jump (Ramey & Williams 1985). A mean peak vertical GRF at front foot impact of 9 BW was reported for javelin throwing (Deporte & Van Gheluwe 1988). These levels show why athletes must not constantly repeat these activities, otherwise overuse injuries will almost inevitably occur.

Take-off and landing forces in gymnastics have also been well researched. A study by Panzer et al. (1988) reported peak vertical GRF on each individual lower limb of 8.8–14.4 BW on landing after a double back somersault. Brüggemann (1987) recorded peak vertical take-off forces of 3.4–5.6 BW for a back somersault following a round-off or flicflac. He calculated that internal forces approaching 10 000 N or 16 BW may be experienced by the Achilles tendon. Miller and Nissinen (1987) also recorded peak single limb vertical GRF at take-off for a running forward somersault of 13.6 BW. It is not, therefore, surprising that athletes involved particularly in jumping activities or in gymnastics must be very careful to avoid overuse or even misuse injuries.

Studies by Elliott and Foster (1984) and Foster et al. (1989) on fast bowling in cricket reported peak vertical GRF at front foot impact of approximately 5 BW. A prospective study over a 12 month period of 82 young fast bowlers (15–20 years of age) found that 38% of these bowlers sustained at least one disabling injury during that season. Eleven per cent of the players sustained a stress fracture to the lumbar vertebra(e) (Fig. 2.16) while 27% sustained a soft tissue injury to the back region that caused them to miss at least one match. These injuries were shown to be related to poor technique and/or overuse.

Biomechanical research requires relationships to be drawn between the kinetics of an activity, the incidence of pain, and the site and type of injury. Potential causes of stress include overuse, misuse through poor technique, poor physical preparation and/or genetic predisposition. There is still much to be learned about the optimal loading of the human body.

Equipment design is another area where biomechanics can be useful in not only enhancing performance but reducing the likelihood of injury.

THE ROLE OF BIOMECHANICS IN EQUIPMENT DESIGN AND LOAD MODIFICATION

The physical properties of sporting equipment have a direct bearing on how movements are performed.

Fig. 2.16 A lumbar vertebra (L5) stress fracture in a 16 year old fast bowler.

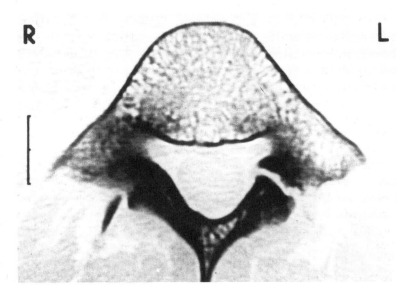

Biomechanics has played an important part in the development of sporting equipment and this has not only decreased the likelihood of injury but often also improved performance.

Protective helmet testing, usually with the aid of an instrumented human headform, has been used to design headgear in American football, ice hockey, baseball and boxing (Norman 1983). Similar techniques have also been used in the development of protective face masks and eyewear, particularly in squash and racquetball (Bishop *et al.* 1982; Easterbrook 1982). Research into tennis racquet design and the performance characteristics of different string types and varying tensions has been directed at improving performance while also reducing the likelihood of injury, particularly lateral epicondylitis or 'tennis elbow' (Brody 1985).

There is little doubt that the 'sport shoe' has been researched more than any other item of sporting equipment. The *'Running Shoe Book'* by Cavanagh (1980) and the book *'Biomechanics of Running Shoes'* edited by Nigg (1986) provide excellent reviews of the influence of load on running mechanics. The general thrust of this research has moved from the testing of materials which comprise the shoe, to testing the shoe with the performer being an integral part of the testing protocol.

Other research studies by McMahon and Greene (1979) on the relationship between track compliance, the kinematics of gait and running velocity, and Hay *et al.* (1979) on design characteristics for the uneven bars in women's gymnastics, are just a few instances where research has been of assistance to both the coach and athlete. Excellent review papers by Reilly and Lees (1984) on 'Exercise and sports equipment: Some ergonomic aspects' and a review by Norman on the 'Biomechanical evaluations of sports protective equipment' (1983) provide very comprehensive background reading in this area.

Biomechanical research into equipment design has not always been directed at the able sports performer. Biomechanical approaches into prosthetic limb construction, taking the forces transmitted at different joints into consideration, have been done by Paul (1976), while research into the design of wheelchairs has been completed in an endeavour to make these chairs more efficient for a number of movement purposes (Rudwick 1978; Cooper 1989).

The Role of Physical Capacities and Body Morphology

The influence of the physical capacities of an athlete during movement has already been discussed in Chapter 1. Several modification strategies were reviewed for each capacity, with the aim of enhancing sport performance and reducing the potential for injury.

It is important to realize, however, that poor technique and overuse, in addition to inappropriate body morphology and/or poor physical preparation all combine to predispose an athlete to injury, which occurs primarily as the load on particular parts of the body is increased. In this respect the biomechanics of movement and the functional anatomy of the athlete are interrelated. Successful development therefore requires the modification of the athlete's physical capacities, in combination with a biomechanically sound technique. If this can be achieved, then the athlete's skill performance will be enhanced.

REFERENCES

Alexander R. McN. & Bennet-Clark H. C. (1977) Storage of elastic strain energy in muscles and other tissues. *Nature* **265**, 114–117.

Bishop P. J., Kozey J. & Caldwell G. (1982) Performance of eye protectors for squash and racquetball. *Physician and Sports Medicine* **10**, 63–69.

Bosco C. & Komi P. V. (1979) Potentiation of the mechanical behaviour of the human skeletal muscle through prestretching. *Acta Physiologica Scandinavica* **106**, 467–472.

Brody H. (1985) *Science made Practical for the Tennis Teacher*. USPTR Instructional Series VI, Philadelphia, PA.

Brüggemann G. P. (1987) Biomechanics in gymnastics. In Van Gheluwe B. & Atha J. (eds) *Current Research in Sports Biomechanics*, pp. 142–176. Karger, Sydney.

Cavanagh P. R. (1980) *The Running Shoe Book*. Anderson World, Inc., Mountain View, CA.

Cooper R. A. (1989) Racing wheelchair crown compensation. *Journal of Rehabilitation Research and Development* **26**, 25–32.

Daish C. B. (1972) *The Physics of Ball Games*. The English Universities Press Ltd, London.

Deporte E. & Van Gheluwe B. (1988) Ground reaction forces and moments in javelin throwing. In de Groot G., Hollander P., Huijing P. & van Ingen Schenau G. J. (eds) *Biomechanics XI-B*, pp. 575–581. Free University Press, Amsterdam.

Easterbrook M. (1982) Eye injuries in squash and racquetball players: An update. *Physician and Sports Medicine* 10, 47–57.

Elliott B. C. & Foster D. H. (1984). A biomechanical analysis of the front-on and side-on fast bowling techniques. *Journal of Human Movement Studies* 10, 83–94.

Foster D., John D., Elliott B., Ackland T. & Fitch K. (1989) Back injuries to fast bowlers in cricket: A prospective study. *British Journal of Sports Medicine* 23, 150–154.

Hay J. G. (1985) *The Biomechanics of Sports Techniques*, 3rd edn. Prentice-Hall, Englewood Cliffs, NJ.

Hay J. G., Putnam C. A. & Wilson B. D. (1979) Forces exerted during exercises on the uneven bars. *Medicine and Science in Sport* 11, 123–130.

Hennig E. & Lafortune M. (1989) Tibial bone acceleration and ground reaction force parameters during running. In Gregor R., Zemicke R. & Whiting W. (eds) *Biomechanics XII*, pp. 226. University of California Los Angeles Press, Los Angeles.

Komi P. (1990) Relevance of *in vivo* force measurements to human biomechanics. *Journal of Biomechanics* 23, 23–34.

Kyle C. (1979) Reduction of wind resistance and power output of racing cyclists and runners travelling in groups. *Ergonomics* 22, 387–397.

McMahon T. A. & Greene P. R. (1979) The influence of track compliance on running. *Journal of Biomechanics* 12, 893–904.

Miller D. I. & Nissinen M. A. (1987) Critical examination of ground reaction force in the running forward somersault. *International Journal of Sports Biomechanics* 3, 189–207.

Nigg B. M. (1986) (ed.) *Biomechanics of Running Shoes*. Human Kinetics Publishers, Champaign, IL.

Nigg B. M., Denoth J. & Neukomm P. A. (1981) Quantifying the load on the human body: Problems and some possible solutions. In Morecki A., Fidelus K., Kedzior K. & Wit A. (eds) *Biomechanics VII-B*, pp. 88–99. University Park Press, Baltimore, MD.

Nigg B. M., Denoth J., Kerr B., Luethi S., Smith D. & Stacoff A. (1984) Load sports shoes and playing surfaces. In Frederick E. (ed.) *Sport Shoes and Playing Surfaces*, pp. 1–23. Human Kinetics Publishers, Champaign, IL.

Norman R. W. (1983) Biomechanical evaluations of sports protective equipment. *Exercise and Sports Science Reviews* 11, 232–274.

Panzer V. P., Wood G. A., Bates B. T. & Mason B. R. (1988) Lower extremity loads in landings of elite gymnasts, In de Groot G., Hollander P., Huijing P. & van Ingen Schenau G.J. (eds) *Biomechanics XI-B*, pp. 727–735. Free University Press, Amsterdam.

Paul J. P. (1976) Approaches to design: Force actions transmitted by joints in the human body. *Proceedings Royal Society London* 192, 163–172.

Ramey M. R. (1970) Force relationships of the running long jump. *Medicine and Science in Sport* 2, 146–151.

Ramey M. R. & Williams K. R. (1985) Ground reaction forces in the triple jump. *International Journal of Sports Biomechanics* 1, 233–239.

Reilly T. & Lees A. (1984) Exercise and sports equipment: Some ergonomic aspects. *Applied Ergonomics* 15, 259–279.

Rudwick L. (1978) New equipment for wheelchair sports. *Sports 'N Spokes*, **December**, 5–11.

Wilson G., Elliott B. & Wood G. (1991) The effect on performance of imposing a delay during a stretch–shorten cycle movement. *Medicine and Science in Sport and Exercise* 23, 364–370.

CHAPTER 3

BIOMECHANICAL ANALYSIS

R. N. Marshall and B. C. Elliott

Biomechanical analysis is the evaluation of technique, whether in sports, industry or everyday life. Methods of analysis used in biomechanics vary from those requiring expensive and complex equipment to techniques utilizing little else than an acute eye and an understanding of the mechanics of the movement.

The previous chapter discussed loads on (or in) the body, the movements which cause them, and their relationship to injury and performance in sport. This chapter will outline methods for determining those body motions and loads, as well as procedures commonly used to assess athletic performance.

Analysis methods in biomechanics may be classified under three general areas, namely *subjective*, *objective* and *predictive* techniques. Most coaches and paramedical professionals use a variety of subjective evaluation techniques during their normal interaction with athletes or patients. They watch a subject, for example, to determine whether there are any gross abnormalities in the range of movement at a joint during walking. Objective techniques in biomechanics refer to the collection, measurement and evaluation of data from the activity of interest. Thus, the gait clinician may use a device to measure the instantaneous angle or the actual range of motion of the knee joint of a patient, in order to evaluate progress in a rehabilitation programme. Similarly, a coach may measure the forces a high jumper exerts on the ground during the take-off by

using a force platform to determine the effect of a change in approach velocity. Predictive techniques attempt to answer the 'What if . . . ?' questions. For example, what effect would reducing the moment of inertia of a below-knee prosthesis have on the swing phase of an amputee's gait?

SUBJECTIVE ANALYSIS METHODS

Subjective, or qualitative, biomechanical analysis involves a non-numerical evaluation of a skill and is most frequently performed during direct observation of the movement. Although a seemingly 'natural' characteristic of good coaches or clinicians, this is a skill which can be learned and improved through practice. The importance of the development of this skill in coaches/clinicians is often underrated, although it is the most common biomechanical analysis technique employed by them. Recent work to refine the techniques and structure of qualitative analysis (Hay & Reid 1988; McPherson 1988) have produced systems which clarify this previously 'intuitive' approach (Fig. 3.1).

These authors propose the employment of a pre-observation phase, where a 'model' of the skill to be analysed is developed, and the mechanical variables concerned and their relationships are described (for examples of these models and their construction, see Hay & Reid 1988). Not all of the features of these models are of the same importance and therefore critical variables must be identified (e.g.

the run-up velocity in the high jump, or the racquet face angle in a tennis topspin forehand drive). An acceptable range for the run-up variable may be between 6 and 8 m·s⁻¹, while a racquet face angle, with reference to the court, of between vertical and 5° forward of this vertical may be acceptable. Objective data reported in applied sport and exercise science research studies usually provide such ranges of acceptability. From this model, the critical variables in the movement are determined and a method for observing these characteristics during the subject's performance is planned. This plan usually involves repeated observations from selected viewpoints and may utilize a recording device such as a videotape recorder. Factors which may be used to

enhance the viewer's perception of the skill should be considered and may include attention to sounds, hand/footprints, or other clues to the way a subject performs a movement. The next phase in this subjective evaluation is the observation of the movement, and a comparison between the observed response and the previously determined desired response. This is followed by the determination of primary errors, from which error correction strategies are communicated to the athlete or patient (Fig. 3.1).

The aim of this approach is to determine the causes of the problem, as opposed to the effects, and to determine the best way to correct those faults. Attempts to correct the effects, such as a diver's incorrect entry, are generally of little value, as they are frequently distanced in time and position from their causes (e.g. body position and forces generated at take-off from the diving board). Another common problem facing observers of motion is the tendency to see what they think they should see, as opposed to what actually occurs in the performance. Like other skills, however, observation becomes better with practice.

OBJECTIVE ANALYSIS METHODS

At any level of movement analysis there is a need for interaction between the coach/clinician and biomechanist if maximum performance is to be achieved. Objective evaluation of movement requires that a permanent record be collected for a number of trials so that each can be viewed and analysed.

Recording of permanent data on movement may take a number of different forms, for example cinematography, electromyography (EMG), accelerometry, dynamometry or electrogoniometry. While some of these techniques may not be available for general use, a more informed reading of the scientific biomechanics literature can only occur if the reader understands how objective data are derived. Such an understanding should also assist the health or coaching professional to ask more pertinent questions on the causes of specific body movements.

An illustration of a biomechanical data acquisition system can be seen in Fig. 3.2, which shows the

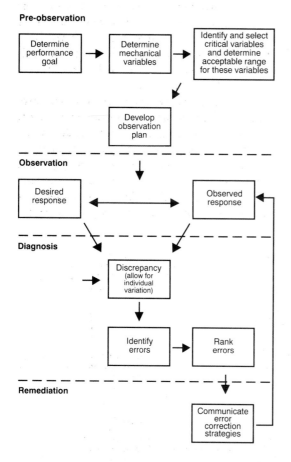

Fig. 3.1 An approach to subjective skill analysis (modified from McPherson 1988).

general components of data collection and recording situations. Typically, a transducer is used to convert changes in the variable of interest into an analogue, or continuous, electrical signal. This signal is then amplified, passed through a signal conditioner which frequently converts it to a numerical (or digital) representation, and recorded. In this example, the force platform is a transducer, converting ground reaction forces into an electrical signal. This signal is then amplified, passed to an analogue-to-digital (A–D) converter (a signal conditioner), and the digital information which represents the characteristics of the ground reaction forces is recorded by the computer. Other transducer–amplifier–signal conditioner–recorder systems may also be seen in Fig. 3.2. The process of recording body movement characteristics on film, through to the production of segmental angular positions, velocities and accelerations represents another system, while the attachment of electrodes to selected muscles, and the subsequent amplification, A–D conversion and recording of the EMG signals illustrates a third.

Three techniques are used to convey the analogue signal from the transducer to the signal conditioner and computer. Frequently the transducer is 'hard wired' to the signal conditioner and computer by being physically connected via a wire. This is often referred to as an 'umbilical cord' and has the advantage of providing high-signal integrity. In some situations, however, the effects of the length and weight of the umbilical cord on the subject may need to be considered. For situations where the subject moves over a large area and an umbilical cord is impractical (such as with a runner), researchers have utilized a telemetry system, where the signals from the transducer(s) are transmitted using radio waves to a receiver and then to the signal conditioner/computer. This requires the subject to carry a small transmitter, but eliminates the problem of an umbilical cord. Unfortunately, some telemetry systems have sampling frequency limitations which introduce the potential for 'aliasing' of the signal. A third alternative is to use a device known as a 'data logger'. Essentially this is a miniature portable computer (usually weighing less than 1000 g), consisting of a microprocessor with a substantial amount of electronic memory. The microprocessor controls the sampling frequency and the data are stored in the memory. The subject carries the data logger in a backpack during their activity and afterwards the researcher transfers the information to their computer.

In the following sections, measurement procedures will be discussed primarily in isolation, although it is common, and often preferable, to use more than one technique during an experiment to gain additional information and thereby provide greater insight into the characteristics of a particular movement. Additional detail regarding equipment used in biomechanics can be obtained from the

Fig. 3.2 A general data acquisition system in biomechanics.

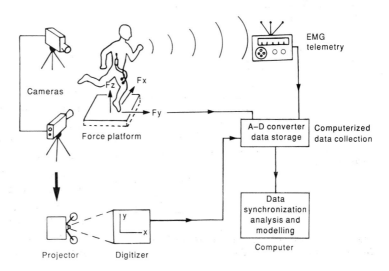

International Society of Biomechanics or the International Society of Biomechanics in Sports. A few textbooks also list suppliers or manufacturers of specialist equipment for biomechanics, and the reader may wish to refer to them (e.g. Whittle 1991; Biewener 1992) for further information.

Image Analysis Techniques

Image analysis techniques, including both movie photography and videography, provide the opportunity to capture complex movement sequences on film or videotape so that a detailed analysis can be performed. However, an understanding of sampling frequency relative to photography or videography is needed prior to discussing different image analysis techniques, as both are sampling processes that record information at discrete points in time during a continuous motion.

The sampling rate needed for an accurate representation of movement must be at least twice the value of the highest frequency component contained in the movement (Shannon's sampling theorem), although many researchers believe sampling rates of five to 10 times the maximum frequency component are necessary. Excessive sampling either increases the cost when using high-speed photography or limits the choice of cameras when using high-speed videography. Under-sampling will cause vital movement characteristics to be missed, or distortions to arise.

At the subjective level of analysis, film or video techniques may be used to record movement and allow general comments to be made on the observed characteristics. At an objective level it is not sufficient to just record and observe movement, as detailed measurements must be completed and inferences drawn with reference to the movement. Specific equipment and procedures must be used if accurate objective data are to be collected using image analysis techniques.

MOVIE PHOTOGRAPHY

In high-speed cinematography a motor-driven camera capable of providing frame rates up to approximately 500 Hz ($c \cdot s^{-1}$) and exposure times up to approximately 1/10 000 s is needed to accommodate movement and sport skills of differing speeds. In a golf drive for example, the ability to clearly record the impact of the ball and club head would require an exposure time of approximately 1/3600 s and a frame rate of 400 Hz. The 400 Hz frame rate ensures that the moment of impact is captured on film, while the exposure time guarantees that no blurring of the image occurs. For an analysis of jogging, an exposure time of 1/800 s would provide a clear image of the leg, while a frame rate of 100 Hz is sufficient to sample leg movement at the required frequency.

The collection of data from film for analytical purposes (digitizing) is the most time-consuming and tedious aspect of cinematographic research. A stop-action projector is needed to control film movement so that an operator can move an X–Y coordinate system until a pointer, pen, light or

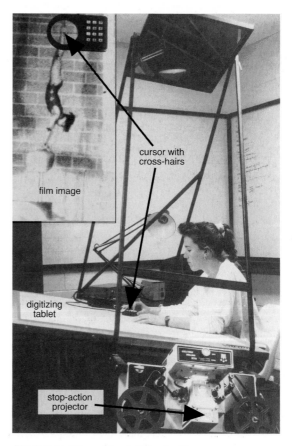

Fig. 3.3 A 16 mm film digitizing facility.

Table 3.1 The information yield from a film motion analysis system

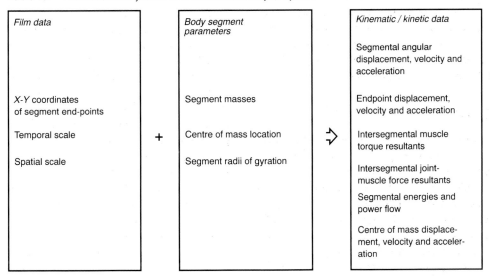

Film data	Body segment parameters	Kinematic / kinetic data
X-Y coordinates of segment end-points	Segment masses	Segmental angular displacement, velocity and acceleration
Temporal scale	Centre of mass location	Endpoint displacement, velocity and acceleration
Spatial scale	Segment radii of gyration	Intersegmental muscle torque resultants
		Intersegmental joint-muscle force resultants
		Segmental energies and power flow
		Centre of mass displacement, velocity and acceleration

cross-hairs lie over the desired anatomical landmark to be digitized (Fig. 3.3).

The coordinates of this point are then stored on a computer. In order for the anatomical landmark to be located, it must be clearly marked on the subject being filmed, so that an accurate identification of the segment end-point or joint centre is possible (see inset to Fig. 3.3). These coordinate data are then smoothed (this topic is discussed later in this chapter) prior to being mathematically manipulated in the calculation of kinematic and kinetic data (Table 3.1).

As is evident from Table 3.1, information additional to the coordinates of the selected landmarks is required. A large sweep-hand clock may be included in the photographic field to establish the actual frame rate of the camera. Alternatively, internal camera lights which flash at a set rate may be used to mark the film and allow film speed calculation. A spatial scale, such as a large metre rule, must also be filmed in the plane of action to convert film scale measures to real values.

Data from film are usually collected in a number of formats and are as follows.

Single camera planar analysis

Sagittal plane cinematographic data supplemented with EMG information from below-knee amputees showed modifications to their gait patterns, such that kinematic, kinetic and EMG asymmetries were recorded during walking (Winter & Sienko 1988). Descriptions of these gait patterns were then able to provide a clear picture of how below-knee amputees walk, and an assessment of the compensations they performed to cater for their altered locomotor characteristics.

Multi-camera planar analysis

Fast bowlers were filmed both laterally and from above while bowling, so that their front foot impacted a force platform during the delivery stride in a study by Foster et al. (1989). Data from these two planes of motion were used to identify biomechanical correlates of back injuries to fast bowlers in cricket.

Multi-camera three-dimensional (3D) analysis

A common practice in cinematographic analysis is to perform 3D spatial reconstructions from 2D film images, using a technique such as the Direct Linear Transformation (DLT) method, which has been adapted from analytical close-range photogrammetry (Marzan & Karara 1975). In this method two or more cameras initially film a reference structure containing markers of known coordinates in space encompassing the field of movement. The reference structure is then removed and the subject filmed in the same area without altering camera position or settings. The 2D images of both the reference structure and subject are then digitized and the unknown 3D coordinates of each of the subject's landmarks are then determined. Inaccuracies in 3D reconstruction are likely to occur if the digitized movement lies outside the reference structure distribution space (Wood & Marshall 1986) and the use of control points distributed around the outside rather than within the space to be calibrated produces superior results (Challis & Kerwin 1992). Subsequent development of 3D filming procedures has seen the refinement of computer software so that panning is possible (de Groot *et al.* 1989) and less reliance placed on large 3D reference structures (Woltring *et al.* 1989).

Elliott *et al.* (1989) provide an example of 3D cinematographic data collection where they described the mechanics of the multi-segment and single unit topspin forehand drives in tennis. A greater understanding of the mechanics, particularly of the multi-segment stroke, will assist coaches to teach this technique with correct body mechanics and thus reduce the potential for upper limb injury.

High-speed photography therefore permits a relatively flexible approach to data recording, with acceptable accuracy and minimal interference to the subject's movements from the attachment of external measuring devices. However, film costs and time delays caused by processing and digitizing may make film less than a perfect medium to study motion. Advances in electronic image analysis technology now permit other techniques, which are frequently videotape based, to compete with film as a convenient, accurate and cost-effective tool to collect objective data on movement.

Video photography

For videography to be used as an objective rather than subjective analysis tool, cameras had to be developed which provided a variety of frame rates and exposure times. In general, the addition of mechanical or electronic shutters reduced the exposure time and removed the problem of blurring in the recording of fast moving images, while an increase in frame rates from 25 up to 2000 frames

Table 3.2 Sample papers from the Book of Abstracts, XII International Society of Biomechanics Congress (University of California at Los Angeles, Los Angeles, 1989) illustrating the use of various videography techniques

---

Opto-electronic measurement systems
    Stokes V. P. Walking-vs-racewalking: 3D kinematic patterns for the trunk (Selspot II).
    Eng J. J. & Pierrynowski M. R. Effect of foot orthotics on the kinematics of the knee-joint (Watsmart)
Closed-circuit TV image analysis
    Bulgheroni M. & Frigo C. A three-dimensional model for leg and foot kinematic studies (Elite)
    Ang E. J. *et al.* Effects of load carriage on the lower limbs (Vicon)
Video image analysis
    Rash G. S. *et al.* Spectral analysis of lower body kinetics during selected activities (ExpertVision)
    Smith S. L. & Werner S. L. Comparative analysis of decathlete and elite javelin throwers (Peak Performance)
    Zhang Y. Three dimensional analysis of the snatch technique for two world record creators at the 6th national athletic meeting of PRC, 1987 (Ariel)

---

per second or more illustrate other recent advances in video technology.

The collection of data from these approaches for analytical purposes is far quicker than in film analysis. Three different types of systems currently being used in video analysis are described below. Table 3.2 lists papers presented at the XII International Society of Biomechanics Congress (Los Angeles, 1989), which illustrate an application of each system.

Optoelectronic measurement systems (e.g. Selspot II, Selective Electronic Inc., Sweden; Watsmart, Northern Digital, Canada). In these systems light-emitting diodes are attached to the subject, and then video-like cameras, a marker detection module and a computer track the diodes in space almost instantaneously. They are geared primarily for laboratory analysis and experience substantial performance reduction when used outdoors. If a recorded image of the performance is required, a video-based analysis system may be preferable.

Closed circuit TV image analysis (e.g. Elite, BTS Bioengineering Technology and Systems, Italy; Vicon, Oxford Metrics Ltd, UK). With this approach,

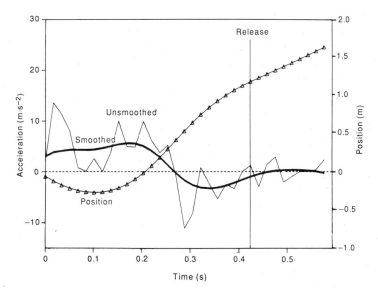

Fig. 3.4 The horizontal position of a ball during and after a throw, and accelerations derived from position–time data, both with and without initial data smoothing.

processing of computer-stored TV images is carried out, but these are not usually recorded on video-tape. Again these systems are primarily geared for the laboratory setting, and their performance may be degraded when used outdoors.

Video image analysis (e.g. Expert Vision, Motion Analysis Corp., USA; Ariel Performance Analysis System, USA; Peak Performance, Peak Performance Technologies, Inc., USA). Like the two previous groups, these systems enable the user to analyse 2D or 3D motion patterns, but record the images from the camera(s) on videotape. This provides not only an image which can be viewed at a later date, but also the opportunity to modify and re-analyse the recording of the motion, a feature not available with the optoelectronic systems discussed pre-viously. By producing a video image this method provides a wider user base in the area of sport biomechanics.

DATA SMOOTHING

Data are usually collected in biomechanics by sampl-ing an analogue, or continuous signal at discrete points in time. The signal of interest may be the

motion of an athlete, and a movie or video camera might collect samples of this every 1/100 s (100 Hz). Alternatively, a computer and A–D converter might sample the EMG activity from a muscle at 1000 Hz. However, due to problems such as the inaccurate digitizing of joint centres, or the sampling of a signal which because of electrical interference is noisy, the data will frequently contain measurement errors. For this reason, particularly if other measures are to be derived from these data (such as velocities and accelerations from position–time information), allowances and corrections must be made for these inaccuracies. For example, small errors in position–time measures will be drastically amplified during the process of numerical differentiation to obtain velocity and acceleration values. There have been many techniques recommended for the removal of noise; however, the two data smoothing procedures most frequently used in biomechanics are least squares approximations using splines (piece-wise polynomials) and digital filtering.

Figure 3.4 shows the smoothed horizontal position–time data for a ball prior to and after release in a throwing action. Also included on the graph are two other curves, one showing the acceler-ation derived from unsmoothed position–time values and the second the accelerations after smooth-ing using a digital filter. The accelerations obtained from the unsmoothed position–time data are obviously of dubious value, as they do not show the smoothness expected in a movement of this nature. Indeed, the horizontal acceleration of the ball after it leaves the hand is known to be virtually zero as shown by the smoothed curve (except for air resistance effects), and that is hardly the case with the unsmoothed curve. Unfortunately, a yard-stick of this nature is not always available to the researcher to indicate the degree of smoothing required. As over-smoothing data may result in significant information loss, several algorithms which determine an optimal level of smoothing based on the inherent statistical properties of the data are commonly used (Woltring 1985). It is beyond the scope of this chapter to provide a detailed account of data smoothing and differen-tiation techniques used in biomechanics, and the interested reader is referred to Wood (1982) or Winter (1990) for further information.

Non-imaging Kinematic Measurement Techniques

Cinematography or videography are the most com-mon objective data collection techniques used in biomechanics because they provide a permanent and visual record of performance. There are, how-ever, other non-imaging measurement procedures that provide valuable biomechanical data for the objective analysis of movement. It may be preferable at times to measure some of the kinematic aspects of a movement directly, rather than derive the measurements from film or videotape. Two types of devices are commonly used for this: an acceler-ometer or an electrogoniometer.

An accelerometer, as the name suggests, measures the acceleration experienced by the object to which it is attached. They are typically either piezo-electric or strain gauge devices, and the reader is referred to the section in this chapter on dyna-mometry for an explanation of their operational principles. Accelerometers can be used to monitor the accelerations sustained by a body segment, such as at impact of the foot during walking or running. Results are usually reported as multiples of the acceleration due to gravity (1 g), and thus in Fig. 3.5 we see an impact shock of 14 g in barefoot

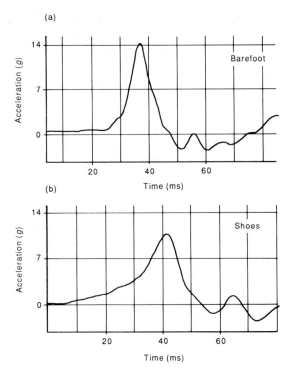

Fig. 3.5 Accelerometer signals recorded on the lower portion of the tibia while running (a) barefoot and (b) in shoes.

running reduced to 10 g over a lengthened time period while running in jogging shoes. Acceler-ometers are also used to measure impact acceleration or vibration characteristics of sports equipment, or the movement characteristics of limbs, for example during reaching or pointing motions. The major advantage of using an accelerometer is the direct measurement of acceleration, without the need for double differentiation of position–time data. It should be noted that velocity and displacement can be obtained by integration of the sampled acceler-ations. The main disadvantages of these devices are in the difficulty experienced in accurate calibration for accelerations greater than 2 g, in the contamin-ation of single axis accelerometer data due to rota-tions of the limb about other axes, and in the need to have cables between the subject and recorder. Some accelerometers are also relatively fragile and care is needed during testing. Another disadvantage is the difficulty experienced in determining limb position after a period of time without resorting to a complex multiple accelerometer measurement.

Accelerometers were used by Voloshin and co-workers (1981) to examine the shock-absorbing capabilities of the joints of the body during walking. They recorded the heel strike impact simultaneously from the tibial tuberosity and the forehead, in both normal subjects and subjects with degenerative joint disease. Their results showed a considerable difference between the abilities of the two groups to attenuate transient impact forces through the locomotor system, with the normal subjects achieving an average of 23% greater force reduction between the ankle and the forehead. These authors suggested that degenerative joint disease reduced that particular joint's shock absorption ability, leading to overloading of the next joint in the system, and that this process may be implicated in the development of osteoarthritis.

There are, however, problems associated with the measurement of acceleration where an accelerometer is fixed to a body segment during rapid movement. Ziegert and Lewis (1979) reported that measured acceleration was affected by the method of attachment of the accelerometer to the tibia, particularly because of skin movement. Lafortune (1991) was able to avoid such problems by measuring

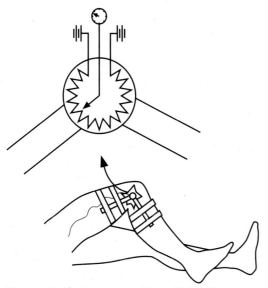

Fig. 3.6 A simple elgon, showing typical positioning on a knee joint and the basic electrical configuration.

tibial acceleration directly during walking and running by attaching a triaxial accelerometer to a Steinmann pin inserted into the lateral condyle of the tibia.

An electrogoniometer is an electrical version of a goniometer, and is a device to measure the angular displacement of a joint. It usually consists of a variable resistor (potentiometer) located over a joint axis of rotation with arms fixed to the long axes of the limb on either side of the joint (Fig. 3.6). Elgons vary from simple, single joint and single plane models to self-aligning 3D versions (Triax, Chattecx Corp., USA). A recent development has been the use of an elgon with a flexible transducer element, which is inexpensive, self-aligning and relatively insensitive to variables such as skin stretch and long axis limb rotation (Penny & Giles, UK).

Elgons can provide rapid and accurate measurement of joint angle (including 3D orientation), providing they are correctly aligned and attached securely. Their major disadvantages include the need for an exoskeleton when using some elgon systems (which may inhibit natural movement), and the need to either have cables connecting the recording system and subject, to carry a data logger or to introduce the additional complexity of telemetering the data. In addition, elgons provide only the relative angle between two segments and therefore do not permit the definition of the absolute position of segments in space.

The advantages of direct and instantaneous measure of limb rotations was noted by Isacson et al. (1986) in their evaluation of free speed walking using bilateral 3D hip, knee and ankle elgons. They noted the technique was a simple and efficient tool for recording and studying gait, giving immediate, accurate and reproducible results which were particularly suited for clinical situations. The method also provides opportunities for studying the co-ordination and symmetry of motion among the major lower extremity joints.

Dynamometry

Dynamometry refers to the measurement of force. While it is possible to estimate both internal and external forces (i.e. bone-on-bone and ground reaction, respectively) from a combination of segment position, velocity and acceleration data obtained from cinematography and anthropometry, it is preferable to measure the actual force or forces if possible.

The direct measurement of external forces, generally collected using a force platform, when combined with cinematographic and anthropometric data, permit more accurate estimates of internal forces to be calculated than with the previously described cinematographic technique. An understanding of internal forces is essential in sports medicine, as they are one of the key factors in the cause of many sports injuries, particularly those related to overuse. It is possible, although not always practical, to measure *in vivo* (internal) forces by attaching a transducer to selected parts of the body, such as tendo calcaneus, and have the subject perform various activities so that forces in this tendon can be measured. Komi (1990) attached a buckle transducer to the Achilles tendon and recorded forces associated with walking, running and jumping. The loading of this tendon in some cases reached values as high as 9000 N, corresponding to 12.5 times bodyweight (BW).

Dynamometers are composed of a transducer which transforms mechanical deformation (strain) into an electrical signal that is proportional to the applied force (stress). As with accelerometers these transducers are generally of a strain gauge or piezo-electric type.

In a strain gauge, very thin electrically resistive elements are bonded to a stiff yet elastic support material and then one or more of these are attached to the object where the force is to be applied. These gauges are then used to measure small deformations caused by an applied force in terms of a change in electrical resistance. Piezo-electric transducers, however, rely on the electrical properties of certain crystalline materials such as quartz, where the deformation caused by the applied force results in a change in electrical resistance. With this type of transducer the crystalline structure is enclosed in a 'load cell', which can be mounted between a fixed surface and the applied force. The small changes in resistance in both these types of transducers require amplification prior to the recording of the signal.

Strain gauge dynamometers have been used in a wide variety of biomechanical studies, some of which are mentioned below:

- The *in vivo* measurement of force in the Achilles tendon was calculated during stretch–shorten cycle activities; these forces provide insight into the potential of a selected activity to cause injury (Komi 1990)
- In equipment design, where maximum forces recorded during actual performances on the asymmetric bars in women's gymnastics were measured using strain gauges; these force levels were then used in the design of this equipment (Hay *et al.* 1979)
- The forces generated by a rower were measured within a competitive environment by attaching strain gauges to the oarlock of a racing shell; these results were then used to assess the force profile of the subject during each stroke cycle so as to match rowers on opposite sides of a shell (Dal Monte & Komor 1989)

FORCE PLATFORMS

The most common dynamometer used in biomechanics is the force platform, which is usually set in concrete, mechanically isolated from its environs and mounted so that it is flush with the laboratory floor (Fig. 3.7a). The transducers may be either piezo-electric or strain gauge, and typically in these platforms three force transducers oriented at right angles to each other are positioned under each of the four corners of a rigid plate. From these 12 force measures the three perpendicular components of the resultant ground reaction forces (F_z, F_y and F_x) are calculated. Further, the point of resultant force application (CP_x, CP_y) with reference to the centre of the platform, a position commonly referred to as the centre of pressure, and a moment (M_z') about a perpendicular axis through the centre of pressure can also be derived.

These measures are used to assist in the understanding of many human movements, and the following examples illustrate this:

- The external forces and centre of pressure data are often used to determine load on the body (see Chapter 2 for a further explanation of this)

- The measures may be used to assist in the monitoring of changes in gait characteristics, particularly for patients following an operation or following periods of intervention
- The centre of pressure movement, although *not* a measure of the motion of the centre of gravity of the body, has been used as an index of postural sway in activities such as archery, rifle-shooting or balance tests

The force platform measures in Fig. 3.7c and d show that fast bowling in cricket is certainly an

impact sport, where the bowler experiences a series of minor 'collisions' during the run-up, followed by two major collisions when the back foot and front foot impact with the ground. Peak vertical (F_z) and horizontal (F_y) ground reaction forces of 3.0 BW and -0.7 BW, respectively, at back foot strike and 4.0 BW and -2.0 BW, respectively, at front foot impact, certainly indicate that this is a potentially dangerous activity, as these impact forces must be absorbed by the body while the trunk is extending, laterally flexing and rotating in an endeavour to achieve maximum power in delivery. Further, the large twisting moments (M_z') under the back foot which occur initially away from the batsman (peak of 40 N m at back foot impact) and later toward the batsman (peak after front foot impact of 35 N m) are indicative of both the level and reversal in direction of trunk rotation during the delivery stride, a factor which researchers have found to be related to the incidence of stress fractures.

Fig. 3.7 Ground reaction forces: measures from a force platform (a); the centre of pressure (F_R) under the foot of a fast bowler at front foot impact in the delivery stride contrasted with one 'frame' of pressure mat data (b); ground reaction force and moment data at back foot (c); and front foot (d) impact during the delivery stride of fast bowling.

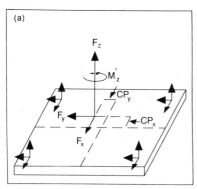

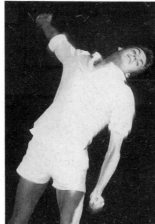

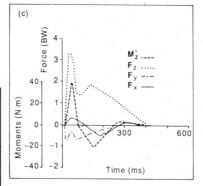

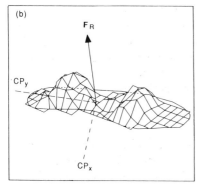

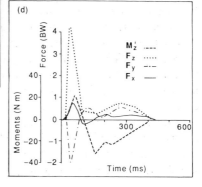

PRESSURE MATS

The centre of pressure information derived from a force platform merely provides the coordinates of the location of the resultant force. In many situations it is more important to know how these forces are distributed under the foot, and for this reason pressure mats are used. These consist of a large matrix of miniature transducers (<5 mm diameter) recording pressure at discrete points on the contact surface. These have been constructed as innersoles which may be placed in shoes to monitor pressures under the foot, or as a mat which may be placed on the contact surface for more general applications. The pressures sensed by the transducers during a movement are captured on computer, and a graphical display is typically used to provide an indication of the time history of the distribution of pressure over the contact surface. Figure 3.8 shows a single 'frame' of pressure mat data obtained from under the foot of a cricket bowler during delivery, as well as the corresponding resultant force and the (misleading) centre of pressure information from a force platform. This figure shows how the force platform centre of pressure information is in reality an average of the pressures on the plantar surface, and may occur at a point where there is little or no actual pressure. A good example of the utility of these devices can be seen in the work of Cavanagh et al. (1985), who have used pressure distribution measurements obtained from the plantar surface of the foot as a prophylactic procedure in the management of diabetics' feet.

STRENGTH-MEASURING DEVICES

Strength is the ability of a muscle or muscle group to generate force, but it is often difficult to measure the actual forces produced. What is usually measured in humans is the torque or moment of force produced about a joint. Evaluation of the mechanics of an athlete's performance is often aided by a knowledge of his or her muscular strength characteristics. Force generation characteristics of muscles may be tested isometrically (with a fixed joint angle and virtually no muscle shortening) or dynamically, where dynamometers are used to measure force production during movement. Methods used to assess the dynamic characteristics of muscle have commonly taken two forms: controlled shortening velocity protocols where a limb segment moves at a constant angular velocity or where muscle is required to shorten at a constant rate; and controlled loading protocols where muscle is loaded with a constant mass and then required to produce its maximal shortening velocity. Current trends favour the first protocol, and often assess strength and power of a muscle group acting about an isolated joint at a variety of joint angular velocities using an 'isokinetic' dynamometer (more properly described as an isokinematic dynamometer). While most dynamometers developed specifically for muscle function testing use this mode, other types of dynamometers are available, and isokinetic machines are only one form of accommodating resistance devices. Both concentric (muscle shortening) and eccentric (forced muscle lengthening) actions may be assessed with a number of the commercially available dynamometers. These provide information on the dynamic properties of muscle, which may be more appropriate to an athlete's or patient's performance than information on isometric strength at specific angles (Fig. 3.9).

The mechanical characteristics of some dynamometers may cause artefacts to be generated and recorded. These may arise, for example, as the

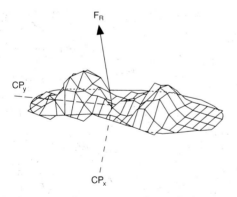

Fig. 3.8 One 'frame' of pressure mat data recorded under the front foot of a bowler during delivery (the higher the 'hill' the greater the pressure). The location of the centre of pressure measure given by a force platform is also shown, and is seen in this instance to be quite meaningless as an index of plantar surface loading.

result of impacts between the limb and the dynamometer as the limb reaches the pre-set speed and is decelerated abruptly (resulting in a 'torque overshoot'); as interactions between the limb and the dynamometer's velocity–feedback system; or as a result of the dynamometer's acceleration or deceleration at the extremes of the range of movement. These all influence the recorded torque, and thus care is sometimes needed in the interpretation of the results.

Strength testing has often been used in conjunction with other biomechanical techniques in the evaluation of subjects, and this was the approach taken by McNair *et al.* (1989). They examined the jogging gait of subjects with anterior cruciate ligament (ACL) deficiency, and used an isokinetic strength-testing dynamometer to assess concentric quadriceps and hamstring muscle group torque generation capabilities. The strength differences between the ACL-deficient and normal limbs were then integrated with EMG and movement information to evaluate the techniques used by subjects to compensate for their knee condition. The subjects demonstrated symmetric interlimb kinematic patterns, but had significantly increased EMG activity in the quadriceps of the ACL-deficient limb immediately before and after heel strike when compared with the normal limb. On the surface this would

appear to be disadvantageous to these subjects, as excessive quadriceps activity in that phase of the gait cycle would exacerbate the ACL deficiency problems. However, when the strength results were included in the analysis and it was noted that the quadriceps were significantly weaker on the ACL-deficient limb, the authors suggested an alternative explanation. They proposed that the quadriceps on the ACL-deficient limb were not in fact producing excessive forces at an inappropriate time, but rather that they were working at a higher proportion of their maximum ability in order to enable interlimb symmetry.

Strength dynamometers have also been used to examine some of the mechanical characteristics of muscles, such as compliance and force–velocity relationships. Marshall *et al.* (1990) collected data on torque, angular velocity and angular position during maximal knee-extension trials and combined this with information on the geometry of the knee joint to determine the linear force, velocity and muscle length characteristics of the knee-extension exercise. These data were then presented as 3D surfaces of muscle function (see Fig. 3.10a and b). Figure 3.10a shows the angular data, and the surface illustrates the general characteristics of both the force–velocity and tension–length relationships discussed in the previous chapter. In the torque–

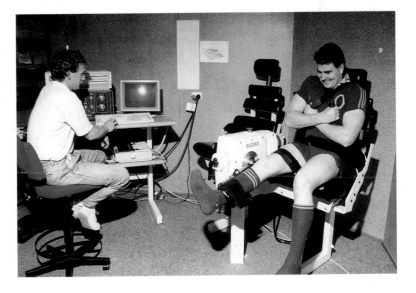

Fig. 3.9 Isokinetic dynamometers provide data on strength characteristics throughout a range of movement. This is important for both the coach and the clinician interested in improving performance through strength development.

angular position plane the curve is reasonably symmetrical, with peak torques recorded at about 65°. Similarly, the torque–angular velocity relationship shows peak torques at or near zero velocity, with torques decreasing with increases in speed. However, substantial differences between the linear and angular surfaces can be seen. The major variation is in the position of maximum recorded torque compared with the position at which the maximum muscle force was generated. The linear data (Fig. 3.10b) indicated that maximum forces were produced considerably earlier in the knee-extension movement than shown in the angular data. The authors suggested that the angular information provided directly from many of the commercially available dynamometers may not be a good indication of the actual forces generated by the knee extensors.

Electromyography

Muscle action is initiated by electrical activity, and the detection and recording of these signals is a technique known as electromyography. The recording is known as an electromyogram (EMG) and shows the changes in electrical potential, which occur as electric currents are propagated along the muscle membranes. These fluctuations in current, or action potentials, are produced by the transfer

Fig. 3.10 (a) 3D surface illustrating joint torque–angular velocity–angular position relationships in a maximal effort knee-extension exercise. (b) This surface illustrates the above data after the inclusion of the knee joint geometric relationships to convert the data to muscle linear force–velocity–length information.

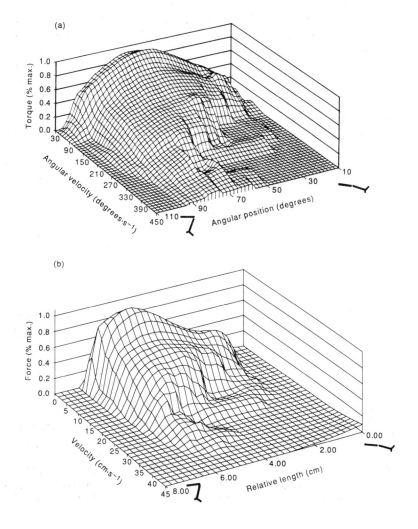

of ions across the muscle cell wall following electrical stimulation. As such, they are only indirectly related to the overall tension produced by a muscle, a point which must be kept in mind during the interpretation of an EMG. At a basic level of analysis, the EMG provides only an indication of activity or non-activity, and comparisons of levels of EMG activity either within or between muscles must be made with caution. The size of the EMG signal recorded from a muscle depends on a variety of factors. The electrode type, size, preparation and placement all affect the recording of the signal, as do factors such as muscle fibre length and arrangement, rate of fibre length change and type of muscle action. Only under carefully controlled conditions can the EMG recording be used as an indicator of the forces produced by a muscle. The factors which affect the force developed in a muscle, such as motor unit firing rates, are also important considerations in the interpretation of an EMG signal.

A variety of electrodes is available for recording muscle activity. Fine wire or needle electrodes may be used to record voltage changes from single muscle cells or single motor units, respectively. However, in sports biomechanics it is more common to use a larger electrode placed on the skin surface overlying a muscle, and to record the activity of many motor units simultaneously (Fig. 3.11 for an example of a typical recording from surface electrodes). Technical guidelines for EMG recording and research reporting have been compiled by the International Society of Electrophysiological Kinesiology (ISEK) and published in various places (e.g. Dainty & Norman 1987), and the reader is directed to these for more specific information.

The lower left portion of Fig. 3.11 shows a simple muscle model that includes the major elements, which contribute to the overall tension produced. The spring-like character of the series and parallel elastic elements (muscle tendon and sheath, respectively, for example) affect the force or rate of force development, while the viscous element has an effect on the speed with which muscle forces change. All of these factors modify either the magnitude or the time course of the forces generated by the contractile element, which is the only component of the muscle associated with EMG activity.

Figure 3.12 depicts the surface EMG activity of selected muscles of the lower extremity during stationary cycling. The rectus femoris (RF), repre-

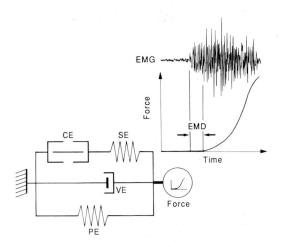

Fig. 3.11 A muscle model showing the mechanical elements which influence force production [contractile element (CE), series elastic element (SE), viscous element (VE), parallel elastic element (PE)]. EMG is only associated with the contractile element, and because of the effects of the other components there is always some electromechanical delay (EMD) between the onset of EMG and the externally measured force.

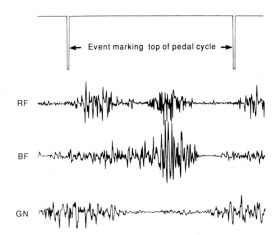

Fig. 3.12 Phasic EMG activity in lower extremity musculature during stationary cycling. (RF = rectus femoris, BF = biceps femoris, GN = gastrocnemius.)

sentative of the knee extensors, shows two bursts of activity. One begins just after the top of the pedal stroke and ends slightly before the knee is fully extended at the bottom of the stroke cycle. A second burst is seen starting at about the bottom of the stroke and finishing about half-way through the recovery (upward) movement. The knee flexors, represented by the muscle biceps femoris (BF), show slight to moderate activity during the propulsive (downward) stroke, and a major burst at the start of the recovery movement. Initially, this might appear to be an inefficient muscle activation pattern, as both knee flexors and extensors are active simultaneously. This apparent conflict of the RF and BF muscles during cycling and walking as well as running is an example of Lombard's Paradox. However, as both RF and BF are two-joint muscles, and have effects at the hip joint as well, perhaps their activity is not so paradoxical. One explanation is that the moment arms of RF and BF at the hip and knee joints change throughout the cycle, giving precedence to one muscle at one stage, and then the other in a later phase. Other factors, such as the actual change of muscle length during the motion are also involved, and interested readers are referred to Andrews (1987) for a more detailed discussion. The gastrocnemius muscle assists with the final aspect of knee flexion prior to the top of the cycle, and is then active in the early part of the propulsive phase in either producing plantar flexion, or in ensuring good force transmission through to the pedal by holding the foot in a static position.

Changes in the magnitude of an EMG are usually indicative of an alteration in the tension produced, although the complexity of the EMG signal has hampered many researchers' efforts to determine useful relationships. One common method of quantifying an EMG signal is to perform an integration procedure (see Winter 1990 for a review of techniques). One approach involves converting all the negative voltages to positive ones (a process referred to as full-wave rectification), followed by an operation which smooths the EMG (low-pass filtering) and accumulates this signal to provide an indication of the total activity (the 'linear envelope'). The typical relationship found between the load lifted and the integrated EMG (IEMG) is a non-

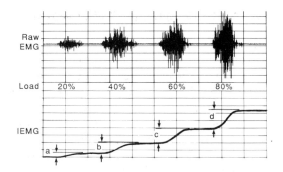

Fig. 3.13 Changes in EMG activity with increasing load during knee extension. Both raw and integrated EMG (IEMG) signals are shown. IEMG levels are seen to exhibit a non-linear increase for constant load increments.

linear one, with increasing levels of IEMG seen for constant increases in load. This relationship is shown in Fig. 3.13, where the raw and integrated EMG data recorded from the RF during knee extension are seen. The non-linear relationship is evident from the increases in magnitude of the IEMG (Fig. 3.13a–d) for constant load increases (from 20 to 80% of maximum).

Researchers are also developing and using other techniques to extract more information from the EMG signal. For example, during a sustained muscular effort an EMG will often exhibit consistent changes in the magnitude and frequency of its action potentials, and these changes can be used as an indication of underlying neuromuscular proesses. In order to see these effects, the EMG signal is transformed from the time domain into the frequency domain using spectral analysis, which gives information on the amplitude and frequency content of the signal. A fast Fourier transform is typically used for this, and produces a 'power spectrum' showing the strength of the signal over a frequency range.

Other researchers interested in quantifying the EMG have had some success in calculating the force produced by a muscle, using the EMG signal and a model of the muscle's contractile and elastic properties. While the technique has some limitations, good results have been shown for several types of muscle contractions: isometric, isotonic, concentric and eccentric (Hof 1984).

PREDICTIVE ANALYSIS METHODS

The previous sections have outlined the major qualitative and quantitative data collection techniques used in biomechanics, and this section reviews some of the predictive approaches. Computer simulation and optimization techniques have been applied widely in studies of sport and human movement. As 'simulation' and 'optimization' often have a variety of connotations, for the purposes of this discussion they will be defined as follows:

- Computer simulation is the use of a validated computer model (a set of mathematical equations describing the system of interest) to evaluate the response of the model to changes in the system parameters
- Optimization is the iterative use of a computer simulation to determine parameter values or control variables which optimize (minimize or maximize) a specified criterion (the performance objective)

The general aim of work in this area is, by using a computer model of a person or piece of equipment (the 'system'), to predict changes which would occur in a movement as a consequence of alterations to the input parameters. That is, one aims to answer the question, 'What would happen to the movement if this factor was changed to . . . ?' The advantages of using computer simulation or optimization include the complete safety of the subjects, an increased speed of assessing changes, the potential for prediction of optimal performance and reduced expense compared with building physical models (Vaughan 1984). Limitations of this approach include the following:

- The frequent need to simplify the 'real-world' system to make it amenable to modelling while attempting to maintain validity
- The expertise and computer power necessary to develop and run the simulation/optimization, and
- Difficulties with the translation of the results into practical terms

Simulation

Computer simulation has been used to evaluate the biomechanics of a wide variety of equipment and body movements, from an equally wide variety of approaches. It is beyond the scope of this chapter to list and comment on the approaches used and the systems modelled, but they vary from the consideration of the human body as a point mass representing the centre of gravity, to a simulation of the 3D muscle mechanics and skeletal dynamics of the lower limb during walking. Most of these programs were written specifically for the system under consideration, although the use of generalized simulation packages, such as symbolic manipulation programs, is increasing (see, for example, Van den Bogert *et al.* 1989).

Schneider and Zernicke (1988) used a validated head–neck–torso model to simulate head impacts in soccer heading in order to estimate the injury risk. Critical output variables were the linear and angular acceleration of the head, and these were compared with standard head-injury tolerance levels. They concluded that head-injury risk can be reduced most effectively in all subjects by increasing the mass ratio between the head and the ball. They stressed that children should therefore use only smaller and lighter soccer balls.

Considerable controversy exists over the techniques used by divers and gymnasts to produce twists in somersaults. Yeadon (1988) simulated twisting somersaults to determine the contribution of asymmetrical arm, chest and hip movements to aerial twists. He demonstrated that sustained twists are most frequently produced by asymmetrical arm movements and further, that even in situations where twist was evident at take-off, the major contributions were still made by aerial techniques.

Computer simulation approaches are also being profitably applied to animals. Van den Bogert and co-workers (1989) have simulated locomotion in the horse, and examined the influence of a therapeutic horseshoe on the distribution of tendon forces in the hind leg. In order to reduce the load on the deep digital flexor (DDF) muscle, horse trainers frequently employ a shoe which raises the heel of the hoof. The simulation showed the forces in the DDF to be substantially reduced, but due to the polyarticular nature of this muscle, the movements of several joints were changed and therefore the loading patterns of other tendons were also altered. They suggested that while the heel rise effectively reduced loads in the DDF, its side-effects on other tendons may not be favourable.

Optimization

Optimization research may be categorized into two general procedures. Parameter optimization refers to those studies where parameters are successively modified to produce an optimal result, such as described in the javelin study below. Optimal control refers to the technique of altering variables which control or determine the output of the system, and an example of this is the cycling study discussed later in this chapter. Interpretation and appraisal of results from optimization studies are guided by the same considerations as for simulation studies, with the added need to evaluate the appropriateness of the performance objective.

Changes made in 1986 by the International Amateur Athletics Federation to the rules for the construction of the men's javelin prompted Hubbard and Alaways (1987) to simulate the flight of the new rules javelin and to determine optimum release characteristics. They discovered that the range of the new javelin was decreased, and that it was less sensitive to release conditions when compared to the old one. They also showed that the optimal release conditions were velocity-dependent, and concluded '. . . the javelin throw has been changed from an event in which finesse and skill were important . . . to one for which strength and power are once again pre-eminent'.

Hull *et al.* (1988), as part of an ongoing project aimed at maximizing cyclist performance, examined the relationships between pedalling rate and the forces in 12 lower limb muscles while pedalling with a constant power output. For steady-state cycling, their results showed an optimum pedalling rate of 95–100 $r \cdot min^{-1}$ which is in close agreement with rates normally observed in cyclists, but in contrast to the 65 $r \cdot min^{-1}$ optimum found by previous researchers.

CONCLUSIONS

Biomechanical evaluation of performance for the purpose of improving technique in sport or aiding in clinical diagnosis is still in its developmental stages. A great deal of progress has been made in the techniques available for data collection and analysis, but the application of biomechanics for the enhancement of sporting performances is not yet commonplace. While biomechanists have been criticized for being preoccupied with methodology and description, the perceived lack of application to improve performance cannot be blamed entirely on them. The failure of coaches and clinicians to come to grips with basic mechanics and the language of technique evaluation has created a minor barrier to communication. It is not always possible to describe the techniques of elite athletes in simple terms, and it is the responsibility of both the coach/clinician and the biomechanist to create a situation where an exchange of information and ideas is possible. The potential for profitable interaction between biomechanists and coaches, clinicians, athletes and patients is enormous and future developments in this arena will be exciting.

REFERENCES

Andrews J. G. (1987) The functional roles of the hamstrings and quadriceps during cycling: Lombard's Paradox revisited. *Journal of Biomechanics* **20**, 565–576.

Biewener A. A. (1992) *Biomechanics: Structures and Systems.* IRL Press, Oxford

Cavanagh P. V., Hennig E. M., Rodgers M. M. & Sanderson D. J. (1985) The measurement of pressure distribution on the plantar surface of diabetic feet. In Whittle M. and Harris D. (eds) *Biomechanical Measurement in Orthopaedic Practice*, pp. 159–168. Clarendon Press, Oxford.

Challis J. & Kerwin D. (1992) Accuracy assessment and control point configuration when using the DLT for photogrammetry. *Journal of Biomechanics* **25**, 1053–1058.

Dainty D. A. & Norman R. W. (1987) *Standardising Biomechanical Testing in Sport.* Human Kinetics Publishers, Champaign, IL.

Dal Monte A. & Komor A. (1989) Rowing and sculling mechanics. In Vaughan C. L. (ed.) *Biomechanics of Sport*, pp. 53–119. CRC Press, Boca Raton, FL.

de Groot G., de Koning J. & van Ingen Schenau G. J. (1989) A method to determine 3-D coordinates with panning cameras. In Gregor R. J., Zernicke R. F. & Whiting W. C. (eds) *Proceedings XII International Congress of Biomechanics*, Abstract 297. UCLA Press, Los Angeles, CA.

Elliott B., Marsh T. & Overheu P. (1989) A biomechanical comparison of the multisegment and single unit topspin forehand drives in tennis. *International Journal of Sport Biomechanics* 5, 350–364.

Foster D., John D., Elliott B., Ackland T. & Fitch K. (1989) Back injuries to fast bowlers in cricket: A prospective study. *British Journal of Sport Medicine* 23, 150–154.

Hay J. G. & Reid J. G. (1988) *Anatomy, Mechanics and Human Motion*, 2nd edn. Prentice-Hall, Englewood Cliffs, NJ.

Hay J. G., Putnam C. A. & Wilson B. D. (1979) Forces exerted during exercises on the uneven bars. *Medicine and Science in Sports* 11, 123–130.

Hof A. L. (1984) EMG and muscle force: An introduction. *Human Movement Science* 3, 119–153.

Hubbard M. & Alaways L. (1987) Optimum release conditions for the new rules javelin. *International Journal of Sport Biomechanics* 3, 207–221.

Hull M., Gonzalez H. & Redfield R. (1988) Optimization of pedalling rate in cycling using a muscle stress-based objective function. *International Journal of Sport Biomechanics* 4, 1–20.

Isacson J., Gransberg L. & Knutsson E. (1986) Three-dimensional electrogoniometric gait recording. *Journal of Biomechanics* 19, 627–636.

Lafortune M. A. (1991) Three-dimensional acceleration of the tibia during walking and running. *Journal of Biomechanics* 24, 877–886.

Komi P. (1990) Relevance of in-vivo force measurements to human biomechanics. *Journal of Biomechanics* 23, 23–34.

Marshall R. N., Mazur S. M. & Taylor N. A. S. (1990) Three dimensional surfaces for human muscle kinetics. *European Journal of Applied Physiology and Occupational Physiology* 61, 263–270.

Marzan G. T. & Karara H. M. (1975) A computer program for direct linear transformation solution of the collinearity condition and some applications of it. *Symposium on Close Range Photogrammetric Systems*, pp. 420–476. American Society of Photogrammetry, Falls Church, VA.

McNair P. J., Marshall R. N. & Matheson J. A. (1989) Gait of subjects with anterior cruciate ligament deficiency. *Clinical Biomechanics* 4, 243–248.

McPherson M. N. (1988) The development, implementation and evaluation of a programme designed to promote competency in skill analysis. PhD thesis, The University of Alberta, Edmonton, Canada (unpublished).

Schneider K. & Zernicke R. (1988) Computer simulation of head impact: Estimation of head-injury risk during soccer heading. *International Journal of Sport Biomechanics* 4, 358–371.

Van den Bogert A. J., Sauren A. & Hartman W. (1989) Simulation of locomotion in the horse: Principles and applications. In Hubbard M. and Komor A. (eds) *Proceedings of the Second International Symposium on Computer Simulation in Biomechanics*, pp. 22–23. Department of Mechanical Engineering, University of California, Davis.

Vaughan C. L. (1984) Computer simulation of human motion in sports biomechanics. In Terjung R. L. (ed.) *Exercise and Sport Science Reviews* 12, pp. 373–416. Collamore Press, Lexington, MA.

Voloshin A., Wosk J. & Brull M. (1981) Force wave transmission through the human locomotor system. *Journal of Biomechanical Engineering* 103, 48–50.

Whittle M. (1991) *Gait Analysis — An introduction*. Butterworth Heinemann, Oxford.

Winter D. A. (1990) *Biomechanics and Motor Control of Human Movement*, 2nd edn. Wiley Interscience, Toronto.

Winter D. A. & Sienko S. E. (1988) Biomechanics of below-knee amputee gait. *Journal of Biomechanics* 21, 361–367.

Woltring H. J. (1985) On optimal smoothing and derivative estimation from noisy displacement data in biomechanics. *Human Movement Science* 4, 229–245.

Woltring H. J., McClay I. S. & Cavanagh P. R. (1989) 3-D Calibration without a calibration object. In Gregor R. J., Zernicke R. F. and Whiting W. C. (eds) *Proceedings XII International Congress of Biomechanics*, Abstract 197. UCLA Press, Los Angeles, CA.

Wood G. A. (1982) Data smoothing and differentiation procedures in biomechanics. In Terjung R. L. (ed.) *Exercise and Sports Science Reviews* 10, pp. 308–362. The Franklin Institute Press, Philadelphia, PA.

Wood G. A. & Marshall R. N. (1986) The accuracy of DLT extrapolation in three-dimensional film analysis. *Journal of Biomechanics* 19, 781–785.

Yeadon M. (1988) Techniques used in twisting somersaults. In de Groot G., Hollander A. P. Huijing P. A. and van Ingen Schenau G. J. (eds) *Biomechanics* XI-B, pp. 740–741. Free University Press, Amsterdam.

Ziegert J. E. & Lewis J. L. (1979) The effect of soft tissue on measurement of vibrational bone motion by skin-mounted accelerometers. *Journal of Biomechanical Engineering* 101, 218–220.

SECTION 2

PHYSIOLOGY AND NUTRITION
APPLIED TO SPORT

CHAPTER 4

PHYSIOLOGY OF TRAINING

Allan G. Hahn

Historically, many sports coaches have achieved outstanding results without a knowledge of exercise physiology. They have developed effective training methods by trial and error, with evaluation based on the results achieved by their athletes. It can be argued that research in exercise physiology over the past 60 years has served largely to provide a theoretical rationale for what coaches were already doing in practice. However, the existence of a theoretical rationale is important, as it offers a foundation for logical change aimed at making training methods progressively more efficient. It permits informed surmise as to which components of previous training programmes may have contributed most to success. Understanding the basics of metabolic energy transfer allows clearer analysis of the demands imposed by various sporting events and assists in the planning of systematic training. Thus the recent research in exercise physiology has, at the very least, accelerated the evolution of effective training methods.

This chapter attempts to provide a physiological basis for the analysis of sporting activities and the design of training programmes. Some attention is also given to the monitoring of athletes through measurement of various physiological characteristics and capabilities.

ENERGY TRANSFER DURING EXERCISE

The energy required for muscular contraction is released by the breakdown of adenosine triphos-phate (ATP) to adenosine diphosphate (ADP) and inorganic phosphate (P_i). This reaction occurs at enzymatically active sites on the cross-bridges of myosin myofilaments and enables cross-bridge movement. The stores of ATP in skeletal muscle are very small and even during exercise lasting only a few seconds, must be constantly replenished and used again. The replenishment of ATP involves recombination of ADP and P_i. In direct contrast to ATP breakdown, this process requires energy. The requirement is met through the contributions of specific aerobic and anaerobic energy pathways.

General Characteristics of Aerobic Energy Transfer

The aerobic energy pathways involve breakdown of fatty acids, carbohydrates and (to a much lesser extent) amino acids in the presence of oxygen. This occurs largely in the mitochondria of the muscle cells. Through a series of chemical reactions, the substrate molecules are progressively stripped of electrons. These reactions are catalysed by enzymes that depend on either nicotinamide adenine dinucleotide (NAD^+) or flavin adenine dinucleotide (FAD) as coenzymes. NAD^+ and FAD are synthesized from B-complex vitamins. The former is structurally similar to nicotinic acid, while the latter is related to riboflavin. Both are capable of accepting electrons. In reactions catalysed by enzymes associated with NAD^+, the coenzyme accepts two electrons and one proton from the substrate molecule. This situation can be represented as follows:

$$NAD^+ + 2e^- + H^+ \rightarrow NADH$$

In accepting electrons, NAD^+ is said to be reduced, while the substrate molecule, in losing electrons, is considered to be oxidized. Energy released through oxidation of the substrate is captured through reduction of NAD^+. A similar function can be performed by FAD. This coenzyme can accept two electrons and two protons from a substrate molecule. In so doing, it is reduced to $FADH_2$. Electrons are subsequently stripped from NADH and $FADH_2$ (which are thereby oxidized) and passed into an 'electron transport chain' consisting of six discrete molecules on the inner mitochondrial membrane. The first molecule in the chain is an enzyme and the second is coenzyme Q. The remaining four molecules are iron-containing proteins called cyto-

chromes and are identified in order as b, c_1, c and a. The electrons released from NADH and $FADH_2$ move along the chain in a series of reactions involving reduction and then oxidation of each molecule. There are three points at which oxidative energy release is sufficient to allow resynthesis of ATP from ADP and P_i. However, electrons derived from $FADH_2$ enter the chain beyond the first of these points. Thus, for every molecule of NADH donating electrons to the chain, three molecules of ATP are formed, while the yield from a molecule of $FADH_2$ is two molecules of ATP. At the end of the chain, the electrons are accepted by an oxygen atom, which is then able to combine with two protons from the surrounding area to form water. It is important to realize that the operation of the electron transport chain (depicted in Fig. 4.1) is absolutely dependent on availability of oxygen as the final electron acceptor.

Aerobic Breakdown of Fatty Acids

The various substrates are broken down by somewhat different chemical processes. Fat metabolism depends partly on diffusion of fatty acids into the muscle cells from the circulating blood and partly on their release from intracellular triglyceride stores. The process is schematically illustrated in Fig. 4.2. Initially, the fatty acid molecules are converted to a slightly different form. They are then able to pass into the mitochondria in a reaction catalysed by carnitine palmityl transferase. Here, in the presence of coenzyme A, they undergo a process known as β-oxidation. This involves loss of some electrons to NAD^+ and FAD and the formation of acetyl coenzyme A. β-oxidation of a typical fatty acid (palmitic acid) yields 14 pairs of electrons (seven combining with NAD^+ and seven with FAD) and eight molecules of acetyl coenzyme A. Each molecule of acetyl coenzyme A then enters a second oxidative pathway known as the Krebs' cycle and is subject to removal of a further four pairs of electrons (three combining with NAD^+, one with FAD). There are two points in the Krebs' cycle at which a molecule of carbon dioxide is produced. At another point sufficient energy is released to allow formation of a molecule of ATP from ADP and P_i. Because

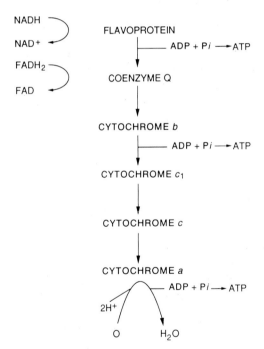

Fig. 4.1 A schematic representation of the electron transport chain. Electron pairs are passed along the chain and at several points the energy release is sufficient to allow re-formation of ATP from ADP and P_i. At the end of the chain, the electrons are accepted by an atom of molecular oxygen and, with the addition of two protons from the surrounding environment, water is formed.

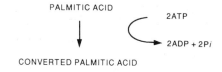

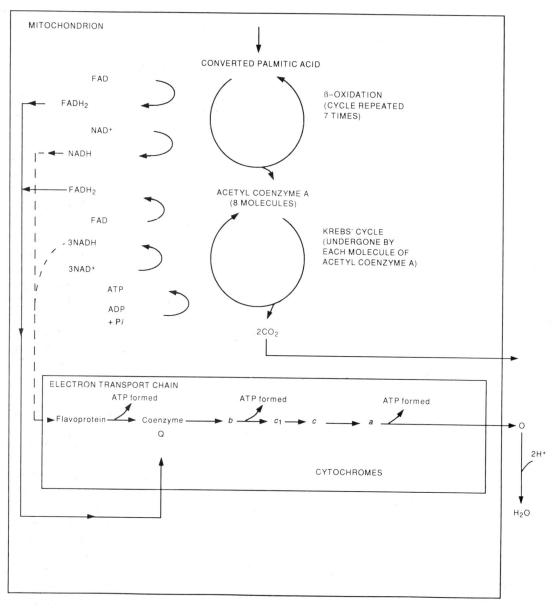

Fig. 4.2   A schematic diagram of the processes involved in the oxidation of fatty acids.

Table 4.1 The number of ATP molecules produced through the complete breakdown of one molecule of palmitic acid

Process	No. ATP molecules
Conversion of palmitic acid before entry into mitochondrion	− 2
Electron transport chain processing of 7NADH formed during β-oxidation	21
Electron transport chain processing of 7FADH$_2$ formed during β-oxidation	14
Substrate level phosphorylation during Krebs' cycle	8
Electron transport chain processing of 24NADH formed via Krebs' cycle	72
Electron transport chain processing of 8FADH$_2$ formed via Krebs' cycle	16
Total	129

this occurs outside the electron transport chain, it is termed 'substrate level phosphorylation'.

In regard to the oxidative breakdown of fatty acids, the following points are particularly worthy of note:

- The process consumes oxygen and produces ATP, carbon dioxide and water
- Complete oxidation of one molecule of palmitic acid results in the formation of 131 molecules of ATP (as can be easily calculated from the above; Table 4.1). In fact, the final yield is only 129 molecules, as two molecules of ATP are used in the conversion of the fatty acid before its entry into the mitochondrion
- The breakdown of palmitic acid involves delivery of 46 pairs of electrons to the electron transport chain. Consequently, 46 oxygen atoms are needed at the end of the chain. This is equivalent to 23 molecules of oxygen
- Krebs' cycle breakdown of the eight acetyl coenzyme A molecules formed in β-oxidation of palmitic acid produces a total of 16 molecules of carbon dioxide

Thus it can be seen that the oxidation of palmitic

acid results in the formation of 5.6 molecules of ATP for every molecule of oxygen consumed. The ratio of carbon dioxide production (16 molecules) to oxygen consumption (23 molecules) is approximately 0.70. This ratio is known as the respiratory quotient. It varies only slightly between different types of fatty acid.

Aerobic Breakdown of Glucose

The steps involved in the aerobic breakdown of glucose are summarized in Fig. 4.3. On entering a muscle cell, each molecule of glucose is converted to glucose-6-phosphate in a process requiring breakdown of one molecule of ATP. It is then either metabolized directly or converted to glycogen and stored for later use. Glycogen is essentially a composite of many glucose molecules linked together in long, highly branched chains. It can be converted back to glucose-6-phosphate in a reaction catalysed by the enzyme glycogen phosphorylase. From glucose-6-phosphate, fructose-6-phosphate is formed and under the influence of the enzyme phosphofructokinase, this is subsequently converted to fructose 1,6-diphosphate. The conversion requires expenditure of another molecule of ATP. Fructose 1,6-diphosphate is broken down to produce two three-carbon fragments, glyceraldehyde 3-phosphate and dihydroxyacetone phosphate. The latter is then enzymatically transformed to produce a second molecule of the former. Each molecule of glyceraldehyde 3-phosphate is oxidized through a series of steps culminating in the formation of pyruvate. Along the way, one pair of electrons is picked up by NAD$^+$ and two molecules of ATP are formed from ADP and P$_i$. The process by which glucose is eventually transformed to pyruvate is known as glycolysis. Pyruvate can pass into the mitochondria, where each molecule is converted to acetyl coenzyme A through reactions involving loss of an electron pair (to NAD$^+$) and the formation of one molecule of carbon dioxide. Acetyl coenzyme A is then oxidized in the Krebs' cycle, just as in the case of fatty acid metabolism. Again, for each molecule of acetyl coenzyme A passing through the cycle, four pairs of electrons are gained by NAD$^+$ (three pairs) and FAD (one pair), two molecules of carbon dioxide

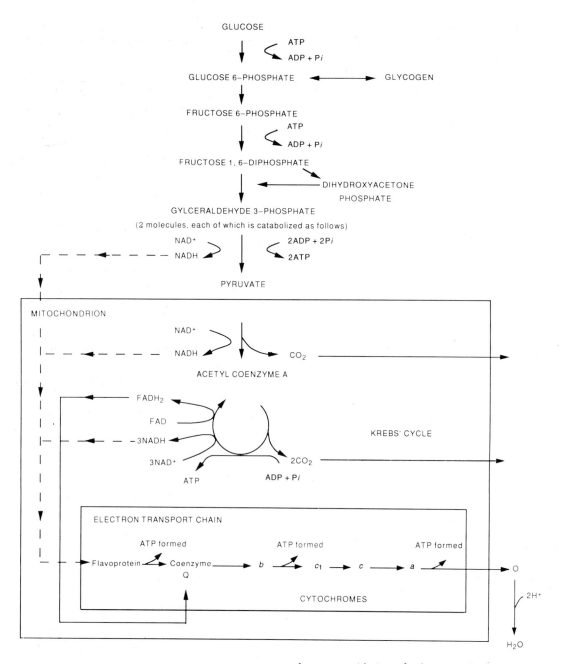

Fig. 4.3 A metabolic pathway for the aerobic breakdown of glucose.

are produced and one molecule of ATP is formed by substrate level phosphorylation. However, it is important to realize that the breakdown of glucose yields only two molecules of acetyl coenzyme A,

whereas β-oxidation of palmitic acid produces eight. The following points should be noted in regard to the aerobic breakdown of glucose:

- Conversion of glucose to pyruvate through glycolysis occurs in the cytoplasm of the muscle cell outside of the mitochondria

- As with fatty acid metabolism, oxygen is required and the final products are ATP, carbon dioxide and water
- For every glucose molecule, 40 molecules of ATP are produced. However, two molecules of ATP are broken down in the early stages of the glycolytic pathway. Consequently, the net yield is 38 molecules (Table 4.2)
- A total of 12 pairs of electrons are delivered to the electron transport chain, necessitating the presence of 12 oxygen atoms at the end of the chain. This is equivalent to six molecules of oxygen
- For each pyruvate molecule converted to acetyl coenzyme A and subsequently oxidized in the Krebs' cycle, three molecules of carbon dioxide

are formed. Therefore, the breakdown of one glucose molecule yields six molecules of carbon dioxide

It can be easily calculated that the aerobic breakdown of glucose produces 6.3 molecules of ATP for every molecule of oxygen consumed. This greatly exceeds the yield provided by oxidation of fatty acids. The respiratory quotient associated with aerobic glucose metabolism is 1.00, as the number of carbon dioxide molecules produced is the same as the number of oxygen molecules consumed.

Anaerobic Breakdown of Creatine Phosphate

Muscle ATP can be replenished through two different mechanisms that do not require oxygen. The muscle cells contain stores of creatine phosphate (CP), which can be broken down to creatine and P_i under the influence of the enzyme creatine phosphokinase. The reaction releases considerable energy, permitting very rapid resynthesis of ATP from ADP and P_i (Fig. 4.4). However, the muscular stores of CP are exhausted after only 5–8 s of maximal exercise. It is widely believed that, on cessation of exercise, CP is quickly replenished.

Table 4.2 The number of ATP molecules produced through the complete aerobic breakdown of one molecule of glucose

Process	No. ATP molecules
Conversion of glucose to glucose 6-phosphate	−1
Conversion of fructose 6-phosphate to fructose 1,6-diphosphate	−1
Electron transport chain processing of 2NADH formed in conversion of glyceraldehyde 3-phosphate to pyruvate	6
Substrate level phosphorylation during conversion of glyceraldehyde 3-phosphate to pyruvate	4
Electron transport chain processing of 2NADH formed in conversion of pyruvate to acetyl coenzyme A	6
Substrate level phosphorylation during Krebs' cycle	2
Electron transport chain processing of 6NADH formed via Krebs' cycle	18
Electron transport chain processing of 2FADH$_2$ formed via Krebs' cycle	4
Total	38

The ATP/creatine phosphate (CP) anaerobic
energy pathway

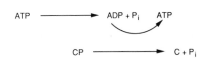

The anaerobic glycolytic pathway

This pathway is identical to that for aerobic breakdown of glucose up to the point at which pyruvate is formed. In anaerobic glycolysis, pyruvate, instead of entering the mitochondrion, undergoes the following reaction:

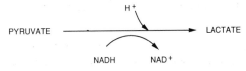

Fig. 4.4 A schematic representation of the anaerobic energy pathways.

This belief is based on studies involving depletion of CP stores in resting muscle by tourniquet ischaemia. It has been found that, following removal of the tourniquet, the CP stores return to normal in only 3–4 min, with the recovery half-time being approximately 30 s. However, recent work has shown that restoration of CP stores after intensive exercise can take more than 10 min (Sapega *et al.* 1987). This has important implications for the planning of sports training programmes.

Resynthesis of CP from creatine and P_i requires energy and this is provided by the breakdown of aerobically generated ATP. Thus, following any intervention causing CP depletion, mitochondrial activity must be elevated for some time. Muscle ADP levels are thought to be important in stimulating mitochondrial respiration. During heavy exercise, the need for rapid ATP regeneration may lead to an increase in reactions between ADP molecules to form ATP and adenosine monophosphate. Consequently, muscle ADP levels may be relatively low at the beginning of the recovery period. This may limit mitochondrial activity and the rate of CP restoration (Sapega *et al.* 1987).

Anaerobic Glycolysis

The other mechanism permitting ATP resynthesis in the absence of oxygen is anaerobic glycolysis. It has already been pointed out that, in the process of glycolysis, glucose is broken down to two molecules of pyruvate. Anaerobic glycolysis involves one further step. Pyruvate, instead of entering the mitochondrion, accepts two electrons and a proton from NADH (which is thereby oxidized to NAD^+). It also obtains a second proton from the surrounding environment and is converted to lactate. The conversion is catalysed by the enzyme lactate dehydrogenase.

To understand the metabolic importance of anaerobic glycolysis, it is necessary to realize that electron transport mechanisms can sometimes fail to keep pace with the stripping of electron pairs from substrate molecules. This occurs, for example, under conditions of oxygen lack. It eventually leads to inhibition of all cellular reactions which depend on the electron transport system for regeneration

of NAD^+ and FAD from NADH and $FADH_2$. The various mitochondrial processes are included in this category. By contrast, glycolytic synthesis of ATP outside the mitochondria can continue, because the conversion of pyruvate to lactate involves oxidation of NADH and so provides the NAD^+ needed for further pyruvate formation. When electron transport mechanisms are severely restricted, anaerobic glycolysis becomes very important in maintaining cellular activity. Although it gives a net production of only two ATP molecules for every molecule of glucose broken down, the amount of ATP produced per unit time can be quite substantial.

It is often claimed that lactic acid is formed in anaerobic glycolysis and that its subsequent dissociation is responsible for the accumulation of hydrogen ions during heavy exercise. In fact, it is lactate and not lactic acid, that is produced. The major cellular source of hydrogen ions is the breakdown of ATP. In aerobic metabolism, the number of hydrogen ions required for resynthesis of ATP is exactly equivalent to the number released in its breakdown. The same does not apply to anaerobic glycolysis, which therefore does result in hydrogen ion build-up (Walsh & Banister 1988). This can contribute to fatigue. Exercise involving absolutely maximal rates of anaerobic glycolysis can usually be maintained for only 30–90 s.

Under aerobic conditions, lactate can be reconverted to pyruvate for breakdown in the mitochondria. Lactate diffusing out of one muscle cell may be taken up and used by another, either in the same immediate area or (through the agency of the circulating blood) elsewhere in the body. Slow twitch muscle fibres play a major role in the uptake and disposal of lactate and cardiac muscle fibres also contribute. Some of the lactate produced during exercise is transported to the liver, where it is converted to glucose through a process known as gluconeogenesis. It is important to realize that mechanisms for lactate removal are operative during exercise as well as afterwards.

The fate of hydrogen ions accumulating as a result of anaerobic glycolysis is complex. Muscle cells contain a number of substances capable of binding hydrogen ions to buffer increases in acidity.

These substances include carnosine (a dipeptide), CP and P_i. Hydrogen ions that pass from muscle cells into the circulating blood can be bound by haemoglobin or by plasma proteins. Alternatively, they may react with bicarbonate to form carbonic acid, which immediately breaks down to carbon dioxide and water. The carbon dioxide can be eliminated through the lungs, so that the buffering reaction is not inhibited by accumulation of end-products. While the various buffering mechanisms inhibit rise in hydrogen ion concentration, they do not actually remove hydrogen ions from the body. This function is ultimately performed by the kidneys.

Regulation of Energy Transfer Mechanisms

In recent years, substantial knowledge has been gained concerning factors controlling physiological utilization of the various energy transfer mechanisms. At a gross level, neuromuscular recruitment patterns have an important influence. In general, slow twitch muscle fibres are well-adapted for aerobic metabolism, while fast twitch fibres have greater anaerobic capabilities. Substrate availability also affects the process of energy transfer. There is evidence that increasing the plasma free fatty acid concentration leads to increased metabolism of fatty acids during exercise (Costill et al. 1977). Similarly, elevation of muscle glycogen stores results in increased breakdown of glucose by both aerobic and anaerobic means (Richter & Galbo 1986). Even under resting conditions, augmented glucose availability causes a rise in muscle lactate concentration (Sahlin et al. 1984).

However, it appears that the most important regulatory mechanisms are based on the relative concentrations of various phosphate compounds. During rest and light exercise, the demand for ATP resynthesis can be easily met. Consequently, the intramuscular ratio of ATP to ADP and P_i remains fairly high. This favours aerobic metabolism of fatty acids, with glycolysis being minimized through an inhibitory effect on the enzyme phosphofructokinase (and perhaps glycogen phosphorylase). As exercise becomes more intense, ATP is broken down more rapidly. The resultant fall in the $[ATP]/[ADP][P_i]$ ratio promotes breakdown of CP stores, while increased ADP concentration acts to stimulate mitochondrial respiration. These changes lead to a higher rate of ATP resynthesis. Reduction in the ratio of CP to P_i is believed to stimulate both the reformation of glucose from glycogen and an increased flux through the glycolytic energy pathway. Thus, as exercise intensity is raised, glucose metabolism (both aerobic and anaerobic) makes a progressively increasing contribution to total energy release. It should be noted that, in absolute terms, the contribution of fatty acid metabolism apparently remains constant (Callow et al. 1986).

There are at least two other aspects of metabolic control that warrant consideration. First, it seems that a certain minimal amount of carbohydrate is required for effective function of the Krebs' cycle. As a result, depletion of muscle glycogen stores is associated with subjective feelings of exhaustion, despite continuing availability of fatty acids as a substrate. Second, the general belief that anaerobic glycolysis is eventually limited by fatigue resulting from intracellular hydrogen ion accumulation is open to some doubt. In studies involving perfusion of isolated muscle preparations with solutions of low pH, decrements in maximum isometric tension have been much less than those observed at a similar muscle pH following intensive exercise (Meyer et al. 1983). This suggests that other factors must be at least partially responsible for fatigue in the exercise situation.

INVOLVEMENT OF THE ENERGY PATHWAYS IN SPORTING ACTIVITIES

The involvement of the various energy pathways in particular sports cannot be precisely quantified. It can differ substantially among athletes competing in the same event, due to the influence of such factors as muscle fibre composition. Even for an individual, there may be variation from day to day in accordance with substrate availability, the tactics employed and a range of other considerations. However, it is possible to gain a general indication as to which energy pathways are most important in specific sports. There are at least three different ways in which this can be achieved, as discussed below.

Physiological Assessment of Athletes During Actual or Simulated Competition

Most studies aimed at assessing the contributions of the different energy pathways have been conducted in laboratories, using ergometers which allow simulation of sports performance (Fig. 4.5) and enable accurate measurement of the total amount of work accomplished. Determination of oxygen uptake during the activity permits close estimation of the amount of energy released by aerobic mechanisms. If consideration is given to the typical mechanical efficiency of the activity (i.e. the percentage of the released energy converted to work as opposed to heat), the aerobic contribution to total

work output can be estimated. Of course, the anaerobic contribution can then be calculated as the residual. Assume, for example, that a person exercises on a cycle ergometer at 350 W for 10 min, with an average oxygen uptake of $3.80 \ L \cdot min^{-1}$. Remembering that watts are equivalent to joules per second, the total amount of work done would be 210 kJ. To accurately determine the amount of energy released for each litre of oxygen consumed, it is necessary to know which substrates are being utilized. Measurement of the respiratory exchange ratio (volume of carbon dioxide produced relative to volume of oxygen consumed) provides some information in this regard. It should be noted, however, that the respiratory exchange ratio is not necessarily equivalent to the average respiratory quotient of the active muscle cells, as carbon dioxide is produced in the buffering of hydrogen ions as well as in cellular metabolism. Let us suppose that, in this case, the respiratory exchange ratio is above 1.00. Under such circumstances, it is usually assumed that glucose is by far the predominant substrate. Aerobic breakdown of glucose yields approximately

Fig. 4.5   An assessment of the energy pathways using a rowing ergometer.

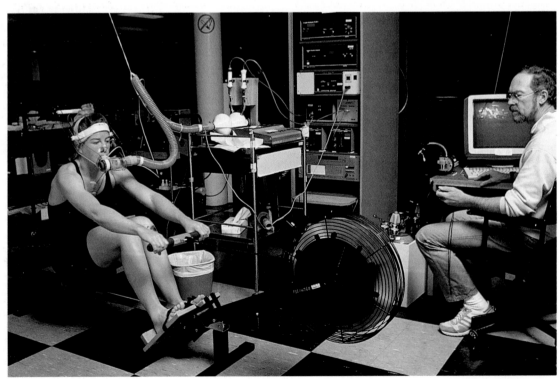

21 kJ of energy per litre of oxygen consumed. Thus it may be calculated that, for our subject, the aerobic energy release over 10 min is 798 kJ. If the mechanical efficiency of cycling is assumed to be 22%, it can be concluded that aerobic mechanisms account for about 175 of the 210 kJ of work done. This is a little more than 83%. The remainder of the work can be attributed to anaerobic energy pathways.

There are several problems with the above approach. In activities involving large variations in exercise intensity, oxygen uptake during the lighter periods is often above the level that might be expected on the basis of the workload. This is due partly to aerobic involvement in the recovery from anaerobic efforts. Calculation of average oxygen uptake over the whole period of the activity can give the misleading impression that the work output is attributable almost entirely to aerobic mechanisms. Apart from this fundamental difficulty, there are some areas of more minor concern. For activities entailing alternation of hard and light efforts, the respiratory exchange ratio is a poor indicator of substrate utilization. Even for exercise at a constant load, there is some doubt concerning the assumption that a respiratory exchange ratio above 1.00 indicates virtually exclusive use of glucose as a substrate. It is likely that, in absolute terms, the amount of energy released through fatty acid metabolism remains constant over a wide range of exercise intensities (Callow et al. 1986). Incorrect assessment of substrate utilization can obviously lead to error in calculating the total amount of work made possible by aerobic energy release. The mechanical efficiency of cycling (and of other sporting activities) varies markedly between individuals. Use of a standard figure is therefore invalid and mechanical efficiency must be separately determined for each athlete. This is a fairly simple matter in the case of cycling. However, there are some sports (e.g. running) for which accurate quantification of work output is much more difficult. As mechanical efficiency is an index of work output relative to total energy release, this is a serious drawback.

A major problem in using laboratory ergometers to study energy pathway involvement in sport concerns the extent to which they really allow simulation of sports performance. Small errors in such factors as resistance to movement might significantly affect the physiological requirements of a particular task. Recognizing this, some researchers have preferred to study athletes in their natural sporting environment. Measurements of oxygen uptake have been made, for example, during rowing, cycling, running and swimming. While the measurements have necessarily been taken during simulated rather than actual competition, they provide a good general guide to the magnitude of the aerobic commitment. Attempts at assessing anaerobic involvement have usually been based on measurement of blood lactate concentrations associated with real or simulated events. This does not permit quantitative analysis, as there is no simple relationship between blood lactate levels and total lactate production. However, it does allow very broad conclusions to be drawn concerning activation of the anaerobic glycolytic pathway.

In some studies, athletes have undergone laboratory testing to enable individual determination of the relationship between oxygen uptake and heart rate. Oxygen uptakes during actual sports performance have then been estimated on the basis of measured heart rates. The results of these studies should be interpreted cautiously, as rise in the core temperature of the body and gradual dehydration during sports performance can lead to substantial elevation of heart rate at a given oxygen uptake. Furthermore, the relationship between heart rate and oxygen uptake during sporting activities requiring intermittent hard efforts may be quite different from that established during laboratory tests entailing successive bouts of continuous exercise.

Physiological Profiling of Elite Athletes

Assessing the various energy pathways in elite athletes from a particular sport provides another means for identifying the pathways of greatest practical importance. If, for example, virtually all outstanding distance runners are found to have well-developed aerobic capabilities, it might be suggested that aerobic mechanisms make a very significant contribution to distance running performance. Conversely, if capacity for anaerobic glycolysis is generally only average, it could be concluded that this pathway is little involved in the sport.

The problem with this approach is that physiological profiles may sometimes reflect the type of training being undertaken, rather than the requirements of the sport itself. Suppose that there is a universal trend for sprint swimmers to participate in a high volume of endurance training. This may lead to a physiological profile typified by high aerobic capability, yet the latter may not necessarily be a critical element in competitive performance.

Estimating Energy Pathway Involvement from the Duration and Pattern of Exercise

The involvement of the different energy pathways in particular sports can be determined with reasonable accuracy from event duration and the typical activity patterns of the competitors. In the 100 m track sprint, which lasts for approximately 10 s, breakdown of CP will obviously provide a significant proportion of the energy needed for ATP resynthesis. The 400 m sprint, with a duration of 45–55 s, demands a substantial contribution from anaerobic glycolysis, though both CP breakdown and aerobic mechanisms for energy release are also involved. In prolonged events, such as the marathon, CP breakdown can provide only a very small fraction of the required energy. Furthermore, the competitors cannot afford to depend too much on anaerobic glycolysis, as this would lead to premature fatigue. The great majority of the energy required for ATP resynthesis (perhaps 95–98%) must therefore be provided by aerobic mechanisms. Many sports require maximal activation of all major energy pathways. These sports include rowing, sprint kayaking, running 1500 m and the 4000 m individual pursuit in cycling. Team games involving brief bouts of activity separated by recovery periods are generally thought to place primary emphasis on CP breakdown and aerobic metabolism. However, moderately high blood lactate concentrations have been observed in both soccer players and water polo players shortly after participation in intensive passages of play. This may be due to the fact that, following heavy exercise, muscle CP stores are not

replenished as rapidly as previously believed (Sapega et al. 1987). With CP stores becoming depleted, dependence on anaerobic glycolysis would tend to be increased.

Expectations based simply on the duration and pattern of exercise are not always confirmed by empirical observation. This is largely because energy pathway involvement is also dependent on the intensity of exercise, which can be difficult to judge.

While none of the methods outlined above is entirely satisfactory, their combined use has contributed to a clearer understanding of energy transfer mechanisms as they pertain to specific sports. This has provided a basis for design of more effective training programmes.

EFFECTS OF TRAINING ON ENERGY TRANSFER MECHANISMS

Training induces adaptations which enhance the function of the energy pathways involved. Endurance training results in improved availability of oxygen to the active muscle cells. This occurs partly through the formation of new capillaries, which facilitate transport of oxygen into the immediate cellular environment. There is also an expansion of total blood volume. In prolonged exercise, fluid is often lost from the circulation due to sweating and leakage from capillaries, particularly in untrained people. Blood volume is thus reduced and may be insufficient to meet the combined demands of exercise and thermoregulation. Consequently, muscle oxygen supply may be reduced. An increase in blood volume through training is protective in this regard. It results from rise in both plasma volume and the total number of red blood cells. With more red cells, there is an increase in total haemoglobin and thus in the overall capacity of the blood for oxygen transport. Plasma volume typically changes by more than the red cell number. Consequently, the viscosity of the blood is reduced, a change which might enable better flow through muscle capillaries and further enhancement of cellular oxygen supply. Red blood cell count, haemoglobin concentration and haematocrit are similarly decreased. This has sometimes led to mistaken diagnoses of anaemia.

Endurance training also improves the capacity of muscle cells to use the available oxygen. Mitochondria become larger and more numerous. At the same time, there is a substantial increase in the activities of various enzymes involved in aerobic metabolism. Movement of fatty acids into the mitochondria for β-oxidation is thought to be rate-limited by carnitine palmityl transferase. This enzyme is extremely responsive to endurance training and the same is true of Krebs' cycle enzymes, such as succinate dehydrogenase (Gollnick *et al.* 1973; Witzmann *et al.* 1978). Mitochondrial adaptation and increases in the activity of aerobic enzymes occur in both slow twitch and fast twitch muscle fibres. Indeed, fast glycolytic (Type IIb) fibres can be converted to fast oxidative (Type IIa) fibres by regular endurance training (Andersen & Henriksson 1977a), so that eventually none of the former remain. The fast twitch fibres of endurance athletes have greater aerobic capacity than the slow twitch fibres of untrained people. It has been reported that changes in enzyme activity with endurance training are subsequent to increased capillarization (Andersen & Henriksson 1977b).

As well as improving both the delivery of oxygen to the muscle cells and their capacity to use it, endurance training increases intramuscular storage of substrates. Resting glycogen levels are substantially elevated, with the effect being about equal for the two major fibre types. Muscle triglyceride stores are also increased, enhancing the immediate availability of fatty acids for aerobic metabolism. This is important, as muscle triglycerides may be the primary source of fatty acids metabolized during prolonged continuous exercise (Carlsson *et al.* 1971). Triglyceride storage is considerably greater in slow twitch than in fast twitch muscle fibres, but the effect of endurance training on the ratio is uncertain.

Training programmes involving brief efforts of high intensity can lead to a slight increase in resting muscle ATP and CP stores and in the activity of the enzyme creatine phosphokinase. However, the changes seem insufficient to account for observed improvements in work output. It is likely that these improvements are at least partly due to an increased amount of myofibrillar protein (an adaptation that contributes to muscle hypertrophy) and

to greater and more synchronous recruitment of motor units.

It is generally believed that appropriate training can greatly enhance capacity for anaerobic glycolysis. However, there has been little research concerning the mechanisms by which this might occur. Resting muscle glycogen stores are apparently increased, but fatigue in anaerobic activities is not normally associated with glycogen depletion. Indeed, it typically occurs in the presence of quite high glycogen levels. Nevertheless, in some studies, glycogen loading through dietary manipulation has improved performance in tasks requiring high work outputs over a few minutes. This could be due to more efficient aerobic metabolism. The amount of ATP resynthesized per litre of oxygen consumed is maximized when glucose is the predominant substrate. On the other hand it is possible that glycogen loading does increase capacity for anaerobic glycolysis. It is known that high-intensity efforts favour recruitment of fast twitch muscle fibres. Owing to the low yield of ATP per unit of glucose broken down under anaerobic conditions, some of these fibres may be rapidly depleted of glycogen. Despite the continuing availability of glycogen in other fibres, the total work capacity of the muscle may be decreased. Glycogen loading could obviously delay this effect.

There is some confusion concerning the effects of anaerobic training on the synthesis of glycolytic enzymes. Glycogen phosphorylase and phosphofructokinase activities have been found to increase substantially in some studies, but have been unchanged in others. This may reflect variations in the training stimulus or in methodological factors. Lactate dehydrogenase activity appears to be unaffected by anaerobic training. On the balance of current evidence, it seems that enzyme changes probably make little contribution to any improvement in the capacity for anaerobic glycolysis.

Anaerobic training may increase the ability of skeletal muscle to buffer hydrogen ions, permitting greater energy release through anaerobic glycolysis before the onset of fatigue. It is believed that muscle buffering capacity depends primarily on the presence of carnosine, a dipeptide containing histidine. Muscular carnosine levels are substantially greater in rowers and 800 m runners than in marathon runners or untrained people (Parkhouse *et al.* 1985). This suggests that regular participation in activities demanding high rates of anaerobic glycolysis may have an adaptive effect. Inadequate dietary intake of protein leads to reduction of carnosine levels. Furthermore, carnosine levels tend to decrease dramatically with age after about 20 years (Parkhouse & McKenzie 1984). This may partially explain the relatively poor capacity of older people for anaerobic glycolysis. Clearly, both dietary factors and age may influence the ability to adapt to anaerobic training.

PRINCIPLES OF TRAINING

To produce the desired physiological effects, training programmes must be carefully planned. Attention should be given to a number of basic principles, as outlined below.

The Principle of Individuality

Even among elite athletes in a single sport, physiological profiles may differ considerably. Any general training programme is likely to be unsuitable for some group members. Wherever possible, the physiological status of each athlete should be assessed in relation to the demands of the sport and individual training programmes designed accordingly. In many sports, opportunity to individualize may be confined to two or three sessions per week. For example, in rowing, training in crew boats requires that all athletes work in a similar way. However, the type of work done during supplementary sessions can be varied on the basis of individual needs. At the very least, athletes can usually be organized into small groups for such sessions, according to perceived strengths and weaknesses.

The Principle of Specificity

In recent years, the specificity of the response to training has become increasingly evident. Many of the adaptations are restricted to the muscles and the energy pathways directly involved. Training at slow speeds of movement may fail to enhance performance at faster speeds. In view of these findings, it is sometimes contended that training should resemble the competitive event as closely as possible. The logical extension of this argument is that competition is the best form of training. Some scientists have scorned the use of high-volume training for athletes whose events last only a few minutes. However, care should be taken in interpreting the specificity data. In fact, it does not imply that all training activities should mirror the demands of competition. Rather, it indicates that training should be specific to the physiological adaptations required at a particular time. If it is thought likely that a middle-distance swimmer could eventually benefit from increased muscle capillarization, a training programme incorporating light sessions of very long duration may be entirely appropriate. If an increase in blood volume is also desired, prolonged cycling might be a useful adjunct, as it stresses physiological mechanisms for blood volume maintenance and should therefore elicit adaptation. At some points in training, it may be advantageous for athletes to take part in a general muscle strengthening programme, rather than concentrating only on the muscle groups most involved in their sports. For many athletes, it is important to develop power at slow movement speeds before progressing to faster work. The skill of a good coach lies partly in identifying the physiological adaptations needed at certain times and in designing training programmes specifically geared to produce them.

The Principle of Progressive Overload

Training effects occur through adaptation to stress. Imposing unusual demands on a physiological system can evoke changes that make the system better able to cope. Consequently, a stimulus that is initially stressful may soon cease to be so and its continued application may fail to produce further change. To gain maximum benefit from training, workloads must be gradually adjusted upwards as adaptations take place. The workloads should not be increased in the absence of adaptation. A physiological system subjected to excessive stress may break down rather than adapting. This may result in illness or injury.

It is important to realize that there are limits to the adaptation of most systems. For example, a point may be reached at which it is not possible to elicit further increase in the maximum rate of aerobic metabolism of a particular athlete. When definite plateaus are encountered, it is often beneficial to turn the emphasis of training towards other physiological systems, while involving the first at a level that is not stressful but just sufficient to ensure maintenance of existing capabilities.

In applying the overload principle, many coaches are now basing their programmes on 2 or 3 week blocks of intensive training separated by 1 week recovery periods during which workloads are substantially reduced. The aim is usually to increase the overall load placed on the athletes from one block to the next. In assessing this load, both the duration and the intensity of the various sessions must be taken into account. The recovery periods between blocks are designed to facilitate successful adaptation, as many of the physiological adjustments to training actually occur in the intervals between heavy workouts. There is accruing evidence that this 'periodization' of training can produce excellent results.

The Principle of Reversibility

Cessation of training results in loss of adaptation. Some effects of training regress more rapidly than others. There is a particularly sharp decrease in the activity of mitochondrial enzymes. Houston *et al.* (1979), studying distance runners, observed a 24% decrease in succinate dehydrogenase activity after 2 weeks of detraining. Similar findings have been reported by others. By contrast, muscle myoglobin levels and capillarization show little change even after 12–16 weeks (Houston *et al.* 1979; Coyle *et al.* 1984). Blood volume is reduced significantly within 4 weeks, compromising oxygen transport capacity. Ability to perform very brief intensive exercise is often improved during the first 2 weeks of detraining and subsequent deterioration is quite slow. The effects of detraining on capacity for anaerobic glycolysis are unclear. Glycolytic enzyme activities apparently show almost no change during the first month after training is stopped, but little is known about alterations in muscle buffering capacity. In general, training effects are lost more quickly than they are gained. Consequently, athletes should be encouraged to continue some form of relevant activity even during the off-season.

BASIC TECHNIQUES FOR MONITORING TRAINING PROGRESS

Testing of athletes provides a basis for initial design of training programmes and allows for monitoring of progress. Used properly, it is not only helpful to coaches but also very motivational for athletes. In most sports science laboratories, techniques allowing close examination of intramuscular events (such as the needle biopsy technique and phosphorous nuclear magnetic resonance) are not available. However, there are various simpler tests that can provide an accurate guide to the physiological status of an athlete. Some of these tests are outlined below.

Tests of Aerobic Power

Aerobic power represents the peak rate at which energy can be released through aerobic metabolism. It is an important characteristic for athletes competing in sports requiring a high-energy output over periods of more than about 90 s. Aerobic metabolism requires the reduction of oxygen to form water at the end of the electron transport chain. Consequently, the maximum rate at which oxygen can be consumed in the active musculature is an index of aerobic power.

Maximum oxygen uptake is easily measured in the laboratory. Athletes are exercised at progressively increasing workloads on · an appropriate ergometer, while breathing through a respiratory valve (Fig. 4.6). Measurement is made of the volume of air breathed and expired air is analysed for oxygen and carbon dioxide content. As the concentrations of these gases in fresh room air are known, it is possible to calculate the total volume of oxygen consumed (and the volume of carbon dioxide produced) over any given period of time. When increase in workload fails to elicit any further rise in oxygen consumption, the maximum oxygen uptake is considered to have been reached. The athlete is typically exhausted at this stage, because once oxygen uptake has reached a plateau, an increase in workload requires that anaerobic energy pathways make a substantially greater contribution to ATP resynthesis. The maximum oxygen uptake may be expressed in either absolute terms (litres per minute — $L \cdot min^{-1}$) or in relation to bodyweight (millilitres per minute for every kilogram of body weight — $mL \cdot kg^{-1} \cdot min^{-1}$). The latter means of expression is preferred for sports in which the bodyweight must be repeatedly lifted, such as running and walking. Elite male distance runners often record values exceeding 80 $mL \cdot kg^{-1} \cdot min^{-1}$, while values for their female counterparts are frequently above 65 $mL \cdot kg^{-1} \cdot min^{-1}$. Corresponding figures for untrained young men and women are about 50 and 40 $mL \cdot kg^{-1} \cdot min^{-1}$, respectively. For weight-

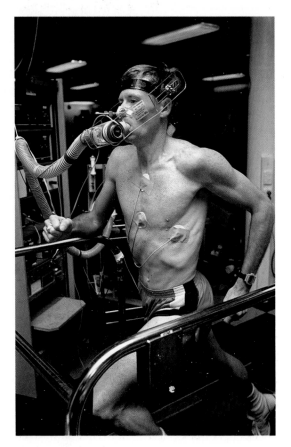

Fig. 4.6 The measurement of maximal oxygen uptake during treadmill running.

supported activities like rowing and kayaking, the absolute values of maximum oxygen uptake are considered more relevant. Readings above 6.0 $L \cdot min^{-1}$ are quite common among elite heavyweight oarsmen and values approaching 5.0 $L \cdot min^{-1}$ may be observed in champion female rowers. Testing of kayakers on a kayak ergometer yields much lower values, due to the smaller mass of muscle actively involved. Kayakers can attain higher oxygen uptakes on a treadmill or arm/leg ergometer than during simulated kayaking. However, the levels attained in the latter situation are more relevant to their sporting performance.

There are numerous simple field tests which permit estimation of maximum oxygen uptake. Some of these are based on the distance an athlete can run in a specified time period, or on the time taken to run a given distance. The results can obviously be influenced by such factors as the nature of the terrain, wind conditions, environmental temperature and humidity and running tactics. Estimates of maximum oxygen uptake derived from these tests have been found to correlate well with directly measured values, but the samples studied have generally been quite heterogeneous. The relationship may be much weaker for groups with a lesser range in maximum oxygen uptake. Other tests allowing estimation of maximum oxygen uptake include those involving measurement of heart rate responses to submaximal exercise on a bicycle ergometer. All of these tests are based on the incorrect assumption that maximum heart rate is relatively constant among individuals of a particular age. As a result, they may be seriously in error and should not be used to categorize athletes in terms of aerobic power.

Tests of 'Anaerobic Threshold'

Anaerobic glycolysis begins making a very significant contribution to muscular ATP resynthesis well before maximum oxygen uptake is reached. Thus, beyond a certain level of aerobic metabolism, there is rapid accumulation of hydrogen ions in the active muscles, seriously limiting the time for which exercise can be continued. This level has traditionally been called the 'anaerobic threshold', although it is now clear that anaerobic mechanisms participate in the process of energy release even under resting conditions. 'Anaerobic threshold' can be expressed in terms of either oxygen uptake or workload. For sports such as distance running, road cycling and cross-country skiing, it is considered more important than maximum oxygen uptake as a determinant of performance. This is because it indicates the load that can actually be maintained over a long period.

There are several techniques for estimating 'anaerobic threshold' in the laboratory. They generally involve the assumption that change in intramuscular concentrations of metabolites leads directly to a change in the blood concentrations. Some assume further that the blood changes have a direct influence on respiratory parameters. Serial blood samples can be collected during a number of prolonged steady-state exercise tests to enable determination of the highest workload that can be maintained without progressive reduction in pH (increase in hydrogen ion concentration) or rise in lactate concentration. This is time-consuming and often impractical. Consequently, sports scientists have devised methods for estimating 'anaerobic threshold' from physiological responses to brief incremental tests. A common protocol involves the athlete completing a series of efforts, each lasting 3–5 min, at successively higher workloads. After each effort, a blood sample is drawn and analysed for lactate concentration. A curve showing the rise in lactate with increasing intensity of effort is then constructed, and a 'breakpoint' indicating the commencement of rapid increase in blood lactate is identified by either visual inspection or mathematical analysis (e.g. Stegmann & Kindermann 1982; Cheng *et al.* 1992). The workload associated with this breakpoint is considered indicative of the threshold. Because the breakpoint is often difficult to discern, some researchers have preferred to determine the threshold workload as that associated with attainment of a blood lactate concentration of $4 \, \text{mmol} \cdot \text{L}^{-1}$ (Heck *et al.* 1985). This seems questionable, as activities involving a relatively small muscle mass may fail to cause much rise in blood lactate concentration even when the muscle concentration is quite high. There is considerable evidence that

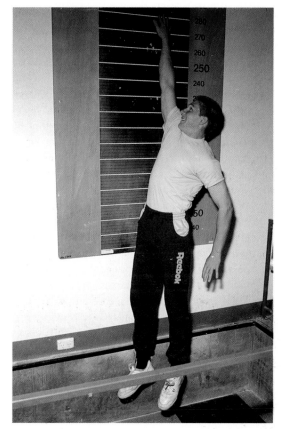

Fig. 4.7 The vertical jump test.

use of a fixed blood lactate criterion can lead to substantial inaccuracy in some cases (Stegmann & Kindermann 1982; Urhausen *et al.* 1993).

As hydrogen ions move from muscle cells into the blood, activation of the bicarbonate buffering system results in production of additional carbon dioxide. It is believed that hydrogen ions and carbon dioxide act on the carotid bodies to stimulate an increase in ventilation. Thus, beyond the 'anaerobic threshold', there should be a disproportionate rise in ventilation relative to oxygen uptake. Respiratory changes have been widely used in estimation of the threshold. However, the point of non-linear increase in ventilation is often difficult to detect. Furthermore, it is now evident that such increase may not be entirely due to the effects of hydrogen ions and carbon dioxide. Increase in plasma catecholamine levels can have a similar effect, as can elevation of arterial potassium concentration (Walsh & Banister 1988). Both are typical responses to exercise. Consequently, it is perhaps not surprising that estimates of 'anaerobic threshold' obtained by respiratory analysis often fail to concur with those derived from measurement of blood lactate concentrations.

Italian researchers have developed a field test for 'anaerobic threshold' based simply on the heart rate response to incremental exercise (Conconi *et al.* 1982). This test (generally known as the 'Conconi test') is now in widespread use. Heart rate normally increases in direct linear relationship to workload until 80–90% of maximum heart rate is attained. Beyond this level, it rises much more gradually. On the basis of studies on many different athletes, it has been claimed that the workload at the 'deflection point' (i.e. the point of departure from linearity) correlates very highly with the threshold workload obtained by measuring blood lactate responses to progressive exercise (Droghetti *et al.* 1985). However, recent studies on competitive runners (Tokmakidis & Leger 1992) and swimmers (Harrison *et al.* 1992) have failed to confirm this relationship. It appears that the estimates of 'anaerobic threshold' provided by the Conconi method are frequently too high.

It should be noted that the 'anaerobic threshold' is not synonymous with the lactate threshold (LT). The latter can be defined as the workload (or oxygen uptake) at which the blood lactate first begins to increase above resting levels, whereas the former represents the point beyond which there is a *rapid* rise in lactate. Many researchers use the LT as an additional reference point for determination of appropriate training intensities and various mathematical techniques have been developed for its identification (Lehmann *et al.* 1983; Beaver *et al.* 1985; Aunola & Rusko 1988). The LT has sometimes been called the 'aerobic threshold' or 'AT1'.

Measuring the Oxygen Cost of Submaximal Exercise

Performance in endurance events is influenced not only by aerobic power and 'anaerobic threshold', but also by exercise economy. All else being equal,

an athlete who requires less energy to perform a given exercise task is obviously at an advantage. Consequently, it is often useful to measure the oxygen cost of exercise at a set submaximal workload. For the purposes of such testing, the exercise intensity must be low enough to exclude the possibility of a large contribution from anaerobic mechanisms. Otherwise, the oxygen cost may not be indicative of total energy expenditure. The exercise equipment must allow close simulation of the actual sporting activity and the athletes should be well accustomed to its use. Dietary factors and muscle glycogen levels are also important, as oxygen cost is partly dependent on substrate utilization. Studies conducted on cyclists at the Australian Institute of Sport have shown substantial increase in the oxygen cost of submaximal work during periods of heavy training. If the potentially confounding variables are controlled, measurement of the respiratory exchange ratio during regular submaximal exercise tests may allow detection of the effects of training on substrate use.

Tests of Peak Anaerobic Power

Peak anaerobic power may be defined as the maximum rate of energy release that can be achieved by anaerobic mechanisms at any instant in time. It is a major determinant of performance in sports requiring rapid production of large muscular forces. Because it can be fully expressed in very brief efforts, it is often thought to depend exclusively on breakdown of muscular ATP and CP stores. However, there is now evidence that anaerobic glycolysis might contribute significantly to energy release from the outset of intensive exercise (Jacobs *et al.* 1983). Thus, from a practical viewpoint, it may not be possible to separately determine the power of the two anaerobic energy pathways.

A review of various anaerobic tests has been published by Vandewalle *et al.* (1987). One common test of peak anaerobic power requires the subject to run as rapidly as possible up a flight of several stairs. The time taken to raise the body through a given vertical distance is electronically recorded. The work done is calculated as the product of the vertical distance and body mass. Division by the time provides a result in units of power. Although this test has been widely used, it is unsatisfactory in several ways. The resistance encountered is often not high enough to allow attainment of true maximum power. Loading subjects with extra weights generally results in higher power scores. The optimal load differs between subjects, due to individual variation in the force–power relationship. Performance on the stair climb test may sometimes be inhibited by fear of injury. With the gradient constant, running up a ramp leads to better scores than stair running.

Vertical jump tests (Fig. 4.7) are often used to assess anaerobic power. Vandewalle *et al.* (1987) have pointed out that the height jumped is more a measure of work than a measure of power, as it is unrelated to time. Nor can the power be accurately calculated from the duration of the ascending phase of flight, as this is not the period during which force is actually developed. Precise results can be obtained only through use of a force platform. Nevertheless, height jumped has been found to correlate very highly with peak anaerobic power as determined from biomechanical analysis. Minor variations in test protocol can greatly affect the height jumped. A counter-movement before the jump and swinging of the arms can each improve performance. However, strict adherence to any one protocol allows for good test–retest reliability.

Another approach to the estimation of peak anaerobic power involves cycle ergometer tests. One such test, performed on a Monark friction-braked ergometer, is designed to allow assessment also of anaerobic capacity. It is generally known as the Wingate test. Subjects are required to pedal as rapidly as possible for 30 s against a resistance determined on the basis of bodyweight. Power outputs are measured over successive 5 s periods and the highest is considered representative of peak anaerobic power. For athletes involved in sports which emphasize the upper body musculature, a similar test can be performed with the arms. The determination of peak power by averaging over 5 s is questionable. Substantial change in power output could occur during this time, masking the true peak. Requiring subjects to pedal for 30 s might inhibit full expression of power in the early stages

of the test. Furthermore, the resistance which permits a true maximum power output does not represent the same proportion of bodyweight for all subjects. Vandewalle *et al.* (1987) suggest that several much shorter tests, performed against different levels of resistance, might be preferable. In Australia, Repco air-braked cycle ergometers are often used to assess anaerobic power. The standard test involves 10 s of 'all-out' effort. A specialized work monitor unit allows recording of peak power over a period of about 300 ms. The gearing of the cycle is constant and therefore almost certainly unsuitable for some individuals. As with the Wingate test, determination of peak power is based on the peak velocity of the ergometer flywheel and not flywheel acceleration. This may cause the power to be underestimated. The results of cycle ergometer tests may be influenced by the constraints imposed on the subjects. Higher power scores are obtained if subjects are permitted to stand during the test. Characteristics of the ergometer, such as crank length, may also have an effect. Nevertheless, if procedures are standardized, test–retest reliability is good.

For many athletes, estimates of peak anaerobic power based on stair climb, vertical jump or cycle ergometer tests lack specificity. To allow detection of training effects, the estimates must relate directly to the muscles involved in the sporting activity. Specific ergometers are now available for numerous different sports. Their use in testing for peak anaerobic power entails problems generally similar to those outlined for the cycle ergometer tests. While the absolute validity of the results is thus uncertain, the reliability seems in many cases to be quite acceptable. Furthermore, it appears that specific ergometer tests can indicate changes induced by training, at least when the changes are large. Peak anaerobic power during running can be estimated from measures of acceleration over very short distances. However, these measures require the use of highly accurate timing devices, such as light gates.

Tests of Anaerobic Capacity

Anaerobic capacity refers to the total amount of energy that can be released by anaerobic pathways during intensive exercise to exhaustion. It seems accepted that, for any individual, this amount will be the same over a range of exercise durations extending from about 60 s to 10 min. Clearly, the breakdown of given quantities of ATP and CP should yield the same amount of energy. However, for anaerobic capacity to be constant, it must also be assumed that muscular exhaustion is always associated with a given total contribution from anaerobic glycolysis. Implicit here is the unproven notion that change in intramuscular pH during intensive exercise depends more on the total production of hydrogen ions than on the rate of production.

Attempts to assess anaerobic capacity have sometimes been based on measurement of peak blood lactate concentration after exhaustive high-intensity exercise. This is an unsatisfactory approach for several reasons. The movement of lactate from muscle cells to the blood seems to depend on an active transport mechanism, which has a rather low maximum rate. Consequently, lactate efflux is not directly proportional to muscle lactate production. Furthermore, blood lactate concentration is determined not only by the efflux, but also by the rate at which lactate is removed from the blood (Brooks 1985). This rate may differ markedly between individuals, being particularly rapid in those with a high proportion of well-capillarized slow twitch muscle fibres. It may also vary for one individual across time, as it is thought to be responsive to training. Finally, it should be noted that blood volume affects the concentration resulting from the presence of a given quantity of lactate in the blood.

Oxygen uptake remains elevated above the normal resting level for a considerable time after exhaustive supramaximal exercise. This has been considered due largely to aerobic involvement in the replenishment of muscle ATP and CP stores and the removal of lactate. The total magnitude of the excess post-exercise oxygen uptake has often been used as an indicator of anaerobic capacity. Logically, a greater contribution from anaerobic pathways during exercise should lead to a larger excess post-exercise oxygen uptake in order to allow for recovery. It has been argued that it is even possible to separately estimate the volumes of oxygen devoted to ATP–CP restoration and lactate removal, thus gaining an indication of the specific capacities of the two anaerobic pathways. This argument is based on the dual assumptions that muscle ATP and CP stores are almost completely replenished within 3 min of exercise cessation and that very little lactate is removed during this time. However, it is now evident that neither assumption is true. Muscle CP restoration can take more than 10 min (Sapega et al. 1987) and there is substantial lactate removal even in the immediate post-exercise period (Gaesser & Brooks 1984). Partitioning of the excess post-exercise oxygen uptake into specific components is therefore invalid. Even without such partitioning, the excess post-exercise oxygen uptake is a poor indicator of anaerobic capacity. It is influenced by factors other than the need for ATP–CP repletion and lactate removal. Increased body temperature, elevated heart rate and an increase in circulating catecholamines all contribute to maintenance of oxygen uptake above the resting level. Test–retest reliability for the measurement of excess post-exercise oxygen uptake is low (Vandewalle et al. 1987).

It has been suggested that anaerobic capacity can be accurately quantified in terms of the amount by which the measured oxygen uptake during exhaustive supramaximal exercise falls short of the calculated oxygen requirement (Medbo et al. 1988). The oxygen requirement of the exercise must be separately determined for each athlete, by extrapolating from the measured oxygen costs of various submaximal workloads. Estimates of anaerobic capacity based on total oxygen shortfall (generally termed the 'maximum accumulated oxygen deficit') have revealed large differences between subjects. However, repeated assessments on the same subjects indicate that the results are quite reproducible (Medbo et al. 1988). The method assumes that the oxygen requirement remains the same throughout a supramaximal exercise bout performed at constant load and can be precisely predicted from the linear relationship between oxygen uptake and workload at submaximal levels. Bangsbo et al. (1993) have raised doubts concerning the second assumption and have provided evidence suggesting that the maximum accumulated oxygen deficit may vary according to the test protocol used for its determination. However, Craig et al. (1993) found maximum accumulated oxygen deficit to be a useful predictor of track cycling performance.

In many laboratories, anaerobic capacity is assessed only on the basis of total work output during an 'all-out' exercise test of 30–90 s duration. This is not strictly valid, as aerobic pathways can make a significant contribution to energy release even during tests lasting only 30 s. Longer tests lead to proportionally greater aerobic involvement (Withers et al. 1993). The optimal duration of ergometric anaerobic capacity tests is a matter for debate.

Discussion is usually centred on the time needed to permit full expression of the anaerobic capacity. This is generally greater for discontinuous activities, such as rowing. However, Vandewalle et al. (1987) have noted that, in bicycle ergometer studies, work outputs achieved during longer and shorter anaerobic tests are very highly correlated. It therefore seems that there is little extra information to be gained by exposing athletes to the discomforts of the more prolonged tests. It is sometimes argued that the decrement in power output during relatively long tests is an interesting physiological characteristic in itself and might be an indicator of muscle fibre type. However, it appears that the test–retest reliability of the power decrement is generally quite poor (Vandewalle et al. 1987).

FROM PRINCIPLES TO PRACTICE — DEVELOPMENT OF TRAINING PROGRAMMES

In practice, many coaches and athletes make extensive use of physiological data in the development of their training programmes. In the sport of rowing, for example, physiological studies have shown that maximum oxygen uptake, anaerobic capacity and muscular strength may all influence competitive performance. Of these parameters, maximum oxygen uptake appears to be the most important, as there is evidence that aerobic pathways account for approximately 80% of the energy release required during a standard 2000 m race.

Maximum oxygen uptake may be limited by either the rate at which oxygen can be delivered via the circulation to the active musculature or the diffusion of oxygen from the red blood cells in the muscle capillaries to the muscle mitochondria (Wagner 1992). The latter is probably dependent on both muscle capillarity and the number and size of the mitochondria.

For purposes of planning, each rowing season can be divided into four distinct phases, termed preparatory, pre-competitive, competitive and post-competitive. The preparatory phase normally lasts for at least 12 weeks, the pre-competitive phase for 6–10 weeks and the competitive phase (which incorporates the build-up to the major regatta of the season) for about 6 weeks. The post-competitive phase, during which the emphasis is on physical and mental recovery, should be from 2 to 4 weeks.

In the preparatory phase, the primary aim of the training programme is the development of capillarization and muscle respiratory capacity. The volume of training is very high, entailing more than 20 hours per week on the water during the 'heavy' weeks of the periodized training cycle. However, the intensity of training is generally low, with more than 80% of the work being performed at a level in the lower half of the range between LT and 'anaerobic threshold'. This is termed 'U2' pace. Typically, about 10% of the work is performed in the upper half of the range between LT and 'anaerobic threshold' (U1 pace), while a further 5% is performed right at or very close to the 'threshold' (AT) pace. Only about 5% of the training is performed above this pace. There is very little supramaximal work — usually less than 1% of the total volume.

As the season progresses, there is a gradual shift towards an increased intensity of training. Early in the pre-competitive phase, this is accomplished merely through a 5–10% increase in the volume of work at U1 intensity and a concomitant decrease in the volume of U2 work. However, by the end of the pre-competitive phase, as much as 25% of the training is performed at the U1 level, 6–7% at AT and 7–8% above AT. The aim is to place increased stress on the physiological mechanisms involved in circulatory transport of oxygen to the active muscles and hence to elicit positive adaptation of these mechanisms.

During the competitive phase of the season, the volume of training is markedly decreased and there is a sharp increase in the percentage of work performed above AT (11–12% is not unusual). As much as 2–3% of the training may be supramaximal, involving 'all-out' efforts over short distances. The purpose here is to maximize the adaptation of oxygen transport mechanisms while also improving other physiological parameters which contribute to the competitive performance, such as muscle buffering capacity (and therefore anaerobic capacity). The development of correct neuromuscular sequencing patterns is also considered highly important. The competitive phase of training incorporates a 'tapering' period leading into the major regatta. During this period, which usually lasts 10–14 days, the volume of training is very low, but intensity is maintained. The aim is to ensure complete elimin-

ation of residual fatigue. An example of a training programme of a rower over the course of a season is shown in Fig. 4.8. It does not include the strength training component, which is usually treated quite separately.

It should be noted that other endurance sports use different terminologies in describing training programmes, but the major reference points for determining training intensities (i.e. LT and 'anaerobic threshold') are common to many. The same is true of the general principles involved in construction of the programme.

The rationale for the progression in training intensity during the season is based on the dual premises that intensity is the major determinant of the stress placed on the athlete and that for optimal adaptation stress should be increased only gradually. It also reflects the conventional wisdom of coaches

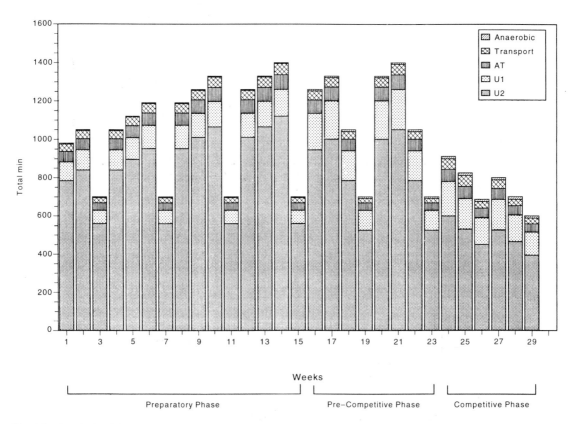

Fig. 4.8 A typical training programme for an elite rower. Note that the 'Transport' category refers to work performed between anaerobic threshold and maximum oxygen uptake. See text for definition of other categories.

that intense training early in the season can lead to premature 'peaking' and subsequent loss of form.

Fig. 4.9   Relationship of blood lactate (- - -) and pH (——) to workload for a male rower performing a progressive rowing ergometer test. The lactate threshold, determined mathematically, is indicated by the arrow. The vertical line indicates the 'anaerobic threshold' point.

From the above, it should be evident that the ability to accurately regulate training intensity is crucial to the success of the training programme. Data from physiological tests can provide coaches and athletes with this ability. Figure 4.9 shows the relationship between blood lactate and rowing ergometer workload (and also between blood pH and workload) for an elite male rower tested at the

Training zone calculations

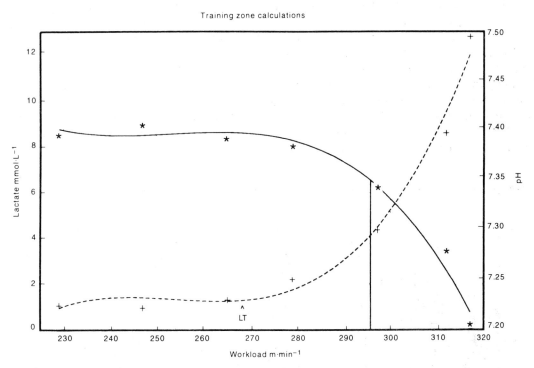

Training HR (pH,fit=0.99)		HR	%$\dot{V}O_2$max
Recovery	<153	125	53
		130	55
U2	153–163	135	58
U1	164–173	140	60
AT	174–176	145	65
Transport	>176	150	69
		155	73
		160	77
Training HR (lactate,fit=0.99)		165	80
Recovery	<153	170	84
U2	153–163	175	88
U1	164–173	180	92
AT	174–176	185	95
Transport	>176	190	99

At LT   Work=268, $\dot{V}O_2$=4.03, %$\dot{V}O_2$max=72
At AT (pH)   Work=295, $\dot{V}O_2$=4.93, %$\dot{V}O_2$max=88
At AT (lactate) Work=295, $\dot{V}O_2$=4.93, %$\dot{V}O_2$max=88

Australian Institute of Sport. The workloads and oxygen uptakes at LT and 'anaerobic threshold' are clearly indicated, having been determined by mathematical techniques. By using these reference points and taking account of the observed relationship between workload and heart rate, it is possible to determine the heart rate ranges corresponding to the various training zones (U2, U1, AT, etc.) included in the structure of the training programme. By monitoring heart rates during on-water sessions (Fig. 4.10), it is possible to ensure that the athlete is working at the required intensity. For sports such as swimming, where the conditions encountered by the athletes show little variation from day to day, it is possible to establish training zones based directly on pace rather than heart rates. For many other sports, the power output required to maintain a given pace can vary markedly according to wind conditions and other environmental factors. Under these circumstances, the use of heart rates is preferable.

The relationship of blood lactate concentration to workload can also change dramatically with training, particularly in the early stages of the season. Consequently, there can be large changes in the workloads and oxygen uptakes corresponding to LT and 'anaerobic threshold'. Heart rates at these points can show an even larger alteration, as heart rate itself is very responsive to training. Consequently, for training zones established through physiological testing to retain practical value, it is necessary for the testing to be repeated at regular intervals. Of course, other physiological parameters with direct relevance to performance should also be repeatedly assessed, in order to allow full evaluation of the response to training and to provide a basis for individualizing the subsequent programme.

MONITORING OF ATHLETES TO PREVENT FAILING ADAPTATION

In their desire for competitive success, athletes can sometimes train too hard. This can result in failure of adaptation, as manifest by fatigue, dramatically decreased performance and occasionally even illness. Much research has been conducted with a view to the early detection of overtraining, so that the situation might be quickly rectified. As yet, however, no single diagnostic test has been developed.

Susceptibility to overtraining is apparently related to the overall level of stress encountered by the athlete, regardless of the source. Lack of sleep, examination pressures or personal problems may cause failure to adapt to a training programme that would otherwise be tolerable. Some types of training are more stressful than others. Intensive anaerobic work may pose a particular risk. In studies carried out at the Australian Institute of Sport, lymphocytes taken from trained cyclists 6 h after a 1 min 'all-out' ergometer test showed reduced ability to respond to challenge. This suggested that immune function was temporarily compromised. By contrast, studies on neutrophils have indicated that an hour of moderate aerobic exercise may lead to a transient improvement in immune function. The effect of training on immune function is discussed elsewhere in this book.

Several physiological changes have been mooted as possible correlates of overtraining. It has been suggested that consistently high blood levels of creatine phosphokinase (an enzyme normally con-

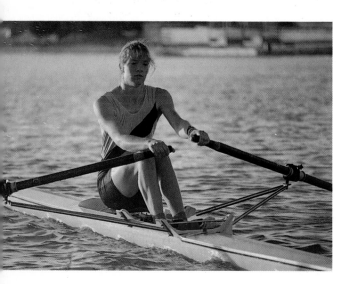

Fig 4.10 In the field, athletes can use heart rate monitors to regulate training intensity. In this photo the display unit is located on the rower's left wrist.

fined to muscle cells) might indicate muscle fibre breakdown and a need for rest. However, high levels may be present for some time after a single weight training session and are not necessarily accompanied by subjective symptoms of overtraining. Conversely, subjective symptoms may occur in the absence of elevated creatine phosphokinase levels. Urhausen *et al.* (1987) made weekly measurements of the resting serum testosterone and cortisol levels of competitive rowers over a period of 7 weeks. They reported that the ratio of testosterone to cortisol was depressed during intensive phases of training and recovered during regenerative phases. This indicates changes in anabolic–catabolic balance. It is thought possible that routine monitoring of the ratio might provide a guide as to when training loads should be reduced. However, further research is needed to evaluate this possibility. At a conference held at the Australian Institute of Sport in 1988, it was argued that many of the symptoms of overtraining may be due to chronic glycogen depletion resulting from a failure to adjust dietary intake to the energy requirements of training. Failure to adapt to training may sometimes be due to specific vitamin or mineral deficiencies. These are discussed elsewhere in this book.

At a practical level, there are some readily observable indicators of failing adaptation. These include constant respiratory tract infections or sore throat, swelling of lymph nodes, stiffness or soreness of joints, sudden loss of weight, insomnia, persistent elevation of basal heart rate and unusual irritability. Recently, Snyder *et al.* (1993) have suggested the concurrent use of physiological and psychological indicators for detection of excessive fatigue in athletes. They have found that, with intensive exercise, the ratio of blood lactate concentration to an index of perceived exertion is depressed when athletes are 'overtrained'.

CONCLUSIONS

In this chapter, an attempt has been made to provide a theoretical framework for the design and monitoring of sports training programmes. It is hoped that the concepts presented might stimulate thought and perhaps lead to innovation. There is little doubt that the study of exercise physiology can point the way in the development of increasingly more effective training methods, thus improving the performance of athletes in the future.

REFERENCES

Andersen P. & Henriksson J. (1977a) Training induced changes in the subgroups of human type II skeletal muscle fibres. *Acta Physiologica Scandinavica* 99, 123–125.

Andersen P. & Henriksson J. (1977b) Capillary supply of the quadriceps femoris muscle of man: Adaptive response to exercise. *Journal of Physiology* 270, 677–690.

Aunola S. & Rusko H. (1988) Comparison of two methods for aerobic threshold determination. *European Journal of Applied Physiology* 57, 420–424.

Bangsbo J., Michalsik L. & Petersen A. (1993) Accumulated O_2 deficit during intense exercise and muscle characteristics of elite athletes. *International Journal of Sports Medicine* 14, 207–213.

Beaver W. L., Wasserman K. & Whipp B.J. (1985) Improved detection of lactate threshold during exercise using a log–log transformation. *Journal of Applied Physiology* 59, 1936–1940.

Brooks G. A. (1985) Anaerobic threshold: Review of the concept and directions for future research. *Medicine and Science in Sports and Exercise* 17, 22–31.

Callow M., Morton A. & Guppy M. (1986) Marathon fatigue: The role of plasma fatty acids, muscle glycogen and blood glucose. *European Journal of Applied Physiology* 55, 654–661.

Carlsson L. A., Ekelund L. G. & Froberg S. O. (1971) Concentrations of triglycerides, phospholipids and glycogen in skeletal muscle and of free fatty acids and β-hydroxybutyric acid in blood in man in response to exercise. *European Journal of Clinical Investigation* 1, 248–254.

Cheng B., Kuipers H. & Snyder A. C. *et al.* (1992) A new approach for the determination of ventilatory and lactate thresholds. *International Journal of Sports Medicine* 13, 518–522.

Conconi F., Ferrari M. & Ziglio P. G. *et al.* (1982) Determination of the anaerobic threshold by a noninvasive field test in runners. *Journal of Applied Physiology* 52, 869–873.

Costill D. L., Coyle E. & Dalsky G. *et al.* (1977) Effects of elevated FFA and insulin on muscle glycogen usage during exercise. *Journal of Applied Physiology* 43, 695–699.

Coyle E. F., Martin W. H. & Sinacore D. R. *et al.* (1984) Time course of loss of adaptations after stopping prolonged intense endurance training. *Journal of Applied Physiology* 57, 1857–1864.

Craig N. P., Norton K. I. & Bourdon P. C. *et al.* (1993)

Aerobic and anaerobic indices contributing to track endurance cycling performance. *European Journal of Applied Physiology* 67, 150–158.

Droghetti P., Borsetto C. & Casoni I. *et al.* (1985) Noninvasive determination of the anaerobic threshold in canoeing, cross-country skiing, cycling, roller and ice-skating, rowing and walking. *European Journal of Applied Physiology* 53, 299–303.

Gaesser G. A. & Brooks G. A. (1984) Metabolic base of excess post-exercise oxygen consumption: A review. *Medicine and Science in Sports and Exercise* 16, 29–43, 1984.

Gollnick P. D., Armstrong R. B. & Saltin B. *et al.* (1973) Effect of training on enzyme activity and fiber composition of human skeletal muscle. *Journal of Applied Physiology* 34, 107–111.

Harrison J. R., Dawson B. T. & Lawrence S. *et al.* (1992) Non-invasive and invasive determinations of the individual anaerobic threshold in competitive swimmers. *Journal of Swimming Research* 8, 11–17.

Heck H., Mader A. & Hess G. *et al.* (1985) Justification of the 4.0 mmol/l lactate threshold. *International Journal of Sports Medicine* 6, 117–130.

Houston M. E., Bentzen H. & Larsen H. (1979) Inter-relationships between skeletal muscle adaptations and performance as studied by detraining and retraining. *Acta Physiologica Scandinavica* 105, 163–170.

Jacobs I., Tesch P. A. & Bar-Or O. *et al.* (1983) Lactate in human skeletal muscle after 10 and 30 s of supra-maximal exercise. *Journal of Applied Physiology* 55, 365–367.

Lehmann M., Berg A. & Kapp R. *et al.* (1983) Correlations between laboratory testing and distance running performance in marathoners of similar performance ability. *International Journal of Sports Medicine* 4, 226–230.

Medbo J. I., Mohn A-C. & Tabata I. *et al.*, (1988) Anaerobic capacity determined by maximal accumulated oxygen deficit. *Journal of Applied Physiology* 64, 50–60.

Meyer R. A., Kushmerick M. J., Dillon P. F. & Brown T. R. (1983) Different effects of decreased intracellular pH on contractions in fast versus slow twitch muscle. *Medicine and Science in Sports and Exercise* 15, 116.

Parkhouse W. S. & McKenzie D. C. (1984) Possible contribution of skeletal muscle buffers to enhanced anaerobic performance: A brief review. *Medicine and Science in Sports and Exercise* 16, 328–338.

Parkhouse W. S., McKenzie D. C., Hochachka P. W. & Ovalle W. K. (1985) Buffering capacity of deproteinized human vastus lateralis muscle. *Journal of Applied Physiology* 58, 14–17.

Richter E. A. & Galbo H. (1986) High glycogen levels enhance glycogen breakdown in isolated contracting skeletal muscle. *Journal of Applied Physiology* 61, 827–831.

Sahlin K., Henriksson J. & Juhlin-Dannfelt A. (1984) Intracellular pH and electrolytes in human skeletal muscle during adrenaline and insulin infusions. *Clinical Science* 67, 461–464.

Sapega A. A., Sokolow D. P., Graham T. J. & Chance B. (1987) Phosphorous nuclear magnetic resonance: A non-invasive technique for the study of muscle bio-energetics during exercise. *Medicine and Science in Sports and Exercise* 19, 410–420.

Snyder A. C., Jeukendrup A. E. & Hesselink M. K. C. *et al.* (1993) A physiological/psychological indicator of over-reaching during intensive training. *International Journal of Sports Medicine* 14, 29–32.

Stegmann H. & Kindermann W. (1982) Comparison of prolonged exercise tests at the individual anaerobic threshold and the fixed anaerobic threshold of 4 mmol·l^{-1} lactate. *International Journal of Sports Medicine* 3, 105–110.

Tokmakidis S. P. & Leger L. A. (1992) Comparison of mathematically determined blood lactate and heart rate 'threshold' points and relationship with performance. *European Journal of Applied Physiology* 64, 309–317.

Urhausen A., Kullmer T. & Kindermann W. (1987) A 7-week follow-up study of the behaviour of testosterone and cortisol during the competition period in rowers. *European Journal of Applied Physiology* 56, 528–533.

Urhausen A., Coen B. & Weiler B. *et al.* (1993) Individual anaerobic threshold and maximum lactate steady state. *International Journal of Sports Medicine* 14, 134–139.

Vandewalle H., Peres G. & Monod H. (1987) Standard anaerobic exercise tests. *Sports Medicine* 4, 268–289.

Wagner P. D. (1992) Gas exchange and peripheral diffusion limitation. *Medicine and Science in Sports and Exercise* 24, 54–58.

Walsh M. L. & Banister E. W. (1988) Possible mechanisms of the anaerobic threshold: A review. *Sports Medicine* 5, 269–302.

Withers R. T., Van Der Ploeg G. & Finn J. P. (1993) Oxygen deficits incurred during 45, 60, 75 and 90-s maximal cycling on an air-braked ergometer. *European Journal of Applied Physiology* 67, 185–191.

Witzmann F. A., Fink W. J., Foster C. C. & Ivy J. L. (1978) Changes in muscle lipid metabolism during endurance training. *Medicine and Science in Sports* 10, 41.

CHAPTER 5

NUTRITION AND ENERGY SOURCES

V. Deakin and J. R. Brotherhood

While there is a long history of *ad hoc* experimentation with dietary practices in the hope of enhancing athletic performance, systematic scientific evaluation of the relationship between diet and sports performance did not begin in earnest until the 1960s. Although this area of research is expanding, many questions remain unanswered. This is largely due to the complex chemistry of food and the variability of individuals in their physiological, psychological and genetic responses to it. Many athletes and coaches are poorly informed about nutrition because they are susceptible to misleading and often conflicting claims and exaggerated testimonials from their peers about the unique properties of specific foods, supplements and dietary programmes.

The purpose of this chapter is to provide a background of the available scientific evidence for good nutritional practices, as well as practical information on the nutritional concerns of athletes.

THE ROLE OF NUTRITION IN SPORT

Three fundamental questions may be posed about the role of nutrition in sport:

- Can nutrition be a limiting factor in physical performance — if so, how and why?
- Is there any evidence of sports-specific or exercise-specific nutritional stresses that make the nutritional requirements of athletes quantitatively and/or qualitatively different from those of non-athletes?
- Is there any evidence for ergogenic effects of food?

Two main lines of scientific inquiry provide the answers to these questions and are as follows:

- Fundamental investigations of the physiological and biochemical nature of the metabolic stresses and strains of exercise and how these may be modified by different foods or dietary practice (e.g. carbohydrate (CHO) and protein requirements)
- Epidemiological evidence of sports-related nutritional deficiencies (e.g. iron deficiency)

Generally, empirical experiments studying the effects of foods, supplements or dietary manipulation are unlikely to provide useful information. Whether food can have ergogenic effects depends on the outcome which is desired. At the present time there is no good evidence that food can boost maximal exercise capacity, strength and power. However, limited body energy stores can limit endurance and appropriate dietary manipulation and nutritional support during exercise can certainly extend endurance, thus improving performance in events which last over long periods of time such as the marathon. Moreover, if the appropriate dietary considerations are not observed, performance both in training and competition will suffer.

The majority of the information in this chapter is based on objective physiological research. Much of it has been carried out under laboratory conditions on highly motivated subjects, not all of whom have been highly trained or are elite athletes. The practising athlete, sports scientist and coach are therefore advised to follow the dietary principles that are indicated but also, within the guide-lines, to experiment for themselves to find the best practice for the individual athlete.

There are three aspects of athletic activity to which nutrition and dietary practice should be applied:

- Training, recovery and the long-term health status of the athlete
- Preparation for competition
- Nutrition while exercising (competition and training)

BASIC NUTRITIONAL REQUIREMENTS FOR TRAINING AND RECOVERY FROM TRAINING

Traditionally athletes place too much emphasis on pre-competition nutrition, thinking that last minute modifications to their diet will boost their performance. If the correct training diet is ignored, dietary imbalances may restrict the ability to train effectively and ultimately to perform at maximum potential. While athletes tend to eat more food than sedentary people, the nature of the diet they should follow is virtually the same as that recommended for the general population.

General Dietary Guide-lines for Athletes

EAT A WIDE VARIETY OF NUTRITIOUS FOODS

The first guide-line for athletes to meet a good training diet is to consume a wide variety of foods across the range of core food groups (Table 5.1). This helps to promote a sufficient supply of essential nutrients. Elimination of foods from one or more core food groups for an extended period of time without replacement of the missing nutrients places an athlete at risk of nutrient depletion and, ulti-

mately, deficiency. For example, people who avoid eating dairy products, a major food source of calcium and riboflavin, may have difficulty meeting their requirements for these nutrients. Because of their higher requirement and turnover of some nutrients, athletes who eat poorly from a limited range of foods are likely to be at higher risk of nutrient deficiency than the general population.

The core food groups for Australians were developed using a population approach based on food availability, Recommended Dietary Intakes (RDI) and food composition data (Cashel & Jeffreson 1995). The final core groups and proposed quantities recommended for each group showed a close approximation to the actual food consumption practices of Australian adults and schoolchildren (Cashel & Jeffreson 1995). The portions suggested in Table 5.1 show the quantities of food necessary to provide approximately 70% of the RDI of most nutrients for most adult people (Cashel & Jeffreson 1995). Athletes expending a lot of energy on training or competition may need two to three times this amount to meet their energy requirements.

EAT PLENTY OF BREADS AND CEREALS (PREFERABLY WHOLEGRAIN), VEGETABLES (INCLUDING LEGUMES) AND FRUITS

The available evidence suggests that relatively high-dietary CHO intakes (about 600 g CHO per day) can restore muscle glycogen depleted from the demands of training (Costill et al. 1981). Wholesome or complex CHO foods provide a higher concentration of nutrients including fibre, B vitamins, iron and zinc compared with refined or simple sugars. For many athletes, diets high in wholesome CHO foods, because of their relatively low-energy content and high-satiety value, aid in weight control. For others with high-energy requirements, this bulking effect may result in inadequate food intake to sustain weight. CHO contributes only 16 kJ of energy for every gram consumed, which is almost half the energy content of the same amount of fat. For these athletes, energy needs can more easily be met (provided a well-balanced diet is consumed), by adding more sugar or, in some cases, adding fats that are predominantly polyunsaturated or mono-unsaturated rather than saturated in composition.

Table 5.1 The core food group plan for adults

Groups	Suggested daily amounts		
Bread and cereals	7 Servings		
Includes breakfast cereals, all breads, pancakes, rice, spaghetti and other pasta	*1 serving*	=	1 slice bread
		or	1 serve cereal, ready to eat (30 g)
		or	¾ cup cooked pasta or rice
		or	4 large cracker biscuits
		or	1 small plain cake
Fruit	2 Servings		
Includes all varieties and their juices, fresh, cooked, frozen and canned	*1 serving*	=	1 medium apple or orange or banana
		or	½ cup fruit juice
		or	¾ cup stewed fruit
Vegetables	5 Servings		
Includes all varieties, fresh, cooked, frozen and canned	*1 serving*	=	½ cup green leafy vegetables
		or	1 cup salad vegetables
		or	½ cup corn, peas
		or	1–2 medium potatoes
Meat and meat alternatives			
Meat, fish, nuts, poultry, eggs, lentils or beans	*1 serving*	=	85 g meat (cooked weight/volume)
		or	1 very small steak
		or	1 chump lamb chop
		or	1 chicken leg
		or	¾ cup cooked dried beans
		or	4 tablespoons peanut butter
		or	80–90 g nuts
		or	3 eggs
Dairy group	450 mL milk or equivalent		
Includes whole, low fat or skimmed milk drinks, yoghurt, ice cream, milk puddings, custard, all types of cheese	*100 mL milk*	=	½ carton yoghurt
		or	20 g cheese (hard)
		or	½ cup cottage cheese
		or	1 scoop icecream
		or	small serve custard

Foods and beverages which don't fit are those that do not provide significant amounts of nutrients. These are frequently high in kilojoules, fat, sugar or salt and should be consumed in small amounts.
Source Cashel & Jeffreson (1995)

EAT A DIET LOW IN FAT AND, IN PARTICULAR, LOW IN SATURATED FAT

Trained athletes use fat as a source of energy to a much greater extent than untrained individuals. Even those athletes with low body fat have a large supply of adipose tissue and do not need to eat extra fat. Fat contains $37 \text{ kJ} \cdot \text{g}^{-1}$ and should be used in moderation, as athletes are susceptible to the adverse health effects of high-saturated fat diets, despite the positive health benefits associated with exercise. Replacement or reduction of saturated fat sources in the diet (e.g. butter, fatty meat, cheese, ice cream, commercial cakes, biscuits, pastry and chocolate) with polyunsaturated or mono-unsaturated margarine) and low-fat dairy products and lean meat, can supply the calories and nutrients with low levels of fat and is a better alternative.

CONTROL YOUR WEIGHT AND MAINTAIN A HEALTHY BODYWEIGHT

The achievement and maintenance of a suitable bodyweight are important aspects of sports performance. For most sports, excess bodyweight stored as fat decreases an athlete's speed, agility and endurance. Conversely, extreme leanness well below usual levels, if brought about by consistent dieting and poor food selection, may also compromise an athlete's nutritional status, strength and endurance capacity and favour injury.

An ideal or healthy bodyweight is difficult to define for an individual athlete or even for groups of athletes. The best method for determining the ideal body type is to estimate body composition using skinfold thickness measures in combination with weight and girth measures and then to compare these with reported reference data. These data are available for groups of athletes involved in different sports and are reported elsewhere (Ross & Marfell-Jones 1982; Ross & Ward 1984; Telford et al. 1988). The general physique and body composition profiles of athletes best suited to different sports are also described in more detail in Chapter 1.

Some athletes in weight category sports train at a weight more than 3 kg above competitive weight to maximize strength effects. When these athletes must 'make weight' for competition, large and rapid reductions in bodyweight, usually induced by self-imposed methods of dehydration or food deprivation, are practised. These practices are associated with unwanted side-effects, which are described in more detail later in the chapter. A desirable bodyweight should be achieved slowly during the off-season and be maintained 1–2% above competitive weight (Burke & Reid 1993) to avoid the need for large and rapid weight losses.

LIMIT ALCOHOL CONSUMPTION

Although alcohol contains a relatively high-energy content (29 kJ·g^{-1}), available evidence suggests that it is not utilized to any significant extent during exercise. Alcohol consumption is associated with many sports as part of the tradition and ritual. The acute adverse effects of alcohol on motor performance, thinking processes and emotional behaviour are well documented. Physiologically, alcohol inhibits gluconeogenesis with resultant hypoglycaemia and may offer increased risks of dehydration during exercise. Hypoglycaemia, in association with alcohol intake, can lead to impaired temperature regulation and when exercising in cold weather, a decrease in body temperature. However, little research has been conducted on athletes concerning the health hazards or benefits associated with intermittent social drinking.

EAT ONLY MODERATE AMOUNTS OF SUGARS AND FOODS CONTAINING ADDED SUGAR

Refined sugar or foods containing added sugar should be limited in the diet basically because the athlete benefits from the minerals, vitamins and fibre associated with the unrefined CHO in fruit, vegetables, grains and legumes.

Some evidence suggests that oral feedings of sugar in the form of glucose, fructose, sucrose or glucose polymer are useful in the speedy recovery of fuel reserves if consumed in the first 2 h after strenuous exercise (Ivy et al. 1988). Eating soon after hard exercise is thought to replace glycogen in depleted muscle almost three times faster than if eaten more than 2 h after exercise. Other CHO-rich foods which have a moderate to high-glycaemic index (GI; e.g. breakfast cereal, bread, fruit and fruit juice) and are readily absorbed, may have similar effects to sugar in promoting greater storage of muscle glycogen in the post-exercise recovery period (Coyle 1991; Burke et al. 1993).

CHOOSE LOW SALT FOODS AND USE SALT SPARINGLY

Contrary to popular belief, athletes do not need to eat salty food or add salt to their food. The case for a high-salt intake or salt tablets as a preventive treatment for cramp has never been substantiated and can exacerbate a dehydrated condition.

Generally, the affluent or Western-style diet is high in sodium with intakes between 130 and 200 mmol·day^{-1}. Recommended daily intakes for sodium between 40 and 100 mmol·day^{-1} are adequate for most athletes. In practical terms, this means that few athletes need to add salt to their food. Even those who sweat heavily every day require no more than is provided by the usual salt content of Western-style diets.

A BALANCED TRAINING DIET

At present, diets recommended for training and recovery from training for most sports are all modifications of the basic balanced diet recommended for the general population. Athletes do not require special foods, supplements or special diets to meet their training needs or improve their performance. A well-balanced diet which is high in CHO-rich foods, relatively low in fat and contains moderate amounts of protein-rich foods can meet the needs of most athletes. The recommended training diet should supply:

- Greater than 55% of total energy from CHO, mostly wholesome CHO foods (cereals, bread, rice, pasta, vegetables and fruit). Individuals involved in exercise for more than 60–90 min·day^{-1} would benefit by increasing the proportion of CHO to 60–65% of the total energy consumed (Brotherhood 1984) or meeting an intake of 9–10 g of CHO per kg of body mass per day (Costill 1988)
- Less than 30% of total energy from fat sources, such as fatty meats, oils, margarine, butter, pastry, full cream dairy products, croissants and fried foods
- 12–15% of total energy from protein, which is found in foods such as lean red meat, chicken (no skin), fish (no batter), eggs and lentils or beans such as soya or baked beans. Despite slightly higher protein requirements for athletes compared with their untrained counterparts, a protein intake of 12–15% of total energy is usually adequate, provided a minimum of 5000 kJ (1200 kcal) is consumed by women and 6200 kJ (1500 kcal) by men (American Dietetic Association 1987)

Frequency of Meals

Athletes often need help in meeting their high energy needs from a low fat, high-CHO diet, as such a diet requires consumption of a large quantity of food. Wholesome high-CHO diets are bulky and therefore filling and need to be spread over several meals, with frequent snacks. Athletes involved in rigorous training schedules have limited time to prepare and digest foods and often resort to frequent snacking of readily accessible convenience foods. Typical choices are high in energy value but usually low in nutrients (e.g. soft drink,

chocolates, ice cream, cakes and take-away foods). Individuals consuming a large portion of their daily energy input from these foods are at risk of acquiring a nutrient deficiency.

Dietary Status of Athletes

In most industrialized countries the average diet is too high in fat and too low in CHO to meet the increased energy demands for regular strenuous exercise. This kind of diet has also been linked to diseases such as heart disease, high blood pressure, bowel disease, diabetes, obesity and certain types of cancer (McMichael 1991). Food consumption practices of athletes are proportionally very similar to national averages except for total energy intake, which is usually higher. Several surveys show that few athletes follow the best dietary pattern for optimal sports performance as they eat too much fat and protein at the expense of CHO (Brotherhood 1984).

Despite a generally higher energy intake compared with non-athletes, suboptimal micronutrient intakes have been reported in some athletic groups. Endurance athletes are potentially one of the most at risk groups for micronutrient deficiencies due to the gruelling demands of their training and competition. Low intakes of iron, some B group vitamins, zinc and calcium are the most commonly reported. Barr (1987) and Deakin and Inge (1994) have written comprehensive reviews of the nutrient intakes of female athletes, including an interpretation of these data, which considers the limitations inherent in dietary assessment methods. Barr (1987) concluded that some groups of women athletes presently have energy intakes that are inadequate, given their activity level.

Assessing Nutritional Status

The purpose of assessing nutritional status is to determine whether an athlete is ingesting a diet that adequately meets the stresses of training. An unbalanced diet or a diet inadequate in nutrients can lead to lethargy or early fatigue, lack of concentration, irritability, poor training and competitive performance. The development of many nutrition-related problems could be prevented through the early detection of symptoms and informed nutritional intervention.

Several methods of assessing nutritional status are utilized including:

- Dietary evaluation
- Clinical observations/medical history
- Biochemical analysis (e.g. blood or urine)
- Physical (anthropometric) measurements

DIETARY EVALUATION

Estimating food intake data using a recall or self-reporting technique is the preferred method in free-living individuals. Recall methods comprise diet history, 24 h recall of foods eaten and records of how often specified foods were consumed. These methods can be used for making qualitative or semi-quantitative measurements. Self-reported recording involves estimating or measuring weights of all foods consumed over a 1–7 day period and is more suitable for quantitative determination of nutrient intakes. The choice of method depends on the objective and the availability of resources to assess the food intake and the compliance and competence of the athlete.

Some athletes may have difficulty in remembering the amounts and types of foods consumed if asked to recall their eating patterns. Others may give biased responses by recording foods which are not typical of their usual eating patterns. The accuracy of self-reporting relies heavily on the diligence and honesty of individuals in recording or recalling foods eaten.

A quick way of assessing dietary status from food records or a 24 h recall is to check if the core food groups are adequately represented as outlined in Table 5.1. As foods are grouped according to nutrient content, assessing dietary status is based on the assumption that diets containing foods from each of the core food groups will probably provide adequate nutrition.

When more detailed quantitative information is required (e.g. vitamin, mineral, fibre, cholesterol, protein, fat and CHO content) the food intake data can be analysed using tables of food composition. Computer software is readily available for this purpose.

Nutrient intakes can be compared against standards such as the RDI or recommended daily allowance (RDA). RDI give values for the average daily amount of nutrients that population groups should consume. As these values are formulated from population data, they should not be confused with individual nutrient requirements or recommendations. Theoretically they cannot be reliably applied to the assessment of nutrient intakes of individuals. Despite this limitation, RDI remain the most frequently used reference when evaluating the adequacy of an individual's diet and have been used extensively for interpreting the dietary status of athletes. In practice, the application of RDI to individual assessments can only be justified as a probable indicator of risk of deficiency if individual intakes are averaged over a sufficiently long period (National Research Council 1989).

CLINICAL OBSERVATION AND MEDICAL HISTORY

The purpose of the clinical examination is to uncover any medical conditions or physiological factors that interfere with food intake, digestion and metabolism. Recent or chronic illness, anxiety, depression and some drugs can interfere with absorption of nutrients and thus affect nutritional status. Diarrhoea, loss of appetite, gastrointestinal disturbances and weight loss may be associated with an underlying illness.

BIOCHEMICAL ANALYSIS

The interpretation of low blood or serum levels of some nutrients is complicated by the fact that they may exhibit some diurnal variation (Vitamin C, B-group vitamins, magnesium, iron and zinc) or they may be redistributed to other tissue. Serum ferritin measures are believed to accurately represent iron storage. Pilon *et al.* (1981) found that for a given individual serum ferritin values varied less from day to day than did serum iron and per cent iron saturation. In most cases, the use of values from a single determination can be misleading. For instance, dehydration at the time of testing is associated with false elevations in blood measures. In contrast, increases in blood volume reported in athletes as a response to training may create a dilutional effect resulting in low blood measures. Furthermore, reference ranges for evaluating biochemical measures in athletes are currently based on population standards. These values may be inappropriate for athletes but serve as the only alternative until further research is available.

PHYSICAL (ANTHROPOMETRIC) MEASUREMENTS

Physical dimensions such as height, weight and skinfold measures can be used to indirectly estimate body composition and calculate energy requirements.

The application of population standards such as height/weight charts or the Body Mass Index (BMI) to determine acceptable bodyweights for athletes may be inappropriate as they do not provide any information on body composition. For example, an athlete with a large frame and muscle mass may be considered overweight using these standards despite carrying little body fat. Athletes should be assessed within their own subpopulation. Chapter 1 has already covered this area in detail.

In summary, some athletes with apparently adequate diets may exhibit biochemical and clinical indicators of nutrient deficiency or dietary imbalance. Conversely, others with suboptimal intakes may show no evidence of deficiency or effect on performance. Failure to detect biochemical or clinical evidence of a deficiency, in conjunction with low intakes, may be a reflection of the time required to deplete nutrient reserves. Chronically low intakes of nutrients increase the risk of developing nutritive problems, which can ultimately affect health and performance. Single measurements of each component of assessment of nutritional status are of limited value. Regular monitoring of nutritional status including a vitamin–mineral supplement history, throughout a training programme is essential to encouraging compliance with a consistent balanced eating pattern.

NUTRIENT NEEDS OF ATHLETES

For most sports the recommended balanced diet for athletes is basically the same as that recommended for the general population, the only difference being a greater energy intake. A nutritionally adequate diet will, in most cases, provide the necessary nutrients (CHO, fat, protein, vitamins, minerals and water) and energy to meet the metabolic needs for optimal functioning of the body.

Energy

DAILY ENERGY REQUIREMENTS

Daily energy requirements are made up of the sum of the 'resting' metabolic rate, dietary-induced thermogenesis and the energy demands of occupational, domestic and recreational activities as well as the energy expended in training or competition. For most adults with typical sedentary or light occupational work, daily energy expenditure in everyday activities is in the order of 10 500–12 500 kJ (2500–3000 kcal) for men and 8400–10 500 kJ (2000–2500 kcal) for women. It is not uncommon for training to increase the daily energy expenditures of athletes by 30% or more. In addition, both dietary thermogenesis and resting metabolic rate may be increased for some hours during recovery from prolonged strenuous exercise. Thus athletes generally have higher energy requirements than non-athletes. However, it is not simply their extra energy expenditure, but also the nature of their energetic lives that determines athletes' special dietary requirements. The high-exercise intensities that are characteristic of training and competition impose specific nutritional stresses which clearly set apart the dietary requirements of athletes from those of less active individuals.

ENERGY EXPENDITURE IN 'DYNAMIC' EXERCISE

The energy cost of basic activities such as walking, running, cycling and swimming are well known. In these activities energy expenditure in training or competition is largely determined by the individual athlete's aerobic capacity. Most endurance athletes train at 70–75% and compete at 80% or more, of their maximum oxygen uptakes (Brotherhood 1984).

There is little information available about energy expenditure in team sports and individual games because of the technical difficulty of measuring oxygen uptake during training and competition. However, prolonged bouts of continuous or intermittent activity are effectively endurance exercise and energy expenditure in these sports can be predicted from Table 5.2. In general, energy expenditures for games players would be lower than for endurance athletes because the aerobic capacities of this group tend to be lower, although greater body mass results in high-energy expenditure in some individuals. During competition in these sports, average exercise intensity would almost certainly exceed 75% $\dot{V}_{O2max}$. During training, however, the intermittent nature and lower demands of skill practice might reduce overall energy expenditure.

Table 5.2 shows estimates of energy expenditure in training and competition in relation to absolute maximal aerobic power. Energy and nutrient requirements in relation to body mass are likely to vary between different types of athletes. For example, a footballer and an endurance runner may have similar absolute $\dot{V}_{O2max}$ (5.00 L $O_2 \cdot min^{-1}$); the footballer due to a moderate maximal power/weight ratio (56 mL $O_2 \cdot kg^{-1} \cdot min^{-1}$) and large body mass (90 kg); the endurance runner due to high power/weight ratio (77 mL $O_2 \cdot kg^{-1} \cdot min^{-1}$) and smaller body mass (65 kg). Thus, both athletes may have similar absolute exercise energy expenditures but in relation to body mass the runner's is greater than the footballer's.

Few athletes are capable of expending more than 5000 kJ $\cdot h^{-1}$ (1200 kcal $\cdot h^{-1}$). On the other hand some cyclists and swimmers, by training for long periods, may expend more than 12 500 kJ (3000 kcal) per day (Costill 1988).

ENERGY EXPENDITURE IN RESISTANCE TRAINING

It is well known that the average energy expenditure in resistance training is lower than in aerobic exercise. A number of reports give similar values for strength training of 33–38 kJ $\cdot min^{-1}$ (8–9 kcal $\cdot min^{-1}$) for men, and about 24 kJ $\cdot min^{-1}$ (6 kcal $\cdot min^{-1}$) for women; the equivalent in both sexes of about 33 kJ (8 kcal) $\cdot kg^{-1}$ lean body mass $\cdot h^{-1}$. Exercise intensities are moderate and average 40–50% of $\dot{V}_{O2max}$. Thus, although resistance training demands short bursts of high-power output, overall energy expenditures are usually not high, because of the intermittent nature of the activity and because only small amounts of muscle are utilized in some exercises. Nonetheless the high loads on individual muscles will result in marked depletion of local energy stores (muscle glycogen).

Table 5.2 Estimates of athletes' energy expenditure, carbohydrate combustion (CHO) and sweat water losses during training and competition, according to aerobic power ($\dot{V}_{O2max}$) and exercise intensity

$\dot{V}_{O2max}$ L·min⁻¹	Exercise intensity					
	Training 75% $\dot{V}_{O2max}$			Competition 85% $\dot{V}_{O2max}$		
	Energy kJ·h⁻¹	CHO g·h⁻¹	Water L·h⁻¹	Energy kJ·h⁻¹	CHO g·h⁻¹	Water L·h⁻¹
5.5	5200	244	1.8	5890	331	2.1
4.5	4253	199	1.5	4820	271	1.6
3.5	3308	155	1.2	3749	211	1.3
2.5	2363	111	0.8	2678	151	1.0

Energy expenditure is proportional to $\dot{V}_{O2max}$ and CHO combustion is proportional to exercise intensity. Energy expenditure is estimated assuming that the energy equivalent of 1 L of oxygen consumed is 21 kJ.

CHO combustion is estimated assuming that at 75% and 85% $\dot{V}_{O2max}$, 75% and 90%, respectively, of energy is derived from CHO and that 1 g of CHO supplies 16 kJ.

Sweat water loss is estimated assuming that 85% of energy output is dissipated by the evaporation of sweat and that the evaporation of 1 L of sweat dissipates 2400 kJ.

Carbohydrate

Recognition of the crucial role that CHO metabolism plays in the performance of high-intensity exercise has made a major contribution to the science and practice of sports nutrition. The correct supply of CHO in the diet is essential to provide the appropriate muscle fuel for rigorous training and maximal performance in competition.

While about half of the energy for everyday activities is supplied by fat, CHO is the major energy substrate during strenuous exercise and is essential for high-intensity exercise. At the high-exercise intensities typical of athletic training ($>70\%$ $\dot{V}_{O2max}$), free fatty acid (FFA) uptake by the muscle cells is too slow because it is limited by the plasma FFA level. Consequently, at least 70% of the energy output arises from CHO combustion. In competition, when exercise intensity of more than 85% $\dot{V}_{O2max}$ must be endured, FFA metabolism is inhibited and virtually all the energy must be derived from the muscle glycogen.

Clearly, as a result of the amount and the intensity of their exercise, athletes have large CHO requirements. Table 5.2 shows estimates of the CHO expenditure during training and competition. In 90 min of hard training an endurance athlete's CHO combustion may be as great as the total daily glucose metabolism (about 300 g) of a sedentary person. When CHO reserves are depleted to low levels high-intensity exercise cannot be performed.

Most of the CHO that is utilized during hard training and competition is provided by intramuscular glycogen. In endurance exercise, increased blood glucose uptake by the muscles also increases demands on the liver glycogen reserves. At the onset of exercise the increased energy production is almost entirely supplied by muscle glycogen. As exercise proceeds muscle glycogen declines and an increasing proportion of energy is supplied by FFA, or if it is available, glucose from the blood. When muscle glycogen levels are close to exhaustion, performance deteriorates. Blood glucose is maintained by the liver, but when liver glycogen is depleted gluconeogenesis may not be fast enough to maintain the blood glucose during hard exercise. Thus, when liver and muscle glycogen levels are near depletion, fatigue and hypoglycaemia occur; both will occur prematurely if glycogen reserves are low at the start of exercise.

The liver glycogen reserves are reduced to about half postprandial levels by the overnight fast and are exhausted within 24 h, even at rest, by fasting or a low-CHO intake. Muscle glycogen stores are more stable at rest and show little change after a number of days of CHO deprivation or starvation. During hard exercise, however, both muscle and liver glycogen are depleted rapidly. At the near-maximal exercise rates endured during competition, muscle glycogen depletion sufficient to impair performance can occur in less than an hour. Following the overnight fast or similar period without food, liver glycogen is restored within an hour or so by a meal containing 100–150 g of CHO. Restoration of the liver and muscle glycogen stores depleted by prolonged strenuous exercise, on the other hand, may take from 24 to 48 h, even with a high-CHO diet.

The maintenance of muscle and liver glycogen stores and therefore the capacity to sustain high-performance exercise on a daily basis, is dependent on the CHO content of the diet. The relationship between dietary CHO and muscle glycogen levels and exercise endurance, was demonstrated in a classical series of experiments by Bergstrom et al. (1967), the results of which are summarized in Table 5.3. All the recommendations relating to CHO requirements that are fundamental to optimal nutrition for athletes are based on these observations.

Higher than average CHO intakes are essential for full recovery from daily strenuous training. If athletes eat less CHO than they utilize during training, their muscle glycogen is not fully restored between sessions and their ability to sustain hard exercise deteriorates over successive days.

Studies on athletes have demonstrated that glycogen is not restored from day to day in the quadriceps and soleus muscles of runners or in the deltoid muscles of swimmers or in the quadriceps muscles of American Football players and soccer players if their diets contain less than 40% of the total energy as CHO. On the other hand, if their diets are rich in CHO their muscle glycogen and

Table 5.3 Relationship between carbohydrate intake and restoration of liver and muscle glycogen after prolonged hard exercise and the effect on subsequent exercise endurance

	CHO content of the diet as % of total energy intake		
	Low (<10%)	Normal (40–50%)	High (>80%)
Liver glycogen (g·kg⁻¹)	6	42	78
Muscle glycogen (g·kg⁻¹)	7	20	37
Exercise time (min)	60	115	170

Liver and muscle glycogen contents are expressed as $g \cdot kg^{-1}$ of liver and $g \cdot kg^{-1}$ of the muscle engaged in the exercise respectively. In a 70 kg male approximately 20 kg of muscle would be engaged in running or cycling.

endurance capacity are fully restored from day to day (Costill 1988; Coyle 1991). Endurance athletes training hard require a diet in which 60–65% of the energy is supplied by CHO (Brotherhood 1984): for example about 550 g for an energy intake of 14 700 MJ (3500 kcal)·day⁻¹. As discussed under daily energy requirements, nutritional requirements in relation to body size depend on the athlete's aerobic power. For sports with moderate total energy expenditures and exercise intensities a CHO intake of 50–55% of energy intake is probably sufficient for daily training.

A CHO-rich diet does not boost performance by enabling the athlete to exercise at higher intensities. Rather, by ensuring an optimal supply of energy substrates, it delays the onset of fatigue in prolonged strenuous exercise. All athletes should be aware that deterioration in performance over a period of intensive training is likely to be due to progressive depletion of muscle glycogen. Similarly, athletes who have to compete at least once every week as well as training or who have to compete daily for a period of time, must take special care to ensure that they have an adequate CHO intake.

CARBOHYDRATE FOODS AND THEIR GLYCAEMIC INDEX

The rate at which glucose enters the blood from the intestine and the consequent glycaemic impact or effect on blood glucose level that follows their ingestion, varies with different CHO-containing foods. This variability is described by the GI, which ranks foods according to their glycaemic

impact compared with that of glucose or white bread (Jenkins et al. 1984).

At rest, the ingestion of glucose results in a rapid rise in blood glucose that induces an increase in insulin secretion. The insulin facilitates the uptake of glucose by the muscles and liver and the blood glucose quickly returns to normal. Eating white bread results in almost the same responses to glucose.

The GI does not correspond with the classification of CHO into simple or complex. It is determined by the rate at which glucose is released by digestion. For example, some complex CHO such as breakfast cereals, bread, rice, potatoes and carrots have high GI similar to glucose, while pasta has a moderate GI and legumes and some fruit have low GI. In contrast, fructose, a simple sugar, has a low GI because it is not actively absorbed in the intestine and must pass through the liver to be converted into glucose (Jenkins et al. 1984, 1988).

Stomach emptying also influences GI. Thus, while the GI of some foods on their own might be high, when combined with other foods, in particular fat, the GI of the meal may be different from its constituents. For example, the GI of bread and butter may be lower than for bread and jam without butter. Processing and cooking may also change the GI of a food.

The GI may have practical implications for sports nutrition because it can influence the rate of storage, utilization and availability of energy substrates. High-GI foods prior to competition may not be ideal. The hyperinsulinaemia following their ingestion promotes glycolysis and also inhibits lipolysis thus limiting the availability of FFA. Under these conditions muscle glycogen may be depleted more rapidly in the early stages of exercise and consequently long-term endurance may be reduced. In contrast, low-GI foods do not induce hyperinsulinaemia and appear to provide a steady supply of glucose during exercise without inhibiting lipolysis (Thomas *et al.* 1991).

High-GI foods promote glycogen storage and appear to expedite muscle glycogen restoration following exercise (Kiens *et al.* 1990; Burke *et al.* 1993). They may also be useful to boost muscle glycogen rapidly before exercise in circumstances of inadequate recovery from previous exercise (Coyle 1991).

Protein

Protein is not primarily a source of energy so that the quantity required in the diet is much smaller than for fat and CHO. The basic protein requirement for healthy adults, to cover the metabolic losses of nitrogen associated with body protein turnover and losses from the skin and intestine, is about $0.6 \ g \cdot kg^{-1}$ body mass $\cdot day^{-1}$. International recommendations (FAO/WHO/UNU 1985) on daily allowances (RDA, RDI) or 'safe levels of intake' for protein are $0.75 \ g \cdot kg^{-1} \cdot day^{-1}$ for adults and $1.0 \ g \cdot kg^{-1} \cdot day^{-1}$ for children and adolescents. They are higher than basic requirements because they incorporate adjustments to allow for individual variability and growth. The protein required for growth, averaged over a long period of time, is not much greater than for maintenance, but recommendations for children include an additional factor of 50% to cover likely peak requirements during growth spurts.

Almost any kind of diet supplying these amounts of protein will contain adequate amounts of the indispensable ('essential') amino acids. The recommended safe levels of intake, which are not linked to energy requirement, correspond to protein contributing about 9% of the energy content of the diet of moderately active individuals. In comparison, protein consumption in many parts of the world exceeds 10% of daily energy intake.

Although the recommended intakes allow for individual variability, physical activity has generally been considered to have only minor effects on protein requirements. Recent research re-examining the relationship between protein metabolism and exercise has suggested that current recommendations for protein intake may not be sufficient for athletes and other physically active people (American College of Sports Medicine 1987).

ATHLETIC ACTIVITY AND PROTEIN METABOLISM

Many athletes and people who work physically hard believe that protein is a particularly important part of their diet and that if they do not have a high-protein intake, which might include supplements, their performance will suffer. To substantiate this belief, which is not wholly supported by scientific evidence, it would be necessary to demonstrate that regular training or hard work has substantial effects on protein metabolism.

Protein metabolism is complex and is affected in both the long- and short-term by the energy content as well as the protein content of the diet. The nature, intensity and duration of exercise also influences protein metabolism. Thus study of the relationships between protein metabolism and sports performance requires careful design, sophisticated techniques and often, extended periods of measurement. Furthermore, even though exercise may affect protein metabolism and muscle and other body structures, it cannot be claimed to increase protein requirements unless it also causes the body to either lose or retain nitrogen (Lemon 1991a,b).

PROTEIN METABOLISM AND ENDURANCE EXERCISE

During exercise protein synthesis decreases and protein breakdown increases. The amino acids which are thus released could be used as fuel. On recovery, provided the diet contains adequate energy and protein, these processes are reversed so that there is not a progressive decline in lean body mass (LBM) with repeated exercise (Lemon 1991a).

With hard exercise lasting more than about 1 h certain amino acids may be oxidized and others may contribute to gluconeogenesis. In these circumstances urea production also increases, suggesting that protein is used as a fuel. Furthermore, amino acid oxidation increases with increasing exercise intensity and is greater when glycogen reserves have been depleted by exercise or a low-CHO intake. Thus, protein catabolism and protein requirements are likely to be increased in athletes engaged in heavy endurance training, particularly if their CHO intake is low.

Protein catabolism during prolonged exercise may amount to 5–10% of the energy expended. While this is a small contribution to overall energy supply, in terms of effect on protein requirement, it represents a significant increment. Nitrogen balance studies show that endurance athletes in training require protein intakes greater than about 0.9 g·kg^{-1}·day^{-1} (Meredith et al. 1989, Tarnopolsky et al. 1988). Current evidence suggests that the protein requirements of male endurance athletes are greater than those of females and that the requirements of both are greater than most current national recommendations for protein intakes (Phillips et al. 1993).

PROTEIN AND RESISTANCE TRAINING

The effects of dietary protein and the specific protein requirements associated with developing muscle mass and strength are not clear. A high-protein intake alone will not increase muscle mass because heavy resistance exercise is required for muscle hypertrophy. Overall energy expenditure in resistance training may not be high nor is there clear evidence that such training results in nutritionally significant muscle breakdown. Therefore, there are no immediate indications that resistance training per se increases protein requirements. Nitrogen balance studies have shown that the protein requirement of experienced bodybuilders during maintenance training, when there is no change in muscle mass, is not much greater than that of sedentary adults (Tarnopolsky et al. 1988). On the other hand, the protein needs of novice bodybuilders in intensive training may be nearly twice as great as currently recommended allowances (Lemon et al. 1992; Tarnopolsky et al. 1992).

Resistance training increases muscle protein synthesis (Chesley et al. 1992) and may result in remarkable degrees of muscle growth; presumably when it does so protein requirements are increased.

In addition to the evidence from nitrogen balance studies already mentioned, estimates of protein requirements could be made from the changes in LBM that occur with resistance training. Published reports indicate that increases in LBM of up to 3 kg can occur during a 10 week programme (Forbes 1985). Assuming that about 20% of the new lean tissue is protein such growth indicates a protein retention of about 9 g·day^{-1}. There have been some claims that LBM can be increased by as much as 10 kg at a rate of 2.5 kg·month^{-1}. This seems unlikely, but if such growth did occur presumably it would involve an average daily protein retention of 15–20 g.

Sufficient energy and CHO intakes, as well as protein, are essential to successful body building and strength programmes. This is because energy is required for the efficient utilization of dietary protein in the development of muscle mass (Forbes 1985; American College of Sports Medicine 1987) and glycogen depletion impairs muscle endurance and strength. When anaerobic/strength athletes such as wrestlers and weight-lifters reduce body mass 'to make weight' they generally lose lean mass as well as fat. A high-protein intake may minimize this loss, but a high-CHO intake may be more important to minimize deterioration in muscle function (Walberg et al. 1988).

RECOMMENDED PROTEIN REQUIREMENTS FOR ATHLETES: CURRENT GUIDELINES

Controversy is likely to continue about the precise protein requirements of athletes. The most recent evidence suggests that the protein requirements of well fed athletes undergoing rigorous training may be about 50% greater than internationally RDA. Protein intakes of about 1.5 g·kg^{-1}·day^{-1}, equivalent to about 10–15% of energy intake, are likely to be sufficient for most athletes, including growing children. Recent recommendations for daily protein allowances, based on nitrogen balance studies, are 1.6 g·kg^{-1}·day^{-1} for endurance athletes and 1.2 g·kg^{-1}·day^{-1} for bodybuilders on maintenance programmes; novice bodybuilders' requirements may be as high as 1.7 g·kg^{-1}·day^{-1} (Lemon et al. 1992; Tarnopolsky et al. 1988, 1992).

In practice, dietary custom means that many

athletes are likely to consume about 15% of their energy intake as protein and so, with their high-energy intake, consume as much as a third more protein than the most generous recommendation. Inadequate protein intakes are therefore extremely unlikely in athletes who eat a good variety of foods.

Although athletes do not require extraordinary amounts of protein they are advised to eat some meat, fish, eggs and dairy products because they are also good sources of other essential nutrients such as iron, zinc, riboflavin, Vitamin A and calcium. High-CHO consumption need not result in an inadequate protein intake because cereal-based foods, starchy vegetables, legumes and nuts also contain protein.

EXCESS PROTEIN

Power and strength athletes traditionally favour high-protein intakes; some individuals consuming as much as 30% of their energy as protein (Brotherhood 1984). Nitrogen retention increases with high-protein intakes but is not accompanied by improvements in muscle size and strength (Lemon *et al.* 1992). Amino acids from protein eaten in excess of the essential needs may be stored, or oxidized or converted into glucose and thus contribute to energy supply. Although very high-protein intakes are probably not harmful they have no known advantages and may even have some disadvantages for the following reasons:

- They are expensive
- They may displace more important CHO-rich foods from the diet
- Excess fat may be associated with animal protein
- The resulting extra nitrogen excretion increases urinary water losses that add to water stress
- High-protein diets may disturb acid/base balance and impair high-intensity exercise performance (Greenhaff *et al.* 1988)

Vitamins and Minerals

There is a common belief that physical activity increases vitamin and mineral requirements and that subsequently supplementation with these nutrients will produce an improvement in per-

formance. A survey on supplementation practices of 4604 Australian athletes indicated that 47% of respondents had used supplements at some time within the last 5 years (Australian Sports Medicine Federation 1983); therefore, it is apparent that vitamins such as Vitamin C, multivitamins and B-complex were taken daily by a large percentage of athletes. Vitamins A, B_{12} and E and the minerals iron and calcium were also used but to a lesser extent. These statistics raise four main questions about the justification for the use of vitamin or mineral supplements:

- Do athletes involved in regular intensive training have higher vitamin and mineral requirements than sedentary people?
- Do athletes consume an adequate diet with regard to vitamins and minerals?
- Do additional vitamins and minerals have an ergogenic effect?
- Have adverse effects been reported from chronic or 'megadose' use of vitamins and minerals?

EVIDENCE FOR AN INCREASED REQUIREMENT FOR VITAMINS AND MINERALS

Despite extensive use of supplements among athletes, there are no reliable research findings indicating that athletes' requirements for vitamins and minerals are excessively higher than sedentary people.

Although additional B vitamins, (thiamin, riboflavin and niacin) are required with increased CHO intake, these needs are usually met by athletes through increased energy intake. Vitamin C needs can easily be met by the regular consumption of fruit juice, fruit and vegetables. Certain risk groups, particularly young women and endurance athletes, may require special attention to ensure a sufficient iron and calcium intake.

EVIDENCE FOR VITAMIN/MINERAL DEFICIENCY IN ATHLETES

Suboptimal indices of vitamin and mineral status have been reported in athletes and are as follows.

Biochemical abnormality

Some studies have reported altered plasma levels of vitamins and minerals, most commonly B-group vitamins, Vitamin C, magnesium, copper, zinc and iron in athletes. These values may reflect losses in sweat and urine, diurnal variation or redistribution to other tissues. Even in the presence or absence of clinical symptoms, prolonged nutrient deficiency and a disease state, interpretation of these values, therefore, requires caution.

Dietary deficiency

Inadequate nutrient intake is not frequently reported among athletic groups. Of the nutrients analysed, less than optimal intakes of thiamin (Vitamin B_1), Vitamin B_6, Vitamin A and iron have been reported in some groups of male and female athletes, particularly in endurance sports and sports where a very LBM is desirable. A number of studies of female athletes including runners, gymnasts, ballet dancers and team sports (hockey, basketball and volleyball) report intakes of iron and calcium to be less than the recommended allowances (Barr 1987; van Erp-Baart et al. 1989). Calcium and iron intake is usually related to energy intake and might be a problem for those athletes on low-energy intakes or weight-reducing diets.

Presumably, the longer the intake continues below the RDI, the greater is the risk of deficiency. Deficiency diseases due to habitually low intakes of a particular vitamin or mineral still persist in some risk groups in the population but in most athletes, consuming a well-balanced diet, overt clinical deficiencies are rare.

Does a deficiency affect performance?

It is well established that subclinical deficiencies of some nutrients impair performance, strength and neuromuscular skill. For some nutrients (e.g. iron) even marginal deficiency has been reported to impair performance, even though the symptoms of clinical deficiency are absent.

Van der Beek (1985) concluded that restricted intakes of B-complex vitamins, individually and in combination, at approximately 35–45% of the RDA may lead to a decreased endurance capacity within a few weeks. Studies on athletes with depleted Vitamin C and fat soluble Vitamin A indices have not indicated a decrease in endurance capacity. Where performance capacity was affected, some groups responded favourably to dietary manipulation or supplementation of the deficient nutrient, while others showed no improvement.

Do vitamins and minerals exert an ergogenic effect?

Numerous claims have been made that B-complex vitamins and Vitamins C, E and B_{12} improve physical work capacity; however, the research in this area is confusing and contradictory. Most research has considered nutrients separately and therefore the interaction between nutrients, particularly the trace minerals, has been overlooked. Many of the studies, including those for and against supplementation, are difficult to interpret due to poor experimental design.

Adverse effects of 'megadose' use of vitamins and minerals

The prolonged use of vitamin and mineral supplementation in amounts that are considered megadoses (10 times the RDI) can lead to inhibition of nutrient absorption, medical complications and potentially toxic effects.

Adverse effects have been reported with Vitamins A (retinol), B_6, C and D and thiamin, niacin and pantothenic acid in the general population. Several cases of toxicity in adults have been reported with Vitamin A (retinol) supplements of 25 000–50 000 IU. Large doses of Vitamin C ($>$2000 mg·day^{-1}) have been associated with gastritis, increase in urinary oxalate excretion and interference with copper absorption, while prolonged use of large doses of Vitamin B_6 (greater than 500 mg·day^{-1}) may induce sensory neuropathy.

Overdosing with minerals is less prevalent than with vitamins, except in the case of iron. Potential problems arising from prolonged use of excess iron supplements are outlined later in this chapter.

Water and Electrolytes

WATER

Water losses in sweat and CHO combustion are the two most important nutritional stresses imposed by hard exercise (Table 5.2).

Considering the importance of minimizing dehydration during exercise, there are remarkably few reports about the magnitude of fluid losses incurred during sports training and competition (see Chapter 6). However, some attempt at estimating sweat losses can be made. About 80% of the energy produced during exercise is released as heat; in moderate thermal conditions most of this heat will be taken from the body by the evaporation of sweat. The evaporation of 1 L of sweat from the skin results in the loss of approximately 2400 kJ (580 kcal) from the body. The sweat losses shown in Table 5.2 represent likely rates of sweat production for athletes wearing light sports clothes exercising outdoors in moderate temperatures of 15–25°C. In cooler conditions sweat rates may be about 25% lower. Elite endurance athletes, in training as well as in competition, may sweat in excess of 1.5 $L \cdot h^{-1}$. In warm and humid conditions, or if much protective equipment is worn, large or well-acclimatized athletes may lose more than 2 $L \cdot h^{-1}$ of sweat.

Thus, athletes have much greater daily water requirements than sedentary people. Athletes must be well hydrated before they exercise because even minor dehydration (>2% body mass; 1–1.5 L) may impair thermoregulation and put them at risk of heat illness and collapse.

ELECTROLYTES

Sweat contains water soluble vitamins and trace minerals, but in such minute amounts that even repeated daily heavy sweating does not increase dietary requirements. In contrast the sweat content of electrolytes, particularly sodium, can be relatively high; however, sweating alone is unlikely to result in electrolyte deficiencies in athletes (Table 5.4). Potassium, magnesium and calcium losses in the sweat are not great. In athletes the daily losses of these ions are unlikely to exceed 1% of the body content and they are readily replaced by a diet that contains a variety of foods (Costill 1984). Similarly, sodium deficiency is unlikely to occur. With repeated strenuous exercise, especially in warm conditions, athletes become heat acclimatized which, among other adaptations, results in a reduction of the sodium content of the sweat. In well-acclimatized people, sweat sodium concentration may be 10–20 $mmol \cdot L^{-1}$, one-third of that in the sweat of untrained and heat unacclimatized people. Furthermore, in response to heat exposure or prolonged exercise there is an increased production of aldosterone which promotes the renal conservation of sodium (Costill 1984).

Summary of Nutritional Recommendations for Training and Recovery

The following summary outlines the nutritional recommendations for athletes in hard training:

- The recommended diet for athletes in general is no different to that recommended for the sedentary population, except that energy, CHO, protein and some minerals and water-soluble vitamin requirements may be marginally higher
- A healthy individual who eats a balanced diet usually receives all the necessary nutrients for physical conditioning provided energy needs are met

Table 5.4 Electrolyte concentration and losses in sweat and dietary intakes

Electrolyte	Sweat Concentration mmol·L⁻¹	Loss per 5 L	Dietary intake mmol·day⁻¹
Sodium	20–80	100–400	85–340
(NaCl g·L⁻¹	0.5–5.0	2.5–25	5–20 g)
Potassium	4–6	20–30	50 (65)–100
Magnesium	0.2–0.8	1–4	17–35

Sodium concentration in sweat is reduced by heat acclimatization and training to the low end of the normal range.

- Athletes with high-energy requirements need to spread food over several meals and ensure that snacks are nutritious
- A high-CHO intake is essential for the maintenance of rigorous training schedules
- CHO-rich foods with a moderate to high GI are recommended after training to promote quick restoration of glycogen reserves in depleted muscles
- Athletes at risk of nutrient deficiencies in the absence of any disease include: those on fad diets, unplanned vegetarian diets or unsupervised weight loss programmes; those consuming low-energy intakes; those living alone or financially disadvantaged; those consuming mostly convenience foods; and those following rigorous training schedules
- In the absence of a diagnosed clinical deficiency, supplementation with vitamins and minerals is not recommended
- A diagnosed deficiency or suboptimal intake of a vitamin/mineral may warrant supplementation only if dietary intervention has been ineffective
- The excessive use of vitamin and mineral supplements does not provide any advantage and may even be harmful
- There is no conclusive evidence to suggest that vitamin and mineral supplementation improves performance in athletes who have normal biochemical indices achieved by consuming a well-balanced diet
- Athletes have greater fluid requirements than sedentary people. However, extra salt or electrolytes are usually not necessary even for athletes on low-salt diets. Low levels of electrolytes and CHO in combination, as found in sports drinks, enhance uptake of fluid. Where water losses are large, consumption of sports drinks or dilute fruit juice or dilute cordial as soon after exercise as possible may be of benefit

NUTRITIONAL PREPARATION FOR COMPETITION

Preparation for competition is the most misunderstood aspect of sports nutrition. Correct dietary preparation for competition, as well as appropriate nutrition during training, is critical for maximal competitive performance. For most sports events the aim of pre-competition nutrition is to enable the athlete to perform at optimal levels throughout the competition independent of external energy supplies.

The major nutritional effects of hard exercise are the rapid combustion of the limited stores of glycogen in muscles and liver and large water losses. For events involving continuous exercise for more than an hour sustained performance depends on the initial levels of glycogen in the liver and muscles and the level of hydration. If athletes train hard, but do not consume adequate CHO, their muscle glycogen will be progressively depleted and become inadequate for competition (Costill 1988). Even with high CHO intake full glycogen recovery from an exhausting training session can take at least 20 h (Coyle 1991). Nutritional preparation for competition must, therefore, ensure:

- Complete recovery from the demands of training or previous competition
- The establishment of optimal muscle glycogen levels and full liver glycogen stores
- Full hydration

Appropriate preparation requires careful consideration of the demands of the event and thus the nutritional objectives. The main factors to be considered are the nature, intensity and duration of the activity. Events lasting less than an hour require only normal CHO reserves. Competition that involves strenuous intermittent or continuous exercise for 90 min or longer requires well-filled glycogen stores, while endurance events that last 2 or more hours require super-filled glycogen stores.

Some foods, particularly those which ferment in the large bowel resulting in gas formation and flatulence may cause gastrointestinal discomfort and should be avoided 6–12 h prior to competition.

ATHLETIC TRAINING AND GLYCOGEN STORAGE

Exercise enhances greatly the ability of muscles to store glycogen. Consequently, athletes have a high potential for glycogen storage. If they reduce their exercise and eat large amounts of CHO they will acquire large glycogen stores. At the same time, however, they may gain weight as water is also stored with the glycogen.

PREPARATION FOR MAXIMAL POWER OUTPUT EVENTS

Energy for maximal aerobic and anaerobic power production is exclusively derived from CHO so that adequate muscle glycogen is essential for very high-intensity exercise. For short (<30 min) high-power output events, however, extraordinary CHO reserves are not required and in events that involve movement of the body against gravity, the gain in mass associated with large glycogen and water storage is likely to be a disadvantage. Athletes in such events, while moderating their training load in the days before competition, should avoid very high CHO intakes (>50% of energy intake) in order to minimize gains in body mass associated with excess glycogen storage.

A predominantly high protein and fat intake in the days before competition is also undesirable. A high-protein/low-CHO intake may reduce plasma buffering capacity and therefore be detrimental for events that have either a high anaerobic component or are performed at near-maximal aerobic capacity (i.e. racing for up to 30 min; Greenhaff *et al*. 1988).

Preparation for Endurance Events

For the purposes of dietary preparation, any competitive activity that involves strenuous exercise for between 1 and 2 h can be considered to be an endurance event. Glycogen reserves greater than those required for routine training are essential. These can be achieved with a high-CHO diet (about 60% of total energy intake as CHO) and a reduction in training intensity and duration. Adequate time is essential and preparation should start 24–48 h before the event.

Carbohydrate Loading

Daily endurance training and a diet supplying 50–60% of total energy intake as CHO result in muscle glycogen stores sufficient for about 20–25 km of running or 90 min of continuous exercise at competitive rates. But, because endurance training and a high CHO intake increases CHO storage, endurance capacity can be nearly doubled by 'CHO loading'.

Early recommendations for CHO loading required preliminary depletion of muscle glycogen by a bout of prolonged exercise (2–3 h) followed by 2 or 3 days of continued training and a very low CHO diet (<10% of total energy intake) to maintain muscle glycogen at a low level. This was followed by 3 or 4 days of reduced training and a very high CHO diet (>80% of total energy intake). The procedure boosted muscle glycogen to levels at least twice normal. Unfortunately, the depletion phase can have effects similar to starvation, with water and sodium loss, hypoglycaemia and ketosis and their attendant symptoms of marked physical and mental fatigue.

This extreme regimen is too disruptive for use by athletes before competition, but it may be useful for non-athletes in preparation for activities such as long cycle rides or hikes. Nonetheless, endurance athletes can boost their glycogen reserves before competition without extreme changes to their diet and with less disturbance to their training. Continued normal training, which could include a long session and a normal mixed diet (40–50% of total energy intake from CHO) for 2 or 3 days during the depletion phase, followed by reduced training and a high CHO (80% of total energy) intake for 2–3 days before competition, results in similar boosts to muscle glycogen content (Costill 1988). Table 5.5 gives an example of a 12 800 kJ (3000 kcal) menu plan with about 80% of the total energy in the diet from CHO sources.

The three important considerations for successful CHO loading are:

- Adequate time on the high-CHO phase; not less than 2 days
- Adequate CHO, about 80% of energy intake and a plentiful water intake
- Rest

Muscle glycogen resynthesis is impaired in injured muscles so that recovery from the micro-trauma of

Table 5.5 Carbohydrate loading meal plan

Total energy	=12 800 kJ (3000 kcals)
	Proportion of total energy
	Protein 75 g = 10%
	Fat 25 g = 8%
	Carbohydrate 645 g = 82%
Breakfast	2 cups breakfast cereal with skim milk and 2–3 teaspoons sugar
	1 banana
	1 muffin/crumpet or 2 pieces toast (no butter)
	2 tablespoons jam/honey
	Glass fruit juice
Snack	Large glass sweetened fruit juice
Lunch	Large bread roll or 2 sandwiches, with banana or salad vegetables (no meat or butter)
	Fruit salad
	Fruit bun/pancake with honey
	Weak tea/coffee
Snack	1 piece light cake
Dinner	2 cups pasta
	1 cup vegetable or lentil sauce
	1 small serve apple crumble and custard made with skim milk
	Weak tea/coffee
Snack	2 crumpets/muffins (no margarine)
	2 tablespoons honey/jam
	1 glass sweetened fruit juice or soft drink

Source English & Lewis (1992)

hard daily training is essential. For athletes, especially runners, who engage in heavy training the best preparation for competition lasting 2 or more hours may be 2–3 days of rest or light exercise and a diet rich in CHO.

As the purpose of CHO loading is to increase energy reserves, an energy intake in excess of energy expenditure is required and an increase in body mass should occur. About 500–600 g of glycogen may be stored. This is accompanied by a gain in body mass of about 2 kg because about 2.7 g of water is also stored with each gram of glycogen. For endurance competition the extra water store provides an advantage because as the glycogen is metabolized during exercise it becomes available to offset the sweat water losses.

Pre-competition Meals

A meal before competition is generally advisable. When athletes are well rested and have had sufficient time to ensure that their muscle glycogen stores are adequate for their event, a pre-competition meal has three essential functions:

- To replenish liver glycogen stores depleted during the overnight fast
- To ensure full hydration
- To prevent hunger and nausea

The meal, eaten 3–4 h before competition and accompanied by fluids, should be low in fat and protein and supply 100–200 g of moderate to high GI CHO. Foods that cause gastrointestinal discomfort should be avoided. Table 5.6 shows some examples of suitable pre-competition meals.

High-GI food eaten in the hours prior to exercise may influence CHO and fat metabolism during exercise. Generally, in order to minimize the effects of hyperinsulinaemia, athletes should aim to complete the major part of their nutritional preparation at least 12 h prior to competition and apart from their pre-competition meal avoid high-GI 'quick energy' CHO prior to exercise.

Recent research has shown that if muscle glycogen is depleted, significant increases in glycogen that extend endurance can be achieved even in the hours before exercise by consuming large amounts of CHO (Coyle 1991). This could be relevant when athletes have to compete in events >30 min more than once on the same day or on consecutive days and who consequently have limited opportunity and time to replenish glycogen between events. In these circumstances 300 g of high GI CHO (maltodextrins) with fluids in the 6 h prior to competition have been shown in the laboratory to improve performance in extended cycling exercise. Some athletes may find it difficult to consume such large amounts of CHO in a few hours prior to competition.

For endurance events lasting >2 h, CHO loading in the days prior to competition is essential. In addition, CHO ingestion during these events may also extend endurance, but is often difficult to achieve. Low GI CHO foods pre-competition may therefore be beneficial. Low GI foods do not induce hyperinsulinaemia (Jenkins *et al.* 1984) and provide a steady supply of glucose during exercise without inhibiting lipolysis (Thomas *et al.* 1991).

Liquid Meals

Some athletes, perhaps due to anxiety, do not tolerate food before competition and prefer to fast. This puts them at risk of hypoglycaemia and premature fatigue. These people can benefit from liquid meals, which may be more rapidly emptied from the stomach and quickly absorbed making them easier to tolerate than solid food. The nutrient composition of these meals should be as for conventional pre-competition meals — predominantly high in CHO and low in fat. Many liquid supplements are supplied in powder form and so have the advantage of portability. They can provide an excellent alternative to conventional meals for the travelling athlete who has difficulty obtaining usual food choices when away from home.

Table 5.6 Pre-competition meals

Excellent choices	Poor choices
Breakfast	
Cereal or pancakes	Bacon and eggs/steak/sausages
Toast	Full cream milk
Low fat or skim milk	Soft drink
Fruit, fruit juice	
Weak tea/coffee	
Light meal	
Lean meat, chicken (no skin)	Meat pie and chips
or fish sandwich with salad	Milkshake
Fruit juice or fruit	Chocolate
Low fat fruit yoghurt	Pastries
Light cake/muffin	
Main meal	
Pasta/rice/potato	Pizza, fried chicken, roast potato
Lean meat and vegetables	Apple turnover
(not fried), baked beans	
Apple crumble	
Pancakes	

Carbohydrates Immediately before Exercise

In the 1980s it was recommended that large amounts of sugar should be avoided close to exercise. Recent research has revised this view (Coyle 1991). As much as 50 g of high GI CHO (sugar) may be ingested within 15 min of the start of exercise without ill-effect (Coyle 1991). In these circumstances the usual rapid rises in blood glucose and insulin are suppressed by the exercise. Hypoglycaemia does not occur and glycolysis is not accelerated (Costill 1988). The extra CHO helps to maintain blood glucose during exercise, contributes to muscular metabolism and may delay fatigue. Such a feeding may even enhance the effect of the pre-game meal.

CHO supplements improve performance not by enabling the athlete to perform at a higher intensity but by delaying fatigue.

NUTRITION DURING EXERCISE

For health, safety and performance, largely related to effective thermoregulation, replacement of the water lost in sweat is the primary aim of nutrition during exercise; particularly in warm and humid environments. In addition, CHO ingested during exercise maintains blood glucose levels, is metabolized and may help to extend endurance. Electrolyte replacement is not required. Electrolyte losses are minimal and inconsequential and because sweat is dilute compared with the blood, heavy sweating results in increased concentrations of electrolytes in the body fluids.

Opinions on the best form of nutrition during exercise have changed in recent years. Water absorption from the stomach is minimal, but occurs rapidly in the intestine. Stomach emptying, which has a maximum rate for plain water of about 1 $L \cdot h^{-1}$, is therefore the major limitation to fluid replacement during exercise. As CHO/electrolyte solutions, especially if hypertonic, slow stomach emptying, plain water or hypotonic solutions have previously been recommended as the best form of nutrition during exercise. Recent investigations, however, have shown that an exclusive recommend-

ation for plain water can no longer be justified (Lamb & Brodowicz 1986; Murray 1987; Maughan & Noakes 1991). In fact, if there is a need for water, CHO will almost certainly also be of benefit.

Significant muscle glycogen depletion can occur within 30 min of sustained high or intermittent very high-intensity exercise. In many individual and team sports, performance may be impaired by glycogen depletion before the end of competition. Similarly, CHO depletion often limits the quality of performance in any hard exercise lasting longer than 2 h. The question therefore arises as to whether CHO taken during exercise can delay fatigue.

Carbohydrate Replacement

CHO ingestion during exercise can prolong endurance and can be achieved without impairment of thermoregulatory and cardiovascular function (Lamb & Brodowicz 1986; Murray 1987; Coyle 1991).

During competition of less than 60 min CHO intake is unlikely to be of benefit, partly because of the delay in absorption. Water is all that is required. Athletes in events of this duration must commence competition fully hydrated and with well filled glycogen stores. They may also benefit from taking CHO immediately before exercise.

In games such as football and hockey lasting up

Table 5.7 Beverage formulation for water and energy replacement during prolonged exercise

Sodium	Replacement not essential
	Promotes water absorption
	in the small intestine
	Improves palatability
	Optimal sodium content: 15–20 mmol·L⁻¹
	NaCl 0.5 g·L⁻¹
Potassium	Replacement not required
	Improves palatability
	(Potassium content: 2–5 mmol·L⁻¹)
Carbohydrate	Maintains blood glucose,
	extends endurance
	Improves palatability
	Optimal content: Glucose 5–10% w/v

(Glucose polymer — no advantage; Fructose —
  gastrointestinal upsets)
Temperature 5–15°C

to about 90 min, CHO taken during the game may reduce deterioration in performance towards the end of the game. At least 30 min must be allowed for absorption. In cool conditions, supplementing CHO may be more beneficial than water replacement so that relatively concentrated CHO (10–20%) solutions may be used (Maughan & Noakes 1991). Alternatively, CHO immediately before play may be effective and more convenient.

Table 5.7 provides broad guide-lines for beverages suitable for competition. Although gastric emptying may be slowed by CHO/electrolyte solutions, water absorption in the small intestine is enhanced from fluids containing low concentrations of glucose and sodium. The addition of glucose, sodium and flavour also improves palatability and promotes higher fluid intakes, thus reducing the degree of involuntary dehydration.

Beverage formulations should be kept within these guide-lines. But they can be varied and may prove for the individual to be a matter of taste and tolerance. Formulations could also be varied according to the nature and conditions of competition. As a general principle, for shorter and more intense activity less water is required and greater concentrations of CHO may be beneficial; while for longer events water uptake should be optimized with greater volumes and lower CHO concentrations (Maughan & Noakes 1991; Gisolfi and Duchman 1992).

The optimal CHO intake during exercise to prolong endurance has not been determined, but at least 30 $g \cdot h^{-1}$ is probably required, although there may be no increased advantage in intakes exceeding 60 $g \cdot h^{-1}$. CHO solutions up to 10% w/v are generally well tolerated, although for some athletes they may be too sweet, or induce thirst or abdominal discomfort. The form of the CHO does not seem to be important; solid, sugar and glucose polymer (maltodextrins) solutions are all equally effective in enhancing endurance. Glucose polymers have the advantage of being less sweet than the simple sugars. Fructose is of no benefit. It is poorly absorbed, contributes less than glucose to energy metabolism and may cause gastrointestinal discomfort.

The mechanism by which CHO feeding during exercise prolongs endurance is not entirely clear. It is not universally due to glycogen sparing. However, as muscle glycogen declines with exercise, ingested CHO boosts the blood glucose to a level that increases the glucose uptake by the muscles, thus allowing high-intensity exercise to continue when muscle glycogen levels are low (Coyle et al. 1986; Coyle 1991).

Water Replacement

The importance of being fully hydrated before exercise, whether it be training or competition, particularly in warm weather, cannot be overstated. To help ensure this, water intake should continue after the pre-competition meal. Three hundred to 500 mL of water should be drunk 5–20 min before the start of exercise.

Although it is usually recommended that athletes should drink sufficient during exercise to replace their sweat losses, complete water replacement is rarely achieved. During exercise thirst is not sufficient stimulus to ensure that fluid intake fully replaces sweat water losses, so that, even when water is freely available, dehydration usually occurs (often referred to as 'voluntary dehydration'). At high-sweat rates maintenance of full hydration may not be possible because water losses may exceed the maximum rate of gastric emptying. Athletes in endurance events usually do not replace more than about half their sweat losses. Despite this, well-trained athletes who start competition fully hydrated rarely suffer serious impairment of thermoregulation (Noakes et al. 1988).

Some water deficit during hard exercise can be tolerated. Significant impairment of performance and thermoregulation does not occur until dehydration of at least 2% of body mass is incurred. Furthermore, because the water associated with glycogen and the water of combustion are released during hard exercise, the true degree of physiological dehydration is less than the sweat losses suggest (Noakes et al. 1988).

For conventional sports in moderate temperatures (15–25°C), fluid intakes that replace about half the sweat loss will be sufficient. Fluid intakes of 150–250 mL every 10–20 min providing up to about 1 $L \cdot h^{-1}$ will be adequate for most athletes and situations. In hot and humid conditions well-acclimatized athletes may sweat at rates >2 L·h⁻¹ and greater water intakes may be possible, be absorbed and be beneficial.

In ultra-long endurance events that continue for many hours, exercise rate and so the rate of sweat secretion, is lower than with shorter and more intense exercise. Total sweat loss, albeit at a slow rate and the associated sodium loss, however, may be considerable. In these circumstances, in some people, continuous water intake greater than their sweat loss and low sodium intake may lead to hyponatraemia or 'water intoxication' (Noakes *et al*. 1985; Gisolfi & Duchman 1992). Thus, in these events fluid intakes should not greatly exceed the expected sweat losses and participants should not attempt to drink at the high rates required for shorter, faster events. In addition, sodium should be added to drinks.

NUTRITIONAL RECOVERY AND REHYDRATION FOLLOWING EXHAUSTIVE EXERCISE

Recovery from exhausting exercise requires at least the replenishment of glycogen, water and electrolytes. Generally, this is achieved with the athlete's usual eating pattern of regular meals and a plentiful supply of CHO. But it takes time as well as food and water.

Following 1 or 2 h of exhaustive exercise only about 5–7% of the muscle glycogen utilized is resynthesized each hour, thus full glycogen restoration may take at least 20 h (Coyle 1991). Glycogen resynthesis proceeds at an optimal rate with a CHO intake of about 25 g·h⁻¹. Both moderate and high GI CHO are suitable and glycogen restoration is similar whether CHO is consumed with several small meals or two or three large meals (Coyle 1991).

An adequate water intake is vital. Rehydration after exercise, however, involves more than simply drinking water. Even after exercise, a large water intake without sodium replacement is likely to result in an increase in urine excretion rather than effective correction of dehydration. A water deficit of 2.5 L, which is easily acquired in 90 min of hard exercise in warm conditions, might take more than 6 h to make up. Water is only absorbed from the intestine. At rest, the maximum rate that water

leaves the stomach is about 1 L·h⁻¹ and this may be reduced three to four times by the presence of food. Furthermore, because water is also stored in association with glycogen, food, particularly CHO, is required for full recovery from exercise-induced dehydration. Despite their large water losses athletes can rehydrate adequately from day to day and generally do so. However, many of them do not drink sufficient fluids to replace their sweat losses until many hours after exercise.

When recovery time is limited, for example, repeated competition on the same day or on successive days, or between sessions of an arduous training regimen, a specific dietary strategy should be used to expedite recovery. High GI CHO which promote the fastest rate of glycogen resynthesis (Kiens *et al*. 1990; Burke *et al*. 1993) should be consumed as soon after exercise as possible when glycogen resynthesis is also at its maximum rate and to allow the longest possible time for resynthesis (Coyle 1991). Sodium, which can be taken as salt added in palatable amounts to food, or in drinks as shown in Table 5.7, is also required to help retain water. Formulated sports drinks (Table 5.7) may therefore be effective aids to hastening recovery.

SPECIFIC DIET-RELATED CONCERNS FOR ATHLETES

Weight Control

The necessity for developing safe and effective methods of losing weight, gaining weight and then maintaining competitive or ideal weight is a matter of concern for athletes, coaches and health professionals. Many athletes are preoccupied with the issues of weight and body fat, usually through pressure from coaches, peers and parents to attain a particular weight or body composition. The focus of weight control should be on body composition rather than on weight as there are no definitive or rigid standards for either weight or body fat in individual athletes. The physique characteristics of successful athletes vary widely from sport to sport and within sports (see Chapter 1). These measurements are useful as guide-lines for groups of athletes, but do not necessarily apply to individuals.

It should be pointed out that sportsmen and

sportswomen are vulnerable to unusual weight control practices, which are aimed at achieving weight goals that are often unrealistic and detrimental to physiological processes, health and performance.

Weight Loss

For the majority of sports, a low body fat and for some sports (gymnastics, ballet dancing) a low bodyweight is desirable for appearance and optimal performance. Sports imposing weight limits for competition, such as judo, horse-racing, light-weight rowing, wrestling and boxing, may involve repeated periods of weight fluctuations. Weight loss and regain among these groups is usually frequent, rapid and involves large weight changes.

Unfortunately, the methods used by many athletes to achieve weight loss are often nutritionally inadequate, potentially dangerous and frequently ineffective. These methods may range from sensible eating to severe and restrictive dietary practices including prolonged fasting, fad diets and even the use of purgative substances or behaviours. Those athletes 'making weight' for competition often practise a combination of severe dietary restriction, excessive exercise and various dehydration techniques ranging from severe prolonged fluid restriction, saunas and diuretic abuse. Donation of blood for weight reduction has also been reported (Hursh 1979).

Inappropriate weight loss methods are associated with inadequate glycogen stores, muscle weakness, dehydration, irritability, anxiety, fatigue, gastro-intestinal upset and malnutrition. These effects lead to decreases in aerobic power, speed, co-ordination, strength, poor health status and ultimately disappointing performances and training sessions.

Effects of Rapid Weight Loss

SHORT-TERM EFFECTS

Rapid weight loss does not always result in desirable changes in body composition. Substantial losses of water, electrolytes, minerals and LBM, including protein within fat-free tissues occurs, accompanied by rapid depletions in liver and muscle glycogen.

There is an obligatory water loss of 2.5 $g \cdot g^{-1}$ of glycogen. Therefore 2–3 kg of weight can be lost in a few days due to glycogen depletion and dehydration. During short-term energy restriction, the loss of LBM is high compared with fat loss and the risk of impairment of strength, endurance and thermoregulation is high.

LONG-TERM EFFECTS

During prolonged reduction diets with severely restricted energy intake, adequate CHO intake to support training and minimize loss of lean tissue stores is crucial. In the long term, a weight reduction diet that is low in CHO and too restrictive in energy may lead to significant losses in body protein. Reductions in blood volume and body fluids, accompanied by weakness and fainting, are reported in subjects on restricted energy diets. Amenorrhoea can be a consequence of severe energy restriction.

EFFECTS OF EXERCISE ON WEIGHT LOSS

A decline in basal metabolic rate is an adaptive response to starvation. Theoretically, the addition of exercise would exacerbate the total energy drain, leading to a further decline in metabolism (Brownell 1987). This theory could explain why many athletes on low-energy diets have limited success in losing weight, despite their high-energy expenditure. For these athletes energy requirements may be lower than expected in order to maintain normal weight and they are unable to meet nutrient needs.

The magnitude of weight loss and change in body composition is proportional to the frequency, duration and intensity of exercise. Vigorous exercise alone without energy intake restriction accounts for relatively small losses of weight in athletes. However, exercise in combination with a moderate energy restricted diet is the most effective way to lose weight and minimize losses of LBM. Exercise is one of the few factors positively correlated with successful long-term weight maintenance.

Guide-lines for Sensible Weight Loss

The goal in any weight reduction programme is to lose fat not LBM.

Ideally, a weight-reduction programme should be supervised by a nutritionist–dietitian. They can assess target weight or body fat goals, determine a nutritionally sound dietary plan and incorporate a behaviour modification programme to identify and treat undesirable eating habits. Monitoring weight and body composition using skinfold measurements is important to assure the desired direction of change. This is also important for athletes attempting to gain weight. Measuring weight daily is usually not helpful because of the large daily fluctuations in weight. The following guide-lines should be adhered to if the athlete wants to lose weight sensibly:

- A moderate energy restriction of 2000–4000 kJ less than the usual dietary intake is recommended. This results in a smaller loss of water and LBM and is less likely to lead to malnutrition. Diets based on wholesome CHO foods, lean protein sources and a decreased intake of high fat and sugar foods are preferred. High-CHO diets are recommended due to their higher satiety value and to help maintain the fuel reserves for training. Diets that restrict CHO are associated with a negative nitrogen balance (loss of protein), nausea, ketosis and a reduced capacity for work performance and endurance
- The rate of sustained weight loss should be no greater than 1 kg per week. In the first weeks of dieting, weight loss appears more rapid due to accompanying water loss. As the diet continues weight loss usually slows
- Ideally, athletes should train no more than 1–2% of their bodyweight above their racing or competitive weight (Burke & Reid 1993). This strategy avoids adverse reactions and decrements in performance due to the necessity to lose large amounts of weight by dehydration and glycogen depletion in the days preceding competition

Weight Gain

The goal in gaining weight is to gain muscle mass (LBM) and minimize fat deposition and fat mass (FM). Muscle mass increases only after a sufficient period of hypertrophic muscle training and cannot

be increased simply by eating more food, more protein or taking protein supplements.

Athletes engaged in an appropriate weight-training programme must consume a diet that meets their nutrient needs as well as their increased energy CHO and protein requirements. Although protein needs are slightly higher in athletes than their non-trained counterparts, most athletes consume substantially more protein than recommended. For this reason protein supplements are unnecessary.

When athletes increase food intake to gain lean weight, there will undoubtedly be an associated increase in body fat, even when accompanied by vigorous exercise. A weight gain of more than 0.5–0.7 kg per week would favour fat deposition in most athletes.

Diets recommended for training and recovery in this chapter are also recommended for weight gain. Due to the problems associated with the bulk of CHO foods, a slight increase in food intake at meal times and the inclusion of frequent nutritious snacks are helpful to maintain a positive energy balance.

An increase in weight with a maintenance or decrease in skinfold measurements indicates a gain in LBM, whereas an increase in weight with an increase in skinfold measurements indicates some gains in FM (Forbes 1985).

Vegetarian Diets

The emphasis on high-CHO diets for athletes has encouraged the adoption of a diet that eliminates or decreases meat intake and emphasizes plant foods, particularly among endurance athletes and triathletes. Although vegetarian diets usually provide a high-CHO intake, there is a slight risk of developing a nutrient deficiency problem. Nutritional adequacy of vegetarian diets varies, but for adults, only the very restricted diets pose a real threat to health.

TYPES OF VEGETARIAN DIETS

The term 'vegetarian' comprises many varieties of vegetarian-style diets based on a limited range of plant food sources (e.g. fruitarian and macrobiotic) to a large range of plant food sources including

Table 5.8 Types of vegetarian diets

Type	Composition
Fruitarian	No animal foods or animal products (dairy products and eggs) are eaten; only plant sources that have undergone minimal processing are eaten. These include fresh and dried fruit, tomatoes, honey, nuts, seeds and vegetable oils
Macrobiotic	No animal foods or animal products are eaten; unprocessed, unrefined cereals and condiments, such as misu and seaweed are eaten
Vegan	No animal foods or animal products are eaten; includes only plant foods and plant products
Lacto-vegetarian	As for vegan but includes dairy products
Lacto-ovo-vegetarian	As for vegan, but includes dairy products and eggs
'New vegetarian'	Mostly plant foods are eaten but occasionally some groups of animal products are eaten. Unrefined, unprocessed, unfortified cereals and organically grown foods or free-range animal foods are favoured.
'Quasi-vegetarian'	Excludes red meat most of the time; fish and chicken are eaten

some meat (Table 5.8). Being vegetarian does not necessarily imply that all animal foods and animal products are excluded. All animal foods and animal products such as eggs and dairy foods are excluded in the fruitarian, macrobiotic and vegan diets. However, lacto-vegetarian, lacto-ovo-vegetarian diets include some animal products while the 'new vegetarian' and 'quasi vegetarian' diets also include some form of meat in addition to other animal products, such as dairy products and eggs (see Table 5.8).

ADVANTAGES OF VEGETARIAN DIETS FOR ATHLETES

Most vegetarian diets if well planned (except fruitarian and macrobiotic), meet the nutrient and energy requirements of athletes. There is considerable evidence based on population studies that vegetarian diets confer health advantages. Compared with non-vegetarians, vegetarians, especially vegans, have a lower serum cholesterol and coronary disease mortality, weigh less and have less FM.

Nieman (1988) in a review on vegetarian diets and endurance performance concluded that vegetarian athletes are more likely to consume the recommended high-CHO intakes which help maximize body glycogen stores than non-vegetarians. Few studies have compared the athletic capabilities of vegetarians and non-vegetarians. This is largely due to the variety of both types of diet and the confounding influences of varied training and lifestyle.

DISADVANTAGES OF VEGETARIAN DIETS

Fruitarian and macrobiotic diets, because of their limited variety of foods do not meet the nutrient or energy requirements for most people and are therefore not recommended for athletes. Risks of dietary deficiency are higher for vegan than other types of vegetarian diet. Among the common nutrient concerns associated with any unplanned vegetarian diets are inadequate food, protein or energy intake and potentially low intakes and reduced bioavailability of the minerals iron, zinc and calcium and low intakes of Vitamins A and B_{12} and riboflavin.

Athletes following vegan diets are not at any additional risk of protein deficiency provided that the combination of protein sources contains all the essential amino acids. Athletes who are lacto-ovo vegetarians usually consume enough protein because of the high-protein quality of dairy products and eggs.

High-fibre intakes often associated with vegetarian diets may contain naturally occurring phytic acid (components of cereal grains and legumes, soya beans) and oxalic acid (sesame seeds, spinach and rhubarb), which bind to iron, zinc and calcium, reducing availability for absorption. Calcium and riboflavin intakes tend to be lower in vegetarians unless dairy products or sufficient quantities of dark green leafy vegetables are consumed daily. The intake of Vitamins A and D is usually low if the intake of fat or fatty foods is very restrictive. Because Vitamin B_{12} is only found in animal food, deficiency of this vitamin may develop in vegans.

DIETARY RECOMMENDATIONS FOR VEGETARIAN ATHLETES

The following recommendations should be followed by vegetarian athletes:

- Vegan athletes need to eat adequate quantities of wholegrain cereals, dark green and orange vegetables, starchy vegetables and legumes or nuts to obtain sufficient amino acids and energy. To allow sufficient consumption of these important foods, only moderate consumption of fruit and other non-starchy vegetables which have a low protein content is possible
- Special consideration must be given to the provision of key risk nutrients when planning a vegetarian food guide, especially if the preferred diet is vegan. For vegans a multivitamin containing B_{12}, iron and zinc, plus a calcium supplement may be indicated if athletes have difficulty meeting the RDI through food sources. For these athletes regular monitoring of nutritional and biochemical status is recommended

Premature Osteoporosis

Osteoporosis is a disease affecting bone turnover and resulting in a reduction in bone mass due to a progressive loss of calcium. While inadequate calcium intake has been implicated in the aetiology, prevention and treatment of osteoporosis, the association is not unequivocal.

Low bone density which is characteristic of osteoporosis and usually found only in the elderly, has recently been detected in young female athletes with amenorrhoea (see Chapter 23 for further information). An accelerated loss of bone mass occurs in females with low levels of the hormone oestrogen. Low oestrogen levels are evident in athletes who cease menstruating or have delayed or intermittent menstruation induced by dieting or strenuous exercise. Low bone density reported in these female athletes may increase the occurrence of stress fractures and the risk in later life of osteoporotic complications, including hip, wrist and vertebral fractures.

Low body fat and low energy diets associated with inadequate dietary calcium are characteristic of many amenorrhoeic athletes. Amenorrhoeic athletes may need up to 1000–1500 mg of calcium·day^{-1} (almost twice the RDI) to meet their needs (American Dietetic Association 1987). Dairy products, particularly low fat choices such as skim milk or fortified low-fat milk and low-fat yoghurt are excellent dietary sources of calcium, which are readily absorbed by the body. Where dairy foods are unsuitable as in conditions like milk allergy or lactose intolerance, adequate calcium intake is usually difficult to achieve. In these circumstances a calcium supplement in the form of calcium lactate, calcium gluconate or calcium carbonate may be warranted.

Other dietary factors that influence calcium retention or absorption need to be considered to ensure adequate calcium status. Large meat intake, excess salt (sodium) and excess caffeine (coffee, tea, chocolate or cola drinks) in the diet promote calcium loss in the urine. Simultaneous excessive intake of foods that contain naturally occurring substances such as phytic acid (found in unprocessed cereal fibre and many wholegrain foods), oxalic acid (found in tea, spinach and rhubarb) with calcium-containing foods, can bind calcium in the gut, inhibiting its absorption and assimilation into the body. It may be beneficial to consume calcium-rich foods, in the absence of these interfering factors.

As a preventive measure female athletes should ensure adequate calcium intake, particularly in the bone forming years of adolescence and possibly avoid large intakes of substances which may affect calcium absorption or loss. For some athletes oestrogen replacement therapy, often in the form of an oral contraceptive, in combination with a high-calcium diet may be an option for treatment and prevention of osteoporosis.

Iron Deficiency

Iron deficiency with or without anaemia is a well documented but controversial problem in athletes.

Interpretation of iron deficiency observed in many athletes as indicative of true iron deficiency is ambiguous. For some athletes reduced iron status may be due to a physiological adaptation to exercise due to haemodilution associated with an expansion of plasma volume (Newhouse and Clement 1988). Despite this adaptation many studies in athletes report low intakes of dietary iron and blood loss in the gastrointestinal and urinary tract.

Iron deficiency with anaemia may lead to decreased aerobic capacity and immunological response and increased fatigue and lethargy. As well, several symptoms associated with anaemia are often observed in iron deficient subjects without anaemia. These include headache, fatigue, heartburn, changes in appetite, vasomotor disturbances, muscular cramping, dyspnoea and amenorrhagia.

PREVALENCE OF IRON DEFICIENCY

Several studies have reported iron depletion without anaemia on the basis of low ferritin levels in highly trained male and female athletes. Clement and Asmundson (1982) suggest the prevalence of depleted iron stores and consequent risk of iron deficiency may be as high as 82% in female distance runners and 29% in male distance runners. Female and endurance athletes are the most frequently cited risk groups. Serum ferritin is regarded as the most reliable single clinical parameter for determination of iron status. In the non-athletic population the mean serum ferritin concentrations for 174 adult men was 69.2 ng·mL^{-1} and for 152 adult women was 34.0 ng·mL^{-1} (Crosby & O'Neill 1984). Similar values are reported in athletic population groups, although the values appear skewed toward the lower end of the range (Newhouse & Clement 1988). Serum ferritin below 30 ng·mL^{-1} indicates latent iron deficiency and serum ferritin levels of 12 ng·mL^{-1} are designated as a clinical iron deficiency (Crosby & O'Neill 1984).

Anaemia is manifest when both haemoglobin and ferritin levels are below the reference range for normal iron storage (Table 5.9).

SOURCES OF IRON

Iron occurs in red meat, especially liver and kidneys, poultry, fish, egg yolk, wholegrain cereal products and breakfast cereals, dried fruit, legumes and nuts. The best naturally occurring sources of iron in plant foods are in dried fruit (apricots) and legumes (lentils and baked beans; Table 5.10).

Most commercial breakfast cereals are fortified with iron and B vitamins and, if eaten in sufficient quantities, provide a substantial iron contribution to the diet.

Table 5.9 Stages of iron deficiency

Stages of iron deficiency	Serum ferritin (g·mL^{-1})	Haemoglobin (g·dL^{-1})
Normal iron storage	30 W	>12 W
	>110 M	>14 M
Latent	<30	>12 W
		>14 M
Manifest (anaemia)	<10	<12 W
		<14 M

W = Women; M = Men.
Adapted from Crosby and O'Neill (1984)

Table 5.10 Sources of iron

Sources		mg per average serve
Animal sources		
Pâté or liver	(75 g)	8.3
Beef	2 slices (75 g)	2.1
Lamb	2 slices (75 g)	1.9
Egg	1 only (45 g)	0.9
Chicken	1 small breast (75 g)	0.9
Fish	1 average piece (75 g)	0.4
Plant sources		
Breakfast cereals (commercial) (iron enriched)	average serve (60 g)	5.6
Baked beans	½ cup (120 g)	1.7
Cooked dried beans, lentils	½ cup (60 g)	1.5
Wholemeal bread	2 slices	1.4
Prunes	5–6	1.4
Green leafy vegetables	½ cup	1.4
White bread	2 slices	0.7
Orange juice	1 small glass (200 mL)	0.6
Fruit	average piece	0.5

Source English & Lewis (1992).

IRON REQUIREMENTS

Daily iron requirements for different sports have not been established and are likely to be highly variable. The daily iron intake to maintain the body's iron stores for most healthy adults is generally thought to be achieved with the RDI of 7 mg·day^{-1} for men and 12–16 mg·day^{-1} for women. The iron needs of athletes may be higher than this due to losses of iron via sweat, urine, gastrointestinal bleeding and menses. To balance these losses, daily iron intakes for distance runners, one of the highest risk groups, may be as high as 17.5 mg·day^{-1} for men and 23 mg·day^{-1} for normally menstruating women, assuming that 10% of dietary iron is absorbed (Haymes and Lamanca 1989).

DIETARY FACTORS IMPLICATED IN IRON DEFICIENCY

Dietary factors implicated in iron deficiency include limited bioavailability (poor absorption) of iron, inadequate dietary iron intake and low-energy intakes.

POOR BIOAVAILABILITY (ABSORPTION) OF IRON FROM FOODS

Iron in food exists in two forms: haem and non-haem iron. Meat, seafood and poultry contain both forms, while cereals, legumes, vegetables and eggs contain only the non-haem form. Haem iron is absorbed more efficiently than non-haem iron, which is influenced by the presence of interfering or enhancing components in food. Non-haem iron absorption may vary up to 10-fold depending on the dietary content of enhancing and inhibiting components. Australian recommendations for iron intakes in people with no iron depletion assume 15% of total iron presented in the diet is absorbed.

Naturally occurring components in food can inhibit absorption of non-haem iron by forming insoluble complexes, which leads to reduced bioavailability of iron. These include phosphates (legumes, whole grains), phytic acid (unprocessed bran, oatmeal, wholegrains), oxalic acid (spinach, silverbeet, rhubarb, soya bean products) and tannic acid (tea and coffee).

The absorption of iron from non-haem sources can be enhanced by many components, the two most well defined are ascorbic acid (Vitamin C) and the quantity of animal tissue present in each meal. For example, simultaneous consumption of orange juice or vitamin C-rich foods or meat with a meal rich in non-haem iron is likely to be an effective way of increasing the absorption of iron from the non-haem source.

INADEQUATE IRON INTAKES

Iron intakes that are less than the RDI have been reported in athletes from various sports, but particularly where the emphasis is on maintaining a LBM. Major risk groups include endurance runners, ballet dancers, gymnasts, jockeys and adolescent athletes. Athletes, particularly females involved in these sports, frequently consume relatively low-energy diets in order to control or lose fat. Intakes below 8300 kJ (2000 kcal) are often associated with suboptimal iron intake (Roeser 1990). Athletes who follow some vegetarian diets which are generally low in haem-iron and bioavailability are also at risk of iron deficiency. Milk and dairy products have negligible amounts of iron while eggs, frequently reported to be iron-rich are a poor source, as the iron is not easily absorbed.

FOOD SUGGESTIONS TO MEET THE RDI FOR IRON

Table 5.11 presents food suggestions to meet the RDI for iron for men and women. Selection of more iron dense foods that are readily absorbed is crucial to meet the increased requirements of the at risk groups. For most healthy adults, daily diets that provide 30–90 g meat, poultry or fish and vegetarian foods containing 25–75 mg of ascorbic acid (after preparation or processing) provide sufficient iron (Herbert 1987). Athletes who eat little or no animal protein and vegetarians who cook most of the Vitamin C out of their food and do not eat uncooked fruit and/or vegetables or drink fruit juice every day, may require higher intakes of dietary iron sources.

These suggestions in Table 5.11 are likely to be inadequate to balance the iron losses in some distance runners who may need to increase their intake of iron dense foods that are readily absorbed to meet their requirements.

Table 5.11 Suggestions for daily food choices to meet the RDI for iron

		Iron content (mg)
Men (RDI = 7 mg·day⁻¹)		
Breakfast cereals	1 medium bowl (60 g)	5.6
Bread (wholemeal)	3 slices	2.1
Lean steak	1 medium (150 g)	4.7
	Total	12.4
Women (RDI = 12–16 mg·day⁻¹)		
Breakfast cereal	1 small bowl	2.8
Bread	5 slices	3.5
Ham	1 slice (50 g)	0.7
Lean steak	1 small	3.7
Green vegetables	1 large serve	0.8
Potato	1 medium	0.7
Fruit juice	1 glass (200 mL)	0.6
Dried fruit	5–6 apricots	1.2
Total		14.0

Source English and Lewis (1992).

Nutritional counselling to maximize iron intake and bioavailability is warranted in those athletes identified as anaemic or iron deficient. Iron depletion and deficiency can be prevented by recognition of risk groups of athletes, early detection and monitoring of biochemical parameters.

IRON SUPPLEMENTS

Many athletes are self-administering iron supplements regularly to prevent iron stores becoming depleted. Balaban *et al.* (1989) found that women runners taking iron supplements had significantly higher serum ferritin levels than controls who were not receiving supplements. However, as the safety and necessity of iron supplements in the absence of a diagnosed iron deficiency is still questionable, they should be taken with caution. Prolonged use of iron supplements in iron-replete athletes containing more than 50 mg elemental iron per day may increase the risk of iron overload, accumulation in tissue and iron toxicity (Haymes 1991). Intake of iron supplements can also induce depletion of other trace minerals such as zinc and copper (Dawson *et al.* 1989; Yadrick *et al.* 1989). Side-effects associated with iron supplements and iron overload include

diarrhoea and (more often) constipation and an increased risk of infection.

Where an iron depletion is present, increasing iron intake by dietary means alone is not sufficient to improve iron status. At least 60 mg of elemental iron in the form of a supplement, in combination with an increase in dietary iron supply, is needed to increase low serum ferritin levels in iron-depleted athletes (Rowland & Kelleher 1989).

DIETARY STRATEGIES FOR THE PROMOTION OF OPTIMAL IRON INTAKE

- Increase total consumption of iron-rich foods in the daily diet (Table 5.11)
- Eat at least small amounts of lean meat, poultry or fish preferably daily (30–90 g)
- Include foods rich in ascorbic acid (Vitamin C) with each meal such as raw or lightly cooked vegetables or salad, fruit, or fruit juice
- Increase consumption of iron-enriched bread and breakfast cereals
- Avoid consumption of strong tea and coffee with meals or non-haem iron sources
- If vegetarian, ensure plant food choices are iron-dense

CONCLUSIONS

This chapter has demonstrated that there are specific nutritional stresses associated with strenuous athletic training and competition and that incorrect dietary practices can impair performance. On the other hand, conventionally recognized nutrients and foods do not in themselves enhance performance. There is no evidence that vitamin and mineral supplements, or extraordinary intakes of nutrients such as protein, are of benefit to athletes other than in cases of established deficiency.

CHO combustion and water losses from sweat are the major nutritional stresses in heavy athletic training and inadequate CHO intake results in premature fatigue. Dehydration also inhibits maximal performance, but more seriously it impairs thermoregulation and puts the athlete at risk of heat illness. Appropriate CHO and water intakes are important in preparation for competition and high-CHO diets in the days prior to events involving continuous hard exercise, are of benefit in extending endurance, as they boost muscle and glycogen stores. For some events, CHO and water intake during the event are recommended.

Recently, certain nutrition-related problems that appear to be associated with heavy athletic training have been recognized. These are, iron deficiency in both sexes, particularly in endurance runners and osteoporosis in amenorrhoeic female athletes. Poor dietary practices that may affect both performance and long-term health are also observed in some groups of athletes. Usually these are associated with habitual use of fad diets or unplanned vegetarian diets or with incorrect weight control practices.

In conclusion, it can be stated that the dietary guidelines and recommendations for the general population are sufficient to support athletic endeavour and to prevent the occurrence of nutritional problems in the majority of athletes.

REFERENCES

American College of Sports Medicine (1987) Amino acid and protein metabolism in exercise. *Medicine and Science in Sports and Exercise* 19, S150–178.

American Dietetic Association (1987) Position stand on nutrition for physical fitness and athletic performance for adults. *Journal of the American Dietetic Association* 87, 933–939.

Australian Sports Medicine Federation (1983) Survey of drug use in Australian sport. Australian Sports Medicine Federation, Canberra.

Balaban E. P., Cox J. V., Snell P., Vaughan R. H. & Frenker E. P. (1989) The frequency of anaemia and iron deficiency in the runner. *Medicine and Science in Sports and Exercise* 21, 643–648.

Barr S. I. (1987) Women, nutrition and exercise: A review of athletes intakes and a discussion of energy balance in active women. *Progress in Food and Nutrition Science* 11, 307–361.

Bergstrom J., Hermansen L., Hultman E. & Saltin B. (1967) Diet, muscle glycogen and physical performance. *Acta Physiologica Scandinavica* 71, 140–150.

Brotherhood J. R. (1984) Nutrition and sports performance. *Sports Medicine* 1, 350–389.

Brownell K. D., Steen S. N. & Wilmore J. H. (1987) Weight regulation practices in athletes: Analysis of metabolic and health effects. *Medicine and Science in Sport and Exercise* 19, 546–556.

Burke L. M. & Read R. S. D. (1993) Dietary supplements in sport. *Sports Medicine* 15, 43–65.

Burke L. M., Collier G. R. & Hargreaves M. (1993) Muscle glycogen storage after prolonged exercise: Effect of the glycaemic index of carbohydrate feedings. *Journal of Applied Physiology* 75, 1019–1023.

Cashel K. & Jeffreson S. (1995) *The Core Food Groups; the scientific basis for developing nutrition education tools.* Australian Government Printing Service, Canberra.

Chesley A., MacDougall J. D., Tarnopolsky M. A., Atkinson S. A. and Smith K. (1992) Changes in human muscle protein synthesis after resistance exercise. *Journal of Applied Physiology* 73, 1383–1388.

Clement D. B. & Asmundson R. C. (1982) Nutritional intake and hematological parameters in endurance runners. *Physician and Sports Medicine* 10, 37–43.

Costill D. L. (1984) Water and electrolyte requirements during exercise. *Clinics in Sports Medicine* 3, 639–648.

Costill D. L. (1988) Carbohydrates for exercise: Dietary demands for optimal performance. *International Journal Sports Medicine* 9, 1–18.

Costill D. L., Sherman W. M., Fink W. J., Maresh C., Witten M. & Miller J. M. (1981) The role of dietary carbohydrate in muscle glycogen synthesis after strenuous training. *American Journal of Clinical Nutrition* 34, 1831–1836.

Coyle E. F. (1991) Timing and method of increased carbohydrate intake to cope with heavy training, competition and recovery. *Journal of Sports Science* 9 (Suppl.), 29–52.

Coyle E. F., Coggan A. R., Hemmert M. K. & Ivy J. L. (1986) Muscle glycogen utilization during prolonged strenuous exercise when fed CHO. *Journal of Applied Physiology* 61, 165–172.

Crosby W. H. & O'Neill M. A. (1984) A small dose iron tolerance test as an indicator of mild iron deficiency. *Journal of the American Medical Association* 251, 1986–1987.

Dawson E. B., Albers J. & McGarrity W. (1989) Serum zinc changes due to iron supplementation in teenage pregnancy. *American Journal of Clinical Nutrition* 50, 848–52.

Deakin V. & Inge K. (1994) Training nutrition. In Burke L. & Deakin V. (eds) *Clinical Sports Nutrition*, pp. 16–37. McGraw-Hill, Sydney.

English R. & Lewis J. (1992) *Nutritional Values of Australian Foods*, pp. 1–36. Australian Government Publishing Service, Canberra.

FAO/WHO/UNU. (1985) *Energy and Protein Requirements. Report of a Joint FAO/WHO/UNU Meeting.* World Health Organization. Technical Report Series No. 724, WHO, Geneva.

Forbes G. B. (1985) Body composition as affected by physical activity and nutrition. *Federation Proceedings* 44, 343–347.

Gisolfi C. V. & Duchman S. M. (1992) Guidelines for optimal replacement beverages for different athletic events. *Medicine and Science in Sports and Exercise* **26**, 679–687.

Greenhaff P. L., Gleeson M. & Maughan R. J. (1988) Diet-induced metabolic acidosis and the performance of high intensity exercise in man. *European Journal of Applied Physiology* **57**, 583–590.

Haymes E. M. (1991) Vitamin and mineral supplementation in athletes. *International Journal of Sports Nutrition* **1**, 146–169.

Haymes E. M. & Lamanca J. F. (1989) Iron loss in runners during exercise: Implications and recommendations. *Sports Medicine* **7**, 277–285.

Herbert V. (1987) Recommended dietary intakes (RDI) of iron in humans. *American Journal of Clinical Nutrition* **45**, 679–686.

Hursh L. M. (1979) Food and water restriction in the wrestler. *Journal of the American Medical Association* **241**, 915–916.

Ivy J. L., Katz A. L., Cutler C. L., Sherman W. M. & Coyle E. F. (1988) Muscle glycogen synthesis after exercise: Effect of time of carbohydrate ingestion. *Journal of Applied Physiology* **64**, 1480–1485.

Jenkins D. J. A., Wolever T. M. S., Jenkins A. L., Josse R. J. & Wong G. S. (1984) Glycaemic response to carbohydrate foods. *Lancet* ii, 388–391.

Jenkins D. J. A., Wolever T. M. S., Buckley G. *et al.* (1988) Low glycaemic index starchy foods in the diabetic diet. *American Journal of Clinical Nutrition* **48**, 248–254.

Kiens B., Raben A. B., Valeur A. K. & Richter E. A. (1990) Benefit of dietary simple carbohydrates on the early post-exercise muscle glycogen repletion in male athletes. *Medicine and Science in Sports and Exercise* **22** (Suppl.), S88.

Lamb D. R & Brodowicz G. R. (1986) Optimal use of fluids of varying formulations to minimise exercise-induced disturbances in homeostasis. *Sports Medicine* **3**, 247–274.

Lemon P. W. R. (1991a) Effect of exercise on protein requirements. *Journal of Sports Sciences* **9**, 53–70.

Lemon P. W. R. (1991b) Protein intake and athletic performance. *Sports Medicine* **12**, 313–325.

Lemon P. W. R., Tarnopolsky M. A., MacDougall J. D. and Atkinson S. A. (1992) Protein requirements and muscle mass strength changes during intensive training in novice body builders. *Journal of Applied Physiology* **73**, 767–775.

McMichael A. J. (1991) Foods, nutrients, health and disease: A historical perspective on the assessment and management of risks. *Australian Journal of Public Health* **15**, 7–13.

Maughan R. J. & Noakes T. D. (1991) Fluid replacement and exercise stress. A brief review of studies on fluid replacement and some guidelines for the athlete. *Sports Medicine* **12**, 16–31.

Meredith C. N., Zackin M. J., Frontera W. R. & Evans W. J. (1989) Dietary protein requirements and body protein metabolism in endurance-trained men. *Journal of Applied Physiology* **66**, 2850–2856.

Murray R. (1987) The effects of consuming carbohydrate–electrolyte beverages on gastric emptying and juice absorption during and following exercise. *Sports Medicine* **4**, 322–351.

National Research Council (1989) *Recommended Dietary Allowances*, 10th edn, p. 21. National Academy Press, Washington, DC.

Newhouse I. J. & Clement, D. B. (1988) Iron status in athletes: An update. *Sports Medicine* **5**, 337–352.

Nieman D. C. (1988) Vegetarian dietary practices and endurance performance in Proceedings on the First International Congress on Vegetarian Nutrition. *American Journal of Clinical Nutrition* **48**, 754–761.

Noakes T. D., Goodwin N., Rayner B. L., Branken T. & Taylor R. K. N. (1985) Water intoxication: A possible complication during endurance exercise. *Medicine and Science in Sports and Exercise* **17**, 370–375.

Noakes T. D., Adams B. A., Myburgh K. H., Greeff C., Lotz T. & Nathan M. (1988) The danger of an inadequate water intake during prolonged exercise: A novel concept revisited. *European Journal of Applied Physiology* **57**, 210–219.

Phillips S. M., Atkinson S. A., Tarnopolsky M. A. & MacDougall J. D. (1993) Gender differences in leucine kinetics and nitrogen balance in endurance athletes. *Journal of Applied Physiology* **75**, 2134–2141.

Pilon V. A., Howanitz P. J., Howanitz J. H. & Domres N. (1981) Day to day variation in serum ferritin concentration in healthy subjects. *Clinical Chemistry* **7**, 78–82.

Roeser H. P. (1990) Iron. In Truswell A. S. (ed.) Recommended nutrient intakes; Australian papers, pp. 255. Australian Professional Publications, Sydney.

Ross W. D. & Marfell-Jones M. J. (1982) Kinanthropometry. In McDougall J. D. & Green H. A. (eds) *Physiological Testing of the Elite Athletes*, pp. 75–115. Mutual Press, Ottawa.

Ross W. D. & Ward R. (1984) Proportionality of Olympic athletes. In Carter J. E. L. (ed.) *Physical Structure of Olympic Athletes*, Part II, *Kinanthropometry of Olympic Athletes.* Karger, Basel, 110–143.

Rowland T. W. & Kelleher J. F. (1989) Iron deficiency in athletes; insights from high school swimmers. *American Journal of Diseases of Children* **143**, 197–200.

Tarnopolsky M. A., MacDougall J. D. & Atkinson S. A. (1988) Influence of protein intake and training status on nitrogen balance and lean body mass. *Journal of Applied Physiology* **64**, 187–193.

Tarnopolsky M. A., Atkinson S. A., MacDougall J. D., Chesley A., Phillips S. & Schwarcz H. P. (1992) Evaluation of protein requirements for trained strength athletes. *Journal of Applied Physiology* **73**, 1986–1995.

Telford R. D., Egerton W. J., Hahn A. G. & Pang P. M.

(1988) Skinfold measures and weight controls in elite athletes. *Excel* 5, 21–24.

Thomas D. E., Brotherhood J. R. & Brand J. C. (1991) Carbohydrate feeding before exercise: Effect of glycaemic index. *International Journal of Sports Medicine* 12, 180–186.

Van der Beek E. J. (1985) Vitamins and endurance training. Food for running or faddish claims? *Sports Medicine* 2, 175–197.

van Erp-Baart A. M. J., Saris W. M. H., Binkhorst R. A., Vos J. A. & Elvers J. W. H. (1989) Nationwide survey on nutritional habits of elite athletes. Part II Mineral and vitamin intake. *International Journal of Sports Medicine* 10 (Suppl. 1), S11–16.

Walberg J. L., Leidy M. K., Sturgill D. J., Hinkle D. E., Ritchey S. J. & Sebolt D. R (1988) Macronutrient content of a hypoenergy diet affects nitrogen retention and muscle function in weight lifters. *International Journal of Sports Medicine* 9, 261–266.

Yadrick M. K., Kenny M. A. & Winterfeldt E. A. (1989) Iron, copper and zinc status: Response to supplementation with zinc or zinc and iron in adult females. *American Journal of Clinical Nutrition* 49, 145–150.

CHAPTER 6

ENVIRONMENTAL STRESS

F. S. Pyke and J. R. Sutton

The stress associated with training and competition is often exacerbated by the environment. High air temperatures or humidity, for example, can induce competition for blood between the skin and the muscles and decrease endurance performance, sometimes even causing progressive dehydration and collapse. This was clearly evident in the cases of British runner Jim Peters during the 1954 Commonwealth Games men's marathon in Vancouver and Gabriella Anderson-Shiess during the women's marathon in the 1984 Los Angeles Olympics. At high altitude the low oxygen pressure in the air can severely limit the capabilities of the oxygen transport system and endurance performances in the 1968 Olympic Games in Mexico City suffered as a result of this problem. The smog-filled air of many bigger cities can also make breathing difficult and imposes an additional stress on the athlete. It has therefore become important for host cities of major athletic competitions to meet acceptable standards of air quality in order to protect the competitors' health. Moreover, the combination of cold and high altitude or heat and air pollution can affect performance even more negatively and, in some situations, poses a serious threat to health and survival. Travel across time zones, particularly to an unaccustomed climate, can sometimes undo the most carefully planned training programme and have a devastating effect on sports performance. This chapter therefore attempts to describe the physiological responses to each of these environ-

mental stresses. It also offers advice that will assist athletes to optimize their performance in these conditions and briefly addresses the health issues related to exercise in harsh environments.

HOT AND COLD CLIMATES

Principles of Body Temperature Regulation

The human is referred to as a homeotherm and is capable of maintaining a relatively constant internal temperature despite being exposed to a wide range of environmental conditions. The core temperature of the body fluctuates at around 37°C, while the peripheral tissues such as the skin are usually cooler and vary according to the nature of the environmental conditions. Depending on the type of exercise involved, between 80 and 90% of the chemical energy available to move the body is transformed into heat energy and heavy exercise in warm conditions can elevate core body temperature to above 40°C. On the other hand, if the person is inactive and the climate is cold, the body may not produce enough heat to prevent reductions in core body temperature to below 35°C, thus creating a condition known as hypothermia or 'exposure'.

Body temperature is controlled by the hypothalamus, an organ located in the third ventricle of the brain. The hypothalamus not only acts as a thermal sensor but it also integrates information from other parts of body and then produces responses that either conserve or remove heat. Depending on the circumstances involved, these effector responses include constriction or dilation of the cutaneous blood vessels and either shivering or sweating. The hypothalamus is thought to function in the same manner as an electrical thermostat. If the integrated sensory information from the thermoreceptors throughout the body suggests that the body temperature is above the set point of the hypothalamus, there is a discharge of efferent impulses from its anterior portion to effect mechanisms of heat removal, such as cutaneous vasodilation and sweating. Conversely, if the integrated sensory information indicates that body temperature is below the set point, the posterior area of the hypothalamus activates mechanisms that conserve body heat, such as cutaneous vasoconstriction and shivering.

Physical Avenues of Heat Exchange

A body is in thermal balance if the algebraic sum of all avenues of gaining or losing heat equals zero. This is expressed in the partitional heat exchange equation

$$M \pm R \pm K \pm C - E \pm W \pm S = 0$$

where

M = metabolism	E = evaporation
R = radiation	W = work done
K = conduction	S = heat storage
C = convection	

The separate parts of this equation include:

METABOLISM

Metabolic heat production is elevated during exercise (10–20 times resting levels) and by shivering (up to four times resting levels) and represents the total energy released by aerobic and anaerobic processes. It is usually estimated from calculations of respiratory gas exchange.

RADIATION

Electromagnetic energy waves pass between bodies of different temperature. This is the way that the earth receives heat by radiation from the sun. Both solar and ground radiation heat up the marathon runners on a warm day, whereas on a cold winter's day the body radiates heat to the objects surrounding it. Radiant temperature is best measured by a thermometer placed inside a black metal sphere and this is often referred to as the black bulb or globe temperature. Light-coloured clothing absorbs less heat than darker clothing. Moreover the radiating surface area is effectively reduced by 10–15% when a person changes posture from a standing to a sitting position.

CONDUCTION

When objects differing in temperature come into contact with each other, heat is exchanged by conduction. The rate of transfer of heat from one object to another is dependent on the temperature difference between them and their respective thermal conductivities. Because metals are good conductors, the mountaineer can lose heat rapidly to ice axes, metal pitons and cold rocks, and the long-distance runner can gain a small amount of conducted heat from contact with a hot road. Conductive heat loss represents only a small proportion of total heat exchange between the body and the environment; however, the thermal conductivity of the medium in which the body is placed is of vital importance. Because water is a better conductor than air, body heat is lost more quickly in water than in air at the same temperature, which explains why immersion hypothermia can occur very rapidly. When still air is trapped in clothing it provides excellent insulation against the cold.

CONVECTION

Heat exchange by convection requires a medium of fluid or air to move across the body. This occurs when the body is fanned by a breeze or when its movement creates air or water movement, such as in cycling, skiing or swimming. Convective heat loss can become a serious problem in cold climates when a strong wind is blowing. This is known as the wind chill factor. Clothing keeps the air still and warm and minimizes heat loss. On the other hand, in climates when the air is hotter than the body, heat can be gained by convection.

EVAPORATION

The most important avenue of heat loss during exercise in any climate is evaporation. This process occurs when water changes state from liquid to vapour and heat is taken from the body surface. The energy required to do this is called the latent heat of vaporization and amounts to 2428 kJ·L⁻¹ of fluid evaporated. In the human, evaporative heat loss occurs as a result of diffusion of water through the skin (insensible perspiration), secretion of sweat from eccrine (thermally stimulated) and apocrine (emotionally stimulated) sweat glands and water losses from the respiratory tract. By far the most significant source of evaporative heat loss is provided by eccrine sweating, which can occur at rates of up to 2 L·h⁻¹. If the sweating process is not available as a means of heat dissipation in hot conditions the core temperature of a vigorously exercising person (metabolism 2700 kJ·h⁻¹) can rise from 37 to 40°C in only 20 min. As evaporation is greatly reduced when the relative humidity is high, the level of thermal stress is often much higher in hot, humid climates than in hot, dry ones.

WORK

Some of the chemical energy is transformed in the body into mechanical energy or work done. In most cases this is negative for work accomplished against external resistances, but it can also be positive when forces are imposed upon the body, such as in downhill running.

HEAT STORAGE

A gain in body temperature indicates that heat is being stored. This is usually estimated from the

Table 6.1 Partitioning of heat loss to the environment while exercising in different conditions

Air temperature	Radiation Convection Conduction	Evaporation
20°C	50%	50%
25°C	35%	65%
30°C	20%	80%
35°C	0%	100%

change in mean body temperature over a period of time and the specific heat of the body.

Each of the components of partitional heat exchange can be measured during exercise in different environmental conditions. The parts played by radiation, convection and conduction depend on the nature of these conditions as shown in Table 6.1. When the climate is cool (20°C) there is an even proportion of heat lost by radiation, convection and conduction on the one hand and evaporation on the other. As the air temperature increases, the greater reliance on evaporative heat loss becomes clearly evident, as it becomes more difficult to exchange heat by the other physical avenues along a temperature gradient from the body to the environment. The balance achieved between heat gain and heat loss in different climatic conditions is shown in Fig. 6.1.

Body Defences Against Temperature Change

Behavioural rather than physiological factors determine survival in temperature extremes. These

Fig. 6.1 The balance between heat gain and heat loss in different climatic conditions.

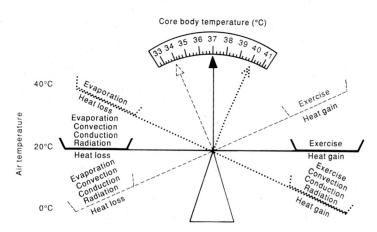

131

include drinking sufficient water, wearing appropriate clothes and seeking shelter from excessive heat or cold. However, the body has some defence against either losing too much heat or overheating. The first line of defence is to alter the flow of blood through the periphery (of the skin). The hypothalamus sends nervous impulses to the vasomotor centre in the brain stem, which controls the smooth muscle of the peripheral arterioles and hence the flow of blood from the core to the surface of the body.

In cold air the blood flow to the uncovered skin is restricted. This occurs in most areas of the body but is particularly so in the extremities which, because of their large surface area/mass ratio, are well adapted for heat exchange. Restriction of blood flow to the skin of the head and face is less well regulated than in the limbs. Thus, the head and face are sites of excessive heat loss. It is therefore important in cold zones to cover the head while hiking or mountain climbing, or to keep the head out of the water during extended periods of immersion.

When the air is warm, blood is directed as a result of cutaneous vasodilation from the core of the body to the surface where heat can be removed. However, this increased blood supply to the skin places a greater strain on the circulatory system, which now distributes blood to a much wider area. Central blood pressure is maintained by compensatory vasoconstriction in the less active vascular beds that supply the intestines and kidneys. Despite this, there is a characteristic rise in heart rate during exercise in hot conditions.

The second line of defence against overheating is the sweating response. Apocrine sweat glands are found on the palms of the hands, soles of the feet, the armpits and the groin and are activated by emotional stimuli. Eccrine sweat glands are distributed more evenly over the body, respond to thermal stimuli and are controlled by the anterior hypothalamus. Eccrine sweating is the principal means of controlling body temperature during exercise in either cool or warm conditions.

The second line of defence of the body to prevent excess body cooling is the involuntary contraction of the muscles known as shivering. While this can elevate resting metabolism four-fold it interferes with skilful movement and is a last resort in keeping the body warm.

Factors to Consider in Hot Environments

CHARACTERISTICS OF THE ENVIRONMENT

Hot/dry or desert conditions are characterized by high air temperatures (35–50°C), low humidity (0–30%) and intense solar radiation. Heat loss by radiation, conduction and convection is difficult, but dry air favours evaporation of sweat. Hot/wet or tropical conditions rarely include air temperatures that exceed 35°C, but as the humidity is high (70%) the loss of heat by the evaporation of sweat becomes less effective as sweat falls from the skin without evaporating.

There are four measurable factors which determine the level of heat stress imposed by the environment: air temperature; radiant temperature of the surroundings; humidity; and amount of air movement. It is essential that all these factors are considered in any assessment, and the importance of each component will vary with the environmental circumstances.

The black bulb, dry bulb and wet bulb thermometers are used to measure radiant temperature, air temperature and relative humidity respectively. Air movement can be measured with either a vane or a cup anemometer. There have been many attempts to include two or more of these factors in a single index of heat stress and, furthermore, to include all four factors together with some consideration of the level of energy expenditure and the clothing of the individual concerned. An excellent summary of these indices is presented by Leithead and Lind (1964).

One useful scale is the WBGT (wet bulb globe temperature) index. In a single value it combines the effects of solar and ground radiation, air temperature, humidity and wind speed. The WBGT index (outdoors) = $0.7X$ wet bulb temperature + $0.2X$ black bulb temperature + $0.1X$ dry bulb temperature. This simple index is very useful for evaluating the amount and level of training which should be administered in hot conditions. In running sports such as athletics, soccer, field hockey, rugby and Australian football it is recommended that caution be exerted when the WBGT index reaches 25°C and that activity be considered unsafe for the poorly conditioned and unacclimatized when it exceeds 28°C. The American College of Sports Medicine position paper (1984) on heat injuries and distance running recommends that such events should not be conducted when the WBGT index exceeds 28°C. During the summer months organizers should try to schedule highly active sports in the early morning or evening rather than mid-afternoon. If this is not possible they should cancel or postpone events until conditions become more suitable.

Another index of thermal strain is the predicted 4 h sweat rate (P4SR). This index expresses, by means of a nomogram the stress imposed by a hot environment in terms of the amount of sweat which would be secreted by fit, acclimatized young men in 4 h. The P4SR has an advantage over other heat indices in that, in addition to air temperature, temperature of the surroundings, humidity and wind speed, it also takes into account the energy expenditure and clothing of the subject. However, the P4SR is quite cumbersome to use and is more appropriate for industrial than sporting situations. The necessary calculations are presented by Leithead and Lind (1964). It is suggested that a P4SR of 4.5 L represents a safe limit of thermal stress for young men but that this should be reduced to 3 L for those aged 45 years and over. These limits should be modified if the duration of exposure exceeds 4 h and are clearly impractical in the sporting arena.

CHARACTERISTICS OF THE INDIVIDUAL

Body build

The index of body build, which has been used most commonly in studies of heat tolerance, is that of the body surface area to mass ratio. A prepubertal child may have a ratio of up to 50% greater than a medium-sized man while for a medium-sized woman it may be 10% greater. However, there are wide individual differences in surface area/mass ratio. Those with a linear physique (ectomorph) have a higher ratio than those who are muscular or fat (mesomorph or endomorph). When working at the same rate a larger person can be expected to produce more heat in relation to surface area than a smaller person. Hence in warm, humid conditions which restrict heat dissipation, the large person will store heat throughout the work period while a smaller person might easily maintain heat balance. In extreme heat (40–50°C) persons with high surface area/mass ratios produce less heat than those with low ratios, but lose their advantage due to greater heat gain by radiation and convection. However, in humid heat, where ambient temperatures (30°C) are below that of the skin, individuals with high surface area/mass ratios have an advantage compared with those with low ratios. This is the result of an additive effect of both lower heat production and a better facility for heat loss by evaporation, radiation and convection. Hence the relationship between physique and heat tolerance is dependent on whether the ambient temperature is above or below the temperature of the skin.

Body composition

The lower heat tolerance of obese compared with lean individuals has been commonly recorded. This response has been attributed to a number of factors. First, the higher surface area/mass ratio of the lean person has already been addressed. Second, the specific heat of fat tissue is considerably lower than that of lean tissue. Hence a given heat load per unit of body mass will produce a higher elevation of body temperature in the obese than in the lean. Third, the cardiovascular fitness level of the obese is usually lower than that of the lean. The resultant cardiovascular strain imposed by hot conditions would therefore be greater in the obese individual.

Age

An indication of the reduced tolerance of older men can be seen in reports on victims of heat stroke. When working in the heat, older men have been shown to have higher rectal temperatures than young men, this difference being greater at higher levels of climatic stress and as the duration of exposure is increased. Wagner et al. (1972) reported that young men (20–30 years) evaporated more sweat per degree rise in rectal temperature and had lower skin temperatures than older men (45–70 years), which indicated an earlier onset of sweating. This reduced the requirement of the young men for skin blood flow in heat transport and therefore minimized the circulatory strain experienced during work in the heat. These observed differences between age groups are complicated by the general deterioration in endurance fitness that occurs with age; however, if fitness is maintained, the tolerance for heat remains high. Bar-Or (1984) gives several reasons for young children being more prone to heat-related injuries than adults. These included a higher body surface area to mass ratio, a higher energy cost of walking or running, a poorer sweating response and a less mature cardiovascular system. Despite these disadvantages, children can acclimatize to exercise in hot conditions, but this is achieved more slowly and to a lesser degree. Interestingly, children do not seem to perceive that they have problems in this area and therefore must be supervised carefully.

Gender

Early research suggested that women were less tolerant than men to work in the heat because of their lower sweating rates. However, this may be somewhat of an advantage in that body water is conserved rather than wasted (Wyndham et al. 1965). More recent studies in which men and women either had an equivalent level of aerobic power or exercised at the same relative work intensity have indicated very little difference in exercise–heat tolerance between the sexes (Drinkwater 1977; Paolone et al. 1977). Hence as in age-group comparisons, it can be strongly argued that aerobic power should be considered as an independent variable when evaluating the differences between males and females. It seems that aerobic fitness is a more important consideration than either age or gender in determining the tolerance for hot conditions.

HEAT ACCLIMATIZATION

Tolerance for heat is improved through acclimatization. It is essential that time is allowed for this to occur if a person is required to exercise in the heat following a sojourn in a cool climate. This process enhances the circulatory and sweating responses which facilitate heat dissipation and minimize increases in body temperature. More specifically, acclimatization is characterized by an increase in the efficiency of the sweating mechanism. Improvements in the capacity to sweat and the ability to commence sweating sooner have been commonly reported, and there are strong suggestions that there is a more even distribution of sweat over the skin surface. These mechanisms increase the temperature gradient between the core and the periphery and permit heat release with a smaller flow of blood required to the skin. The accompanying larger blood flow to the muscles during work allows more energy to be provided aerobically. The acclimatized person therefore produces less lactic acid during intensive submaximal work, and hence work time is extended.

During a standard exercise–heat tolerance test, the acclimatized person will also display an improved circulatory stability (reduced heart rate) and a reduction in core temperature. Increases in plasma volume that have been reported to occur with acclimatization are likely to contribute to this adjustment, which is also accompanied by both renal and sweat gland salt conservation. As an individual becomes acclimatized the sweat progressively contains less salt. However, the acclimatization process is retarded by dehydration and, for optimal adaptation to occur, fluid balance should be maintained during the recovery period between daily bouts of work in the heat.

It is generally agreed that between 60 and 90 min of moderate work per day in hot environments will result in almost complete acclimatization in 7–10 days. The magnitude and rate of de- and re-acclimatization also seems to be dependent on the level of physical fitness of the subject.

Intensive physical training in a cool environment greatly improves thermoregulatory responses but does not produce the full acclimatory adaptation obtained by actually training in the heat. However, the elevation of rectal temperature to nearly 40°C in interval running training sessions thus provides a stimulus for the improvement in circulatory and thermoregulatory responses, which are characteristic of the acclimatized individual.

The procedure of adding extra layers of clothing during winter training as preparation for an event held in the heat has been investigated as a means of promoting acclimatization. However, despite producing elevated thermoregulatory responses during each training session the practice has met with only limited success as a method of artificial acclimatization (Dawson & Pyke 1988).

CLOTHING

Evaporative cooling is seriously restricted by barriers of impermeable clothing. A humid microclimate develops between the skin and the garments, which promotes a rise in skin temperature as well as profuse sweating and fluid loss, without adequate evaporative cooling.

Equipment used in American football impairs body temperature regulation. The heat loss barrier of the uniform prevents evaporation of sweat and results in high skin temperatures in areas covered by the pads and clothing, as well as a higher rectal temperature, sweat rate and heart rate than when wearing shorts alone or shorts and a backpack of equivalent weight to the uniform. There was also a slower decrease of rectal temperature in the recovery period after exercise when still wearing the uniform (Matthews *et al*. 1969). A case is therefore made for removing the uniform to promote cooling after strenuous exercise on the football field. As a result of this research the fish-net jersey is now used by many football teams during late summer practices and early season games in the United States.

Unlike American football uniforms, which are necessary for bodily protection, those used in Australia present very few heat problems if they are made from open weave cotton or woollen fibres rather than close weave synthetic fibres, such as nylon. On extremely hot days evaporation can be enhanced by pulling the jersey out of the shorts during rest periods to expose the skin surface of the abdomen, back and chest. The amount of protective tape used should also be reduced to a minimum. Short-sleeved garments allow a greater surface area to contribute to the process of evaporative cooling but also increase the chance of being

sunburned. In many sports, hats are valuable for protection against the sun. Cricket players can minimize heat problems by wearing hats and white clothing with long sleeves made from natural fibres and allowing frequent breaks in play for drinks.

The rubber sweat suits worn by many people to lose weight are potentially dangerous and have resulted in death from heat stroke (Brahams 1988). Even though sweating is profuse it is not evaporated through the impermeable suit and the body temperature can rise to critical levels.

FLUID REPLACEMENT

If the plasma volume is significantly reduced as a result of dehydration or if the blood flow to the muscles is compromised in any way, as during exercise in hot conditions, endurance performance and temperature regulation are impaired. Performance decrements have been noted following dehydration of 2% bodyweight. At greater levels of dehydration there are dramatic declines in endurance performance and elevations in heart rate and rectal temperature.

In order to prevent these problems it is essential that the body fluids lost in sweating are replaced. In addition to the water and salt lost in sweat, prolonged exercise can produce hypoglycaemia and glycogen depletion, both of which contribute to fatigue. The volume and composition of any replacement fluid then become important considerations in endurance performance.

While the nature of fluid replacement depends to some extent on the individual concerned, the intensity of the effort and the environmental conditions, there are some useful guide-lines to follow. One of the key factors is the emptying rate of the fluid from the stomach into the small intestine where it can be readily absorbed into the bloodstream. While there is great individual variation in this function, the following factors should be considered.

Fluid volume

The optimal rate of fluid intake for attenuating hyperthermia and maintaining performance is not yet clear. During low-intensity exercise, studies show that this is best achieved by a replacement rate that closely matches sweat rate (Pitts *et al.* 1944). However, as there is some gastric discomfort in consuming large volumes during more intensive exercise, in these circumstances it is more usual to only replace between 40 and 50% of sweat loss. While this procedure seems to be adequate its precise effect on both temperature regulation and performance remains unknown. Studies need to be conducted that evaluate the efficacy of replacing a higher percentage (75–80%) of sweat loss during prolonged intensive exercise.

Temperature of fluid

Cold fluids (5–10°C) empty from the stomach faster than warmer ones and are preferred. There is no strong evidence that fluids ingested at cold temperatures cause stomach cramps or electro-cardiogram irregularities.

Fluid composition

Sweat contains many of the constituents of plasma but in much lower concentrations. Principal electro-lytes, such as sodium and chloride, are about one-third as concentrated in sweat as in plasma. These sweat concentrations are usually lower in an acclimatized person and higher during heavy exercise when the sweat rate is higher. Hence, as the body loses more water than electrolytes during exercise, the body fluids actually become concentrated. Therefore there is a greater need to replace water than electrolytes during periods of heavy sweating. However, there may be occasions when drinking solutions containing small amounts of electrolytes can be beneficial (e.g. when there is prolonged repeated exposure to exercise and heat, or a diet that is salt-restricted). Salt tablets should not be used as a substitute for fluid replacement during exercise as water is the primary need.

The addition of carbohydrate (CHO) to fluid replacement beverages can also be beneficial during prolonged exercise when there is an inadequate supply of endogenous CHO to meet energy re-quirements. Glucose, glucose polymers and sucrose are equally effective in this process. On the other hand, fructose is not actively absorbed in humans and can produce gastrointestinal distress.

Hence there are circumstances during prolonged exercise when it is beneficial to ingest fluid con-taining both CHO and electrolytes. This also enhances palatability and is the rationale behind the composition of most commercially available sports drinks.

Key factors such as the emptying rate of fluid from the stomach into the small intestine and the absorption rate from the intestine itself must also be considered. Gastric emptying is influenced by many factors, most noticeably the volume and caloric content of the ingested fluid. Smaller and more concentrated drinks empty more slowly than larger more dilute ones. However, there are great differences between individuals in gastric emptying rates. The rate of intestinal absorption is increased in the presence of glucose and sodium (Mitchell 1988).

The extent of fluid replacement depends on the individual concerned, the intensity and duration of effort, the environmental conditions and the state of training/heat acclimatization. The following provides some useful guide-lines for replacing fluid during sporting events of different durations.

Fluid replacement guide-lines

For events lasting less than 1 h, 300–500 mL of a 6–10% CHO beverage is recommended pre-event (0–15 min), and cool (5–15°C) water in a volume approximating half the subject's sweat rate is recom-mended during exercise. For events between 1–3 h long, 300–500 mL of water is recommended pre-event, and 800–1600 mL per h of a 6–8% CHO solution with 10–20 mEq Na$^+$ is recommended during exercise. For events longer than 3 h, 300–500 mL of water is recommended pre-event, and 500–1000 mL per h of a 6–8% CHO beverage with 20–30 mEq Na$^+$ is recommended during exercise. In recovery, a beverage containing 5–10% CHO with 30–40 mEq Na$^+$ should be ingested in the first 2 h to maximize glycogen repletion (Gisolfi & Duchman 1992).

In summary, in most sport played in warm conditions and involving high rates of sweating, cool water is an ideal replacement. However, low concentrations of CHO (6–8%) and electrolytes enhance palatability and encourage drinking and therefore can be beneficial during prolonged exercise, particularly in warm conditions.

In cooler conditions where sweat losses and the demand for fluid may not be as great, the addition of higher concentrations of CHO (up to 10% CHO) enhance the availability and utilization of blood-borne glucose.

Coaches should encourage participants to drink cold fluid (300–500 mL) 15 min before any contest that relies on endurance capabilities. Regularly scheduled drinks throughout the contest (150–250 mL every 15–20 min) will assist in maintaining the integrity of the circulation and permit the required effort to be continued safely (Fig. 6.2). As the sensation of thirst lags considerably behind a state of negative water balance, thirst should not be used as the signal to drink, as the negative effects of dehydration may be experienced well before a person feels thirsty. Hence, forced and regular drinking rather than *ad libitum* consumption is essential to avoid dehydration (Pitts *et al.* 1944).

Athletes should also be warned that inducing weight loss by sweating does not result in fat loss. Jockeys, rowers, boxers and weight-lifters, who reach weight limits by inducing high sweat losses, are in danger of developing severe medical problems associated with chronic dehydration. Exercising in rubber sweat suits or prolonged sojourns in saunas are also strongly discouraged for the active sportsperson. Coaches should make daily weight checks before and after practice and encourage athletes to regain at least 80% of the weight lost in the previous session before embarking on another training session. Athletes should be encouraged to drink fluids freely between vigorous training sessions conducted in warm conditions. Alcohol is not an option in this respect, as it acts as a diuretic and encourages dehydration rather than alleviates it.

SYMPTOMS AND TREATMENT OF HEAT ILLNESS

Heat cramps

Heat cramps are caused by heavy and prolonged sweating and/or inadequate salt intake and occur in the muscles involved in the exercise. They are relieved by resting in a cool environment, replacing fluid (containing saline) and adding salt to the diet.

Heat syncope

Peripheral vasodilation associated with high environmental temperatures and subsequent pooling of blood in the veins creates instability in the circulation. This can lead to fainting (syncope) and collapse, particularly in older individuals with poor vasomotor tone. The condition is characterized by weakness, fatigue and hypotension, and is most common immediately following exercise when venous return is not being assisted by the action of the muscles. Relief is provided by having the collapsed person lie down in a cool environment, elevating the legs and, when he or she is conscious, providing fluid replacement.

Heat exhaustion and heat stroke

Heat exhaustion and heat stroke are part of a continuum and are caused by heavy and prolonged sweating in hot conditions with inadequate fluid intake or time for acclimatization. It is characterized by dizziness, headache, nausea, rapid pulse, elevated core and skin temperatures and a lack of co-ordination. The patient may progress to fits or loss of consciousness which characterizes severe heat stroke.

The early descriptions of heat stroke incurred during prolonged marches noted a progressive decline in the ability to sweat, accompanied by confusion, delirium, collapse, coma and a hot, dry skin. However, as noted by Sutton *et al.* (1972) in fun runs of short duration, heat stroke with rectal temperatures of 42–43°C may occur without marked dehydration in patients whose skin is moist and cool, thus providing a confusing clinical picture (Fig. 6.3).

Although the exact mechanisms causing heat stroke are unknown, Moseley and Gisolfi (1993) have likened it to septic shock. In susceptible individuals exercising in the heat can result in a relatively ischaemic bowel which causes an impairment of bowel–mucosal barrier function. Gut bacteria are absorbed into the portal and the systemic blood with systemic endotoxaemia resulting. A series of biochemical/cytokine cascades occur, especially interleukin-1 and lipopolysaccharide. This then gives rise to further hormonal activation and

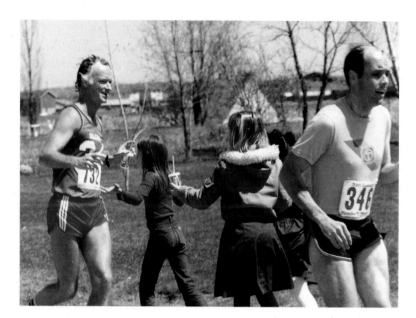

Fig. 6.2 Runners using a drink station in a distance running event.

subsequent multiorgan failure. This sequence is seen diagrammatically in Fig. 6.4.

Treatment must involve immediate attempts to reduce body temperature. This is best accomplished by intravenous fluid administration and by the application of ice-cold sponges, ice packs and cold sprays. The most appropriate means of preventing and treating exercise-induced thermal illness has been reviewed recently by Sutton (1989).

The patient was hypotensive, with a blood pressure of 60 mmHg systolic, a tachycardia of 180 beats·min⁻¹ and appeared cold and sweaty. His oral temperature was low — 35.5°C. Nevertheless, I took his rectal temperature and there it was — 42°C.

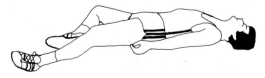

Fig. 6.3 Heat stroke in a runner. Note the difference in rectal and oral temperature.

Factors to Consider in Cold Conditions

CHARACTERISTICS OF THE ENVIRONMENT

Forced air convection increases dramatically with greater air movement around the body. This occurs particularly when the wind is blowing strongly or when the person is moving rapidly. This 'wind chill' factor is such that a temperature of 4°C in still air becomes −9°C if a 40 km·h⁻¹ wind is blowing or if a skier or a cyclist is moving at that speed. In order to retain body warmth it is necessary to wear a windproof overgarment. The hiker, mountaineer or orienteer should be prepared for changes in climatic conditions and therefore should carry extra water and windproof clothing. Similarly, the skier or cyclist should guard against the cold created by travelling at high speeds. This can be a particular problem when cycling after the swim stage of a triathlon for example.

CHARACTERISTICS OF THE INDIVIDUAL

Fat tissue provides insulation against the cold. A combination of cutaneous vasoconstriction and subcutaneous fat offers a thick overcoat of insulated tissue. Swimmers who compete in distance events in cold lakes, rivers and oceans often smear grease

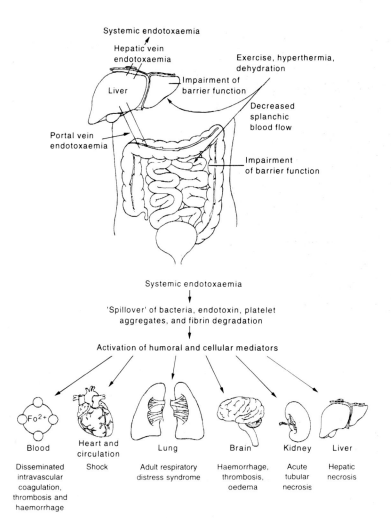

Fig. 6.4 Mechanisms of exercise hyperthermia (Sutton 1994).

on their skin for extra insulation. On the other hand thin pre-adolescent children with a high surface area/mass ratio are very susceptible to rapid cooling while swimming in cold water and core body temperatures below 35°C have been commonly observed in children after swimming in 20°C water temperatures. This is of some concern to swimming coaches who rely on the child's perception of cold to avoid the problem. A lean and ambitious young swimmer could easily become hypothermic while training in an unheated pool and should be watched carefully. Comparisons between the sexes in terms of cold tolerance is complicated by differences in relative exercise intensity, somatotype and body composition.

The level of endurance fitness of the individual is also important in that the fitter person can continue exercise for longer than the less fit, as a high level of fitness assists in maintaining body temperature during prolonged efforts. If a marathon runner slows down towards the end of an event held on a very cold day, heat loss is likely to exceed heat production, resulting in hypothermia or 'exposure'. Such a scenario occurred in a 'go as you please' race in Hobart in 1903 and resulted in the deaths of two competitors (Sutton *et al.* 1972).

COLD ACCLIMATIZATION

There is much less known about acclimatization to cold than to heat. However, until more research is carried out, it is advisable that athletes experience cold conditions for 10 days before competition so as to decrease discomfort and lower their threshold for shivering. The elevation of metabolism by hormonal means in the process of non-shivering thermogenesis has been commonly observed in residents of cold climates but is a longer-term adjustment.

CLOTHING

Insulative clothing traps warm air close to the body and prevents heat loss by convection. One of the problems in sport is that the clothing thickness must vary both with the intensity of exercise and alterations in climatic conditions. More clothing is needed during rest than during exercise in the cold and more clothing is needed during light than heavy exercise. A doubling of the work rate from 3 to 6 METS (1 MET = resting metabolism) performed in 5°C air temperatures requires one-third of the insulation. During hiking in cool weather heavy sweating should be avoided as it can lead to rapid and excessive evaporative cooling when the person ceases to be active. In sub-zero temperatures sweat can also freeze into garments, replacing dead air space and destroying their insulatory value. Sweating can be minimized by reducing the activity level and/or making adjustments to clothing as the situation demands. Clothing insulation is also reduced if clothing such as down becomes wet from external sources. However, this is less of a problem with woollen garments than for the newer polypropylene materials. Waterproof overgarments are useful to maintain the insulatory value of inner layers but ideally should allow some ventilation, such as with cortex type material.

Clothing which permits insulation to be added or subtracted in accordance with the intensity of exercise is the most useful. Jackets that open down the front are more convenient than pullovers. Hoods that can be drawn back are ideal during intermittent activity. Drawstrings that allow clothes to be tightened or loosened at the collar, waist and arm and leg cuffs conveniently vary the insulative value of garments. It is more important to insulate the trunk than the extremities. A ratio of three units torso–two units limbs–one unit hands and

feet has been recommended (Kaufman 1982), and a cap or balaclava reduces heat loss from the head. Inactivity immediately after the heavy sweating induced by vigorous training or competition can invite rapid cooling and a dramatic fall in body temperature. This can occur on the interchange bench after an intensive period of play in a team game or perhaps as a result of an enforced rest during an endurance event. It is important to have warm dry clothing available to arrest any decrease in body temperature in these situations.

Heat loss by radiation can be minimized by curling the body up and reducing the surface area exposed. Such a behavioural response is common when resting in cold conditions. It is recommended that persons waiting to be rescued in cold water should don a life-jacket and adopt this knees-to-chest posture (referred to as HELP — Heat Escape Lessening Posture). In comparison with treading water with the body extended, the HELP posture has been shown to significantly reduce the rate of body cooling and increase survival time. An attempt should also be made to keep as much of the body out of the water as possible, as heat transfer to air is considerably less than to water. Also, the head is a site of considerable heat loss. Treading water or swimming for long periods is not recommended when the swimmer is threatened by hypothermia, as the movement of the limbs in cold water facilitates heat loss by convection. The decision to swim should only be made when the shore is close, otherwise waiting to be rescued is often a better proposition (Hayward et al. 1975).

SYMPTOMS AND TREATMENT OF COLD INJURY

Hypothermia

Hypothermia is characterized by extreme fatigue, shivering, loss of control of movement, disorientation, and poor judgement and reasoning. As the temperature decreases further, shivering ceases and the subject loses consciousness. When the core temperature falls below about 28°C the heart will fibrillate and the patient will die (Fig. 6.5).

The primary objective with an exposure victim is to minimize any further heat loss and add heat to the body. In the field it is important to place the

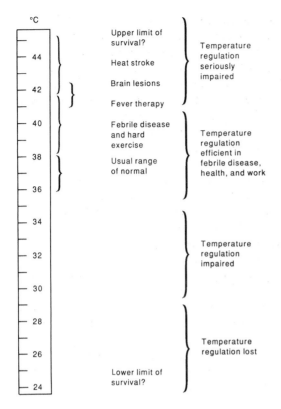

°C

- 44 — Upper limit of survival?

Heat stroke

- 42 — Brain lesions

Fever therapy

Temperature regulation seriously impaired

- 40 — Febrile disease and hard exercise

- 38 — Usual range of normal

Temperature regulation efficient in febrile disease, health, and work

- 36 —

- 34 —

- 32 — Temperature regulation impaired

- 30 —

- 28 —

- 26 — Temperature regulation lost

Lower limit of survival?

- 24 —

Fig. 6.5 Extremes of human body temperatures, defining the zones of temperature regulation (Du Bois 1948).

person out of the wind in the best shelter available, ensure that there is adequate insulation from the ground and replace wet with dry clothing. The individual should be warmed gradually either under blankets or in a preheated sleeping bag, and warm, sugared drinks should be administered. The patient must be kept awake until normal body temperature has been restored. If the patient is unconscious then attention to the airways and the usual management of the unconscious patient will apply. The in-hospital treatment is beyond the scope of this paper and the reader is referred to Mills (1983) for further details.

However, in the case of hypothermia the old maxim of 'prevention is better than cure' is very true. For a well-planned hiking expedition, all members of the party need to be fit and healthy, well briefed and mentally prepared, and must be wearing appropriate clothing and carrying emer-

gency sleeping equipment. Furthermore, if the weather changes it is prudent to seek shelter before the group becomes fatigued or darkness falls. In team games where interchange players are used, the bench should be well provided with warm clothing for insulation against cold, wind and possibly rain, during periods of substitution.

Frost-bite

Frost-bite is relatively common in the northern hemispheres but less so in Australia. It occurs with local cooling but also in the presence of generalized hypothermia, when the core temperature has fallen below 35°C. Tissues become frozen, interstitial crystals form and there is exudation of plasma with blister formation. There are also a number of metabolic changes that may potentiate further constriction and ischaemia. The most vulnerable parts of the body have a large surface-area-to-mass ratio, namely the fingers, toes, nose and ears. Tissues such as nerves, muscles and blood vessels may be damaged by temperatures above freezing. The affected part should be warmed in water heated to 40°C until it has thawed and should then be kept cool to reduce its metabolism and minimize inflammation. The part should then be covered and the person kept warm with blankets. In the field if there is likely to be re-freezing then the limb should not be thawed as the eventual loss of tissue will be much greater than if the limb had remained frozen. Again prevention is better than cure and the hands, feet and head must be kept covered with suitable and effective insulatory garments when exposed to extreme cold (Fig. 6.6).

ALTITUDE

As altitude increases there is a decrease in barometric pressure and the air becomes less dense. This offers some advantage for sprinters, jumpers and throwers who experience less resistance both for themselves and their implements. However, the opposite is true for endurance athletes. While the percentage of oxygen in the air remains constant with increasing elevation, the decrease in barometric pressure causes a reduction in the pressure of oxygen. This can

Fig. 6.6 Various examples of frost-bite. (a) Superficial frost-bite. (b) Deeper frost-bite. (c) Deep frost-bite. (d) Toes amputated because of frost-bite. (e) Fingers amputated because of frost-bite.

(a)

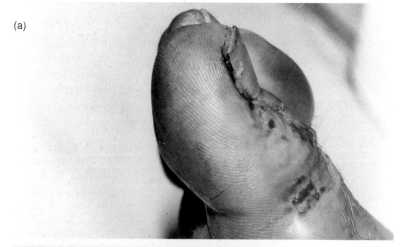

(b)

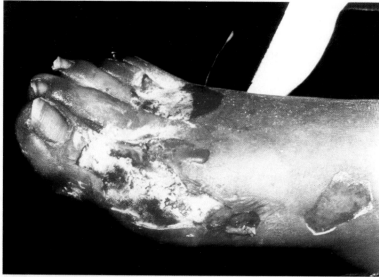

(c)

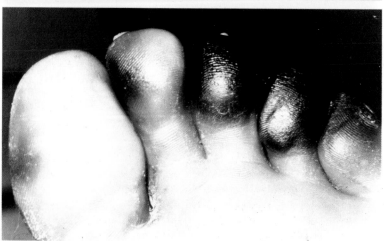

(d)

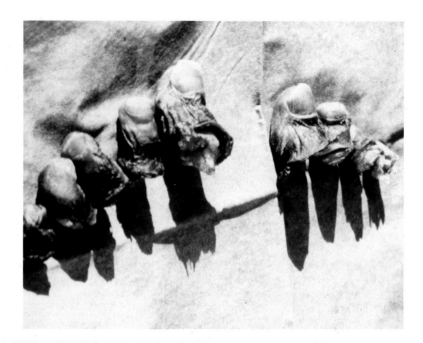

(e)

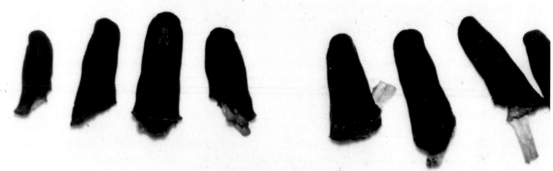

result in the pressure of oxygen in inspired air (P_{IO_2}) falling from about 150 mmHg at sea level to 110 mmHg at Mexico City (2300 m) to 75 mmHg at Pikes Peak (4300 m) and to 43 mmHg at the summit of Mt Everest (8848 m). There is also an accompanying decline in the pressure of oxygen in the lungs (P_{AO_2}) consequently lowering the pressure of oxygen in the arterial blood (P_{AO_2}). It is this pressure that determines the capacity of the blood to carry oxygen, most of which combines with haemoglobin in the red blood cells. The sigmoid shape of the oxygen dissociation curve results in very little change in oxyhaemoglobin saturation from 98% at sea level to 90% at just over 3000 m. However, above this altitude the steeper part of the curve is involved and marked decreases in the

oxygen saturation of haemoglobin occur. On the summit of Mt Everest the P_{AO_2} falls below 28 mmHg and saturation is below 50%. These relationships are summarized in Fig. 6.7.

Acute Responses to Altitude

The immediate response to a lowered P_{O_2} in the arterial blood and a reduction in its oxygen carrying capacity is hyperventilation. This is brought about by the sensitivity to changes in arterial P_{O_2} of chemoreceptors located in the aortic and carotid bodies. This response increases alveolar oxygen pressure and enhances oxygen diffusion into the blood. Also, there is an increase in heart rate and cardiac output, the net effect of which is to maintain

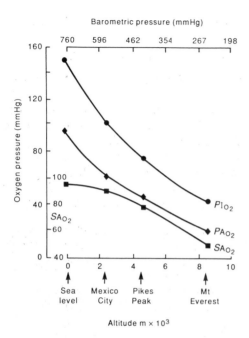

Barometric pressure (mmHg)

Fig. 6.7 Changes in barometric pressure, inspired P_{O_2}, alveolar P_{O_2} and oxyhaemoglobin saturation with altitude.

oxygen supply to the tissues in the presence of a reduced arterial blood oxygen content.

Initial reductions in plasma volume due to dehydration developed in cold, dry air are associated with increases in haemoglobin and haemocrit concentration. However, if this is excessive, greater blood viscosity makes blood flow difficult, decreases venous return and increases the work done by the heart. The concentration of 2,3-diphosphoglycerate, contained in red blood cells, increases during the first day at altitude and assists in unloading oxygen from haemoglobin in the muscle capillaries. This offsets the effect that hyperventilation has in lowering arterial carbon dioxide pressure and shifting the oxygen dissociation curve to the left. An initial increase in blood pH is partially compensated for by increased renal excretion of bicarbonate, although arterial pH always remains alkaline.

However, none of these adjustments is sufficient to overcome the initial shortfall in oxygen transport that occurs during exercise at altitudes above 1500 m. This is shown in values for maximal oxygen consumption which are reduced by approximately

3% for each 300 m above 1500 m. Hence in Mexico City the decrease in maximal oxygen consumption would approximate 10%. However, there is some individual variation in this response and the rate of decrease is more severe at high altitudes. Thus, on the summit of Mt Everest, $\dot{V}_{O_2max}$, for those who can reach that height, is reduced to less than one-third of sea-level $\dot{V}_{O_2max}$.

Altitude Acclimatization

After a period at high altitude some acclimatory adjustments occur. Pulmonary ventilation continues to be elevated and there are progressive increases in red blood cell mass and haemoglobin over several months, which help restore the oxygen content and oxygen transport. Also, there is improved capillarization and concentration of oxidative enzymes in the muscles, which assist in work performance. These adaptive changes improve endurance capabilities but never allow them to reach those achieved at sea level. The time for full acclimation depends on the altitude and the individual. It takes about 3 weeks to acclimate to moderate altitude (2300–2700 m). Despite allowing time for these adjustments at an altitude of 2300 m, maximal oxygen consumption will still fall 6–7% below that obtained at sea level. This means that the acclimation process has provided a 3–4% recovery towards sea-level performance. However, above 6000 m acclimatization is not possible and subjects will deteriorate, losing bodyweight and performance ability with prolonged exposure.

Altitude Training

Because the physiological adaptations to living at high altitude are similar to those resulting from endurance training, it has been suggested that for best results the stresses of altitude and training should be combined. While several studies have demonstrated that the sea-level performance of untrained subjects is improved after training at altitude, the same cannot be said for the well-trained athlete (Adams *et al.* 1975). The major problem with altitude training is that the intensity and volume of work must be lowered in order to cope with the environment. If a coach or athlete wishes to indulge in altitude training it is recommended that the selected altitude is only moderate (1800–2000 m) where the symptoms of mountain sickness are not felt and the work rate can be maintained at a reasonable level. Another strategy is to alternate short periods of training at moderate altitude and at sea level. At higher altitudes, it is unlikely that any of the physiological adjustments will compensate for forced reductions in training intensity. However, further investigation is necessary of the time course for adjustment to altitude training and subsequent sea-level performance and the individual variation in response to training at higher altitudes.

If the competition is going to be held at a higher altitude it is important to undertake some prior altitude training. It is essential to have a high level of aerobic fitness before departure from sea level, then gradually ascend to altitude at a rate of $300 \; m \cdot day^{-1}$ above 1500 m, accompanied by a gradual increase in the intensity of training. Low work intensity and long recovery periods are essential in the first few days at altitude until the symptoms of mountain sickness have disappeared. This is assisted by consuming large amounts of fluid and a CHO-rich diet to offset dehydration and improve exercise performance.

Altitude Illness

Rapid ascent to moderate and high altitude is often associated with several different illnesses.

ACUTE MOUNTAIN SICKNESS

This is a common condition experienced during the first 4–72 h at altitudes above 2000 m. It is associated with symptoms such as headache, irritability, insomnia, dizziness, nausea, anorexia and vomiting, the severity of which depends to a large extent on the speed of ascent. Acute mountain sickness (AMS) can be minimized if: the ascent progresses slowly from low to moderate altitude over several days; fluid and CHO intake in the diet are increased; and the training programme is kept light. Usually, the illness only lasts for 2 or 3 days. Acetazolamide (Diamox) has been demonstrated

to minimize the incidence of AMS (Sutton *et al.* 1979).

HIGH-ALTITUDE PULMONARY OEDEMA

This is a medical emergency and requires immediate treatment and evacuation if possible. The time course is similar to AMS. The predominant symptoms include breathlessness, coughing, chest discomfort and the production of often copious quantities of frothy, blood-stained sputum. The treatment involves resting the patient in an upright position, administering oxygen, frusemide (Lasix) and immediate evacuation, if possible (Fig. 6.8).

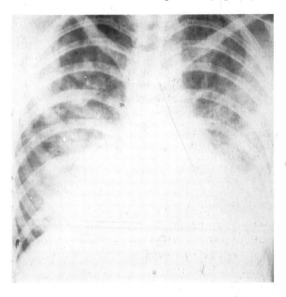

Fig. 6.8 High-altitude pulmonary oedema.

HIGH-ALTITUDE CEREBRAL OEDEMA

This is a rare but life-threatening condition that occurs at altitudes above 4000 m. Its symptoms include severe headache, disorientation, hallucinations and coma, and treatment requires oxygen therapy, intravenous corticosteroids and an immediate return to low altitude. Again the illness can be prevented by allowing time for acclimation during a slow ascent (Fig. 6.9).

HIGH-ALTITUDE RETINAL HAEMORRHAGE

At altitudes above 3500 m small haemorrhages may occur in the retina of the eye. They are usually

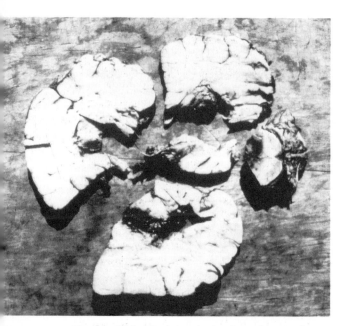

Fig. 6.9 High-altitude cerebral oedema: thrombosis and haemorrhage.

asymptomatic unless located in the macula region when visual disturbances occur (Fig. 6.10).

One might expect seasoned mountaineers to be at greatly reduced risk of incurring these altitude problems, but this is not necessarily so. Even such a great climber as Sir Edmund Hillary suffered several life-threatening high-altitude medical emergencies.

AIR POLLUTION

Air pollution or smog is common in large, densely populated cities and can have a serious effect on physical performance, particularly in individuals who suffer from diseases of the respiratory tract such as asthma, emphysema and chronic bronchitis. The heat of Los Angeles or the altitude of Mexico City can significantly add to the stress offered by polluted air and create a very difficult environment for the endurance athlete.

Constituents of Polluted Air

The primary constituents of smog include carbon monoxide, nitrogen dioxide, sulfur dioxide and particulate matter (dust, ash). Carbon monoxide is produced by incomplete combustion of organic fuel such as wood, petroleum and tobacco. Car exhausts are the major outdoor source of carbon monoxide but it is also contained in high concentrations in cigarette smoke. In a city with an abundance of sunshine such as Los Angeles, nitrogen dioxide emitted by car exhausts is converted by ultraviolet light rays to a form of secondary pollutant called ozone. In cool humid climates such as those experienced in London, sulfur dioxide from the burning of fossil fuels is oxidized in the presence of other air pollutants and sunlight and then reacts with water vapour in the air to form another secondary pollutant, sulfuric acid. This results in acid rain, which has destroyed extensive forests in Europe and more recently, in North America.

The formation of smog in a particular area is dependent on the air temperature and humidity, the wind speed and direction, and the geography of

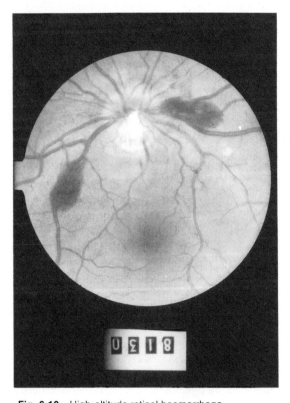

Fig. 6.10 High-altitude retinal haemorrhage.

the region. The pollution is usually worst in times of temperature inversions where a layer of cool air next to the ground is trapped by warmer air above it. Also, prevailing on-shore breezes can trap smog against the backdrop of mountains such as in Los Angeles and the cold, humid climate of some parts of Europe encourages excess burning of oil and coal for heating homes and buildings, thus presenting an ideal environment for the formation of smog.

Physiological Responses to Pollutants

The affinity of haemoglobin for carbon monoxide is more than 200 times greater than for oxygen. Hence, in the presence of carbon monoxide, there are substantial reductions in the oxygen-carrying capacity of the blood. It is not unusual to measure 5% carboxyhaemoglobin levels in persons residing in polluted areas or walking or driving during the 'rush hour' traffic. This is about the same concentration as might be found in a light to moderate smoker (20 cigarettes per day). Also, the binding of oxygen to haemoglobin is much stronger in the presence of carbon monoxide. This makes it more difficult to unload oxygen from haemoglobin in the muscle capillaries, effectively shifting the oxygen dissociation curve to the left and decreasing oxygen utilization.

The other constituents of polluted air all affect the respiratory passages. For example, sulfur dioxide increases airways resistance due to bronchoconstriction. Ozone makes it even more difficult to breathe and has an irritating effect on the eyes, nose and throat. Particulate matter irritates the large airways and stimulates reflex coughing and bronchoconstriction. These effects are much more marked in patients with increased airways reactivity, for example the asthmatic.

These physiological responses to pollutants also affect sports performance. Maximal oxygen consumption is reduced significantly (4–5%) when the carboxyhaemoglobin saturation exceeds 5% and then decreases linearly from this point (Horvath 1982). The detrimental effects of carbon monoxide can be felt within 1 or 2 h of being in a smoggy city containing heavy traffic. Not only does it produce significant reductions in endurance performance but also deterioration in visual acuity and mental functions, which can result in judgemental errors in some sports. Carbon monoxide can also distress athletes by causing headaches, particularly in hot weather.

The respiratory discomfort experienced when inhaling other pollutants is magnified during exercise when the ventilatory volume is increased. This can impair performance when breathing high concentrations of ozone (0.75 parts 10^{-6}). Significant reductions in maximal work rate, pulmonary ventilation, oxygen consumption and heart rate have been observed. There are also detrimental psychological effects associated with the mere smell of ozone that can affect an athlete's willingness to perform. Sensitivity to ozone is an individual matter, some athletes being unaffected while others complain of breathing difficulty, eye and throat irritation and spasms of coughing.

Particles of dust or pollen in the air can also seriously affect the performance of athletes who suffer from allergies. The use of the traditional antihistamine drugs to negate these responses is not recommended as they promote drowsiness and lethargy, but there are newer agents without these effects (e.g. Hismanal). Asthmatics should avoid these environments but, if that is not possible, medication must be optimized.

Combinations of ozone, carbon monoxide and heat can have an additive effect. The circulation contains less oxygen and is often less fluid as a result of heavy sweating. This double demand on the circulation to supply both the muscles and skin with blood requires some compromise and the athlete is forced to reduce the work rate. Athletes should therefore avoid exposing themselves to the substances contained in smog during training and for a 3 or 4 h period prior to competition. In particular they should avoid smoking, smoke-filled rooms and areas containing heavy traffic. Exposure can be minimized by training early in the morning or late in the evening. As there does not appear to be any functional adaptation to smog the wisest strategy is to spend as little time as possible in areas where smog may exist. Also, there is always the possibility that inhaling atmospheric contaminants will pose some long-term risks to one's health.

TRAVEL STRESS
The Travel Problem

Many athletes must travel long distances to compete. The sum of the stresses caused by jet lag, travel fatigue and life-style changes is called travel stress. Jet lag is a problem commonly experienced by athletes who have to travel east or west rapidly across several time zones to participate in competition. The 'competitive edge' can be lost even after crossing one or two time zones and can be significantly affected if greater distances are covered. Jet lag results from a disruption of the body's circadian rhythm (internal clock) by alteration of the sleep–wake cycle. These daily rhythms have been observed for many variables including body temperature, heart rate and hormone secretion, especially melatonin from the pineal gland. They are set by different cues called *zeitgebers* (time-givers), which might include light, meals, clocks and exercise. Reaction times, moods, motivation and thought processes can all be negatively affected by jet lag. When the biological rhythm is altered and competition occurs at a different point in the sleep–wake cycle, the likelihood of optimum physical performance is also reduced.

Added to jet lag is the fatigue associated with the travel experience. The air in jet aircraft is dry and somewhat deficient in oxygen and can cause dehydration and a feeling of lassitude. Some athletes may experience stiffness and constipation due to prolonged sitting. Also there is the need for athletes to adapt to new living conditions after travelling between cities. These life-style changes can be stressful in themselves and lower the potential for peak performance.

Travel Stress and Performance

There are a number of cues that a coach can use to judge how well an athlete is adjusting to travel stress. The best single index is the requirement for sleep. If this is unusually high, particularly during the day, it is likely that the athlete is suffering from travel fatigue. Reduced enthusiasm, attention span and the quality and quantity of performance in training sessions are valuable additional indicators of travel strain.

The extent of disruption from jet lag depends on the individual and the situation. Travellers report less difficulty in recovering from a westbound than an eastbound trip, as there is less loss of sleep. Individuals who adhere to a rigid daily schedule are more affected by jet travel than more flexible persons. Good health and fitness also facilitate adjustments to rapid shifts in time zones. There are a number of procedures that coaches and athletes can follow to reduce the impact of travel stress. These have been adapted from those provided by Fahey (1986). While they have not been submitted to extensive scientific evaluation, these recommendations are observed by frequent travellers.

- Before travelling, attempt to adopt the times of the place of destination. When travelling east arise and go to bed 1 h earlier for the same number of days as the time zones about to be crossed. When travelling west, arise and go to bed 1 h later
- Schedule eastbound flights during daylight hours to arrive at night before normal sleep time. Schedule westbound flights later in the day to arrive just before normal sleep time. Schedule flights so that 1 day per 1–1½ h time difference is allowed for adjustment prior to competition
- Drink plenty of fluids (juices, water, mineral water) during the trip. Avoid alcohol, cola, coffee or tea as they are mild diuretics and decrease body water content. Eat meals that are light and have a high fibre, high CHO content. This will aid digestion and assist in fluid retention. High CHO meals are particularly useful in the evening to stimulate the production of the neural transmitter substance, serotonin, and promote sleep upon arrival. Meals containing a high fat content or unfamiliar foods should be avoided as they may promote gastrointestinal problems.
- Engage in reading, listening to music and chatting during the trip to promote relaxation and avoid idleness
- Take a short walk and stretch and flex the muscles regularly to overcome stiffness and fluid accumulation in the feet
- Only sleep on the plane if travel is overnight and it will be morning at the destination.

Sleeping before an evening arrival will delay adjustments to time zone differences. Upon arrival in the morning try to stay awake and follow the local schedule. Naps taken throughout the day will confuse the internal clock and delay adjustments to time zone changes. If arriving in the evening a light workout is useful to loosen up before going to sleep

CONCLUSIONS

New and harsh environments can play havoc with the capacity of an individual to meet the demands of exercise. When the motivation to continue exceeds one's capacity to do so there is the distinct possibility that health and, in some cases, even life will be threatened. This places the onus on those responsible for prescribing and implementing exercise programmes to understand the impact of environmental extremes on the human body and to undertake the necessary precautions to guarantee safe conditions for the participant.

REFERENCES

Adams W. C., Bernauer E. M., Dill D. B. & Bomar J. B. (1975) Effects of equivalent sea-level and altitude training on V_{O_2max} and running performance. *Journal of Applied Physiology* **39**, 262–265.

American College of Sports Medicine (1984) Position stand on 'Prevention of thermal injuries during distance running'. *Sports Medicine Bulletin* **19**, 8.

Bar-Or O. (1984) Children and physical performance in warm and cold environments. In Boileau R. A. (ed.) *Advances in Pediatric Sport Sciences*. Human Kinetics Publishers, Champaign, IL.

Brahams J. (1988) Death of a soldier: Accident or neglect. *Lancet* i, 485.

Dawson B. & Pyke F. S. (1988) I. Responses to wearing sweat clothing during exercise in cool conditions. II. Training in sweat clothing in cool conditions to improve heat tolerance. *Journal of Human Movement Studies* **15**, 171–183.

Drinkwater B. L., Kupprat I. C. & Horvath S. M. (1977) Heat tolerance of female distance runners. *Annals New York Academy of Science* **301**, 777–792.

Fahey T. D. (1986) *Athletic Training: Principles and Practice*. Mayfield Publishing, Palo Alto, CA.

Gisolfi C. V. & Duchman S. M. (1992) Guidelines for optimal replacement beverages for different athletic events. *Medicine and Science in Sports and Exercise* **24**, 679–687.

Hayward J. S., Eckerson J. D. & Collis M. L. (1975) Effect of behavioural variables on the cooling rate of man in cold water. *Journal of Applied Physiology* **38**, 1073–1077.

Horvath S. M. (1982) Impact of air quality on exercise performance. In Miller D. I. (ed.) *Exercise and Sport Sciences Reviews*, Vol. 9. The Franklin Institute, Philadelphia, PA.

Kaufman W. C. (1982) Cold weather comfort or heat conservation. *Physician and Sports Medicine* **10**, 70–75.

Leithead C. S. & Lind A. R. (1964) *Heat Stress and Heat Disorders*. Cassell, London.

Mathews D. K., Fox E. L. & Tanzc D. (1969) Physiological responses during exercise and recovery in a football uniform. *Journal of Applied Physiology* **26**, 611–615.

Mills W. J. (1983) Accidental hypothermia. *Alaska Medicine* **25**, 29–32.

Mitchell J. B., Costill D. L., Houmard J. A., Flynn M. G., Fink W. J. & Beetz J. B. (1988) Effects of carbohydrate ingestion on gastric emptying and exercise performance. *Medicine and Science in Sports and Exercise* **20**, 110–115.

Moseley P. L. & Gisolfi C. V. (1993) New frontiers in thermoregulation and exercise. *Sports Medicine* **16**, 163–167.

Paolone A. M., Wells C. L. & Kelly G. T. (1977) Sexual variations in thermoregulation during heat stress. *Aviation Space and Environmental Medicine* **49**, 715–719.

Pitts G. C., Johnson R. E. & Consolazio F. C. (1944) Work in the heat as affected by intake of water, salt and glucose. *American Journal of Physiology* **142**, 253–259.

Sutton J. R. (1989) Exercise and the environment. In Bouchard C., Shephard R. J., Stephens T., Sutton J. R. & McPherson B. (eds) *Exercise Fitness and Health*, pp. 165–179. Human Kinetics Publishers, Champaign, IL.

Sutton J. R. (1994) Physiological and clinical consequences of exercise on heat and humidity. In Harries M., Williams C., Stanish W. D. & Micheli L. J. (eds) *Oxford Textbook of Sports Medicine*, pp. 211–238. Oxford University Press, Oxford.

Sutton J. R., Coleman M. J., Millar A. P., Lazarus L. & Russo P. (1972) The medical problems of mass participation in athletic competition. The 'City to Surf' race. *Medical Journal of Australia* **2**, 127–133.

Sutton J. R., Houston C. S., Mansell A. L. *et al.* (1979) The effect of acetazolamide on hypoxemia during sleep at high altitude. *New England Journal of Medicine* **301**, 1329–1332.

Wagner J. A., Robinson S., Tzanhoff S. P. & Marino R. P. (1972) Heat tolerance and acclimatization to work in the heat in relation to age. *Journal of Applied Physiology* **33**, 616–622.

Wyndham C. H., Morrison J. R. & Williams C. G. (1965) Heat reactions of male and female caucasians. *Journal of Applied Physiology* **20**, 357–364.

SECTION 3

SPORT PSYCHOLOGY AND PERFORMANCE ENHANCEMENT

CHAPTER 7

SELF-REGULATION AND GOAL SETTING

A. M. D. Gordon

Applied sport psychology focuses on 'under-standing psychological theories and techniques that can be applied to sport to enhance the performance and personal growth of athletes' (Williams 1993). This working definition captures the essence of both research and practice in this field, which addresses personal development as well as skill development through participation in all physical activities including sport.

An illustration of what applied sport psychology practitioners 'do' is shown in Fig. 7.1, which is a flow chart of the performance enhancement services offered by the Sport Psychology Unit at the Australian Institute of Sport (AIS).

While the nature and content of different pro-grammes alter according to the context (e.g. elite vs. recreational sport), client (e.g. individual vs. team sport athlete) and task (e.g. open vs. closed skills), the AIS model highlights the three most appropriate procedural objectives in applying psy-chological principles to sport. First, to identify and define the mental skill requirements and demands of the activity for clients, through assessment, observation and discussion with coaches, athletes and others; second, to teach the skills required to enhance performance and personal growth; and third, to monitor and refine progress in skill development as clients move through different phases of learning.

The most effective applied sport psychology programmes appear to be characterized by a long-term educational/developmental approach to train-ing appropriate mental skills, which are integrated with the progressions required to develop other performance related skills (e.g. technical, tactical and physical skills). When presented by personable practitioners who have the full support of coaches, such programmes can be invaluable to the majority of athletes in both elite and recreational sport environments. The key component of all mental skills training programmes is self-regulation of behaviour through goal setting. The purpose of this chapter therefore is to describe both the theory and practical applications of both self-regulation and goal setting, using actual case examples from soccer and cricket.

SELF-REGULATION AND GOAL SETTING: THE KEYS TO OPTIMUM PERFORMANCE

The significance of the connection between research and theorizing on self-regulation and sport psy-chology has been emphasized by Kirschenbaum (1984), who defined performance enhancement in sport as a problem in self-regulation. An explanation of this perspective is summarized in the following:

> Whether the sport takes a few minutes to perform in competition or many hours, effort devoted to the solitary pursuit of excellence must far exceed efforts directly influenced or controlled by others. In fact, it seems entirely appropriate to view the outcome of

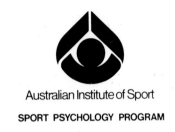

Australian Institute of Sport

SPORT PSYCHOLOGY PROGRAM

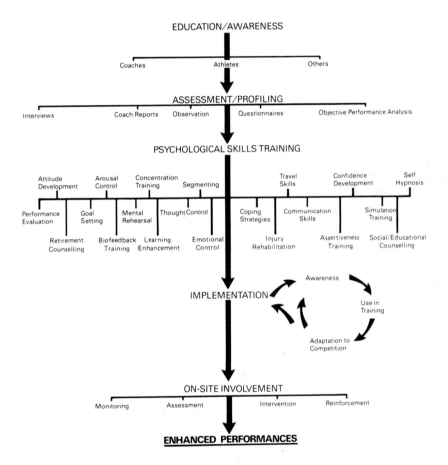

Fig. 7.1   A flow chart of a sport psychology programme.

competition as merely a test of the effectiveness of the athlete's skill in self-directed thinking and behaving (Kirschenbaum 1984).

Kirschenbaum (1984) and his colleagues (e.g. Kirschenbaum *et al.* 1982; Kirschenbaum & Wittrock 1984) have proposed a five-stage model of self-regulation (Fig. 7.2), which relates to the

acquisition of mental skills as well as all other skills concerned with performance enhancement.

The remainder of this chapter will present the concepts and principles associated with Kirschenbaum's (1984) model as they apply to sport, and will describe goal setting as a skilled procedure in self-regulation that can be taught to individuals and groups. Both self-regulation and goal setting have direct influence on performance enhancement and personal growth of athletes, by structuring the mental skill development process.

Self-regulation as a Five-stage Process

PROBLEM IDENTIFICATION

The first phase of the self-regulation process (Fig. 7.2) is problem identification. Athletes can become so task-focused and regimented in their training that improved performance is regarded as almost impossible. This may be particularly true for elite or experienced athletes who become content in the belief that they have already 'peaked' and that further improvements are unlikely. Therefore, the central concern at this stage is to assist each athlete in evaluating the quality of his or her training behaviour and begin working to change and improve it. The emphasis is on behaviour change, that is, changes in routine activities, such as waking, eating and various work habits, as well as mental skills training. In contrast to an athlete's perception of performance ability, behaviour can always be changed and hence may well facilitate improved performance. Problem identification, therefore, does not focus on raw performance and whether or not it can be improved, but instead establishes the fundamental importance of acknowledging that behaviour change is always possible and is a goal worth striving for.

COMMITMENT

Phase 2 is commitment and involves 'acting upon' the decision that behaviour change is possible. Public and written announcements, of both aspirations and plans of action, are associated with

increased commitment and particularly with adherence to sport and fitness programmes of various types. However, neither the expression nor the development of effective plans to achieve desired outcomes may be as critical as establishing whether change is desirable in the first place. Athletes must want change, and by posing the question 'How good do I really want to be?', realistically and responsibly, an athlete is accepting the consequences of behaviour changes. Typical questions might be: 'Am I happy in my role as a non-starter?', 'Have I fully extended myself in my achievements in this sport?', 'Does my personal best reflect the ultimate limit of my talent?' Some athletes who fail to commit themselves fully to behaviour change often manifest psychological symptoms of 'fear of failure' and/or 'fear of success'. They are unable to assume responsibility for perceived negative consequences and do not really desire change. Ambitious athletes, on the other hand, who have a firm and strong intention and commitment to behaviour change, do not evidence these symptoms, and perceive the consequences of behaviour change in a positive light.

EXECUTION

Once a self-regulating problem has been identified and an appropriate level of commitment is formed to modify it, the third phase of self-regulation concerns execution. This refers to the process of achieving behaviour change and begins with monitoring one's behaviour (self-monitoring) and comparing observations with the goal or standard set (self-evaluating). Self-monitoring and self-evaluating are then linked to self-consequating; that is, communicating feedback to oneself. A simple example of positive self-consequation would be 'keep doing what you have been doing, it's working — don't change'; and negative self-consequation would be 'it's not working, change what you are doing, try something else to help you reach your goals'. This circular arrangement of self-monitoring–self-evaluating–self-consequating–self-monitoring, etc. has been described as a cybernetic model (Fig. 7.3) which utilizes a negative feedback loop as the basic functioning unit. This information processing unit is considered 'negative' because its

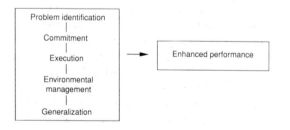

Fig. 7.2 A five-stage model of self-regulation (adapted from Kirschenbaum 1984).

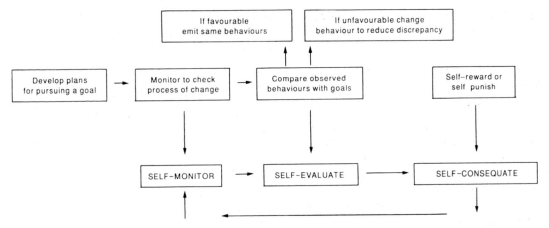

Fig. 7.3 The cybernetic model (adapted from Kirschenbaum 1984).

function is to negate or reduce perceived deviation from a standard of comparison (Kirschenbaum 1984). Four important principles emerge from this cybernetic model and the execution phase of self-regulation.

First, self-monitoring alone will not maintain effective self-regulation. Self-focused attention studies indicate that increasing attention to oneself increases attempts to match behaviour to action plans and goals, and also facilitates a more complete and careful introspection. However, self-monitoring without systematic self-evaluation on a continual basis will not promote self-regulation. In other words, athletes should determine objective and measurable criteria to evaluate their efforts in behaviour change; for example: 'Is snacking between meals consistent with my goal to lose weight?' 'How much extra time have I actually devoted to improving my weaknesses this week?'

Second, as some personality and situational characteristics, and their interaction, can determine most of an individual's behaviour, self-regulatory skills may largely be a function of self-motivation and self-reinforcement style (personality factors), and degree of competence and nature of task characteristics (situational factors). This second principle can dramatically affect the execution phase in the self-regulation process. In simpler terms, self-motivated and talented athletes possess more

important dispositional styles and capacities than coach-motivated and less-skilled athletes. Individual differences, therefore, in the interaction between personality and competence have the potential to affect self-regulated performance.

A third principle relates to self-evaluation and self-consequation. Self-regulation and sport psychology research suggests that attention given to positive expectancies and successes, as opposed to negative expectancies and failures, facilitates performance on tasks that are difficult or poorly mastered. A focus on negative expectancies and failures debilitates self-regulation on these tasks, but not, however, on tasks that are well mastered. On well mastered (easy) tasks a focus on mistakes enhances, rather than inhibits, self-regulation; for example, attention to faulty technique on simple (basic) skills can facilitate improvement more effectively than attention to correct technique. Consequently, mid-field soccer players practising improvement in their vision and setting up attacks (difficult task), should be encouraged and reinforced in all efforts to make penetrating passes behind opposing defenders. The same players, however, should be highly self-critical when practising the basic skills of angling to receive and make passes (easy task). Both strategies, in different practice situations, facilitate self-regulated performance.

The fourth and final principle related to the cybernetic model also relates to the performance of difficult versus easy tasks, but concerns the role of cognition (affect and emotion) on execution. A cognition is merely a thought or series of thoughts

Table 7.1 Examples of thought-stoppage technique in soccer

Stress situation	Self-defeating inner dialogue	Self-enhancing modified inner dialogue
Referee makes bad decision against me	What an idiot! If he makes a bad call again I'm going to 'blow my stack'.	This referee is having a bad day! *STOP.* But we all have bad days and I can't control another's form. Keep your mind on *your* form.
	Consequences: Play focuses on the referee instead of the game. Allows referee to influence emotional control.	*Consequences:* Player rationalizes poor performance of referee and re-focuses on what he has control over, that is personal performance.
Opposition player continually fouls and gets away with it.	That dirty so-and-so! Next time he comes near me I'm going to 'get' him.	What a thug! *STOP.* Keep your cool. He's losing his. Back into the game. The referee's in charge.
	Consequences: Player is again distracted by the play of another. Preoccupied with revenge rather than playing the game.	*Consequences:* Player keeps his focus on the game. Passes control over to the appropriate person (referee). Stays task-oriented.
Opposition player is in dominating form	I'll stop this superstar. I'll show him he can't make me look ordinary.	He's had a great game so far. *STOP.* I need to alter my tactics somehow. What do I have to do here?
	Consequences: Player focuses on dubious tactics that could get him sent off, the team penalized, or the opposition player seriously injured (or all three!)	*Consequences:* Player remains task-oriented and determined to give 100% of his effort. A focus on tactics will likely include assistance from others which will assist the player and the team.

related to an aspect of performance and can be described as an 'inner dialogue'. Research evidence suggests that affect and emotion have a greater effect on the performance of poorly mastered (difficult) tasks as opposed to well mastered (easy) tasks. To reduce negative affect therefore, self-talk can be used to direct attention away from the occasional debilitating sensations experienced during poor performances. For example, self-talk techniques such as 'thought stoppage' can be used to help athletes replace negative, counter-productive and frequently irrational inner dialogues. Examples of 'thought stoppage' for a soccer player with emotional control problems are illustrated in Table 7.1.

In summary, these four principles affecting the execution phase in self-regulation would suggest that athletes first learn how to observe their performances systematically and continually; second, attend to favourable aspects of performance and positive expectancies when tasks are new or difficult; third, focus on errors or problems when tasks become easy or routine; and fourth, use cognitive distractors or other means to reduce negative affect, particularly when tasks are difficult and complex.

ENVIRONMENTAL MANAGEMENT

The fourth phase in self-regulation, environmental management, can affect all other phases, as achievement of behaviour change does not occur in a vacuum and depends largely on the support from many aspects of one's social and physical environment. The potential of these environments to inhibit and/or facilitate efforts in achieving goals cannot be underestimated, and when managed correctly can provide a sustained source of energy. Effective environmental management is achieved through opportunity and support, that is, the opportunity to train, to be coached in appropriate facilities with good equipment and have the financial means to achieve this; and support, from people significant to the athlete, such as team-mates, coaches, family and friends, who provide encouragement for practice and competition. The detrimental effects of, specifically, negativistic coaching, which develops dysfunctional attitudes, both to sport and the self, as well as faulty tech-nique development, cannot be over-emphasized. Research evidence suggests that the alternative, 'behavioural coaching', enhances self-regulation through accurate definitions of skill components (self-monitoring) highly task-specific, non-emotional and positive feedback (self-evaluation), which promote positive expectation and avoidance of negative expectancies (self-consequation).

GENERALIZATION

The fifth and final phase in the self-regulation process is generalization. According to Kirschen-baum (1984), maintenance of self-regulated be-haviour change often fails because individuals allow irrelevant and distracting habits and thoughts to interfere with the accomplishment of goals. A compulsive–obsessive style (characteristic of many elite performers) of self-regulation is therefore advised to sustain efforts over long periods of time. Studies of gymnasts, golfers, wrestlers and divers, who evidence obsessive–compulsive be-haviour are testimony to both effective self-regu-lation and elite performance outcomes. Examples of the generalization process in practice would be the self-imposed withdrawal from others and the highly structured life-styles of some Olympic athletes as they prepare for competition. The highly self-focused and task-oriented atmosphere at sports institutes would also characterize 'generalization'. Unrelated to specific competitions, the practice of mental skills in non-sport as well as sports situ-ations would be an appropriate example of 'gen-eralization'; for example using concentration skills at work or study.

These essential elements and operational prin-ciples of the self-regulation process are inherent in goal setting, which is a performance enhancement tool commonly used in both sport and business settings. The next section of this chapter will describe the theory, techniques and skills of goal setting as they relate to sport.

Goal Setting in Sport: Theoretical and Practical Considerations

Goal setting is a cognitively based, planning, organizational and evaluative tool. It has not only been shown to influence task performance of individuals of varied age and competency levels, but has also been associated with positive changes in significant psychological states, such as motiv-ation, confidence and anxiety. Psychological re-search on goal setting in various laboratory and field settings has been impressive and has produced a consistent pattern of results. In a review of over 100 studies on goal setting, Locke *et al.* (1981) concluded:

> The beneficial effect of goal setting on task perfor-mance is one of the most robust and replicable findings in the psychological literature. Ninety percent of the studies showed positive or partially positive effects.

Although relatively few investigations on goal setting in sport have produced equivocal results, Burton (1989) maintains that where there are inconsistent results in these studies, they can be attributed in large part to methodological limi-tations of designs in sports research. As the leading researcher in goal setting in sport, Burton maintains that it is still widely regarded as an important fundamental skill and technique that athletes, coaches and applied sport psychology practitioners should regularly employ.

BENEFITS OF GOAL SETTING

Carron (1984) has summarized the benefits of goal setting under the following four categories:

- Improvement in coaching climate and general atmosphere for athletes and groups
- Personal growth
- Leadership
- Improvements in group goals and objectives

With regard to climate and general atmosphere, goal setting can address and reform problem behaviour, such as tardiness, laziness and unsports-manlike conduct. It can also improve communi-cation among individuals and enhance empathic understanding in groups by sharing setbacks and successes. Goal setting also cultivates confidence and morale in groups by increasing levels of satisfaction among individuals through meeting new standards and the achievement of small goals. Personal growth and psychological maturity are also facilitated as individuals learn how to self-manage and self-direct their endeavours, which is the key objective in self-regulation. Individuals also learn how to adapt to different situations by improving their coping capabilities, and these strategies and procedures have utility in other aspects of life including personal, social and career affairs. Leadership also becomes more enjoyable, and leadership effectiveness is generally enhanced through goal setting as followers (subordinates) become more motivated, enthusiastic and self-determined in their efforts. Finally, benefits from improvements in group goals and objectives stem from specifying priorities among all group members. Priorities for members may include objectives set for social experiences as well as performance outcomes, thus acknowledging a humanistic focus in applied sports psychology. Furthermore, if sport and competition have social value, then every

participant has the right to be successful, and a comprehensive goal-setting programme facilitates both the attainment of this right and the benefits of this important humanistic perspective.

The benefits of goal-setting programmes for coaches and athletes, are illustrated in Fig. 7.4.

According to researchers (Burton 1983; Carron 1984; Locke & Latham 1985) at least five mechanisms can account for performance changes attributable to goal-setting programmes. First, goals influence important psychological attributes, such as anxiety, confidence and motivation; second, goals direct attention to critical aspects of the tasks and skills being performed; third, goals mobilize greater effort on the part of individuals who work harder to achieve more difficult goals; fourth, goals not only increase immediate effort, they prolong effort and promote persistence; and finally, goals motivate individuals to develop new learning strategies and plans of action for training. These five mechanisms represent both cognitive and organizational theoretical explanations for the performance/goal-setting relationship and are illustrated in Table 7.2.

Fig. 7.4 The benefits of goal-setting programmes (adapted from Coaching Association of Canada 1979).

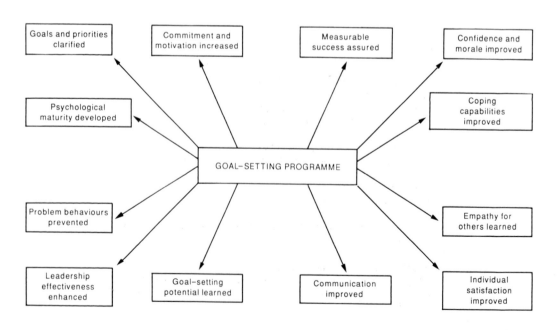

Table 7.2 Motivational mechanisms associated with goal setting

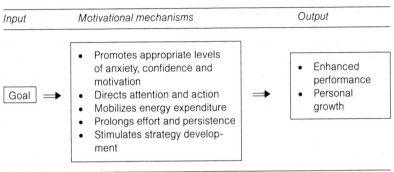

Input	Motivational mechanisms	Output
Goal ⟹	• Promotes appropriate levels of anxiety, confidence and motivation • Directs attention and action • Mobilizes energy expenditure • Prolongs effort and persistence • Stimulates strategy development	⟹ • Enhanced performance • Personal growth

Adapted from Carron (1984).

GOAL-SETTING PRINCIPLES AND GUIDE-LINES

The notion that goal setting is an easy skill to learn and use is perhaps the first mistake athletes and practitioners can make. The basic guiding principles of goal setting are summarized by Gould (1993) in Table 7.3.

All problems in goal-setting can be attributed to faulty or complacent self-regulation processes (Fig. 7.2) over which individuals have direct control, and Gould (1993) has identified six of the more common and frequently encountered problems. These are briefly described as follows:

Setting too many goals, too soon
Coaches and athletes often fail to prioritize goals, and end up as a result not achieving set standards and performances. A focus on only one or two goals at a time is advised, which will enable proper monitoring of progress and a greater likelihood of the accomplishment of the goal or goals.

Setting goals that are too general
'Improve my ball control', 'score more goals than last year' and 'concentrate better' are goals an inexperienced soccer player may make — but they are too vague. More effectively stated they could be changed; for example 'I want to improve my first touch on the

Table 7.3 Goal-setting guide-lines

Set:
- Specific goals in measurable and behavioural terms
- Difficult but realistic goals
- Short-range as well as long-range goals
- Performance goals as opposed to outcome goals
- Goals for practice and for competition
- Positive goals as opposed to negative goals (e.g. 'be enthusiastic/supportive' vs 'must not get angry/frustrated')

Identify:
- Target dates for attaining goals
- Goal achievement strategies

Record:
- Goals in written form once they have been identified: 'ink it, don't just think it'

Provide for:
- Feedback and evaluation of goals
- Support for goals from family, friends, coaches and team-mates

From Gould (1993).

Table 7.4 How to set goals: concentration in elite cricket. Long-term objective: 'To improve my concentration on the field'

Question	Probable answer(s)
Step 1: Task analysis	
What do I have to do?	• Develop an awareness of symptoms of lapses in concentration
	• Learn skills to address these lapses when they occur
How am I going to do this?	• Learn and develop 'switch-on' and 'switch-off' strategies to maximize periods of optimum concentration
	• Develop 'checklists' and 'triggers' and build these into a pre-delivery routine so that I can concentrate on the right things at the right time
	• Use and refine these at practice
Step 2: Measuring performance	
How can I measure improvement?	• Record the number of concentration lapses in each session during 4 day games, and when they occur, record them in a diary
	• Record the number of times I have to use 'switch-on' strategies in each session
How will I know that I have improved?	• When I record fewer lapses in concentration during sessions of play in a 4 day game
	• Feedback from team-mates, captain and coach
When do I want this to happen?	• Over the next 4 games (1 month)
Step 3: Support for goals	
Who can help me achieve my goals and objectives?	• The mental skills coach can teach me how to develop pre-delivery techniques (checklist/triggers), how to 'switch-off', and how to record my progress
	• My team-mates can assist me at the nets and in games by observing my efforts to develop and improve these skills

ball', 'I want to improve the quality of strikes at goal (heading and different types of shooting) and frequency of getting into scoring positions', and 'I want to develop an awareness of concentration lapses and learn skills to address these during a game'. Goals must be measurable and specific.

Failing to modify unrealistic goals
Goals need to be re-evaluated periodically during a season in order to raise or lower standards. Athletes usually have little difficulty raising goals but they often fail to lower them and subsequently they can become unrealistic because of illness, injury or external factors. Unrealistic goals can effectively inhibit motivation during a season and negatively affect confidence.

Failing to set performance goals
Athletes often can't stop themselves thinking about outcome goals, that is, winning, gold medals and end results. However, it is critical that they focus instead on performance goals and the process of achieving outcome goals. Athletes have little or no direct influence on outcomes but they have direct control over their performances. For example, a focus on 'session by session' and ultimately 'ball by ball' in a 5 day cricket Test match helps players concentrate on performance as opposed to outcome goals. By focusing on the process of playing a Test match the outcome looks after itself. Similarly, coaches, team-mates and friends can promote performance goals by asking 'How did you play?', which is performance oriented, as opposed to 'Did you win?', which is outcome oriented. This is related to the next common problem.

Failing to create a supportive goal-setting environment
By informing team-mates, coaches, family members and friends of their goals, athletes not only create a network of support and encouragement for their achievements, they also develop greater personal commitment to their own efforts by declaring their

Table 7.5 Examples of long-term objectives and short-term goals in six goal areas for a test bowler in international cricket

Goal area	Long-term objective	Short-term goal*
Technical goals (performance-related goals)	To improve and sustain my strike rate	Execute my stock ball and at least one other type of ball, on demand Maintain line and length consistently well
Tactical goals (strategy concerns)	To pre-plan my performance against opposition batsmen	Determine and record (in a diary) observations of opposing batsmen (weaknesses/strengths) Prepare (with captain) to expose weaknesses of the opposing batsmen
Physical goals (fitness and health goals)	To improve and sustain my endurance, flexibility and strength	Improve timed runs on fixed distances Develop and maintain a daily flexibility and strength programme
Mental goals (e.g. concentration and visualization skills)	To improve my concentration and technique through visualization	Obtain video recordings of my performance to enhance my external imagery ability Develop written scripts of kinesthetic cues for performance to enhance my internal imagery ability
Behavioural goals (e.g. observable individual and group behaviour)	To improve my levels of enthusiasm and determination throughout the tour	Record (in a diary) negative body language characteristics 'communicated' during entire games Modify body language through active practice at nets and games
Environmental goals (e.g. personal and domestic concerns)	To structure effective time with my wife and family each day before and during the tour	Prioritize my activities for periods in each day and include scheduled family time Accommodate team responsibilities and commitments without compromising family time each day

*Only two goals are presented as examples.

goals publicly. Quite often it is the encouragement from non-sport related associates that can spur an athlete to ultimate goal accomplishments.

Failing to recognize individual differences
Coaches need to realize that not all athletes will be interested in setting goals and some may actively rebel against the idea. Furthermore, group goals may be simply unattainable for some individuals whose subsequent performances may drop dramatically due to lack of confidence or lack of motivation. The key for coaches is first to introduce goal setting as an option so athletes don't feel it is forced or imposed upon them; and second, to preserve the importance and significance of individual accomplishments as well as group accomplishments — this relates directly to the fundamental principles of self-regulation.

All of the above problems are easily detected and therefore easily controlled and avoided. Recog-

nition of problems, usually at the beginning of a goal-setting programme, should be an expected and built-in component of the goal-setting process.

HOW TO SET GOALS

A single goal has been defined as 'attaining a specific standard of proficiency in a task, usually within a specified time limit' (Locke *et al.* 1981). Goals are therefore regarded as small and specific steps towards fulfilling a larger purpose which can be regarded as an objective. The relationship between goals and objectives can be likened to a staircase. At the top of the staircase is the ultimate objective and each step represents a goal. An example of a long-term objective is an elite cricketer who wishes to improve his or her concentration in the field (fielding). To determine appropriate short-term goals this individual must heed at least three steps and respond to the questions illustrated in Table 7.4.

Using the same procedure and sets of questions, cricketers can set goals related to longer-term objectives in at least six goal areas. A real life example of short-term goals and long-term objectives for a bowler in international cricket preparing for a Test series is illustrated in Table 7.5.

CONCLUSIONS

Applied sport psychology concerns performance enhancement and personal growth of athletes through the acquisition and development of mental skills as they relate to sport situations. Performance enhancement has been defined as a problem in self-regulation, which first involves identifying possibilities of behaviour change and, at the individual level, structuring commitment and efforts to maintain change. Research findings from both self-regulation and sport psychology suggest that self-regulation is a five-stage process which incorporates pedagogical and cognitive principles of learning and development.

There is strong empirical, experiential and anecdotal support for using goal setting in sport. As a tool it not only facilitates performance enhancement and personal growth of athletes, it also affects the self-regulation process, which is fundamental to the field of applied sport psychology. Self-regulation and goal-setting principles promote attention to the process of achievement, not outcomes or end results. Guide-lines on how to set goals in six areas have been presented, which illustrate how self-regulation principles can be applied to different achievement situations. The focus in the chapters that follow, on mental skills training for individual and team sport athletes,

builds on the goals set for learning and developing mental skills. Self-regulation and goal-setting principles are regarded, therefore, as the major keys to optimum skill performance.

REFERENCES

Burton D. (1983) Evaluation of goal setting training on selected cognitions and performance of collegiate swimmers. PhD thesis, University of Illinois, Urbana (unpublished).

Burton D. (1989) The impact of goal specificity and task complexity on basketball skill development. *The Sport Psychologist* 3, 34–47.

Carron A. V. (1984) *Motivation: Implications for Coaching and Teaching.* Sports Dynamics, London.

Coaching Association of Canada (1979) *National Coaching Certification Program: Level 2 Coaching Theory.* Coaching Association of Canada, Ottawa.

Gould D. (1993) Goal setting for peak performance. In Williams J. M. (ed.) *Applied Sport Psychology: Personal Growth to Peak Performance*, 2nd edn, pp. 158–169. Mayfield Publishing Company, Palo Alto, CA.

Kirschenbaum D. S. (1984) Self-regulation and sport psychology: Nurturing an emerging symbiosis. *Journal of Sport Psychology* 6, 159–183.

Kirschenbaum D. S. & Wittrock D. A. (1984) Cognitive–behavioral interventions in sport: A self-regulatory perspective. In Silva J. M. & Weinberg R. S. (eds) *Psychological Foundations of Sport*, pp. 81–97. Human Kinetics Publishers, Champaign, IL.

Kirschenbaum D. S., Tomarken A. J. & Ordman A. M. (1982) Specificity of planning and choice in adult self-control. *Journal of Personality and Social Psychology* 41, 576–585.

Locke E. A. & Latham G. P. (1985) The application of goal setting to sports. *Journal of Sport Psychology* 7, 205–222.

Locke E. A., Shaw K. N., Saari L. M. & Latham G. P. (1981) Goal setting and task performance: 1969–1980. *Psychological Bulletin* 90, 125–152.

Williams J. M. (ed.) (1993) *Applied Sport Psychology: Personal Growth to Peak Performance*, 2nd edn. Mayfield Publishing Company, Palo Alto, CA.

CHAPTER 8

THE INDIVIDUAL ATHLETE

J. W. Bond

This chapter examines a multidimensional psychological model which has been derived from experience with elite athletes across many different sports and recommended for use by various practitioners, coaches and athletes as a framework for:

- Psychological profiling of individual athletes
- The development of mental skills training programmes for the individual athlete and/or coach
- For decision-making concerning appropriate interventions in the competitive situation

The model is based on a series of psychological antecedents which may influence the athlete's ability to produce and maintain an ideal performing state. They include various attitudes associated with commitment and professionalism, the importance of a task as opposed to an outcome focus, the establishment and maintenance of life-style balance and sport-specific self-confidence.

Five categories are presented as representative of the major psychological explanations of performance decrement. These include various cognitive, psychophysiological, attentional, emotional and organizational factors.

The information is relevant and applicable to male and female athletes in individual sports and to individual athletes in team sports who wish to improve their training and competitive performances. Because successful coaching is dependent on well developed psychological skills, the applied model is directly relevant to those coaches and sports psychologists who seek to improve the consistency and quality of their interactions with athletes, as well as the effectiveness of their own decision-making in stressful competitive situations.

This model is not being proposed as a 'panacea for all ills'; it does not cover all the factors which may be relevant for a given athlete, and it is not a recipe for a 'one programme fits all' approach to sports psychology. Rather, it should be considered as a framework for more effective decision-making in the individual situation.

The development and application of a sports psychology programme as suggested by this model assumes that the athlete and coach are also taking part in similar programmes, that is skill development, specific training, nutrition and sports medicine. This approach is based on the premise that an athlete will only ever be as successful as his or her greatest weakness and it is common to observe unsuccessful athletes being let down by such a weakness when it is apparent that they have very well developed skills in other areas. Structured observations at many major international competitions reinforce the importance of the constant need for athletes and coaches to work diligently in the total preparation which is necessary for success in elite sport. There is a common saying in sport: 'It is not necessarily the best athletes who win, it is the best prepared athletes who win.'

The concept which is stressed throughout this

chapter, is that athletes and coaches must be totally 'professional' in their pursuit of excellence in all aspects of a well-rounded training and competition programme.

THE IMPORTANCE OF 'IDEAL' PERFORMING STATES

There has been a great deal written about the arousal–performance relationship in the sports psychology literature. Despite a number of proposed variations including drive theory (Rushall 1979) and reversal theory (Kerr 1985), it would appear that the original inverted U hypothesis proposed by Yerkes and Dodson (1908) remains an acceptable general explanation of this relationship. Figure 8.1 provides a general outline of the arousal–performance relationship for the sports psychology practitioner, coach and athlete.

There is a good deal of evidence, both experiential and research (Landers 1980; Ravizza 1984; Csikszentmihalyi 1990; Jackson & Roberts 1992), as well as intuitive support for the notion of an 'ideal' performing state. This hypothesis maintains that an athlete may sometimes be under- or over-aroused for a particular task. Under-aroused states are uncommon for elite athletes; however, they can occur as a result of overconfidence or fatigue. The individual may feel somewhat lethargic, less intense and perhaps struggling to maintain an

appropriate attentional focus, with non-specific or non-challenging goals for the performance. Under these conditions it is common for athletes to experience underachievement.

In the over-aroused state it is more common for the serious elite athlete to report the following stress symptoms: feelings of tightness; changes in normal breathing patterns; an overly narrowed or overloaded concentration span; quick shifts in emotional states; rapid reversals; positive–negative in self-talk and images; and/or decreased control over pacing and rhythm. It is not difficult to forecast a performance decrement occurring when these symptoms of stress are present.

At the optimal level of arousal, athletes report feelings of total control, focused and yet relaxed concentration, ample decision-making time, feelings of being 'in synch' or 'in flow'. These experiences are typified by positive self-talk and images, extreme self-confidence and quality self-management. One of the primary tasks for the serious elite athlete is the consistent production and maintenance of these optimal arousal states.

Information absent in the original arousal–performance relationship hypothesis includes the specificity of the antecedents involved in arousal shifts and the individual reactions to these shifts, that is specific functional breakdowns which contribute to the performance decrement. The antecedents must be viewed both in terms of:

- Individual characteristics, such as level of skill, level of anxiety, self-confidence, competition performance, attitudes and other possible personality characteristics
- Situational factors, including specific arousal-related features of the performance environment, such as crowd size and noise levels, physical risks such as excessive speed or height and situational task demands

There are also the complex interactions which occur between the above and the interaction model, as shown in Fig. 8.2.

The absence of specificity information also relates to the individual reactions or responses experienced by the person. While one athlete may find a particular level of arousal positive, the next one may

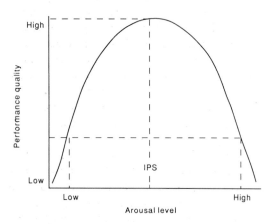

Fig. 8.1 The Yerkes-Dodson inverted U (adapted from Yerkes & Dodson 1908).

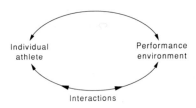

Fig. 8.2 The interaction model.

find it quite negative. It is probably true to say that for every athlete there is a 'turn-over' point in the arousal curve, that is, there is a point where even the most experienced athlete will become over-aroused with adverse effects on his/her performance. However, there are many and varied individual responses to a similarly damaging state of over-arousal. This individual specificity requires that there be some form of framework within which accurate interpretations can be made, in order to develop more effective intervention strategies.

The following description of a multidimensional model is an attempt to assist in this area. It describes a method for psychologically 'profiling' individual athlete responses prior to and during training and competition. This profile can be of significant benefit to the athlete in terms of enhanced self-awareness, to the coach who is concerned about better coaching interaction and to the allied health professionals who also interact with the elite athlete.

THE DEVELOPMENT OF AN APPROPRIATE ATTITUDE BASE

In sport it is both necessary and common for athletes with a commitment to excellence to spend many years perfecting their technical and/or their physiological capacities, yet applied sports psychologists are often confronted with athletes and coaches who are looking for the 'quick fix', or the 'psych-up' just before the grand final or important performance.

What they are essentially asking for is that the sports psychologist 'wave a magic wand' and not only teach them the necessary mental skills in a short period of time, but teach them so well that

the skills will hold up under the pressures which typically exist in high-level competitive sport. This is a request that few sports psychologists could ever be expected to achieve, as there are no short-cuts in the field of mental skills development. Time must be spent in identifying and practising the skills required for enhanced performance. There are of course some short-term interventions which can help 'turn athletes around' in times of critical stress, but it must be remembered that these interventions have questionable long-term effects.

The multidimensional model presented below is based on the need for the initial development of specific attitudes towards training, preparing for competition and competing. Without these attitudes it becomes increasingly difficult for an athlete to continue to make the sacrifices necessary to consistently produce the high quality training and competition standards required for success in sport. It is also difficult for athletes to maintain ideal levels of arousal prior to and during performances. These attitudes are based on a number of essential requirements.

PROFESSIONALISM

There is a need for high performance athletes who aspire to international success to develop a very high level of commitment and 'professionalism.' These attitudes are responsible for, and in some cases are derived from, these long-term goals or dreams associated with ultimate success in sport. Those athletes who win Olympic gold medals or set new world records have dreamed about achieving their ultimate goal for many years. They are obsessive about this dream, they plan around it and most of all they believe that they will achieve this level of success. These goals also provide a sound base for the development or conditioning of what might be called 'elite behaviours' in non-sporting, training and competition environments.

There is a school of thought existing among some elite coaches that a committed and dedicated attitude cannot be instilled or developed and that an athlete either 'has it or does not'. This approach reflects the belief that winning athletes are 'born rather than made'. By contrast, sports psychologists believe that many of our attitudes are formed early in life, but that they can be modified by learning and experience through well-designed coaching and sports psychology training programmes.

For example, the Australian 1987 Wimbledon Men's Champion actually began his final assault on this prestigious event from his hospital bed. He had suffered a serious back injury which had forced him off the professional circuit for approximately 6 months. It was during this time that he realized he needed to be strong in every area of his physical, psychological and technical preparation if he was to regain his ranking and achieve his ultimate dream of winning at Wimbledon. The forced lay-off and the seriousness of his injury actually proved to be a bonus for this player. He had the time and some extra objectivity, away from the rigours of the professional circuit, to contemplate where he was, where he wanted to be and how he was going to get there. Instead of his injury being the negative influence it might have been for many athletes, it in fact turned his career around.

At the Seoul Olympic Games in 1988, the author spent a good deal of time with a young male swimmer who had not managed to qualify for the team. He had unfortunately been diagnosed as suffering from leukaemia after failing to make the team at the trials, but he was able to attend the Games, reside in the Olympic village and observe the competitors in action. These observations and associated discussions made him realize exactly what he wanted to do with his life and future athletic career. He went back to his home city and prepared for the inevitable bone marrow transplant and chemotherapy programme. His treatment progressed exceptionally well, probably due in part to his very positive attitude, and he set his sights on not only competing, but winning at the 1992 Olympics. Not only had he seen the champions in action, he had met and talked with them. His statement that he now 'knew what he had to do and exactly what was required for success in the Olympic arena', set him on a path which one hopes will gain him the success he desires.

Standard goal-setting programmes, based on ultimate, long-term, intermediate and short-term objectives, rely on adherence by the athlete, and

this only comes from the existence of 'professional' attitudes and a clear 'dream' of ultimate success. The work of Orlick and Partington (1986) in surveying Canadian Olympic athletes reinforces the use by high level athletes of specific goal setting for training and competitions. It is important to note here that goal-setting programmes must include a variety of goals specifically in the short-term and intermediate phases covering the following:

- Performance goals
- Techniques
- Psychological skills
- Physiological capacities
- Self-management routines

Table 8.1 provides an example of specific, multi-dimensional short-term goals used by a tennis player

Table 8.1 An example of short-term goals from an elite tennis match evaluation

Technical	Forehand	12345678910
	Topspin backhand	12345678910
	Slice backhand	12345678910
	Approach shots	12345678910
	First service	12345678910
	Second service	12345678910
	Volleys	12345678910
	Overhead	12345678910
Physical	Hustle	12345678910
	Footwork	12345678910
	Recovery	12345678910
	Presence	12345678910
	Speed	12345678910
	Endurance	12345678910
Mental	Concentration	12345678910
	Imagery	12345678910
	Emotional control	12345678910
	Recovery from errors	12345678910
	Self-talk	12345678910
	Arousal control	12345678910
	Attitude	12345678910
	Rhythm	12345678910
Organizational	Pre-match preparation	12345678910
	Pre-match warm-up	12345678910
	Pre-match hit-up	12345678910
	Equipment	12345678910
	Food	12345678910
	Timing	12345678910
	Between points routine	12345678910
	End change routine	12345678910

as a means of preparing for a particular tennis match, for maintaining focus during the match and for post-match debriefing. The lower ranked scores achieved by this player are then 'rolled over' to the next match or practice session. They become the specific focus for the subsequent practice sessions and competition and the process continues after the next competition evaluation.

Paradoxically, sometimes an abundance of 'natural' talent in sport coincides with a lower level of commitment. These athletes appear to have accomplished good results in youth sport through exceptional abilities, without having to work hard and develop dedicated attitudes. Once these habits have set in, it is often very difficult to inculcate 'professional' attitudes in these athletes. Most coaches will readily attest to the frustration which accompanies their efforts to extract consistent, hard work from exceptionally talented individuals. These are the athletes we refer to as having 'great potential', which they rarely achieve because of the absence of appropriate attitudes and commitment.

A number of elite sports programmes at the Australian Institute of Sport (AIS) have attempted to overcome this problem by inviting small numbers of less talented athletes to accept an AIS scholarship, in the hope that these 'harder workers' with more professional attitudes will gain success and influence the adoption of similar attitudes and work ethics by the more talented members of the team. In many cases this approach has paid dividends, as some of these so-called less talented athletes have trained in such a dedicated manner that they have won Olympic and Commonwealth Games medals. Further, they have influenced the adoption of more professional attitudes by some of the more talented individuals. The combination of high levels of physical talent with a positive and professional attitude, has made for consistent and superior sporting performances.

A PROCESS FOCUS

The sporting and social culture which surrounds international elite performance encourages the development of 'outcome' related cognitions and beliefs by athletes and coaches. The essential concept is that there are only two kinds of people in the world: winners and the rest, and that the only measure of success in sport is winning. Sports psychologists and coaches observe substandard performances in comparison with training and previous competition expectations, as a result of poor attitudes and behaviours in athletes and coaches. These in turn contribute to increased levels of anxiety and 'fear of failure' thoughts prior to and during elite competition performances.

This phenomenon appears to occur at all age groups for both sexes across all sports. As a 1984, 1988 and 1992 Australian Olympic team sports psychologist, the author was able to gain first-hand experience of this tendency to focus on possible outcomes and other extrinsic influences. The majority of athletes actually underachieve in major competitions at this level and this was true for many members of the 1984, 1988 and 1992 Winter and Summer Australian Olympic Games teams. These athletes do not underachieve because they deserve to; on the contrary, to have qualified for an Olympic Games team speaks highly of the athletes' dedication, years of hard training, physical qualities and personal sacrifice.

Underachievement more often than not occurs because each athlete has an area of 'susceptibility' or 'weakness'. The examples presented below are only two of many which could have been selected but were chosen because they involved questionable levels of psychological training in what was otherwise an excellent preparation programme.

Included among the members of the 1984 Australian swimming team was a young female swimmer who at the time of the Olympics was ranked second in the world in her main event. She had undergone a rigorous physical and technical preparation and had posted the best training performance times ever for an Australian in this event. Moreover, the number one ranked swimmer was from the eastern bloc and would not be competing in Los Angeles. This effectively meant that she was the highest ranked swimmer in the event and seemed in a good position to win a gold medal.

In consultations (which should have taken place much earlier) with her sports psychologist, the swimmer discussed her fears about the pressure she would experience coming from her coach, other members of the team, the media and the general public, who were all expecting her to win the gold medal. She felt that it would be critical for her to be able to maintain a task-oriented focus and to shield herself from the influence of others who would be likely to transfer their expectations to her. Although it was late in her preparation, a situation was devised in an attempt to assist her to maintain the focus and type of control over her final preparation that she considered necessary. This included discussions with her coach about the potential dangers associated with an undue emphasis on possible race outcomes, such as winning a gold medal.

On the day of the event, her coach, who felt that she was very well prepared, gave her his pre-race advice. His words to her were in effect that she had the gold medal in her hands, all she had to do was to reach out and take it! Up until this time the swimmer had maintained good self-control; but this was more than she could cope with. Her focus shifted involuntarily from her prepared pre-race and race plan (task) to the exciting possibility of a gold medal and also the embarrassing consequences of failure (outcome).

Despite her very best intentions, she did not make the final and swam a time which was far below her previous training swims, let alone competition times. During the course of a post-race debriefing session she described the classic symptoms of an athlete who had lost control over arousal levels, positive emotional state, attentional focus, self-talk, confidence and general self-management skills. In the water for the start of the heat reflecting on her coach's words, she reported feeling slow, heavy, extremely anxious and confused. She emphasized the incredible pressure she felt when her attention involuntarily focused on the expectations about her winning the gold medal, a situation that had been identified earlier, but a 'weakness' which had been her downfall.

The second example is also from swimming, this time in Seoul in 1988, and concerns the performances of a very talented and hard-working young athlete who won a gold medal and broke the existing world record. He and his coach planned the 'perfect race' for this swim. He was seeded in the lane next to the current world champion but managed to maintain his attention on his plan (a process focus) and swam to a comfortable victory.

In his next race 2 days later which was his preferred event and the one he was actually trained for, he again had a chance to capitalize on his excellent preparation and the confidence gained from his previous gold medal win. This time, however, a decision was taken that he should 'swim off' his greatest rival for the gold medal (an outcome focus). During the race he executed the plan perfectly; however, although he touched in ahead of his main rival, another swimmer touched in ahead of them both! In post-race debriefing it was revealed that he had swum a little below his capabilities and that the plan to focus on the position of another competitor during the race perhaps cost him a second gold medal. Had he focused on producing his own best-ever swim during that race, a process focus, he may have won the event.

Performance Attitude

The competition performance attitude proposed in this section is consistent with a large proportion of 'successful' elite athletes whose cognitions and behaviours have been labelled a 'process' or 'task focus'. This attitude predisposes the athlete to maintain an orientation towards the actual functions or processes to be executed prior to and during the performance and is in contrast to a focus on the possible outcomes or consequences. It is also important to note that athletes dominated by a process focus more easily maintain a level of arousal consistent with successful performances.

Although it may appear to some that this 'process' focus may be contrary to the primary purpose for competing, which is in fact to win, it merely represents an alternative and entirely compatible approach which assists the athlete and/or coach to maintain a focus on the quality of execution rather than the potentially distracting outcomes of winning or losing.

This is not to suggest that there is no place for an outcome focus. On the contrary, many elite athletes use this type of focus very successfully, but in training rather than during an actual competition. On cold, wet and windy mornings when it is tempting to remain in a warm bed, athletes can use outcomes as an incentive to make that extra effort and sacrifice. Reminding oneself of the need to defeat a particular opponent, to prove something to someone through winning, or to remind oneself of the excitement and satisfaction associated with standing on the winner's dais at a major competition all have their place, but not at the precise time one has to produce a 100% high quality performance.

LIFE-STYLE BALANCE

It is also necessary for elite athletes to manage their life-styles in a manner conducive to 'survival' in training and competition environments. Given the special requirements and demands on an athlete's time and energies arising from current training regimens and competitive schedules, matters of life-style quality and balance become critical. There is mounting case study evidence that less successful athletes have considerable difficulty in maintaining this life-style balance as compared to their more successful counterparts.

A decision taken at the AIS in 1981, that athletes on scholarship should be encouraged to maintain an involvement in part-time studies or other employment, appears to have been made in consideration of a commitment to the athletes' future career prospects, as well as the view that athletes should not be focused on their sport for 24 h each day. This policy recognizes that it is psychologically beneficial for athletes to 'switch off' their sport and maintain adequate 'rest'/work ratios. Not all athletes would agree that study or some form of part-time employment is a form of rest; however, these activities do provide opportunities for the athlete to focus on things other than the stresses of their training and competition schedules, thus representing a form of 'psychological rest'.

The same can be said for the need for athletes to maintain some form of hobby and social interest. Athletes who are training 5 or 6 h each day as well as studying or working, lead quite eccentric life-styles by normal standards. They obviously have a great need for normal rest and recovery, and they typically claim to have little if any time for social activities or hobbies. It is quite common for sports psychologists to find that athletes experiencing poor motivation report diminished or non-existent social activity and hobbies. These other facets of an athlete's life assist with the management of the stress to which most elite athletes must subject themselves if they are to reach high international standards.

There are several other individual factors which may influence an individual athlete's ability to consistently produce and maintain quality states of readiness in terms of optimal levels of psycho-physiological arousal. These include the following.

General Personality Style

Sports psychology research indicates that it is extremely difficult to predict performance success from general personality style information (Morgan 1980). However, most of the available data indicates that athletes are more extroverted than introverted (Nideffer 1989), a finding which is consistent with the intuitive notion that sports competition environments generally increase arousal for athletes. This would indicate that introverts have a neurological system that is already highly aroused, hence the tendency for them to shy away from highly stimulating situations. It appears that further arousal increases make them uncomfortable and they have difficulty in maintaining optimal levels of arousal in competitive sport situations. Applied clinical experience supports the observation that highly introverted athletes quickly become over-aroused in important competitions. Conversely, the typically extroverted athlete shows a tendency to seek out excitement, social settings, etc. (Eysenck & Wilson 1975). These athletes appear to be able to tolerate highly stimulating competitive environments without being so quickly over-aroused.

There are exceptions to this commonly held belief, as some world class athletes are introverted; however, it seems that these people have learned some very effective techniques for controlling undesirable arousal increases under competitive conditions.

Trait Anxiety

This is another individual characteristic which serves as an important antecedent in arousal control (Borkovec 1976). Spielberger's (1971) work on trait and state anxiety has served as a stimulus for a great deal of research in sport settings. Athletes with high levels of trait anxiety are more likely to have problems with arousal control in competition. These athletes typically report problems with over-arousal and associated performance decrements. The treatment of high trait anxiety has long-term implications, as compared to the development of strategies for the shorter-term state anxiety, which is commonly experienced by elite athletes in competitive settings (Mahoney & Meyers 1989).

Sport-specific Self-confidence

This characteristic can significantly influence an athlete's ability to produce optimum levels of arousal during competitive performances. Specific self-confidence, or self-efficacy as it is sometimes called, is itself influenced by more general levels of self-esteem. Many athletes experience considerable self-doubt and hesitancy immediately prior to and during sporting competitions.

Sports psychologists are often called in by coaches or consulted by athletes seeking some 'magical' formula for immediate increases in self-confidence. While there are some intervention strategies, which will enhance self-confidence in the short term, it is necessary to incorporate self-esteem and self-confidence training into the total preparation programme. The establishment of re-inforcement and incentive systems for quality performances in training (Bandura 1969), goal setting, daily diaries, high quality imagery pro-grammes, simulated competitions, assertiveness training, etc., based on a truly 'professional' approach to the development of programmes in all the areas previously mentioned, are all important factors in developing self-confidence.

PSYCHOLOGICAL FACTORS ASSOCIATED WITH PERFORMANCE DECREMENTS

In the earlier part of this chapter it was suggested that performance decrements may occur under poor arousal control conditions for individual athletes for a number of psychologically related reasons. If we assume that an athlete has a high level of technical skill and an appropriate level of physiological conditioning, then it is probably true to say that performance decrements may occur primarily through a lack of control over arousal, affecting one of a number of the additional psycho-logical factors discussed below.

Cognitive Factors

These include the appropriate use of self-talk and imagery strategies as part of the contribution towards maintaining a positive and confident attitude and a focus on the quality of the per-formance. At or close to the ideal performing state, the athlete more often than not uses positive affirmations, successful images and self-instructions associated with achieving successful, high quality performance. At either end of the arousal con-tinuum, and for the elite competitor, particularly at the over-arousal end of the inverted U curve, considerable negative self-talk, self-doubt and images associated with errors in the performance are commonly reported experiences.

It is proposed that the development of these 'controllable' cognitive skills can be achieved through the utilization of one or more of the cognitive behaviour therapies (Unestahl 1982) or through various behaviour conditioning strategies (Rushall 1979).

Applied experience with elite athletes would indicate that it is possible to enhance the vividness and accuracy of mental rehearsal or imagery using the following:

- Specific instruction and attentional cueing
- The creation of a conducive environment incorporating quality relaxation and restricted environmental stimulation

- Graduated learning techniques including specific training in the use of multiple sensory modalities, imagery from a performance perspective both inside and outside the skill, and experimentation with the timing of the rehearsal sequence (Suinn 1984)

Self-talk strategies can be learned through the use of techniques such as performance segmenting, and various cognitive 'programming' approaches, including hypnosis (Morgan 1980; Clarke & Jackson 1983), rational emotive therapy (Ellis 1966), salt water flotation (Bond 1987) and other counselling techniques (Fig. 8.3). For example a female tennis player who consulted the author with a specific performance decrement, responded very well to a short programme of self-hypnosis. This athlete described a problem with her volley. She was a very good serve and volley player, but her volley was consistently letting her down on important points and she had tried the traditional increased dose of volleying practice without success. Under hypnosis she reported that she had begun to consistently say something negative to herself when approaching volley situations in matches. This resulted in a tensing of her upper body so that she experienced a subsequent difficulty in hitting the volley with authority. Using hypnosis as a tool she replaced the negative self-talk with a positive instruction linked to a specific part of the volley preparation. The new positive self-instruction restored quality both in her volleys and general match play.

Self-confidence is a very complex cognitive issue for the athlete, sports psychologist and coach (Marsh 1990). Athletes who are able to maintain an ideal performing state in terms of level of arousal consistently report high levels of self-confidence and a belief that they can accomplish the task they have in front of them. Conversely, athletes who are over-aroused typically begin questioning themselves, their levels of preparation and their ability to win. This is typical of a shift from process to outcome focus. It is therefore imperative that coaches and sports psychologists work consistently to reinforce the multidimensional nature of an athlete's self-confidence through quality programming.

Psychophysiological Factors

These include those mind–body reactions which athletes commonly experience in response to situations perceived as stressful. It is commonly accepted that perceived stress will result in any one of a number of bodily reactions. For some athletes stressful competitive situations will produce such responses as increased heart rate (HR), blood pressure, breathing rate, length of 'normal' breath and deeper breath being taken, muscle tension (which may be specific to certain body sites), muscular tremor and changes in brain wave activity. Common symptoms also include ineffective decision-making, increased reaction time, 'forgetting' and changes in technique. It is this latter point which is so often confusing to the athlete and coach. What appears to be a technical error is often based in a less observable stress reaction, such as increased muscle tension. Further, this reaction is often the result of an 'outcome' focus occurring at a time when the athlete should be focused on a more relevant task-related cue. The traditional response to technique errors is to spend more time 'grooving' or automating the skill, thus moving the skill higher on the learning curve. Sometimes in this situation a repetition of the technique error occurs as soon as the athlete returns to the stressful competitive or training situation. The problem, however, may not lie in the technique area at all, as it may be a complex stress-based reaction which will not be overcome by mere physical practice.

One of the features mentioned earlier which is part of an ideal performing state is best described as 'feel', or sometimes referred to as 'flow'. It is an attempt to describe the controlled but ready and alert, or aware state, which is characteristic of the body's level of functioning at a particular point in time. Some better mentally prepared and more fortunate athletes manage to maintain this 'feeling' state for relatively lengthy periods of time, while others appear to be able to produce it when required. What is clear is that the higher the characteristic level of performance of the athlete, the more consistent is the production of the ideal psychophysiological state. These athletes also recog-

Fig. 8.3 A flotation tank used in elite sport for restricted environmental stimulation therapy.

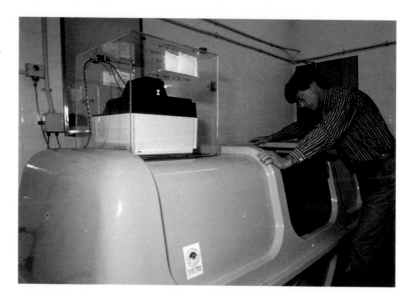

nize inappropriate arousal levels and shifts much more quickly than less successful athletes. They are then able to quickly effect a positive change and move back to the desired state. Conversely, the non-ideal performing state is regularly associated with a number of adverse bodily reactions. The lower level or less experienced athlete generally shows less consistency in maintaining an ideal state, is much slower in recognizing it when a shift has occurred, and often lacks the strategies to return to it.

One intuitive proposition holds that these mind–body reactions are indeed controllable by the athlete and a considerable amount of research in areas of biofeedback support this view (Landers 1980; Zaichowsky & Sime 1982). If the individual is able to control the firing of single muscle fibres (Basmaijan 1977), then it is certainly possible for the majority of athletes to learn to adjust HR, breathing or muscle tension functions. Biofeedback simply establishes a feedback loop which permits the central nervous system to attend to and change a particular aspect of bodily functioning. It is common now in high performance sport for athletes to be exposed to biofeedback techniques usually associated with HR and/or muscle tension in specific areas of the body. The majority of sports psychologists include training for athletes in the

area of arousal control and adjustment in a performance-enhancement programme. Various forms of relaxation training for the reduction of high arousal levels either prior to or during competition, and energizing techniques for increasing low-arousal levels before and during competition, are essential ingredients of the serious athlete's repertoire of psychological skills.

One example of the efficacy of biofeedback training occurred when the author began working with an elite Olympic weight-lifter. This athlete was the Australian champion in his particular weight division, but was 'sidelined' as a result of a knee injury. He was, however, able to ride a bicycle, and it was during one of these training sessions that this lifter experienced the ideal performing state he would like to be able to transfer to the competitive platform. He was subsequently given a portable HR monitor to take on his training rides for the rest of the week. He was instructed to check his HR if and when he reached that particular 'ideal state' during his ride. It seemed that this state was associated with a HR of about 135 beats·min^{-1}. In subsequent biofeedback training the lifter attached the HR monitor and practised reading his HR at different levels. He accomplished this by jogging to raise his HR, or relaxing using a breathing/centring procedure, then returning it to the desired level. In essence the training programme was designed to teach the lifter to be able to 'read' his own HR. He subsequently became very skilled at judging it without the HR monitor attached and to make appropriate adjustments to approximate the 135 'ideal' previously established as the desired target. This was then transferred to practice sessions, simulated training 'competitions' and finally to the competition situation. HR adjustment became an integral part of this lifter's pre-lift routine.

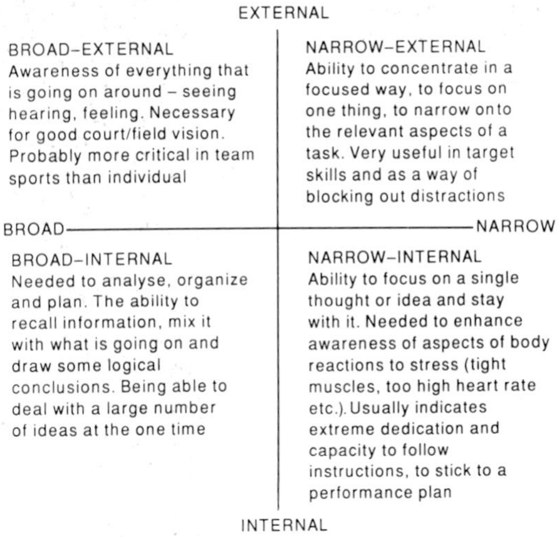

Attentional Factors

Focused concentration is also a feature of the ideal performance state and certainly contributes in a very significant way to performance quality. The work of Nideffer (1976) in developing a theory of attention and a questionnaire (the Test of Attentional and Interpersonal Style) to measure certain aspects of concentration style has been a landmark in this area of sport. Athletes often explain a substandard or super-standard performance in terms of concentration. It is quite typical for athletes and coaches to use an instruction to 'concentrate better, longer or harder'.

Nideffer maintains that an athlete will concentrate effectively and with the necessary flexibility in order to match the rapidly changing demands of the situation at a given point in time with the type of concentration necessary for high-quality performance, given an appropriate level of arousal.

An ineffective level of arousal reduces the athlete's control over attention, resulting in a mismatch of the attentional and situational demands through a return, under conditions of perceived pressure, to the use of an attentional 'strength'. This proposal assumes that each athlete has identifiable attentional 'strengths' and 'weaknesses' based on four types of concentration described in Nideffer's theory of attention in sport (Fig. 8.4). He maintains that concentration types can be described in terms of direction (external or internal) and bandwidth (broad or narrow). This provides at least four types of attention:

- Broad–external — peripheral or field awareness

EXTERNAL

BROAD–EXTERNAL	NARROW–EXTERNAL
Awareness of everything that is going on around – seeing hearing, feeling. Necessary for good court/field vision. Probably more critical in team sports than individual	Ability to concentrate in a focused way, to focus on one thing, to narrow onto the relevant aspects of a task. Very useful in target skills and as a way of blocking out distractions

BROAD ——————————————————————— NARROW

BROAD–INTERNAL	NARROW–INTERNAL
Needed to analyse, organize and plan. The ability to recall information, mix it with what is going on and draw some logical conclusions. Being able to deal with a large number of ideas at the one time	Ability to focus on a single thought or idea and stay with it. Needed to enhance awareness of aspects of body reactions to stress (tight muscles, too high heart rate etc.). Usually indicates extreme dedication and capacity to follow instructions, to stick to a performance plan

INTERNAL

Fig. 8.4 Nideffer's attentional types based on direction and bandwidth (Nideffer 1976).

- Broad–internal — analysis or problem-solving
- Narrow–internal — focused internal awareness or self-coaching
- Narrow–external — focused concentration or targeting

BROAD–EXTERNAL

The athlete with broad–external strength will perform very well in situations where field or court awareness is important or where immediate reactions to external stimuli such as an opponent's movements, are required for success. Under conditions of over-arousal or high levels of self-perceived pressure, these athletes at times 'subconsciously' use this characteristic when it may be inappropriate and become easily distracted by things going on around them. We often see examples of this in professional tennis or golf, when an athlete becomes 'externally distracted' by crowd noise or movement in high-pressure situations.

BROAD–INTERNAL

An athlete with broad–internal strength will perform well under ideal arousal levels in competitive situations which require that the athlete concentrate in an analytical or problem-solving way. These athletes are the 'thinkers' and analysers and they are often creative and can change strategies or develop new ones as required. Under high-arousal conditions they may, however, become overly analytical and react slowly to external stimuli because they are preoccupied with internal thoughts. They typically become caught up with inappropriate self-talk and are then 'internally distractible'.

NARROW–INTERNAL

Athletes with narrow–internal strength are generally very successful under ideal arousal conditions in competitive situations, when required to maintain a narrow focus on a specific coaching point or on a specific bodily feeling or position. They may become inflexible under high-arousal conditions in a self-coaching sense by locking on to a strategy and not letting go, or by narrowing on to an inappropriate internal cue, such as for example, the pain associated with lactate build-up.

NARROW–EXTERNAL

The narrow–external strength athletes perform very well in targeting situations. They are able to block out distractions and remain narrowly focused for long periods of time. Under adverse arousal levels, however, they may focus on an inappropriate external target at the wrong time, becoming too narrow externally and unable to retain attentional flexibility. An example would be an athlete focusing so intently on the ball that he/she loses awareness of an opponent's change of position.

ATTENTIONAL OVERLOAD

Overload may occur either externally, by the athlete becoming confused when trying to concentrate on too many external cues at the one time, or internally through too much self-talk or internal coaching. These overloads occur under increasing pressure for athletes in a way which is analogous to the learner driver becoming confused at a busy inter-section by the other traffic, pedestrians, traffic signals, etc. (external overload), or by focusing on so many driving tips that he/she becomes confused (internal overload). These types of overload are very common for inexperienced athletes competing in major competitions or in competitions which have a great deal of importance for them.

REDUCED FLEXIBILITY

In making the appropriate attentional shifts to match the requirements of a rapidly changing situation, reduced flexibility can also occur for athletes under perceived pressure. Excessive stress or competitive pressure results in concentration being focused internally and becoming so rigid that the person makes ineffective decisions. This is the type of error which is typical in life-threatening situations, such as theatre fires, where people are 'trampled' trying to leave via one door when there are others readily available. For some athletes, the stress of competition, though not 'life-threatening', may be perceived as 'all-important', resulting in a dramatically inflexible concentration capable of producing significant errors in performance.

Nideffer's Test of Attentional and Interpersonal Style remains the most useful applied/educational and clinical profiling instrument for use in areas such as concentration in sport (Bond & Nideffer 1992), despite the criticisms which have been made by various researchers (Van Schoyck & Grasha 1981; Vallerand 1983; Nideffer 1990; Ford & Summers 1992). His model of attention serves as a very useful tool in teaching athletes about their own concentration style, potential mismatches and overloads (Fig. 8.5). The model also gives athletes

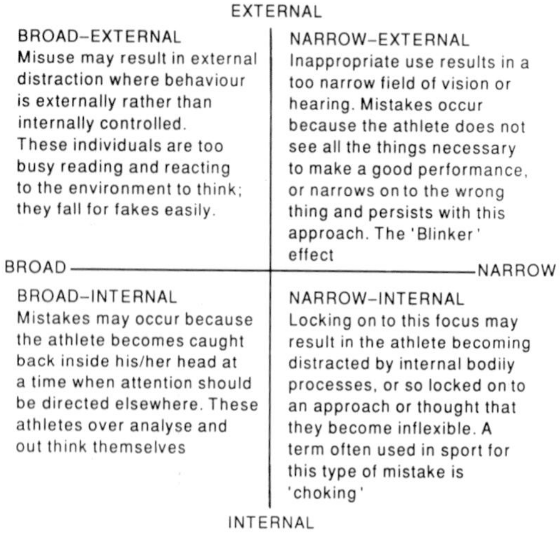

	EXTERNAL	
BROAD–EXTERNAL Misuse may result in external distraction where behaviour is externally rather than internally controlled. These individuals are too busy reading and reacting to the environment to think; they fall for fakes easily.	**NARROW–EXTERNAL** Inappropriate use results in a too narrow field of vision or hearing. Mistakes occur because the athlete does not see all the things necessary to make a good performance, or narrows on to the wrong thing and persists with this approach. The 'Blinker' effect
BROAD	NARROW
BROAD–INTERNAL Mistakes may occur because the athlete becomes caught back inside his/her head at a time when attention should be directed elsewhere. These athletes over analyse and out think themselves	**NARROW–INTERNAL** Locking on to this focus may result in the athlete becoming distracted by internal bodily processes, or so locked on to an approach or thought that they become inflexible. A term often used in sport for this type of mistake is 'choking'.
	INTERNAL	

Fig. 8.5 Nideffer's attentional errors based on the misuse of each of the four types of attention (Nideffer 1976).

and coaches another dimension for analysing performance errors, and provides valuable information necessary for the identification of specific attentional cues for use in developing performance plans.

Emotional States

Mood states or emotions play a significant role in the performances of some athletes (Morgan 1980). Reports of ideal performing states often include descriptions such as feeling 'up' or feeling alert and full of energy or vigour. Reports following poor performances and non-ideal arousal levels often include descriptions of negative mood states. Morgan (1980) popularized a profiling instrument for various aspects of emotion in sport called the Profile of Mood States (POMS; McNair *et al.* 1971). This instrument asks athletes to describe

how they feel given various time frames, according to the following six subsets of emotional state:

- Tension–anxiety
- Depression–dejection
- Anger–frustration
- Vigour–activity
- Fatigue–inertia
- Confusion–bewilderment

Morgan (1980) coined the phrase: 'Iceberg Profile' to describe the shape of the effective mood state profile, which is predictive of subsequent high-quality sporting performances (Fig. 8.6).

Because the POMS is easy to administer, score and interpret, sports psychologists have used it to help athletes become more aware of their mood state, how this may relate to performance quality and how a change in mood state may be introduced during the pre-competition and competition

Fig. 8.6 The typical 'iceberg' athlete profile showing the elevation of the positive mood state with reduced negative emotion (McNair *et al.* 1971).

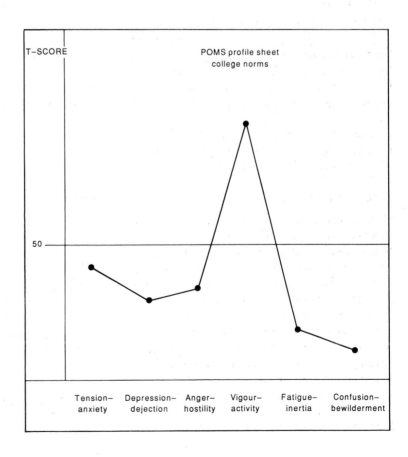

periods. This profile appears to be quite sensitive and predictive.

Information about mood state can be particularly useful for the individual if compared with previously developed baseline data. An interesting exercise is to contrast mood state profiles for high-quality and low-quality competition performances. The POMS profiles taken over a number of situations may indicate which aspect of emotion has a significant influence for a particular athlete. On this basis, change strategies can be planned for and more effective decisions provided for athletes and coaches, about what might be done immediately prior to competition to enhance mood and minimize the potentially harmful effects of an inappropriate emotional state. The use of cue or mood words, mental images, music, physical activity, attentional cueing, humour, social involvement, etc. has considerable intuitive appeal in

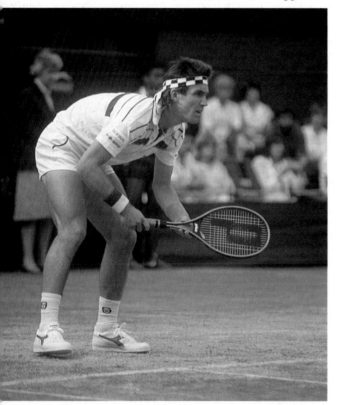

Fig. 8.7 A former Wimbledon champion displaying an intensive on-target attentional focus in readiness for a service return.

creating positive changes in certain areas of mood state.

Performance Routines and Rituals

Ideal performing states and their accompanying high-quality performances are characterized by the athlete adhering to consistent preparatory routines and rituals. The term 'preparatory' refers not only to pre-competition routines, but to specific preparation routines within the sport, such as preparing to serve a tennis ball, start in an event, etc. Very experienced athletes have a well-established and tested set of routines or 'rituals' which they use as part of their efforts to create an ideal performing state. If one observes the world's best tennis players or golfers, it is clear that these preparatory routines are a consistent feature and that they are a very necessary component of a successful performance (Fig. 8.7).

It appears that these routines provide a source of security for the athlete in a high-stress competitive situation, through the control they give over timing and rhythm (Flintoff-King 1992). These routines are part of the 'feel' which athletes describe as important in quality performances.

Well-established routines are also useful in assisting athletes to recover from unexpected interruptions, which may occur from time to time. Sometimes this will take the form of someone approaching them with unwanted advice just prior to the performance. More serious forms include re-scheduling the start of a performance or even tactical distractions by opponents.

The 1980 Moscow Olympics provided an illustration of the importance of preparatory routines. The finalists for the men's 100 m track event were being marshalled in a room under the main grandstand. These athletes were kept under armed guard in a situation having the potential for elevated levels of arousal. One can imagine that some athletes would have been trying to 'psych out' their opponents by 'eyeballing' them, while others were probably trying not to be distracted and to remain relaxed and isolated. Apparently, the competitors were finally summoned to their feet by the armed Russian guard and led out into the daylight down a short tunnel to the track. The extra light and the roar from the crowd as they reached the edge of the track further increased their arousal levels. The armed guard then stopped the group because there was a medal ceremony in progress and marched them back into the marshalling room. Not long after they had resumed their seats, one of the competitors leapt to his feet apparently in some sort of a 'fit'. He fell to the floor amidst a great deal of confusion and shouting, but eventually recovered to retake his seat. Soon after, the group was again marched out on to the track for the start of the final. History records that the very athlete who created the disturbance went on to win the 100 m final!

The point of this story is that many inexperienced athletes do not have well thought-out and established preparatory routines for situations such as marshalling, locker rooms, pre-start routines, etc. Under high arousal and possibly distracting conditions, these athletes are open to control and manipulation by the situation or an opponent.

Poor quality performances are often accompanied by observable shifts in these routines. For inexperienced athletes, these routines may not be well established, and therefore do not permit the athlete to maintain control or 'feel' in stressful situations. Athletes will typically rush their preparation, leave out parts of their preparatory routines or even add new components for no apparent reason.

It is a relatively simple task for a sports psychologist and/or coach to assist an athlete with the development of routines for various aspects of the preparation for and execution of areas of a performance (Bond 1985). This work must be based on a detailed knowledge of the sport, the specific situation in which the athlete is placed and the psychological characteristics of the individual. Table 8.2 is an example from competitive swimming showing some of the immediate pre-race and within-race detail that can be included in such plans.

Once these routines have been detailed, the task is then for the athlete to learn the performance plan so that it will occur more or less 'automatically' in the competitive environment. This learning of

Table 8.2 Competition swim plan detailing attentional cues based on the race plan

Race segments	Attentional cues
Pre-start	One lane pool
	Focus on own lane (imaginary barrier)
	Arousal check (adjust as necessary)
Start	Be alert
	Total concentration on gun
	Explosive reaction, leg and arm drive
False start plan	Longer streamline in dive
	A few easy, long strokes
	Slowly out to side and towel off
	Check arousal (adjust as necessary)
	Refocus on start routine
Dive	Streamline entry (small hole)
	Head down, kick
	Powerful first stroke to surface
	Head up, hold breath for first few strokes
First 25	Reach, stroke rate
	Powerful kick
	2–3 breaths
Second 25	Maintain stroke rate
	Powerful kick
	Check stroke length and rate
Turn	Focus on wall
	Power stroke (accelerate) into wall
	Fast tuck and feet on wall
	Explode off wall, streamline and kick
	Balance stroke, hold breath off wall
Third 25	Maintain speed and stroke efficiency
	Reach, grab and flick
	6 beat kick
Fourth 25	Focus on fast kick
	Reach, grab and flick
	Imagine breaking through the barrier
	Give it everything
Finish	Head down from flags
	Focus on wall and accelerate
	Extra reach
	Super fast last stroke, smash the wall!

routines and plans can be enhanced through the use of audio tapes, mental rehearsal sessions, practice in simulated competition settings, and fine tuning in lead-up competitions.

PERIODIZATION IN THE SPORTS PSYCHOLOGY PROGRAMME

Like other aspects of the athlete's training programme, it is important to consider how various psychological skills might be planned in relation to the timing of competitions, as there are certain psychological skill development programmes which are more appropriate as long-term training components.

Long-term Psychological Skills

Skills which require long-term application and learning are as follows:

- Attitude development
- Goal setting (in its broader context and in relation to training sessions)
- Basic arousal control techniques
- Individual awareness training through psychological profiling
- Emotional state awareness and manipulation
- Life balance skills involving work, rest and regeneration, and time management
- Confidence and self-esteem building
- Basic imagery techniques

These are not areas to be left until immediately prior to competition because improvement will only occur with correct practice over a long period of time. There is no set formula for the amount of practice required to learn these skills because this is dependent on the individual athlete and the situation.

Intermediate Psychological Skills

There are some psychological skills which can be added to the basic or long-term training programme in the period leading up to a major performance. This 'intermediate' skills programme may be introduced and practised or fine-tuned in the month or two prior to a performance. The skills involve those more specifically related to the actual performance and the venue in which the performance is to take place.

Specific mental rehearsal of the performance, including lead-up routines and the actual performance itself, within the context of the actual or perceived features of the venue, is one important example of a shorter-term psychological skill often used by many elite athletes. This rehearsal must be based on specific performance and pre-performance routines worked out by the athlete, coach and sports psychologist. They invariably contain 'contingency plans' as a coping mechanism to be used by the athlete in case things do not go exactly to plan in major competitions. They must take into account the goals set by the athlete, the technical, physical and mental objectives developed by the 'team', and the important features of the competition venue and surrounding environment. This technique is a type of mental 'simulation training' which is better designed to prepare the athlete for the competition performance.

The specific goal setting and performance evaluation programmes are an obvious adjunct to the development of preparation and performance routines and their mental rehearsal. Some athletes develop quite complex evaluation schedules, while others may prefer something more simple (Table 8.1).

Another important factor for athletes and coaches who travel long distances to compete is the area of travel skills (Bond 1986; Horsley 1988). Some athletes are experienced travellers and others are poorly skilled in this area. Applied sports psychologists may need to assist athletes and coaches to identify some of the important skills involved in travelling to and from competitions. This is of significance to the coach or athlete who must arrive ready to fine-tune the tapering or peaking process with the highest degree of quality possible. To be feeling jet-lagged, travel-weary, homesick or to have experienced several days of substandard training immediately prior to a major competition performance is a 'recipe for disaster'. The implications of these travel skills are evident for the individual athlete, as well as for the rest of the team or travelling group. A great deal of the unrest which is common among groups of athletes and coaches travelling long distances to compete is derived from the discomfort experienced by individuals within the group because of poorly developed travel skills; Chapter 21 should be read for further detail.

Short-term or Immediate Psychological Skills

These psychological skills include those which are utilized by the athlete in the competition itself. Included in this group are the specific preparation strategies for use prior to the competition and during the performance. The application of these strategies is dependent on a number of factors which are as follows:

- The athlete's state of long-term and intermediate psychological preparation
- The athlete's attitudinal focus at the competition in terms of process as opposed to outcome focus
- The athlete's state of awareness and self-control prior to and during the performance. This is sometimes referred to by coaches as sporting 'intelligence' on the part of an athlete who seems to have the presence of mind to be able to cope with any situation
- The extent of the athlete's 'bag of tricks' or ready-to-use mental strategies. This is a function of prior preparation training programmes

Immediately prior to competition and during competition, the areas of attitudinal focus and arousal control or regulation assume critical importance. By the time athletes reach the competition, there is little that they can do to significantly improve their technique or fitness if the work on these areas has not already been done. The competitor's capacity to produce the high quality which is necessary for successful performance will depend to a large extent on his or her ability to control the psychological responses which are used to adapt to the competitive situation. The negative aspects of these psychological responses can be minimized if the athlete and coach can avoid focusing on possible end-results and the many other potential distractors which abound at sporting contests, hence the importance of the long-term development of appropriate attitudes towards competition performances. Such an attitude must be so well learned that it is automatic, so as to retain a task focus

which achieves a performance of higher quality than has been previously experienced.

CONCLUSIONS

The multidimensional model presented in this chapter is proposed as a framework within which the coach, athlete and sports psychologist might be better able to 'profile' the individual's response to high-stress performance situations. It may also help to identify some possible features of a psychological skills training programme intervention strategy for use in the competitive environment.

Each individual athlete will have his or her own special blend of important psychological factors which impinge upon performance quality. Some athletes are dominated by emotional states, others by attentional fluctuations, and yet others by cognitive factors, or combinations of all of them. It appears that attitudes to the competition performance are an important prerequisite for many athletes. The emphasis must be on quality 'profiling' if sound decisions are to be made for individual athletes in their own specific performance environments.

The coach or athlete who is attempting to gain a greater understanding of some of the psychological factors which affect competitive performances can achieve a good deal by integrating the multidimensional model presented in this chapter. This model:

- Indicates some of the individualized responses which may occur as a result of perceived high stress in the performance situation
- Provides the athlete and coach with some insight into the sources of performance error which may significantly affect the quality of technique
- Also provides information and a basic framework for those who seek to individualize specific interventions in competition environments

No longer should it be acceptable for an athlete or coach to explain away a substandard performance with statements like the athlete did not 'concentrate hard enough', suffered a 'concentration lapse', did not feel 'in control emotionally', was 'too tight', or was plagued by 'negative self-talk or images'.

These explanations which were at one time considered too complex to understand fully or change, are now well catered for by the model presented in this chapter and the information currently available in the sports psychology literature. The model suggests a set of psychological skills which can be learned and fine-tuned, and furthermore it provides a framework for interpreting what is occurring in the complex interaction between athlete, performance and situation.

The applied sports psychologist who is attempting to unravel the complexities of a performance-related issue which may be confronting an elite athlete ought to be able to utilize the model which incorporates the concepts of:

- Arousal control
- Attitude development
- Cognitive factors
- Attentional factors
- Psychophysiological factors
- Emotional factors
- Routines and rituals

Attention to all these factors is needed so that effective decisions concerning the most appropriate forms of assistance for that individual in that specific situation can be made. This model therefore provides relevant information for better understanding on the part of the athlete and coach, appropriate individualized psychological skills training programmes, and specific forms of intervention which may be required for individual assistance in the short-term. There are also other approaches which are considered by Rushall (1992) and Williams (1993).

REFERENCES

Bandura A. (1969) *Principles of Behaviour Modification*. Holt, Rinehart and Winston, New York.

Basmaijan J. V. (1977) Learned control of single motor units. In Schwartz G. E. & Beatty J. (eds) *Biofeedback: Theory & Research*. Academic Press, New York.

Borkovec T. D. (1976) Physiological and cognitive processes in the regulation of anxiety. In Schwartz G. E. & Shapiro D. (eds) *Consciousness and Self-Regulation Advances in Research*, Vol. 1. Plenum Press, New York.

Bond J. W. (1985) Performance planning or segmenting. Australian Institute of Sport, Canberra.

Bond J. W. (1986) Minimising jet leg and jet stress. Australian Institute of Sport, Canberra.

Bond J. W. (1987) Flotation therapy: Current concepts. *Excel* 4, 2–4.

Bond J. W. & Nideffer R. M. (1992) Attentional and interpersonal characteristics of elite Australian athletes. *Excel* 8, 101–110.

Clarke J. C. & Jackson J. A. (1983). *Hypnosis and Behaviour Therapy: The Treatment of Anxieties and Phobias*. Springer Publishing Company, New York.

Csikszentmihalyi M. (1990) *Flow: The Psychology of Optimal Experience*. Harper & Row, New York.

Ellis A. (1966) A rational approach to interpretation. Paper delivered at a symposium for the American Psychological Association Convention, New York.

Eysenck H. J. & Wilson G. (1975) *Know Your Own Personality*. Macmillan, Melbourne.

Flintoff-King D. (1992) Preparing for Barcelona. Video tape developed for the 1992 Australian Olympic Team, Australian Olympic Committee, Sydney, Australia.

Ford S. K. and Summers J. J. (1992) The factorial validity of the TAIS attentional style subscales. *Journal of Sport and Exercise Psychology* 14, 283–297.

Horsley C. (1988) *Travel Skills*. Australian Institute of Sport, Canberra.

Jackson S. A. & Roberts G. C. (1992) Positive performance states of athletes: Toward a conceptual understanding of peak performance. *The Sport Psychologist* 6, 156–171.

Kerr J. (1985) A new perspective for sport psychology. In Apter M. G., Fontana D. & Murgatroyd S. (eds) *Reversal Theory Applications and Developments*. University College, Cardiff Press, Cardiff.

Landers D. M. (1980) The arousal–performance relationship revisited. *Research Quarterly for Exercise and Sport* 51, 77–90.

McNair D. M., Lorr M. & Droppleman L. F. (1971) *Manual: The Profile of Mood States*. Educational and Industrial Testing Service, San Diego, CA.

Mahoney M. J. & Meyers A. W. (1989) Anxiety and athletic performance: Traditional and cognitive-developmental perspectives. In Hackfort D. & Spielberger C. D. (eds) *Anxiety in Sports — An International Perspective*. Hemisphere Publishing Corporation, New York.

Marsh H. W. (1990) A multidimensional, hierarchical self-concept: Theoretical and empirical justification. *Education Psychology Review* 2, 77–172.

Morgan W. P. (1980) Test of champions: The iceberg profile. *Psychology Today* 21, 92–99, 101–108.

Nideffer R. N. (1976) Test of attentional and interpersonal style. *Journal of Personality and Social Psychology* **34**, 398–404.

Nideffer R. N. (1989) *Predicting Human Behaviour: A Theory and Test of Attentional and Interpersonal Style.* Enhanced Performance Services, Oakland, CA.

Nideffer R. M. (1990) Use of the test of attentional and interpersonal style (TAIS) in sport. *The Sport Psychologist* **4**, 285–300.

Orlick T. & Partington J. (1986) *Psyched: Inner Views of Winning.* Coaching Association of Canada, Ontario.

Ravizza K. (1984) Qualities of the peak experience in sport. In Silva J. M. & Weinberg R. S. (eds) *Psychological Foundations of Sport*, pp. 452–462. Human Kinetics Publishers, Champaign, IL.

Rushall B. S. (1979) *Psyching in Sport.* Pelham, London.

Rushall B. S. (1992) *Mental Skills Training for Sports — A Manual for Athletes, Coaches and Sports Psychologists.* Sports Science Associates, CA.

Spielberger C. D. (1971) Trait-state anxiety and motor behaviour. *Journal of Motor Behaviour* **3**, 265–279.

Suinn R. M. (1984) Visual motor behaviour rehearsal: The basic technique. *Scandinavian Journal of Behaviour Therapy* **13**, 131–142.

Unestahl L. E. (1982) *Better Sport By IMT — Inner Mental Training.* VEJE, Sweden.

Vallerand R. J. (1983) Attentional decision making: A test of the predictive validity of the Test of Attentional and Interpersonal Style (TAIS) in a sport setting. *Journal of Sport Psychology* **5**, 449–459.

Van Schoyck R. S. & Grasha A. F. (1981) Attentional style variations and athletic ability: The advantages of a sport-specific test. *Journal of Sport Psychology* **3**, 149–165.

Williams J. M. (1993) *Applied Sport Psychology: Personal Growth to Peak Performance*, 2nd edn. Mayfield Publishing Company, Mayfield, IL.

Yerkes R. M. & Dodson J. D. (1908) The relation of strength of stimulus to rapidity of habit-formation. *Journal of Comparative Neurology and Psychology* **18**, 459–482.

Zaichowsky L. & Sime W. (eds) (1982) *Stress Management for Sports.* AAHPERD, VA.

CHAPTER 9

TEAM ATHLETES

B. P. Miller

During our lifetime we are all part of formal and informal groups which have a powerful and significant impact on our lives. Since the turn of the century, behavioural scientists have been interested in evaluating, observing and otherwise recording the behaviours within groups. Social psychologists in particular have analysed the interactions between the individual members of a range of groups. In the last 20 years, a great deal of attention has been focused on sporting teams as a source of research data, and psychologists all over the world have examined successful teams, squads and clubs in an effort to determine the 'special factors' that influence sporting performance.

DEFINITION

Shaw (1976) has defined a group as 'two or more persons who are interacting with one another in such a manner that each person influences and is influenced by each other person'. The degree of interaction might well differ among different sporting teams, but it is nevertheless present. In fact, it is this interaction factor that sets apart a group from a mere collection of individuals. A team must have a sense of shared purpose, structured patterns of interaction, interpersonal attraction, personal interdependence and a collective identity. Sport groups can be thought of as a collection of interdependent individuals, co-ordinated and orchestrated into various task-efficient roles for the

purpose of achieving some goal or objective that is deemed important for that particular team (Yukelson 1984).

STEINER'S MODEL OF GROUP PERFORMANCE

What makes a group effective? How can athletes improve the overall performance of their team? Psychologists working in industrial and educational settings have studied productivity or performance for several decades. While their findings may not always be directly relevant to the sporting arena, some of their theoretical models are invaluable. One conceptual framework in current use was developed by Steiner (1972) and has been applied and extended by a number of sports psychologists since then.

The essence of Steiner's model (Fig. 9.1) is that a group's actual productivity is equal to potential productivity, minus losses due to faulty process.

Actual productivity or performance can be defined as the performance that is actually attained. Potential productivity is the group's best possible performance given its resources and the task de-

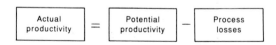

Fig. 9.1 Steiner's model of group effectiveness (Steiner 1972).

mands. The group's resources comprise all relevant knowledge, abilities and skills of the individual members, including the overall level and distribution of these talents. Process, that is everything the group does while transforming its resources into performance, is a critical but less defined part of Steiner's model. Group processes are the steps or actions performed individually or collectively by group members to carry out the group task.

When individuals work in groups, communication, co-ordination, and interaction are necessary. Process losses are subdivided by Steiner (1972) into two general categories, namely co-ordination and motivation losses. Steiner's model is classically described using a hypothetical tug-of-war team. In the case of a two-man team, each individual may be capable of pulling 100 kg. Thus, the potential productivity is 200 kg, but in a controlled trial, the actual performance is only 180 kg. The group has therefore experienced a decrement of 20 kg or 10%, which may be due to the inability of the athletes to co-ordinate their efforts; and/or because each athlete may let the other athlete do more of the work. The result is a process loss of 10%.

This idea of 'process loss' was fundamental to the psychological skills programme developed specifically for the Australian women's Olympic hockey team which won the Gold Medal in Seoul in 1988. A similar programme was utilized by the author with the British women's hockey team which won a Bronze Medal at the 1992 Barcelona Olympic Games. If Steiner's (1972) model is extended into the competitive arena, it becomes obvious that process loss must be reduced. If Team A is to be more effective than Team B, then there are three contrasting scenarios that will make this possible.

- Team A possesses greater relevant resources than Team B, and experiences fewer process losses than the opposition
- Team A possesses greater relevant resources than Team B, but experiences approximately equal process losses
- Team A possesses approximately equal relevant resources, but experiences fewer process losses

In the high-performance sport arena, most of the teams will be fast, strong, powerful and skilful, as well as experienced. They may appear to have comparable relevant resources, but the amount of process loss will be different. The role of the sports psychologist therefore is to work on reducing the amount of process loss that occurs.

GROUP VERSUS INDIVIDUAL PERFORMANCE VARIABLES

Do the Best Individuals Make the Best Teams?

It seems reasonable to assume that the most successful sports groups are those with the better individual athletes. Individual ability has been described by Gill (1986) as, '. . . probably the most important resource for sports groups. Perhaps the most accepted maxim by both researchers and practitioners is that the best individuals make the best team'.

However, the relationship between individual ability and group performance is not always perfect. Social psychologists have shown that there is a positive relationship between individual ability and group performance, but that the relationship is moderate at best and is mediated by task and situational factors. Moreover, the human resources available to any team must be relevant to that particular task. An extreme example, for instance would be an Olympic rowing eight, which may meet the requirements for a rowing championship, but is much less likely to meet those of a gymnastics championship at a high level. In the first instance their somatotype is advantageous in rowing, but in the latter sport it is a distinct disadvantage.

In one of the few studies involving sports teams, Jones (1974) investigated the relationship of team performance (as measured by win/loss records) with individual match statistics for such sports as American football, basketball, and baseball. Correlations ranging from 0.60 to 0.90 led Jones to conclude that group effectiveness was positively related to individual effectiveness in all cases.

The Ringelmann Effect

The above research conducted by Jones (1974) did not, however, take into account any intervening group processes. In other words, he viewed the players as individuals whose performances did not rely upon other individuals. Jones did not attempt to describe or measure the processes taking place between the players.

By comparison, there have been a number of investigations which have examined the so-called Ringelmann effect, which is entirely based upon intervening processes. Over 50 years ago a German psychologist named Ringelmann observed individuals pulling a rope in groups of two, three and eight. Although the groups pulled harder than the individuals, they did not apply as much force as might have been predicted by simply adding the individual forces together. For example, the eight-person groups did not pull eight times as hard as the individuals, but rather only four times as hard, and the average individual force for the eight-person group was only 49%. This decrease in average individual performance with increases in group size is now known as the Ringelmann effect.

More recently Ingham et al. (1974) resurrected the original Ringelmann paradigm with updated controls and modifications. Their results generally supported the findings of Ringelmann, although in their study the percentage decrements were not quite as large. Ingham et al. (1974) concluded that the decreases in average performance were due to motivational losses within groups.

In discussing their findings, Ingham et al. (1974) referred to sports groups that may be susceptible to motivation losses. In particular they quoted rowing statistics from the Olympic Games from 1952 to 1964, which revealed, for instance, that eight-man crews were only 23% faster than pairs. The results from the 1993 World Championships held in the Czech Republic (Table 9.1) also revealed similar findings. Obviously there are other factors

involved in rowing performances which must be taken into consideration such as shell length, crew weight, weather and water conditions.

When measuring the performances of the men's coxed pairs, fours and eights in terms of speed, the eight travelled at more than $1 \text{ m} \cdot \text{s}^{-1}$ faster than the pair, whereas the four-man crew fell almost exactly between the pair and the eight in terms of rowing speed.

Social Loafing

Latane et al. (1979), coined the term 'social loafing' after a series of studies in the period 1979–81 on motivational losses in groups. They found that individual efforts get somehow 'lost in the crowd' and group performance decreases. They also confirmed this as evidence of a robust phenomenon threatening effective collective endeavour across different activities.

Latane et al. (1979) established that social loafing was in part due to a diffusion of responsibility. In other words, when individuals were performing in a group where their precise contribution was hard to identify or measure, the degree of social loafing was greater than when they performed in a task where individual performances or contributions were easily identified. They concluded that identifiability of individual performance is critical and that when individual efforts are lost in the crowd, performance decreases.

Social loafing and individual performance identifiability were also seen as important factors in reducing the amount of process loss surrounding the 1988 Australian women's Olympic hockey team. Using a variety of competitive small-sided games and individual goal setting for training and match-play situations, the coaches worked on providing individual feedback to all team members. The players also took an active part in immediate post-game discussions, with the result that during the 2 year programme the players became more and more aware of their own performance levels and those of their colleagues. This was a relatively new development within the sport of hockey, and helped to reduce social loafing to a minimum. The players took more responsibility for their own actions

Table 9.1 Relative winning performances from the 1993 world rowing championships

Crew	Winning time	Speed (m·s⁻¹)
Pairs	7.01.50	4.75
Fours	6.14.64	5.34
Eights	5.37.08	5.93

both on and off the field, and the coaches used an empowering coaching style which helped the athletes to retain their sense of initiative and self-determination.

Traditional coaching styles are often de-powering in nature. That is, they tend to strip athletes of their initiative and they gradually become dependent on the coach. Players have little or no input regarding training programmes, tactics, competition schedules, etc. and coaches make most of the decisions concerning their development in the sport. This can often cause problems when athletes mature and are competing in a major championship like the Olympic Games. Ultimately, it is the competitor who must compete in this pressurized environment; therefore it is important that they retain their initiative and independence. The empowering style of coaching is geared towards these joint goals.

THE DEVELOPMENT OF INTERACTIVE SKILLS

In general, coaches would agree that there is a need to reduce co-ordination and motivation losses within any team. In a situation where the coach has a choice of athletes available, identifying those who possess individual interactive skills as well as physical talent could greatly reduce the co-ordination losses to which Steiner referred. However, if there is no choice available, coaches need to direct their efforts toward enhancing the team's interactive skills in several different ways by developing a series of specific responses to on- and off-field events.

On-field Strategies

An example of this approach was developed in hockey for the 1988 Olympic Games. It consisted of a strategy for dealing with on-field injuries, which necessitated a break in play while the doctor or physiotherapist came on to the field. A well-defined policy was formulated in which individual players came together as a group during any such short break. One player was asked to look towards the coach on the bench to receive any pre-planned, strategic hand signals, while another was positioned to see the progress being made with the injured

player, so that the team could quickly resume playing positions as soon as the treatment concluded. The rest of the team was taught to listen to the captain's comments, but there was also a 'lookout' who told the other players when to return to the play.

At first sight this tactic may seem trivial and insignificant but it was important that the players felt that they were in control of all of the controllable variables such as the on-field injury programme, warm-up, half-time team talk and post-game discussion. Other factors such as an umpire's decision or an unlucky stick deflection were out of their control and as such were to be ignored.

The Australian victory against the Koreans in the 1988 Olympic women's hockey final provided the team with a good test of this on-field injury strategy. An Australian player accidentally hit the ball into the face of a Korean player and the game was immediately halted. The injury at first looked worse than it actually was; nevertheless the player needed treatment. The Australian team went through their injury routine, coming together as a group, and discussed the state of play. By comparison, all of the Korean players rushed in to help their fallen team-mate. Two coaches and two medical personnel also joined in the throng, and it meant that the Korean players were involved in an undisciplined, unmanaged break in the middle of the biggest game of their lives. In the minutes following this interruption, the Australian players were able to settle into a style and mode of play which allowed them to dominate the game. In contrast, the Koreans were unable to gain control and the number of unforced errors after this incident increased dramatically.

While there are many factors that may have contributed to this situation, there is no doubt that the Australian team was able to focus on the mechanisms of success while the Koreans allowed themselves to be distracted at a crucial time in the game. In other words, there were co-ordination losses occurring and their actual productivity decreased. By careful planning and forward thinking it may be possible to reduce such losses by establishing mutually agreed strategies which form part of a contingency management programme.

Off-field Strategies

There are many off-field strategies available to the coach which will improve the team's performance. Rather than deal with them at this point they will be discussed in the 'How to encourage cohesion' section later in the chapter.

The Importance of Feedback

The coach's goal must be to identify individual behaviours which contribute to group performance and work to increase those behaviours. Once these are identified, strategies to encourage and reinforce them are needed. Most coaches are aware that feedback is a key element in this situation as research has suggested that individuals work harder and more successfully when provided with individual feedback within a group situation.

Gross (1982) examined social loafing and the influence of group and individual feedback on a group motor task. Although four-person groups did not exhibit social loafing, possibly due to identifiability and evaluation potential in the group task, feedback effects were observed. Groups who received feedback of both individual and group times improved performance more than did groups who received only group feedback.

Extrinsic and Intrinsic Motivation Factors

Encouragement and reinforcement can also be used to supplement pure information feedback. However, it is recommended that extrinsic rewards are not emphasized at the expense of intrinsic motivation. According to Gill (1984), 'verbal encouragement and specific, informative evaluations of positive behaviours will likely be more effective and have fewer negative consequences than adding extensive extrinsic reward systems'.

In summary, it is important that coaches identify the individual behaviours that contribute to desired group performance. It is equally important that in order to make actual performance closely reflect potential performance, there is a need to make sure that individual behaviours are recognized and re-warded in order to reduce the process losses within the team situation. While the available research is minimal and often poorly defined, observation of successful coaches across a variety of team sports suggests that this is the most efficient route to performance improvement.

TEAM AND GROUP COHESION

The term cohesion is derived from the Latin word *cohaesus*, which means 'to cling together', so it is not surprising that the term 'cohesion' has been used by social psychologists to describe the behaviour of many groups. Cohesion reflects the strength of the bond among individual members within a group. Cartwright and Zander (1968) developed a model of cohesion, which has been variously modified to suit the sporting context (Carron 1982). Figure 9.2 represents a summary of the forces which have been identified as determining the levels of group cohesion.

Carron (1982) stressed the need to view cohesion as a dynamic process, which is reflected in the tendency for a group to remain united in the pursuit of its goals and objectives. Importantly, Carron's definition suggests that there are at least two important dimensions to team cohesion, namely task cohesion and social cohesion.

Social Versus Task Cohesion

Social cohesion reflects the degree to which the members of a team like each other and enjoy each other's company, while task cohesion reflects the degree to which members of a group work together to achieve a specific and identifiable goal; this is usually associated with the purpose for which the team or group was formed. For example, the 1988 Australian hockey team had the general task of winning an Olympic gold medal, and a specific one of trying to score more goals than the other team in every match they played.

These two types of cohesion can work independently of each other and it is possible that a team with high levels of social cohesion has low levels of task cohesion. For instance, a team of recreational basketballers or a veterans' rugby side are likely to

Fig. 9.2 Carron's conceptual system for cohesiveness in sports teams.

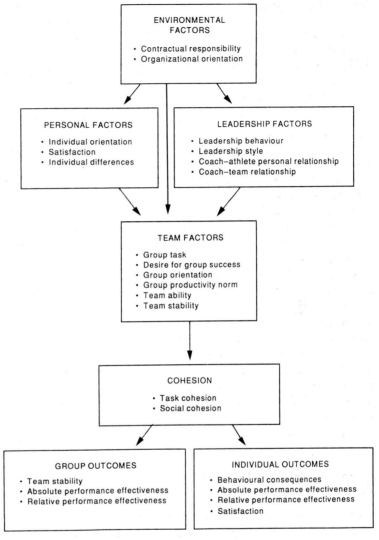

be driven by social goals rather than task goals *per se*. They will, of course, try to win matches, but perhaps they are more concerned with the interactions that occur after the game than during it.

In a similar vein, it is possible that a team will be highly focused on a task goal, but have little interest in social objectives. Indeed, there are many examples of very successful professional clubs who have major social problems, but because of their 'professional' approach to their sport, they are prepared to work together in order to win. The best results, however, will be obtained when social and task cohesion are equally developed.

The Nature of the Cohesion–Performance Relationship in Different Sports

Studies which have examined the effect of cohesion upon levels of performance have failed to produce consistent results. While some research has suggested that successful teams are also more cohesive units, this has not been replicated in all sports. For instance, basketball teams have tended to provide data suggesting a positive link between cohesiveness and performance (Klein & Christiansen 1969; Martens & Peterson 1971; Arnold & Straub 1972).

However, other authors have reported a negative relationship. Lenk's (1969) research with rowing is one example, and McGrath's (1962) work with rifle teams is another. Landers and Luschen (1974) were the first to put forward a theory which could reconcile these differences as they felt that the task structure and its demands could account for the results.

The task dimension originally proposed by Landers and Luschen (1974) was coaching versus interacting. In interacting teams, the total group effort is a product of team-work. This situation has been described by Thomas (1957) as high means interdependence. By comparison, in a coaching situation, the group product is achieved via the summation of individual group members' efforts. This is described as low means interdependence. A track and field or rifle team would be an example of a coaching team, while the major field games for example soccer, rugby, hockey, etc. would typify interacting sports.

According to Carron (1980) it is only within those sports which require interactive dependence, that cohesiveness will contribute to improved performance because of improved co-ordination. In coactive situations, cohesiveness is unrelated to performance success. Carron (1980) summarizes this by stating that

> Sports differ in the degree to which task interdependence is required of participants; the degree of task interdependence present affects the type of co-ordination necessary; and the type of co-ordination necessary affects the degree to which group cohesiveness is a mandatory factor in performance outcome.

The Role of Communication in Cohesion

There are a number of properties associated with cohesiveness, a major one being communication. The level of communication relating to task and social issues increases as the group becomes more cohesive. Group members are more likely to talk openly with one another, and perhaps more importantly, they are more prepared to listen to each other's views. As cohesiveness increases, so does the exchange of useful, relevant task information.

Increasing cohesiveness also encourages greater conformity to group standards for behaviour and performance. As a group improves its cohesiveness, its members place increasing value on social approval and show a greater tendency to adhere to the group norms. This very cohesiveness, however, can make the introduction of new members more difficult within an already successful, cohesive team and specific deliberate strategies have to be adopted in such circumstances in order to reduce the possibility of new players or officials being shunned by the group.

How to Encourage Cohesion: A Practical Example

On a practical level, there are a number of exercises or off-field strategies that can be carried out with any given group of athletes, which can help to promote both task and social cohesion. Traditionally, they take the form of educational sessions and are useful for bridging any real or perceived gaps between the older and younger members of any team or squad.

During 1987 and 1988, the above-mentioned women's hockey team completed a number of exercises in the build-up to Seoul. One such exercise was known as 'The Perfect Hockey Player'. Figure 9.3 is taken from the players' training diaries used on their European tour of 1988, and it formed the basis of the session. Basically, the players were asked to develop a profile of how they thought the perfect or model player would react in certain situations that might affect an international hockey player taking part in the Olympic Games.

The squad was divided into four groups of four, each group including some experienced players. Within each group the athletes nominated a spokesperson and a 'minute taker' to keep notes of their group's discussions. Each group was allowed 30 min in which to summarize their ideas on how the perfect player would react to various hypothetical situations which were common or at least feasible within their sport. Each of the items was developed in conjunction with the coaching staff of the team to ensure a sense of realism.

After the 30 min period, the four small groups

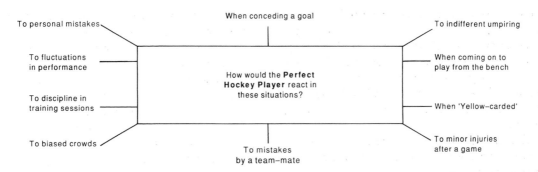

Fig. 9.3 Situational demands on emotional and attentional control in hockey (based on Miller 1988).

came together, and each spokesperson presented that group's opinions. There was a great deal of discussion about acceptable behaviours or strategies for dealing with these situations. A general consensus was reached and it was agreed that this was to be the standard by which the players could justifiably judge one another.

This exercise has been tailored and used by the author with other sports in Australia, New Zealand and Britain. The individual elements have to be changed, for example, with Rugby League reference must be made to the 'sin-bin' and the word 'try' added, but the general principle remains the same. The athletes work in small groups to arrive at a consensus and this is then used as a benchmark for excellence, against which they can assess themselves.

The importance of such an exercise is that players have an opportunity to contribute to the formation of a team strategy. They also have the chance to listen to each other's views and to agree upon an accepted task orientation. Additionally, such sessions are used to help unite team members from a social cohesion point of view and help the younger players settle into a new and challenging situation. In summary, the educational nature of these sessions was useful in providing opportunities for the development of both task and social cohesion.

OTHER METHODS OF DEVELOPING TEAM COHESION

While most researchers stress the need to be able to measure cohesion accurately, most coaches do not

focus on this element, relying rather upon intuition. However, the following methods have been used successfully in the past by this author, and can be employed with athletes from a range of sports, and with a variety of age groups. Some of these are cited in Yukelson's (1984) work on group motivation and they are principles around which the psychological preparation of any sports team can be based. While the research concerning cohesion and performance is somewhat equivocal, there is no doubt that coaches prefer to work with a team that is cohesive and united in purpose. While it is acknowledged that there have been some notable exceptions to the rule, it is generally accepted that sports teams should be cohesive units, particularly with regard to task cohesion (Figs 9.4 and 9.5).

Post-play Debriefing

Another approach designed to promote improvements in both elements of cohesion can also be employed. If a team is involved in a tournament, they will have to play several matches spread over several days, and most World Cup and Olympic competitions are based around such a format. It is important that when one game is completed, players and coaches learn from that game, discuss its implications and then put that game out of their minds as they prepare for the next. It is vital that players are assisted to analyse a performance honestly and accurately. They must learn from it, but win, lose or draw, they must not dwell on it.

Although this strategy may seem logical, it is easier said than done when the athletes are involved in a vital competition. It is very likely that in the face of a disappointment, players may be tempted

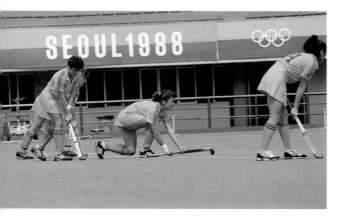

Fig. 9.4 Team co-operation in hockey.

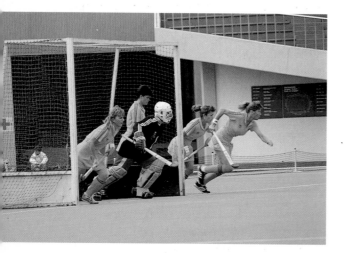

Fig. 9.5 Empowered hockey players striving to attain team goals.

to over-analyse and be overly critical of themselves, their team-mates or the coach. Typically, this does not make a positive contribution to subsequent pre-match preparation, and can lead to the development of cliques or disaffected factions within the group.

It is important that there is always an opportunity for any player to comment on any aspect of the game. Also, after the player input, the coaches must summarize the match. As part of the em-

powering coaching style, it is important not to stifle any player contributions by the coach dictating the theme of the discussion. These sessions, known as post-game analysis (PGA), should be utilized after every practice game, or competition match, irrespective of the result. They allow the players to 'put that game to bed' and concentrate on the next one. This approach helps to improve task cohesion and reduces the opportunities for any destructive social factors to develop.

The Replacement Process

Within every team, squad or club there will be a turnover of athletes. People will move away from the area, or they will simply retire from the sport because of injury, age or changing priorities. Thus, a major problem can exist with the assimilation of new players and coaches and senior athletes need to

Table 9.2 Typical examples of professional goals quoted by Australian athletes

---

'To eat only nutritious food while on road trips.'

'I will try hard to get on with all the other athletes on tour.'

'Use my walkman for recreation and relaxation on long trips during the tour.'

'Ensure I do not react to suspect refereeing in a negative way.'

'Make sure I get a daytime sleep every day.'

'Make sure I do mental rehearsals at least once a day.'

'I will try to be a supportive member of the team, especially when on the bench and when others are feeling a little down.'

'Keep reasonable hours during the trip and be aware of my room-mates' wishes.'

'Accept the desires of the majority of the squad and support their decisions.'

'Ensure I am mentally prepared to train intensely, thereby using each training session as an opportunity to develop.'

'Take the opportunity to learn from the older players.'

'I won't overeat at breakfast, even if they lay on "the works".'

'Set goals for each training session / game and constantly evaluate my progress.'

'Focus on controllables, and stay single-minded.'

---

be aware of the possible effects of the team dividing into 'mature' and 'young' player groups. Such educational exercises as 'the model player', and 'what if . . . ' (Miller 1988) can be helpful in this context, but the attitude of key personnel is probably more important than any one-off psychological team-building session. The replacement process is inevitable within every group, so it is important that disruption is kept to a minimum. It requires a conscious commitment from the existing personnel to achieve a smooth transition.

Open Communication Channels

It is important that effective communication occurs between coaches and athletes. The foundation for this communication is trust and mutual respect and ideally, coaches should strive to establish an atmosphere where individual players feel that their contributions are welcomed and appreciated. Sarcasm and ridicule play no role in this process, and it is important to note that communication is a two-way process. Both the coach and the athlete have a responsibility toward each other to make it work.

Goal Setting

Pride comes from the self-satisfaction that goals set by individuals and the group have been achieved. Goal setting can go a long way towards achieving pride in the team's efforts. Professional as well as performance goals should be established and Table 9.2 includes some of the goals that have been used by athletes in the past.

As well as individual aims, team goals should be discussed and targeted. Typically, they should focus on the process of success, rather than the outcome. Naturally a team wants to win, but that should not be their stated goal. Rather they should be concerned with ensuring that they control all of the controllable variables and take each game as a separate entity. They must focus on the 'here and now', rather than concentrating on the consequences of any one result, such as 'If we win this match today, we will be in the semi-final tomorrow', or 'We only need a draw today to make next week's play-offs'.

The uniqueness of group goal setting has been highlighted by Mills (1984) who noted that a group's goals are not the sum of the personal goals of team members. Findings from Brawley *et al.* (1993) have suggested that the group variable of cohesion is greater among those individuals who perceive that their team engages in group goal setting for competition. Following on from their earlier research (Brawley *et al.* 1992), these authors concluded that 'When groups are less involved in participative group actions such as setting team goals, the degree to which group unity and other group goal-related variables are perceived is correspondingly less'. An important element of the mental preparation of both the Australian and British women's hockey teams in 1988 and 1992, respectively, was to promote this sense of involvement in such activities as team goal setting.

Goal setting for matches and tournaments is now a commonly accepted practice, but using goals for training sessions is slightly more unusual. Most importantly, the goals that are established have to be evaluated and provision must be made for this in a well balanced training programme. The coach is also important in teaching players to self-evaluate themselves and must provide feedback concerning their goals and objectives. It is important that the athletes learn to carry out this process so that they can evaluate their own performance after the coach has given them the method to be used.

Clear Guidelines for Behaviour

Behaviour norms need to be conducive to the goals the group is striving to achieve and it is suggested that the general philosophy on behaviour needs to be stated explicitly. Athletes should be able to discuss the topic and then formulate a plan to which all players agree. Ambiguity and lack of clarity can be disastrous at this stage, and it is important that all personnel strive towards the same clearly stated goal. For example, athletes travelling to foreign venues find many distractions and temptations, and it is important that coaches retain some control over the team's free time. If the athletes slip into a 'tourist mode' over a number of days it can seriously impair performance.

The Role of Praise

Individuals who excel within their designated role should be recognized and verbally rewarded with praise. Some coaches are reluctant to do this within a team context for fear of causing resentment and jealousy. However, the coach's goal should be to have all members of the team fulfilling their individual goals, and thus it is important to let players know that their efforts are appreciated. Such recognition can serve to make athletes ego-involved rather than just task-involved.

At one stage it seemed unfashionable to praise team athletes, and coaches appeared to spend most of their time being critical of their charges and trying to correct faults. Of course, correction is an important part of the coach's role, but it is vital that athletes strive towards a performance that brings with it praise and recognition. The coaching style has a direct bearing on this process.

CONCLUSIONS

Team athletes play their sport within a group. These groups are dynamic and are influenced by many external factors. In order for athletes to achieve their full potential they need to share common goals with their team-mates. The group needs to have an effective communication system that promotes goal achievement.

Any team that seeks to make actual productivity closely related to potential productivity (Steiner 1972) must work to promote cohesiveness within its ranks. Co-ordination losses and motivation losses need to be minimized if a team is to fulfil its potential. By eliminating social loafing and by increasing individual performance, the coach can help to create an efficient working unit. If negative influences are not reduced or removed, the coach will have difficulty in concentrating on the technical and tactical elements of team preparation.

There are a number of principles and techniques that can be employed with sports teams which can help promote a co-operative environment and team cohesion is one of these. Respected West German soccer coach, Franz Beckenbauer (1990) whose team won the 1990 World Cup was quoted before the first round as saying that his team would play well throughout the tournament because

the communication between players is excellent, on and off the field. There are no groups at meal times, as there were in the previous World Cup — a Bayern Munich table here, a Cologne table there. Part of the way to achieve harmony in the squad is in selection. Even our substitutes are in a happy mood and contribute to the morale of the side.

Although research in this field is scant, it appears that there are already some convincing examples in international team sports of the success of the empowering coaching style. If thoughtful coaches develop team cohesion, clear guide-lines and intelligent strategies, they can then greatly improve their team's performance and sense of achievement.

REFERENCES

Arnold G. E. & Straub W. F. (1972) Personality and group cohesiveness as determinants of success among inter-scholastic basketball teams. *Proceedings Fourth Canadian Symposium on Psycho-Motor Learning and Sport Psychology.* Health and Welfare Canada, Ottawa.

Beckenbauer F. (1990) Harmony the keynote of German success. *The Times* **June 19**, 40.

Brawley L. R., Carron A. V. & Widmeyer W. N. (1992) The nature of group goals in sport teams: A phenomenological analysis. *The Sport Psychologist* 6, 323–333.

Brawley L. R., Carron A. V. & Widmeyer W. N. (1993) The influence of the group and its cohesiveness on perceptions of group goal-related variables. *Journal of Sport and Exercise Psychology* 15, 245–260.

Carron A. V. (1980) *Social Psychology of Sport*, p. 249. Mouvement Publications, Ithaca, NY.

Carron A. V. (1982) Cohesiveness in sports groups. Interpretations and considerations. *Journal of Sport Psychology* 4, 123–138.

Cartwright D. & Zander A. (1968) *Group Dynamics: Research and Theory*, 3rd edn. Harper & Row, New York.

Gill D. L. (1984) Individual and group performance in sport. In Silva J. M. & Weinberg R. S. (eds) *Psychological Foundations of Sport*, pp. 315–328. Human Kinetics Publishers, Champaign, IL.

Gill D. L. (1986) *Psychological Dynamics of Sport*. Human Kinetics Publishers, Champaign, IL.

Gross J. (1982) Effects of knowledge of results upon individual performance on a motor task under alone and group situations. PhD thesis, dissertation. University of Iowa (unpublished).

Ingham A., Levinger G., Graves B. & Peckham V. (1974) The Ringelmann Effect: Studies of group size and group performance. *Journal of Experimental Social Psychology* 10, 371–384.

Jones M. B. (1974) Regressing group on individual effectiveness. *Organisational Behaviour & Human Performance* 11, 426–451.

Klein M. & Christianson G. (1969) Group composition, group structure and group effectiveness. In Loy J. W. & Kenyon G. S. (eds) *Sport, Culture and Society*, pp. 397–408. Macmillan, Toronto.

Landers D. M. & Luschen G. (1974) Team performance outcome and the cohesiveness of competitive coacting teams. *International Journal of Sport Sociology* 9, 57–71.

Latane B., Williams K. & Harkins S. (1979) Many hands make light work: The causes and consequences of social loafing. *Journal of Personality and Social Psychology* 37, 823–832.

Lenk H. (1969) Top performance despite internal conflict: An antithesis to a functionalistic proposition. In Loy J. W. & Kenyon G. S. (eds) *Sport, Culture & Society*, pp. 393–397. Macmillan, Toronto.

McGrath J. E. (1962) The influence of positive interpersonal relations on adjustment and effectiveness in rifle teams. *Journal of Abnormal and Social Psychology* 65, 365–375.

Martens R. & Peterson J. (1971) Group cohesiveness as a determinant of member satisfaction in team performance. *International Review of Sport Sociology* 6, 49–61.

Miller B. P. (1988) Touring skills: Learning to cope. *Excel* 4, 3–5.

Mills T. M. (1984) *The Sociology of Small Groups*, 2nd edn. Prentice-Hall, Englewood Cliffs, NJ.

Shaw M. (1976) *Group Dynamics: The Psychology of Small Group Behaviour*, 2nd edn. McGraw-Hill, New York.

Steiner I. (1972) *Group Process and Productivity*. Academic Press, New York.

Thomas E. J. (1957) Effects of facilitative role interdependence on group functioning. *Human Relations* 10, 347–356.

Yukelson D. (1984) Group motivation in sport teams. In Silva J. M. & Weinberg R. S. (eds) *Psychological Foundations of Sport*, pp. 229–241. Human Kinetics Publishers, Champaign, IL.

CHAPTER 10

THE PSYCHOLOGICAL ASPECTS OF INJURY IN SPORT

J. R. Grove and A. M. D. Gordon

Sports injuries occur with alarming frequency, and large numbers of sports performers are treated each year by medical personnel. Although contact sports produce more injuries per participant than non-contact sports, sudden and traumatic incapacitation may occur in either type of activity. In order to fully understand the injury occurrence/recovery process, practitioners must consider both psychological and physiological factors.

Traditionally, the medical literature has focused on the physical aspects of the injury process and de-emphasized the importance of the psychological factors. Recent evidence suggests, however, that psychosocial factors can have a significant impact on injury occurrence and recovery. This evidence can be categorized into four broad areas relating to the psychology of sports injury (Wiese & Weiss 1987):

- Psychological variables as predictors of injury occurrence
- The athlete's psychological response to injury
- Psychological aspects of the rehabilitation process
- Psychological readiness to return to competition

PSYCHOLOGICAL PREDICTORS OF INJURY OCCURRENCE

A number of variables have been examined as potential predictors of injury occurrence in sport.

Early work in this area provided descriptive accounts of the types of athletes thought to be prone to injury and suggested that intrapersonal conflict, anxiety, depression, guilt and low self-confidence were important contributors to injury occurrence (Sanderson 1977). Subsequent research has taken a variety of other factors into account, and the manner in which they interact has been summarized by Andersen and Williams (1988) in their stress-related model of the injury occurrence process in sport. This model, a simplified form of which is shown in Fig. 10.1, provides an excellent framework for examining the psychological precursors to injury.

The Stress Response

At the core of the Andersen and Williams model is the stress response. This response consists of a cognitive component and a physiological/attentional component, both exerting reciprocal influences on each other. Evaluations of the demands inherent in the sports situation, the resources available to meet these demands and the consequences of successful versus unsuccessful coping produce physiological tension as well as attentional deficits. At the same time, these physiological and attentional changes influence the nature of the ongoing evaluation. If the perceived threat is sufficiently strong or recurrent, this response may increase the risk of injury by disrupting co-ordination and flexibility as well as interfering with the detection of important

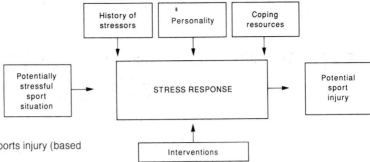

Fig. 10.1 A stress-related model of sports injury (based on Andersen & Williams 1988).

environmental cues: for example, an opposition player moving in from the side to attempt a tackle. A number of identifiable factors have the potential to exacerbate or moderate this response.

Personality

Perhaps the most widely researched mediating variable is the athlete's personality. Unfortunately, very few reliable relationships have been demonstrated between personality and sports injury. A few studies suggest, however, that certain variables are worthy of consideration: for example, several investigations have reported connections between injury occurrence and scores on Factor I (tender-minded vs. tough-minded) and Factor A (reserved vs. outgoing) of Cattell's 16 PF (Personality Factor) Questionnaire. Players scoring near the tender-minded and reserved ends of these scales may be more prone to injury than their more tough-minded and outgoing peers. Similarly, low scores on measures of general self-esteem have been implicated as a precursor to injury by a number of researchers.

Lysens *et al.* (1987a,b) have also reported interesting findings concerning the interaction of personality and the type of injury likely to be experienced. Their data suggest that acute injuries are frequent among competitors with extraverted tendencies and a low sense of responsibility. Overuse injuries, on the other hand, are frequent among competitors with high levels of dedication and responsibility. Research by Banks (1989) also suggests that different personality factors may be implicated in different types of injury. Other personality variables such as

hardiness, the Type A behaviour pattern and optimism/pessimism have not been examined thoroughly in connection with injury, although they have been linked to other health-related outcomes (Rodin & Salovey 1989; Grove 1993).

History of Stressors

A second factor that may influence sports injury indirectly through its impact on the stress response is the athlete's history of stressors. The most frequent finding along these lines has been a positive association between measures of stress from major life events and the incidence of injury. This relationship appears to be strongest in contact sports such as American football where there is a high baseline rate of injury, but it has been observed in other sports as well. There has also been speculation that 'daily hassles' experienced by the athlete may be positively related to the chances of injury. The effect of these chronic, low-level stressors may be cumulative, and they have been shown to influence both mood and general health (DeLongis *et al.* 1988). A final history variable that may be important in producing stress for the athlete is his/her experience of prior injury. Situations which have led to injury in the past undoubtedly have the potential for generating considerable tension and anxiety which may, in turn, predispose the athlete to injury by virtue of physical and/or attentional deficits. These 'situations' could be as general as the point in the season (pre-season, just before finals, etc.), or as specific as the playing surface, the venue, the opponent, or the game circumstances.

Coping Resources

The final general class of mediators in the stress–injury relationship is the nature of the athlete's coping resources. These consist of a variety of behaviours and interpersonal networks which aid the individual in dealing with life's positive and negative events (Andersen & Williams 1988). Research indicates that social support systems are a particularly important coping resource, both in terms of general health and sports injury. These systems consist of coaches/team-mates, partners/spouses, friends/relatives and supervisors/co-workers who provide emotional support to the individual. The quality of the social support system will be determined by the extent to which the athlete believes these people care about him/her, trusts and confides in them and can access them in times of need. A number of studies indicate that high levels of social support are associated with low incidences of injury, and that low levels of social support are associated with high incidences of injury. Although other coping resources have not been studied as extensively as support networks, there is speculation that life-style factors such as diet, sleep habits, exercise regimens and alcohol/drug use could also contribute to the risk of injury (Banks 1989).

PSYCHOLOGICAL RESPONSE TO INJURY

Because injuries will never be completely eliminated from sport, it is important to understand how athletes typically react to injury as well as the psychological factors that might influence this response. Awareness along these lines will help therapists, coaches, administrators, team-mates, family and friends interact with the injured athlete in a more effective and positive manner.

Emotions and Behaviour

There is agreement among practitioners, athletes and researchers that sports injuries have strong emotional and behavioural consequences. In a general sense, this emotion/behaviour syndrome can be viewed as a three-element, repeating cycle comprised of distress, denial and a determination to cope (Heil 1993). Distress and denial tend to peak in the early stages of rehabilitation and then give way to increasing amounts of determined coping in the later stages. However, even in the later stages of recovery, transient periods of distress/denial can be expected to occur in response to specific difficulties, such as pain or lack of progress.

The specific emotions experienced by the injured athlete may be similar to those experienced as part of the grief response (Kubler-Ross 1969). Physical capabilities constitute an important dimension of personal identity for most athletes, and injury can therefore pose a threat to their self-concept. Particularly in the case of a serious injury, the athlete is likely to respond initially with shock, denial and an overly-optimistic belief that the injury is less serious than it appears (Suinn 1967).

This initial numbness is followed by a period of heightened emotionality in which feelings of isolation/loneliness, anger/resentment, depression and anxiety may be experienced (Rotella & Heyman 1993). The athlete may become irritable and/or self-critical at this time, and there may be a loss of interest in usual activities. The athlete may also question the value of treatment and fail to comply with recommended rehabilitation procedures.

Adaptation begins with partial acceptance, which is characterized by a bargaining mentality. The player may become inquisitive about the injury or treatment protocol and may make it known that he/she will comply with the treatment if convinced that the procedures will work and noticeable progress will be made. This bargaining phase may represent an attempt by the athlete to establish personal control over a process that has been, by and large, beyond his/her control. The final phase is one of general acceptance, where the athlete becomes resigned to the limitations imposed by the injury, focuses on what needs to be done to facilitate recovery and becomes actively involved in the rehabilitation process.

Mediating Factors

It is likely that the duration and intensity of emotional and behavioural reactions to injury will depend on a number of factors. At present, however, theoretical models and empirical evidence address psychological factors primarily as predictors of injury occurrence and not as determinants of injury response. Some potential psychological mediators of injury response are presented below, using the Andersen and Williams (1988) model as a guide (Fig. 10.1). A similar approach has been adopted by other researchers who have addressed the psychological aspects of rehabilitation (Grove et al. 1990; Grove 1993; Wiese-Bjornstal & Smith 1993). Coaches, medical practitioners and other support personnel are urged to consider these potential mediators in their work with injured athletes.

Sanderson (1978, 1981) has proposed that the personality dimensions of extraversion/introversion and neuroticism/stability could be important in determining behavioural responses to injury. Extraverts have been shown to be impatient and to have relatively high pain tolerance, so it is possible that highly extraverted athletes would tend to ignore pain and return to competition too soon. Introverts, on the other hand, may not return soon enough because they tend to be apprehensive, indecisive and guarded. High neuroticism scores could also delay progress during rehabilitation because of a tendency to over-react to the injury. As hardiness, dispositional optimism, and explanatory style have demonstrated a relationship to general health, it is suggested that they might also influence reactions to sports injury (Grove 1993). Finally, self-motivation, self-esteem and self-concept, particularly body concept and physical self-esteem, deserve attention as correlates of emotional reactions to injury and behavioural persistence during rehabilitation (Weiss & Troxell 1986).

The athlete's stress history and coping resources are also potentially important mediators of the response to injury. The experience of previous injuries, the trauma associated with them and the success of prior rehabilitation efforts will undoubtedly influence the nature of post-injury stress. There is evidence that general life stress delays recovery from minor illness and injury among athletes (May et al. 1985), and it is reasonable to assume that daily 'hassles' occurring during rehabilitation may produce similar effects. Although it is

difficult to find direct evidence that social support networks or life-style factors influence recovery from sports injury, such an assumption also appears reasonable (Gordon et al. 1991; Ford & Gordon 1993).

Finally, it appears that injury-related factors should be taken into account when analysing the athlete's response to injury. Sanderson (1981) notes that players are likely to react negatively if they feel that their injury occurred as a result of a teammate's illegal or unacceptable behaviour. Similarly, the severity of the injury in terms of pain, persistence and disruption of normal activities may affect emotions and behaviour. The timing of the injury within the season as well as within the athlete's career has also been noted as an important determinant of the response to injury.

PSYCHOLOGICAL ASPECTS OF THE REHABILITATION PROCESS

Once athletes have adapted to their injury and learned to accept their incapacity, the first step towards rehabilitation must be determined. Adherence to physical treatment protocols is necessary; however, in order to facilitate and promote a positive and determined attitude to rehabilitation, certain psychological factors must also be considered. A concomitant mental and physical effort therefore seems necessary for effective rehabilitation to take place.

Two sets of psychological strategies have been summarized by Wiese and Weiss (1987) as having potential to facilitate such an effort. Both are educational strategies, namely communication skills and motivation techniques.

Communication Skills

Health care professionals can facilitate rehabilitation by providing detailed information about all aspects of the athlete's injury (Weiss & Troxell 1986). A detailed description of the nature of the injury and the prescribed rehabilitation programme and a programme rationale should be provided, together with realistic expectations concerning pain, lack of mobility, inconvenience and physical and psychological setbacks. An emphasis on positive attitude and persistence during rehabilitation must be communicated. Heil's (1993) list of factors to be addressed in a comprehensive injury management programme are shown in Table 10.1 and emphasize the educational value and importance of communication.

To achieve effective communication, health care professionals must become responsive listeners with athletes, who may require assistance in dealing with the emotional challenges posed by rehabilitation. While severely troubled or depressed athletes should be referred to licensed psychologists, preferably with sports science training, the majority of non-

Table 10.1 Injury education guide-lines

Basic anatomy of the injured area.

Changes caused by injury.

Description of diagnostic and surgical procedures (if necessary).

Guide-lines for independent use of modalities (i.e. heat, cold).

Purposes of medication with emphasis on consistent use as prescribed.

Potential side-effects of medication with encouragement to report these to the physician.

Potential problems with pain and how to cope with these.

Differentiation of benign pain from dangerous pain.

Active and passive rehabilitation methods.

Mechanisms by which rehabilitation methods work.

Plan for progressing active rehabilitation (e.g. resistance training).

Anticipated timetable for rehabilitation.

Possibility of treatment plateaus.

Rationale for limits on daily physical activities during healing.

Guide-lines for the use of braces, orthotic devices or crutches.

Injury as a source of stress and a challenge to maintaining a positive attitude.

Rehabilitation as an active collaborative learning process.

Methods of assessing readiness for return to play.

Deciding when to hold back and when to go all-out.

Long-term maintenance and care of healing injury.

Adapted from Heil (1993).

professional counsellors who deal with athletes on a daily basis, such as coaches, physiotherapists and parents, can easily learn to communicate effectively with an injured athlete.

Motivation Techniques

The question of motivation during rehabilitation becomes particularly critical during inevitable setbacks and periods of little or no improvement, which will challenge the athlete's motivation and enthusiasm for treatment. Five categories of strategies have been identified that can be employed when assisting athletes to maintain their motivation and persistence (Heil 1993).

GOAL SETTING

The process of goal setting should include goals to follow the prescribed treatment protocol (e.g. attendance at treatment sessions, perseverance with homework exercises) and goals for incorporating psychological strategies (e.g. relaxation, imagery, self-talk) within the rehabilitation programme.

The general principles and guide-lines of goal setting are outlined in Chapter 7. The first step is to set realistic, specific and measurable goals, which should be written down by athletes and re-evaluated frequently. Daily, weekly and monthly goals need to be monitored and updated periodically as progress is recorded. Feedback to the athlete must be provided and based upon objectively determined standards of achievement. The observable improvements should promote motivation as well as healing.

RELAXATION

A relaxed condition facilitates healing by moderating the sympathetic nervous system functions, which are usually activated by stressful situations and conditions. Relaxation therefore helps to conserve vital energy required to promote healing and fight discomfort and disease (Turk *et al.* 1983).

Through regular use of relaxation skills, athletes can facilitate and perhaps accelerate their recovery from injury. Three techniques that could be employed are: progressive muscular relaxation (PMR); autogenic training; and biofeedback. PMR teaches injured athletes to recognize the build-up and release of tension in different muscle groups and is particularly applicable for dealing with pain experiences or sensations, and for preparing for treatment (Turk *et al.* 1983). Autogenic training works through self-suggestion and focuses on both physical relaxation, using sensations of warmth and heaviness, and mental relaxation in the form of visualization. In medical as well as sports studies, the ability of subjects to control blood flow, alter skin temperature and produce hot or cold sensations in different parts of the body has been attributed to autogenic training. Biofeedback can be incorporated into rehabilitation programmes to help individuals train and control their body reactions. Through the use of electromyography or galvanic skin response indicators, both visual or audible, injured athletes can be taught to monitor and control relaxation levels during treatment (Achterberg & Lawlis 1980).

IMAGERY

The 'imagination' can also be used to facilitate the rehabilitation process, particularly when used in conjunction with relaxation exercises. Athletes whose imaginations dwell on 'worst possible' scenarios can be taught to control and channel their images and thus reduce anxiety and fear, as well as enhance healing. Various imagery techniques can be taught to injured athletes and are described below.

Emotive imagery helps athletes feel more positive about themselves and what they can achieve. By using imaginary scenes that the athlete recalls with pride and enthusiasm, for example feelings of pride in having recovered from previous injuries or setbacks, this technique boosts confidence levels. The goal is not to deceive the athlete but rather to evoke positive, composed and calm feelings associated with memorable past experiences (Lazarus 1977).

Body rehearsal is a second technique that facilitates healing, by using positive images. First, the athlete is given details of what has happened internally as a result of the injury, so that he/she can develop a clear picture of the internal damage caused by the injury. Next the intent of the rehabilitation programme is explained, which en-ables the athlete to imagine precisely what is happening internally during the healing process (Rotella 1985).

Mastery rehearsal, in which physicians and physiotherapists explain in specific detail what must occur internally to effect healing, can also be used in concert with body rehearsal. Only successful surgery or recovery is visualized, never setbacks or problems (Mahoney 1979). While this technique may induce confidence levels in athletes and enhance physical performance, mastery rehearsal may not be applicable to certain cases or suitable in dealing with inevitable setbacks in rehabilitation.

Coping rehearsal, on the other hand, teaches athletes to anticipate problems in recovery through the preparation of plans to deal with periods of anxiety, worry and pain. Such preparation might also induce unnecessary anxiety on the part of some athletes who may find anxiety levels overwhelming; however, this technique is generally regarded as a realistic and valuable tool to learn and use (Meichenbaum 1985).

Finally, time projection is an imagery technique which effectively distances injured athletes from their current frustrations, inconveniences or pain. If athletes are taught to picture themselves 2 or 6 weeks in the future, they can attain some instant relief from their present experiences. By planning ahead through time projection on a day-by-day/week-by-week basis, using a range of positive steps, athletes will learn to deal with current crises more effectively (Lazarus 1977).

POSITIVE SELF-TALK

Self-talk differs markedly from the 'power-of-positive-thinking' approach which tends to promote a formula of rote repetition and emotionless patter. While there is an element of positive thinking and self-reliance inherent in self-talk, the latter is unmistakably an active problem-solving approach and not simply a series of verbal palliatives. Injured athletes can benefit enormously from learning a cognitive restructuring programme because they tend to dwell on negative and irrational thoughts and beliefs about themselves and their chances of recovery, particularly during long and painful periods of treatment (Rotella & Heyman 1993).

Table 10.2 Some irrational thoughts after injury and during rehabilitation changed to rational responses

Event	Irrational self-defeating thoughts	Rational self-enhancing thoughts
Injury	'I'm finished! Most players never recover from this injury.'	'I'm seriously injured. But with the advice and expertise of the doctor, I'll be OK. This is the attitude of athletes who recover. I must do my part in the rehabilitative process.'
Rehabilitation	'What do they (doctors and therapists) know? This treatment is a waste of my time and theirs.'	'Therapy is really a drag! But healing won't come unless I give these sessions my best shot. They're doing their best to help me, so I've got to do my part. It's going to take a while, but unless I'm dedicated I'm not going to recover as quickly as I would like.'

From Gordon (1986).

In implementing cognitive restructuring techniques, mental skills consultants would first assist athletes in understanding the nature of their reactions to the stressor (e.g. pain associated with treatment). Athletes would then be shown how automatic and irrational thought processes can negatively affect responses to injury and rehabilitation. Some typical counter-productive thought processes are illustrated in Table 10.2.

Next, athletes would be assisted in breaking down their responses into components and taught how and when to use both cognitive and behavioural coping strategies to deal with each component. An example of this process for an athlete dealing with pain in rehabilitation is illustrated in Table 10.3.

The third stage of implementing a cognitive restructuring programme would involve athletes practising these techniques in a variety of stressful situations during rehabilitation. The primary purpose, therefore, is to teach athletes how to integrate cognitive and behavioural skills and to apply them to all situations perceived as stressful during the rehabilitation process.

One of the easiest cognitive techniques to both teach and learn is thought stoppage, which effectively 'stops' self-defeating inner dialogue and turns it into self-enhancing inner dialogue. Two rehabilitation scenarios are described in Table 10.4 together with examples of thought stoppage interventions that produce both productive and self-enhancing self-talk.

SOCIAL SUPPORT

A final factor that can affect motivation during rehabilitation concerns the influence and support of other individuals. According to Rosenfeld et al. (1989), social support networks can influence stress levels in athletes and involve a unique set of contributions from coaches, team-mates, family and friends. While coaches and team-mates provide technical support for athletes, they are generally not expected to provide as much emotional support as family and friends. Some contrasting evidence exists concerning the level of social support coaches and team-mates can provide to athletes (Gordon & Lindgren 1990); however, such contributions are exceptional and it is usually left to family and friends to provide empathy and emotional support.

Hardy and Crace (1991) have proposed eight distinguishable types of social support that injured athletes could benefit from during rehabilitation. They are as follows:

- Listening support — behaviours that indicate people are listening without giving advice or being judgemental

Table 10.3 Self-instruction training through four stages of dealing with pain

---

Stage 1: Preparing for the stressor (a visit to the clinic)

Purpose of statements:

To combat negative thinking and to emphasize planning and preparation

'This visit is going to be tough and challenging, but I know what I have to do today'

'I can think of many reasons and excuses for not going — no time, too busy, clinic hours are ridiculous, etc. — but I must recognize those excuses and be ready for them'

'To recover from this injury I must always find a way to get my treatment'

Stage 2: Confronting the stressor (pain)

Purpose of statements:

To reassure, control and reinterpret the pain as something that can be used constructively

'Don't think about that machine — just about what you have to do'

'The therapist told me to expect this pain for a certain period of time'

'Relax, take a deep breath — that's better — I'm in control now and I'll help the healing process by keeping my cool!'

Stage 3: Feeling overwhelmed (pain)

Purpose of statements:

To provide encouragement and to focus on concentration

'The pain is getting worse — it's pretty high on my scale of 0–10! but I coped with pain like this before by relaxing these muscles and breathing slowly'

'This is getting too much, but it's a signal of what I have to do — which may, if necessary, include calling the therapists because they will appreciate being told'

Stage 4: Evaluation of personal efforts

Purpose of statements:

To evaluate what worked and what didn't work; to praise self for effort and to self-attribute successful accomplishment

'It's getting better each time I use this procedure. I've got this technique taped'

'Didn't work today but that's OK — What can I learn from my efforts for next time?'

'Good stuff, I handled that well — must tell the therapists (coach, friends or other injured athletes) how it went. I'll do even better next time'

From Gordon (1986).

- Emotional comfort — behaviours that comfort the individual and indicate people care about them
- Emotional challenge — behaviours that challenge the individual to evaluate their attitudes, values and feelings
- Task appreciation — behaviours that acknowledge individual efforts and express appreciation for the work they do
- Task challenge — behaviour that prompts, encourages and challenges the individual to do more and achieve more
- Reality confirmation — behaviours by people with similar experiences, priorities, values and views that reassure the individual during times of stress or confusion and confirm perceptions and perspectives of the situation
- Material assistance — behaviours that provide the individual with financial assistance, products or gifts
- Personal assistance — behaviours that indicate a giving of time, skills, knowledge and/or expertise to help the individual accomplish tasks

The above behaviours represent three generally accepted dimensions of social support: emotional (listening support, emotional comfort and challenge); informational (reality confirmation, task

Table 10.4 Some examples of thought stoppage techniques

Stress situation	Self-defeating inner dialogue	Self-enhancing modified inner dialogue
7.30 a.m. The clinic is closed and the therapist fails to appear for a regular treatment session.	'That idiot! Gives me the lecture yesterday about the importance of regular treatments in rehabilitation and then doesn't show up! She'd better apologize before I show up again. I've had it!' *Consequence*: Athlete assumes no responsibility and fails to realize who is suffering most by not receiving therapy.	'I'm really mad — stop! But this is strange. Something important must have delayed her because I know how punctual and professional she is and how much she wants me to recover. I must get treatment regularly. I'll check back later to see if she can schedule another time for me.' *Consequence*: Athlete rationalizes non-appearance of the therapist. Takes on responsibility for personal efforts to recover.
The athlete experiences great pain and discomfort during exercises and notices no significant improvements to the injury.	'This really hurts! I'm sick and tired of the pain! And there's no improvement! I need a break — they don't give a hoot — and if it really is important they'll call me. This will heal itself in time anyway.' *Consequence*: Athlete benefits little from the token effort expended during treatment. Develops and rationalizes excuses for giving up.	'Boy this hurts a lot — stop! But this pain is what I was told to expect. If it gets too bad I guess I'd better tell them because they'll want to know. But I must persevere and try to get through it. This way I'll soon get out of here and be playing again.' *Consequence*: Athlete gives 100% in a quality session, and prepares for more of the same; expresses difficulties and concerns to the therapists who positively encourage and appreciate this attitude; feels good the rest of the day because personal behaviour is becoming more helpful and less inclined to self-pity.

From Gordon (1986).

appreciation and challenge); and tangible (material and personal assistance) (Hardy & Crace 1993).

Two recent studies investigated various means of improving current provisions of social support for injured athletes within both the medical and sports communities. Ford and Gordon (1993) describe over 50 suggestions sports physiotherapists from Australia and New Zealand perceived as both 'important' and 'practicable' in their treatment of injured athletes. In general, these data suggested that, while in an excellent position to offer informational support, sports physiotherapists can also provide significant emotional and tangible support. By doing so, they will facilitate much more effective communication and feedback between the athlete and his or her rehabilitation team. Ford *et al.*, (1993), in a similar study with 28 elite Australian coaches, also illustrated the case with which emotional, tangible and informational support can

be applied during rehabilitation to motivate athletes and help them deal with their injury more effectively.

Athletes sometimes respond more effectively to injury if two particular strategies to provide support for injured athletes are also incorporated in the rehabilitation programme. First, peer modelling (Weiss & Troxell 1986) involves the interaction of injured athletes with previously injured athletes who have successfully recovered. These 'positive models' can provide support and encouragement to currently injured athletes and, more importantly, provide empathic understanding of the painful and emotional experiences during recovery. Second, injury support groups (Weiss & Troxell 1986) involve regular meetings with trainers or physiotherapists who facilitate discussion among other injured athletes who share their thoughts, emotions and concerns.

While further research is necessary on the nature

and scope of social support systems, all of the above strategies can promote motivation during rehabilitation.

PSYCHOLOGICAL READINESS TO RETURN TO COMPETITION

Although closely related, physical readiness and psychological readiness to return to competition following injury are not synonymous. Unfortunately, however, some health care professionals, coaches and athletes often assume that the latter follows 'naturally' from the former. In some cases this has led to heightened anxiety and fear and loss of confidence on the part of athletes, who subsequently perform poorly when they return to competition or re-injure themselves (Rotella 1985). In order to avoid a repeat of the injury and further loss of confidence in their performance, it is essential that injured athletes be fully consulted about their complete recovery and readiness to return to competition (Heil 1993).

Physical recovery from injury can be determined objectively from the physical signs and symptoms of healing, for example absence of pain, full range of motion, and a return to full strength of the injured body part. However, psychological recovery is a highly subjective phenomenon and ultimately rests with the perceived confidence of injured athletes in meeting the physical demands of full competition.

Although little empirical evidence supports the contention that 'confidence' is significant to the athlete when deciding to return to competition, researchers (e.g. Rotella 1985; Weiss & Troxell 1986; Wiese & Weiss 1987; Gordon & Lindgren 1990; Rotella & Heyman 1993) believe it is vital. The evidence suggests that athletes should only be allowed to return to competition when they themselves consider that they are both physically and mentally ready to do so.

CONCLUSIONS

The psychological aspects of sports injury include psychosocial factors related to injury occurrence, specific emotional and behavioural responses to injury, psychological principles used in rehabilitation programmes and psychological readiness for returning to competition. Although research into psycho-

Table 10.5 Some guide-lines for athletes during the stages of adaptation following a sports injury

Respond positively to the incapacities, pain and weaknesses from the injury:
- Inform the trainer and/or coach immediately
- Denial of injury is dysfunctional to rehabilitation, and may contribute to a premature end of your career

Adapt promptly to the stresses of treatment procedures:
- Accept that hospitals, treatment rooms, orthopaedic devices and rehabilitation timetables will be unsettling and difficult at first
- Adjustments, however, do occur with time

Place trust in medical personnel and encourage communication:
- Diminished trust in professionals in unfamiliar settings can be anticipated; this is normal
- Athletes often feel vulnerable when dependent on others

Maintain an emotional balance:
- Avoid self-blame and/or guilt for accidents (past events)
- Focus on rehabilitation and recovery (present events)

Maintain a healthy self-image:
- Forced inactivity and non-participation is extremely frustrating; few will fully comprehend this emotional challenge
- Keep a healthy and positive perspective on life; loss of mastery, competence and participation is only temporary
- You can return; focus efforts on rehabilitation

Preserve relationships with team-mates, coaches, family and friends:
- With only a little effort athletes can preserve relationships and normal interaction patterns
- Avoid alienating or isolating yourself from associates who may find dealing with your injury difficult

Look forward positively to an uncertain future:
- Surgery and advanced rehabilitation techniques can both raise and destroy hopes of full recovery, but you must do everything you can for yourself
- Always be enthusiastic and positive about full activity and an active life

Accept the limitations and restrictions imposed by the injury and adjust life-style and goals accordingly:
- Focus on what you *can* do, not on what you can't do; learn to accept physical realities
- Keep moving forward in life; looking back with regret is a waste of time

Adapted from Rotella (1985).

social predictors of injury has been criticized for adopting an atheoretical approach, some consistent relationships have emerged. Certain personal, historical and social variables appear to exert weak but reliable influences on the occurrence of injury, and psychologists are now expanding their investigations into the areas of injury response and injury rehabilitation.

In terms of emotional and behavioural responses, athletes appear to exhibit a somewhat predictable reaction to injury. This reaction typically involves an initial tendency to ignore or deny the trauma, as well as a subsequent tendency to experience feelings of anger, depression and anxiety. Although very little research has focused on the factors which may alleviate these reactions among sports performers, it is possible that variables related to the injury itself and/or the athlete's personality are important. Past and present stressors as well as the availability and use of coping resources may also play a mediating role. Awareness of these tendencies and potential moderating factors will help practitioners to understand the injured athlete and to offer advice which is relevant to both the individual athlete and the stage of recovery. Table 10.5 offers some general suggestions along these lines.

It appears that psychological factors play a critical role in rehabilitation performance and are related to those components of the stress model identified in Fig. 10.1. Personality factors, history of stressors and coping resources can all affect mental and physical performance in recovery. Strategies such as communication skills and motivational techniques which athletes can learn and use, can be incorporated in rehabilitation programmes. The physical and mental challenges of lengthy recovery periods can often seem overwhelming; however, with expert assistance, support and commitment to learn these techniques, these problems can be overcome.

Further research on the psychological readiness of injured athletes to return to competition is necessary, requiring both qualitative and quantitative methodological approaches. The common attitude that 'if the body is ready the mind is also' must continue to be challenged, as an athlete's anxiety and fear and lack of confidence must be addressed and alleviated before he or she returns to

competition. This highlights the important role of the mental skills consultant as part of the coaching team who, together with the athlete, can make more informed decisions on complete recovery and readiness to return to competition.

REFERENCES

Achterberg J. & Lawlis G. F. (1980) *Bridges of the Body Mind: Behavioral Approaches to Health Care*. Institute for Personality and Ability Testing, Champaign, IL.

Andersen M. B. & Williams J. M. (1988) A model of stress and athletic injury: Prediction and prevention. *Journal of Sport and Exercise Psychology* 10, 294–306.

Banks J. P. (1989) *Psychological Factors in Sports Injuries Among Elite Hockey Players*. Unpublished master's thesis. The University of Western Australia, Perth.

DeLongis A., Folkman S. & Lazarus R. S. (1988) The impact of daily stress on health and mood: Psychological and social resources as mediators. *Journal of Personality and Social Psychology* 54, 486–495.

Ford I. W. & Gordon S. (1993) Social support and athletic injury: The perspective of sport physiotherapists. *Australian Journal of Science and Medicine in Sport* 25, 17–25.

Ford I. W., Gordon S. & Horsley C. (1993) Social support for injured athletes: The perspective of elite coaches. *Sports Coach* 16(4), 12–18.

Gordon A. M. (1986) Sport psychology and the injured athlete: A cognitive–behavioural approach to injury response and injury rehabilitation. *Science Periodical on Research and Technology in Sport*, Coaching Association of Canada, Ottawa.

Gordon A. M. & Lindgren S. (1990) Psycho-physical rehabilitation from a serious sport injury: Case study of an elite fast bowler. *Australian Journal of Science and Medicine in Sport* 22, 71–76.

Gordon S., Milios D. & Grove J. R. (1991) Psychological aspects of the recovery process from sport injury: The perspective of sport physiotherapists. *Australian Journal of Science and Medicine in Sport* 23, 53–60.

Grove J. R. (1993) Personality and injury rehabilitation among sport performers. In Pargman D. (ed.) *Psychological Bases of Sport Injuries*, pp. 99–120. Fitness Information Technology, Morgantown, WV.

Grove J. R., Hanrahan S. J. & Stewart R. M. L. (1990) Attributions for rapid or slow recovery from sports injury. *Canadian Journal of Sport Sciences* 15, 107–114.

Hardy C. J. & Crace K. R. (1991) Social support within sport. *Sport Psychology Training Bulletin* 3(1), 1–8.

Hardy C. J. & Crace K. R. (1993) The dimensions of social support when dealing with sport injuries. In Pargman D. (ed.) *Psychological Bases of Sport Injuries*, pp. 121–144. Fitness Information Technology, Morgantown, WV.

Heil J. (1993) *Psychology of Sport Injury.* Human Kinetics Publishers, Champaign, IL.

Kubler-Ross E. (1969) *On Death and Dying.* Tavistock, London.

Lazarus A. (1977) *In the Mind's Eye: The Part of Imagery for Personal Enrichment.* Lawson Associates, New York.

Lysens R., Ostryn M., Auweele V. V., Lefevre J., Vuylsteke M. & Renson L. (1987a) A retrospective study of the intrinsic risk factors of sports injuries in young adults. *Proceedings of the Second South African Sports Medicine Association Congress. Medical News Group*, Cape Town.

Lysens R., Ostryn M., Auweele V. V., Lefevre J., Vuylsteke M. & Renson L. (1987b) A one-year prospective study of the intrinsic risk factors of sports injuries in young adults. In *Sports Injuries: Proceedings of the Third International Causation Symposium*, pp. 75–83. Fround, London.

Mahoney M. J. (1979) Cognitive skills and athletic performance. In Kendall P. C. & Hollen S. O. (eds) *Cognitive–Behavioral Interventions: Theory, Research and Procedures*, pp. 423–443. Academic Press, New York.

May J. R., Veach T. L., Reed M. W. & Griffey M. S. (1985) A psychological study of health, injury, and performance in athletes on the US alpine ski team. *The Physician and Sportsmedicine* 13, 111–115.

Meichenbaum D. (1985) *Stress Inoculation Training.* Pergamon, Toronto.

Rodin J. & Salovey P. (1989) Health psychology. *Annual Review of Psychology* 40, 533–579.

Rosenfeld L. B., Richman J. M. & Hardy C. J. (1989) Examining social support networks among athletes: Description and relationships to stress. *The Sport Psychologist* 3, 23–33.

Rotella R. J. (1985) The psychological care of the injured athlete. In Bunker L. K., Rotella R. J. & Reilly A. S. (eds) *Sport Psychology: Psychological Considerations in Maximizing Performance*, pp. 273–287. Mouvement Publications, New York.

Rotella R. J. & Heyman S. R. (1993) Stress, injury and the psychological rehabilitation of athletes. In Williams J. M. (ed.) *Applied Sport Psychology: Personal Growth to Peak Performance*, pp. 338–355. Mayfield, Palo Alto, CA.

Sanderson F. H. (1977) The psychology of the injury prone athlete. *British Journal of Sports Medicine* 11, 56–57.

Sanderson F. H. (1978) The psychological implications of injury. *British Journal of Sports Medicine* 12, 41–43.

Sanderson F. H. (1981) The psychological implications of injury. In Reilly T. P. (ed.) *Sports Fitness and Sports Injuries*, pp. 37–41. Faber & Faber, London.

Suinn R. M. (1967) Psychological reactions to physical disability. *Journal of the Association for Physical and Mental Rehabilitation* 21, 13–15.

Turk D. C., Meichenbaum D. & Genest M. (1983) *Pain and Behavioral Medicine: A Cognitive–Behavioral Perspective.* Guildford, New York.

Weiss M. R. & Troxell R. K. (1986) Psychology of the injured athlete. *Athletic Training* 15, 144–146.

Wiese D. M. & Weiss M. R. (1987) Psychological rehabilitation and physical injury: Implications for the sports medicine team. *The Sport Psychologist* 1, 318–330.

Wiese-Bjornstal D. M. & Smith A. M. (1993) Counselling strategies for enhanced recovery of injured athletes within a team approach. In Pargman D. (ed.) *Psychological Bases of Sport Injuries*, pp. 149–182. Fitness Information Technology, Morgantown, WV.

CHAPTER 11

TALENT IDENTIFICATION AND PROFILING

J. Bloomfield

The previous chapters in this book have dealt with the subdisciplines of sports science and how they can assist an athlete to achieve the ultimate performance. This chapter is oriented towards the application of this knowledge and how it can be applied when identifying talent and profiling athletes.

During the last 50 years coaches have informally identified talent and profiled athletes, but it was not until the early 1970s that eastern European countries began the systematic programmes which were to help them win a large number of medals internationally in the 1970s and the 1980s. Both Alabin *et al.* (1980) and Hahn (1990) suggest that efficient talent identification procedures play a very important part in modern sport and were a major

factor in eastern Europe's domination of many Olympic sports in the past two decades.

Similar programmes emerged in western Europe, North America and some Commonwealth countries in the 1980s, but it is extremely difficult for countries which do not have sports institutes or centres of excellence for sport to compete with those who do. Where such sports systems are in operation, sports scientists and sports medicine specialists have been able to form sophisticated testing teams for talent identification and profiling, gathering systematic information from the athletes and integrating it into scientifically based training programmes for the benefit of both individuals and teams.

TALENT IDENTIFICATION

The majority of talent identification is done at the junior level in sport, although occasionally one hears of individuals who have been advised to change their event or sport when they are already senior athletes. This has occurred because sports science tests have shown that they have certain physical and/or physiological capacities which may enable them to perform at a high level in a particular sport. It is important to point out, however, that late identification is occurring less frequently as international competition becomes more intense.

RATIONALE FOR TALENT IDENTIFICATION

As the aggressive sports systems of eastern Europe have gradually broken down, the stigma of talent identification as being an undesirable practice is fast disappearing. In fact, apart from the use of drugs, which in some of these countries was rampant and cannot be condoned under any circumstances, talent identification was positive in many cases, as young athletes were well catered for both personally and from a sport development viewpoint. Bloomfield *et al.* (1994) stated that the positive features of such programmes are as follows:

- 'Children are directed towards sports, or particular events, for which they are physically and physiologically best suited. This in turn means that they will probably obtain good results and enjoy their training and participation more'
- 'Because of the nature of the programme, their physical health and general welfare are well looked after'
- 'They are usually the recipients of specialized coaching, which is well supported by the sports medical team and sometimes by a sports psychologist'
- 'The administrators of many of these programmes are now concerned about the vocational opportunities for the athletes after the conclusion of their competitive career and cater for them with high quality secondary or tertiary education or vocational training'

THE TALENT IDENTIFICATION PROCESS

Talent identification can be either very simple or highly sophisticated. One may find, for example, a school basketball coach recruiting players simply because they are tall for their age. Or a school swimming coach, who when walking around the playground, may observe the way children are standing; if they have naturally large pronated feet they may be prospectively good breast-stroke swimmers, as this physical capacity is needed for an efficient kick. Sophisticated programmes on the other hand are highly oriented towards sports science and medicine, with a comprehensive test battery used to screen the young athletes.

General Talent Identification Screening

Sports systems or institutions within them which have sophisticated screening programmes examine several parameters which relate to junior athletes and construct a general profile of each subject. The following screening tests and observations illustrate this.

HEALTH STATUS

First a medical examination is normally conducted, during which special attention is paid to the musculoskeletal and cardiovascular systems. Athletes with medical conditions which may at some time in the future limit their training or participation should be very carefully evaluated. Komadel (1988) quoted the diseases which were listed by the Czechoslovak Ministry for Health as contraindications to competition in sport at the highest level. Many Western sports medicine physicians would not totally agree with all of these, citing asthma and diabetes mellitus as diseases which can now be well controlled by high-level athletes with the modern drugs which are currently available.

There would be, however, a general endorsement of the abovementioned list by the majority of sports physicians currently working with elite athletes.

HEREDITARY FACTORS

There are important hereditary factors which should be considered in the selection of talented athletes. As yet no systematic research has been carried out in this area, mainly because the parents of current high performance athletes did not have the opportunities to train as intensively, or to be tested as athletes are today and thus there are very few comparative data. There is little doubt, however, as Sloane (1985) pointed out, that parents who have a personal interest in their children's activities will strongly support them and this will be of great assistance to them while they develop their basic skills. Even without categorical research, however, subjective observation points to the fact that there is often a strong genetic link between parents and their offspring in various sports.

TIME SPENT IN SPORT

It is important to establish how long each athlete has trained for his or her sport and how much coaching he or she has received. In some instances certain children will have been in a particular sport for a much longer period of time than others and will have already received considerably more specialized coaching. In such cases they may not develop much further with their skills and/or their cardiovascular capacity, if these are important selection criteria.

MATURITY

This important factor must be considered in any talent selection procedure. It is well known that early maturers are often taller, heavier, more powerful and faster than their counterparts during the early to mid teenage years. Many coaches have observed that early maturers have an advantage in junior sport and often neglect their skill development, whereas less physically mature athletes are forced to develop their skills earlier to perform well. The latter group when fully matured may have definite advantages over the early developers, because their physical capacity level is just as high, but their skills are better.

Specific Talent Identification Screening

All talent identification programmes must be concerned with every facet of the particular sport or event. The athletes' physical, physiological and psychological capacities must be carefully assessed in order to ascertain the level of their talent; however, it should be understood that not all of the above capacities are needed in equal amounts in various sports or events. Therefore, talent identification screening must be sport specific.

Physical Capacities

SOMATOTYPE (BODY TYPE)

Body type is a general physical capacity, which can be a useful indicator of future elite performance.

The *stability during growth* of the somatotype has been discussed by Malina and Bouchard (1991), who suggested that ectomorphy was reasonably stable during growth, but that mesomorphy and endomorphy in adolescent boys was not as predictable. Because boys experience a marked increase in muscle mass during the adolescent growth spurt as a result of testosterone secretions, it is logical that somatotype variations will occur in this component. However, reasonably accurate forecasts can be made in mesomorphy, from about stage

3.5–4.0 of pubescent development, when a boy's musculature rapidly develops, that is at approximately 14.0–14.5 years of age. The stability of the somatotype components in girls during adolescence is less well understood, but many coaches suggest that adolescent girls from about the age of 12.5–13.0 years tend to steadily increase their endomorphy rating as they develop and that this is accompanied by a drop in their power/weight ratio. This decrease can be detrimental for them in weight-bearing ballistic sports such as gymnastics, basketball, netball and volleyball where powerful movements are essential (Bloomfield *et al.* 1994).

The *most suitable body types* for various sports and events have been discussed by Bloomfield *et al.* (1994) and they state that:

> To be within one component of the mature body type at any time during the adolescent growth period would indicate that the young athlete is generally 'on track' as far as the attainment of an optimal shape is concerned. Well-trained coaches are now aware that special intervention programmes using strength and power training and/or nutrition can alter the primary somatotype components over a 1.5 to 2.0 year period.

BODY COMPOSITION

Like somatotype, body composition is only a general indicator of high-level performance. The *stability during growth* of an individual's body composition has been reviewed by Malina and Bouchard (1991) who suggested that body fat was not particularly stable from birth to 5 or 6 years, or during adolescence. They also stated, however, that 'the mark of excess fatness (in adults) thus appears to be greater for those who have thicker subcutaneous fat measurements during childhood'.

The *most suitable body composition* for young athletes in various sports has not been systematically documented. However, if they are within 1–2% body fat for a male or 3–4% for a female, at about stage 3.5–4.0 of their pubescent development or when they are close to their peak height velocity (PHV), then they are 'on track' for the optimal body composition that is generally required for that sport or event. It should be noted, however, that the demands of some sports to have low-fat levels, for example in field or court sports, are not as great as in other sports such as gymnastics, where power to weight ratios play a significant role in an athlete's performances. As for body typing, coaches who are trying to predict late adolescent and post-adolescent female body composition, particularly fat mass (FM) for sports such as gymnastics, should 'err on the side of conservatism'. This means that they should select girls who have measures below the accepted optimal FM levels, in order to be as sure as possible that they will not increase their FM to the point where it will greatly affect their power to weight ratio. As a general rule this should be about 2% body fat (Bloomfield *et al.* 1994).

As with body type, intervention programmes which use strength and power training and/or nutrition can be used to assist the young athlete to reach accepted body composition levels, both for lean body mass and FM if they are reasonably close to the accepted levels in the first place.

PROPORTIONALITY

This physical capacity can be an important self-selector for various sports and events. Many accurate forecasts with relation to individual and team performances have been made during the last two decades on the measurements of height and body mass alone.

Predictions of height and body mass (weight) have been made reasonably accurately for some time and Lowery (1978) gave several formulae to estimate height. He also quoted the work of Bayley and Pinneau (Bayer & Bayley 1959) who used skeletal age and tables to forecast growth. Another way to estimate final height and body mass is to determine a subject's skeletal age from an X-ray of the hand and wrist using Greulich and Pyle's atlas (1959), then use growth standards (Tanner 1989) for height and body mass to determine the mature measures. This method has been used by some coaches to forecast final heights and body masses of athletes where these variables are important factors, either when the athlete is too large for the event, as in gymnastics, or too small, such as in the throwing events.

Finally, it is important to point out that very little research has been done on the stability of the proportions of the growing child and adolescent. Ackland and Bloomfield (1993) have suggested, however, that various segment widths remain stable throughout adolescence and can therefore be used for predictive purposes. On the other hand they also found that many segment lengths were unstable during adolescence and suggested that these should not be used as prediction criteria in talent identification programmes.

POSTURE

As with proportionality, posture is an important self-selector for various sports and events within them. However, the *stability of posture* during growth has not been examined in a systematic way and again most of the information has been formulated from anecdotal evidence. The general feeling about posture is that it steadily develops during adolescence and becomes more extreme as the individual ages. Perceptive sports scientists and coaches, however, will be able to identify these developments and forecast with some degree of accuracy what the athlete's ultimate posture will be.

The *posture of athletes*, like that of the normal population, varies greatly. However, there are several postures which give athletes immense advantages over their competitors and the majority of them are reasonably obvious before the onset of adolescence. Bloomfield *et al.* (1994) have listed them as follows:

- Individuals with *inverted feet* or 'pigeon toes' have a speed advantage over short distances when compared with those athletes with conventional foot posture or everted feet (Bloomfield 1979). This characteristic is especially valuable where acceleration is needed over short distances in games such as tennis, squash, badminton and volleyball

- In sprint running events, or in games where very fast running is advantageous, athletes with *partial lordosis accompanied by an anterior pelvic tilt* (APT) are at an advantage. If this characteristic is combined with *protruding* or 'high' *buttocks* which are also well muscled, then the athlete is normally a very fast runner, provided that the other physical capacities are present which are important in sprinting (Bloomfield 1979). This posture also appears to assist those individuals who are in jumping-oriented games such as basketball and volleyball, as well as the jumping athletes in the field events

- Agility athletes who possess the overhanging knee joint where there is a small degree of flexion at this joint, appear to have an advantage in sprinting and in events where mobility is necessary
- Distance runners generally have *'flat backs'* with little lordosis, almost no pelvic tilt and flat buttocks. This type of posture assists them to run with a reasonably upright body, which in turn enables them to develop an uncramped stride, thus marginally increasing their stride length
- Female gymnasts with *lordosis* and an accompanying APT are able to hyperextend their spines more easily than competitors with a flat lower back and buttocks. This postural characteristic also appears to enable them to leap higher than gymnasts who lack this feature
- Various postures assist swimmers in different events. It is well known that *'square shouldered'* swimmers with long clavicles and large scapulae, particularly the acromion process, have lower levels of flexion–extension movement of the upper limb and shoulder girdle. Foot and leg postures are also important, with *everted feet* or 'duck feet' being very suitable for breast-stroke swimming, while swimmers with *inverted feet* or 'pigeon toes' are able to perform the dolphin, freestyle and backstroke kicks more efficiently

Coaches need to carefully observe the athlete's posture in order to determine whether or not it is advantageous to the performance. Posture can be partially modified using flexibility and strength training, but this must be done at an early stage in the individual's development because changes are difficult to make during late adolescence and early adulthood (Bloomfield *et al.* 1994).

STRENGTH AND POWER

Strength and explosive power in many sports are essential physical capacities and performances in sport have improved at a rapid rate since they became important components of the modern training programme.

Eastern European coaches have suggested for some time that around the PHV period (approximately 14 years of age) in the adolescent male's growth spurt, is a reasonably reliable time to make future forecasts on mature strength levels. This has been done particularly well in the sport of weightlifting and can probably apply to other sports.

The *importance of strength and power* in the majority of sports is now well accepted and early identification of high strength and power levels can be very helpful to the coach. Strength and power are closely related to body shape, body composition, proportionality and posture, and therefore the coach can observe the more powerful athletes as they develop during adolescence. Athletes can at an early stage continue to develop this important characteristic as part of the normal training programme if they already demonstrate this capacity, but a special intervention programme may be necessary for the young athlete whose skill levels and other physical attributes are high, but whose levels of strength and power are low (Bloomfield *et al.* 1994).

FLEXIBILITY

Flexibility is a very important physical capacity in the majority of modern sports; however, very little research has been done with relation to its *stability during growth*.

Anecdotal evidence suggests that coaches can forecast reasonably well whether the young athlete is flexible enough for a particular sport or event. If flexibility levels naturally decrease at any time, however, and this does occur in some males during stages 3 and 4 of adolescence, then modern flexibility training methods must be used so that optimal levels can be attained.

SPEED

Speed of movement is an essential physical capacity for high levels of performance in many sports. Again very little research has been done in this area except for running speed, which is only one aspect of speed. However, most coaches are aware at an early stage whether their athletes are fast or slow either in running speed or other movements, because they are continually comparing them with other athletes of similar age.

Finally, speed training techniques are now well developed, and intervention programmes are commonplace in modern training, but young athletes should be at least 10 years of age before they embark on such a programme, if high levels of performance are to be reached by the time they become senior athletes (Bloomfield et al. 1994).

Motor Capacities

Various validated tests have been used extensively in talent identification programmes during the last two decades. Various agility tests, standing long jump, vertical jump, reaction time, large or small ball throws for distance and accuracy and 40 yard or 40 m sprints are universally performed. Because of this there are a large number of norms available for comparative purposes, which are useful when coaches wish to compare their athletes with others (Bloomfield et al. 1994).

Physiological Capacities

Physiological tests are important to screen those individuals who must rely fully or partially on cardiovascular endurance. Komadel (1988) suggests that $\dot{V}_{O2max}$ is an important factor in evaluating endurance capacity, while Wilmore and Costill (1994) state that 'many investigators consider the lactate threshold (LT) to be a good indicator of an athlete's potential for endurance exercise'. If this is so, then it should be a useful predictor for endurance-oriented sports. Power output on the other hand, as evaluated by anaerobic power or capacity tests 'does not seem to be useful for the identification of young talent' according to Komadel (1988). He further states that 'muscle biopsies to determine the muscle fibre types predominant in particular muscles do not help ascertain potential talent either, although it seems hopeful from a theoretical point of view'.

Another physiological consideration in talent identification may be the ventilatory response to breathing carbon dioxide (VE/PA_{CO2}). This is a measure of the innate sensitivity of the respiratory centre to carbon dioxide and could provide some indication of a child's endurance or sprint potential. Endurance performers possess a low sensitivity to inhaled carbon dioxide while sprinters exhibit a high sensitivity.

Other factors which might indicate limitations to performance include low haemoglobin and ferritin levels as well as children with low lung function test scores. If a prospective endurance athlete has a severely restricted chest expansion with involvement of the costovertebral joints, then a condition such as ankylosing spondylitis may severely restrict their performance.

Psychological Capacities

Komadel (1988) under a section on psychological abilities has described the general profile which is needed for a young elite athlete to succeed in his or her chosen sport. He says that emotional stability, combined with a low anxiety level, enables the athlete to tolerate a high level of training. It also appears that a low level of neuroticism is important, as this characteristic allows the athlete to better tolerate frustration and to avoid overtraining.

Komadel also emphasizes the importance of self-motivation, so that the athlete can cope with long-term monotonous training. As well, a very high level of sensory motor ability is also an important element in the learning of complex motor skills.

Other factors such as functional intelligence, which is essential for fast information-processing and decision-making, and social skills, particularly in team sports, are also important.

CONCLUSION

In conclusion, the selection of prospective elite athletes using talent identification is a complex problem. Because there is a dearth of knowledge as to how maturity affects the physical, physiological and psychological make-up of the individual, it is often difficult to ascertain whether the results of tests given early in an athlete's life will be useful predictors for the future. With more longitudinal testing of elite groups, the sports scientist and sports physician will be able to predict future success more accurately and in so doing make talent identification a more reliable method of choosing future sporting talent. A further important point was raised by Hahn (1990) who stated that:

Talent identification and talent selection programmes will not of themselves guarantee the emergence of champions. To realize their potential, the people selected must have regular access to top-level coaching, as well as appropriate facilities and equipment. They must (also) have a clear network of support, and, if possible, such additional elements as sports science and sports medicine services.

PROFILING

Athletic profiling has been carried out by coaches in an informal way for many years. During the last two decades formal profiling has steadily developed, first in eastern Europe and more recently in western Europe, North America and some Commonwealth countries. The purpose of this section is to discuss modern sports profiling and how it can aid athletes to produce their best performances.

RATIONALE FOR PROFILING

All high-level athletes are unique individuals with many physical, physiological and psychological strengths, otherwise they would not have reached the elite level. Athletes also have weaknesses which need to be known by the coach, who will then be able to take remedial action to strengthen them, because the old adage that 'a chain is only as strong as its weakest link' is true for an athlete as well.

TYPES OF PROFILING

Two types of profiling should be carried out with high-level athletes, and these are as follows.

General Profiling

General profiling is done in a de-trained state and administered at the commencement of a season. The results of a series of tests will give the coach a general profile of the athlete.

In order to ascertain the individual's actual status within the group, the above results should be evaluated, not only against other high-level athletes in the same sport or event, but also against their own team-mates. The most important comparison will be that which is made against other elite athletes in the same sport or event. However, the individual's status within the team or squad is often of interest to the athlete and is certainly of value to the coach.

When the coach has evaluated the test results with the relevant sports scientists and/or the sports physician, the season's training schedule, with each individual's strengths and weaknesses in mind, can then be planned. Often, this general training plan will also take into consideration skill weakness, so that several team members ranking lower than their team-mates in the various tests will be given an intervention programme in addition to their normal training. It should be kept in mind that general profiling is often more useful for the potential elite athlete in the developmental stages while still at the national junior or youth level, whereas for the senior international level athlete it will not be as valuable.

FREQUENCY OF THE TESTS

Most coaches only profile once each season at this level in order to identify weaknesses. Others have follow-up tests at varying intervals to monitor the general progress of the intervention programmes. Agility athletes in 'closed' sports such as gymnasts and divers are regularly monitored for body composition, because power/weight ratios are crucial factors in their performances.

Specific Profiling

This is usually done with elite senior athletes where events are won by very small margins or times, as in aerobic sports such as swimming, rowing, kayaking, running and cycling, where it is important to accurately evaluate the individual's adaptation to the stress of heavy training at regular intervals.

FREQUENCY OF THE TESTS

In some programmes tests are done as regularly as every 2 weeks, but more often a month apart, which fits in well with a 3/1 training cycle. When a major championship is approaching, some coaches request that only the 'key' stress adaptation tests be done at more regular intervals, which could be as often as every week. With athletes who are more skill oriented, specific profiling will only be done approximately every 6 months, because alterations to the athlete's physical capacities take a longer time to occur.

HEALTH STATUS CHECKS

At the commencement of each season a general health evaluation should be conducted by a sports medicine physician. This can also be followed up in mid-season or at other times which are thought appropriate by the medical and coaching team.

These checks give the sports physician and other specialists such as the nutritionist an opportunity to discuss both at the team or individual level, various personal health problems which the athletes may have. Young athletes in particular feel that such discussions are very valuable.

SPORTS SCIENCE TESTS USED IN PROFILING

Various sports have differing demands, therefore only tests which are highly specific to that sport should be used. It is pointless giving a pistol shooter or archer complex cardiovascular evaluations at regular intervals, because endurance is not an important factor in these events. One should not completely dismiss this point, however, because all athletes need a reasonably high physical fitness level to assist them with other more specific skills and mental tasks, even if there is no specific cardio-vascular component in their event. However, unless there is a definite need for both endurance and skill in an event, it is often a waste of time and money giving a sophisticated test such as a maximal oxygen uptake ($\dot{V}_{O2max}$) to a non-endurance athlete (Bloomfield *et al.* 1994).

Physical Capacity Tests

Several of these tests have been mentioned in the talent identification section of this chapter as well as being discussed in Chapters 1 and 3 of this book.

The following capacities are normally profiled:

- Height and body mass (weight)
- Somatotype and body composition
- Proportionality (body lever lengths)
- Strength and explosive power
- Speed of movement
- Flexibility
- Posture
- Balance and agility

Physiological Tests

These tests are selectively used by sports scientists to suit different types of sports or events and fall into the following categories.

CARDIOVASCULAR TESTS

The following tests are normally used in specific profiling:

- Aerobic power tests utilizing specific ergometers to suit the sport or event in which the individual is competing
- Anaerobic power and capacity tests using specific ergometers where mean power output is calculated and total body load measured

BIOCHEMICAL AND HAEMATOLOGICAL TESTS

The following tests are used in order to identify non-adaptation to training:

- Haemoglobin (Hb)
- Blood haematocrit
- Lymphocyte and neutrophil counts

Table 11.1 Percentile scores of international women tennis players

Variable	Percentile								
	10	20	30	40	50	60	70	80	90
Height (cm)	163.0	164.7	165.7	166.5	167.5	168.5	169.5	171.3	173.0
Body mass (kg)	51.6	53.9	56.5	58.7	60.7	62.7	64.8	67.4	70.9
Body composition									
Body density (g/mL)	1.009	1.022	1.031	1.039	1.047	1.055	1.063	1.070	1.075
Body fat (%)	30.3	28.8	26.2	24.1	22.1	20.1	17.9	15.3	11.8
Triceps skinfold (mm)	17.0	16.1	15.5	15.0	14.5	14.0	13.4	12.8	11.9
Subscapular skinfold (mm)	11.0	10.1	9.5	9.0	8.5	8.0	7.4	6.8	5.9
Supra-iliac skinfold (mm)	14.4	12.9	11.8	10.8	10.0	9.1	8.1	7.00	5.5
Abdominal skinfold (mm)	14.8	13.2	11.6	10.7	10.1	9.3	7.9	7.2	5.4
Proportionality									
Brachial index	73.2	75.2	76.6	77.8	79.0	80.1	81.8	82.7	84.7
Crural index	98.2	100.2	101.6	102.8	104.0	106.1	108.3	109.7	112.0
Relative sitting height (%)	50.3	51.0	51.6	52.0	52.5	52.9	53.3	53.9	54.6
Flexibility									
Arm flexion−extension (degree)	182.2	189.7	195.1	199.7	204.0	208.2	215.9	224.2	235.7
Forearm flexion−extension (degree)	124.6	129.9	133.7	137.0	140.0	143.0	146.2	150.0	155.3
Foot dorsoplantar flexion (degree)	54.7	58.2	60.8	63.0	65.0	67.0	69.1	71.7	75.2
Leg flexion (degree)	107.0	113.2	117.7	121.5	125.0	128.5	132.2	136.7	142.9
Strength									
Grip strength (kgf)	20.9	23.5	25.4	27.1	28.6	30.1	31.7	33.6	36.2
Arm flexion strength (kgf)	14.2	24.8	32.5	39.0	45.0	51.0	57.4	65.1	75.7
Arm extension strength (kgf)	11.8	21.5	28.5	34.5	40.0	45.5	51.4	58.4	68.1
Leg extension torque									
SS3 (ft lb)	16.4	69.2	107.6	140.0	170.0	200.0	232.4	270.8	323.6
SS7 (ft lb)	14.4	54.2	92.6	125.0	155.0	185.0	217.4	255.8	308.6
Power/speed									
Jump and reach (cm)	37.3	39.9	41.8	43.5	45.0	46.5	48.1	50.0	52.6
40 m dash (s)	7.1	6.8	6.6	6.4	6.3	6.1	5.9	5.7	5.4
Agility run (s)	18.7	17.8	17.2	16.7	16.2	15.6	15.1	14.5	13.6

Endomorphy mean = 3.5; mesomorphy mean = 3.5; ectomorphy mean = 3.0.
Source Bloomfield *et al.* 1994.

- Ferritin
- Uric acid
- Urea
- Creatine phosphokinase (CPK)
- Testosterone/cortisol levels

Psychological Tests

A large number of psychological variables have recently been isolated which are known to affect sports performance. They are normally used in general profiling and are as follows:

- Aggression
- Anxiety
- Arousal
- Attention
- Cohesion
- Independence
- Personality — extroversion/introversion
- Leadership
- Mood
- Motivation
- Self-concept/self-esteem

The major psychological inventories which are used to assess the above variables are as follows:

- Coopersmith Self-Esteem Inventory (SEI; Coopersmith 1967)
- Eysenck Personality Questionnaire (EPQ; Eysenck 1968)
- The Group Environment Questionnaire (Widmeyer *et al*. 1985)
- Profile of Mood States (POMS; McNair *et al*. 1971; Morgan 1980)
- Sport Competition Anxiety Test (SCAT; Martens 1977)
- Test of Attentional and Interpersonal Style (TAIS; Nideffer 1976)

For additional information on the application of the above variables and inventories readers are referred to Chapters 7–9.

Skill Evaluation

During the last decade, coaches and sports biomechanists have been developing skill profiles on both their individual athletes and their games players. With the use of high-speed photography or video, coaches are now able to accurately 'pinpoint' technique weaknesses in their athletes. Some coaches still administer skills tests to their competitors, but much less of this is now being done, mainly because an artificial 'laboratory' environment is created and also because modern technique analysis equipment used in a competitive training situation allows for a more realistic assessment.

Further information on skill evaluation can be found in Chapter 3.

When technique errors are located the athlete is placed on a special intervention programme in order to improve one or several skills where the coach feels additional training is needed. This is usually done in separate remedial workouts and not in the scheduled team or squad training sessions.

SETTING UP THE PROFILE

As has been previously mentioned, profiles are normally constructed from data obtained from other elite athletes within the same sport or event. Until recently it has been difficult to obtain international level data for comparative purposes, as there was a dearth of it in published form and because the test protocols sometimes varied from country to country. It is pleasing to note that both these problems are now being overcome and more reliable data are available for comparative purposes.

To develop a profile when one has the data is relatively simple. Norms must first be constructed based on percentile scores, T scores, Z scores, or deviations from the mean of these data. Table 11.1 demonstrates this, giving physical capacity percentile scores for international women tennis players. It is important to note that some psychological profiles are not set up numerically but have rankings from very low to very high on each variable (Table 11.2).

A profile sheet can be used to enter the data then a graph can be constructed from it. Figure 11.1

Table 11.2 EPQ personality scores (1-E scale) of State junior tennis players shown in categories

Category (years)	Males 10–11 (n = 170)	12–13 (n = 208)	14–15 (n = 116)	16–17 (n = 22)	Females 10–11 (n = 103)	12–13 (n = 140)	14–15 (n = 89)	16–17 (n = 18)
Very low	10	9	9	9	8	10	9	9
Low	14	14	14	14	13	14	14	14
Low/medium	16	17	17	17	15	17	17	17
Average	18	19	19	19	17	18	18	18
High/medium	20	21	21	21	19	20	20	20
High	22	23	23	23	21	22	22	22
Very high	24	24	24	24	23	24	24	24
$\bar{x}$	19.2	21.0	20.6	19.7	22.1	19.7	20.2	16.3
s.d.	3.2	11.0	3.6	3.6	15.7	3.7	4.3	5.0

Source Elliott *et al*. 1989.

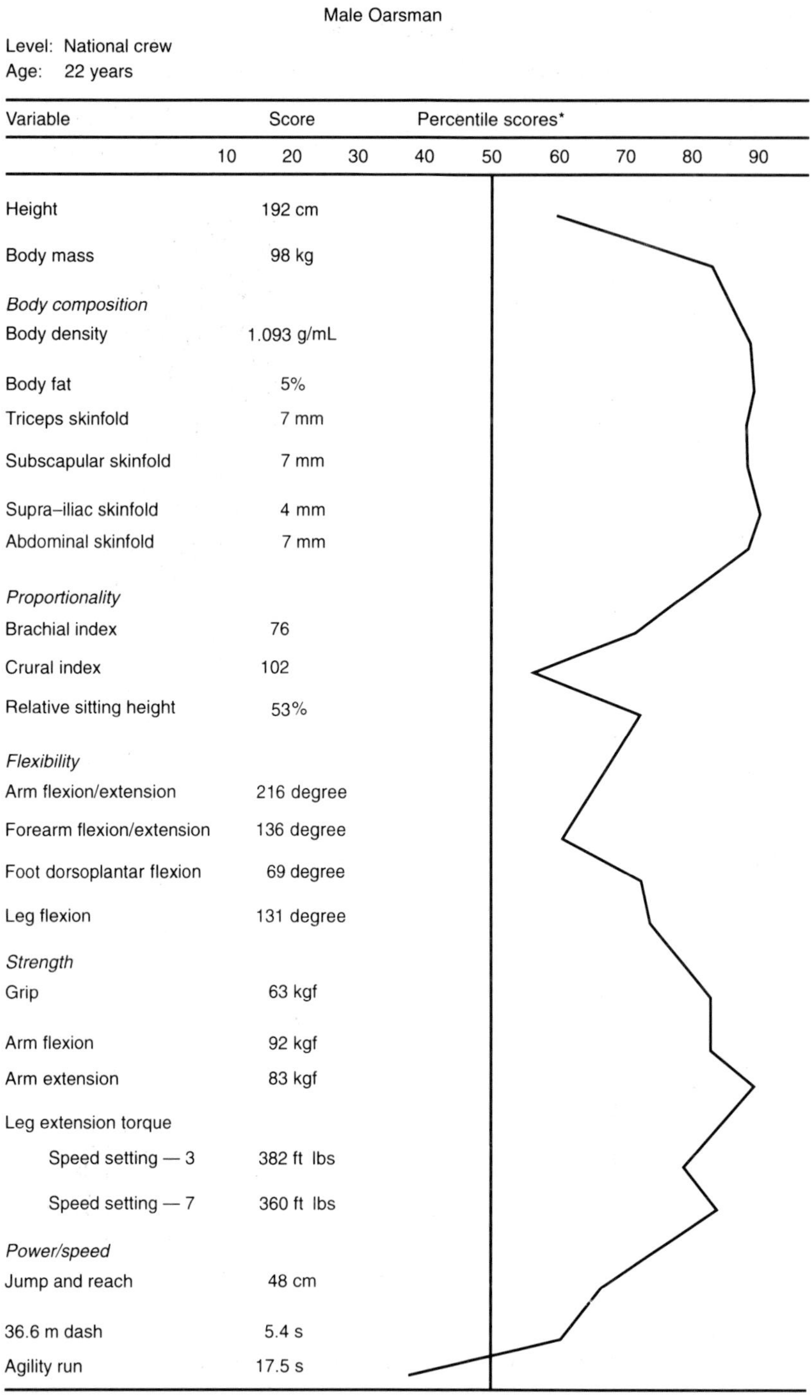

Male Oarsman

Level: National crew
Age: 22 years

Variable	Score	Percentile scores*							
		10	20	30	40	50	60	70	80	90

Height — 192 cm

Body mass — 98 kg

Body composition
Body density — 1.093 g/mL

Body fat — 5%
Triceps skinfold — 7 mm

Subscapular skinfold — 7 mm

Supra–iliac skinfold — 4 mm
Abdominal skinfold — 7 mm

Proportionality
Brachial index — 76

Crural index — 102

Relative sitting height — 53%

Flexibility
Arm flexion/extension — 216 degree

Forearm flexion/extension — 136 degree

Foot dorsoplantar flexion — 69 degree

Leg flexion — 131 degree

Strength
Grip — 63 kgf

Arm flexion — 92 kgf

Arm extension — 83 kgf

Leg extension torque
    Speed setting — 3 — 382 ft lbs

    Speed setting — 7 — 360 ft lbs

Power/speed
Jump and reach — 48 cm

36.6 m dash — 5.4 s
Agility run — 17.5 s

Somatotype:
Endomorphy 1.5; mesomorphy 6.0; ectomorphy 2.5.
* Percentile scores for international level oarsmen.

Fig. 11.1 A profile of an international level oarsman (Bloomfield *et al.* 1994).

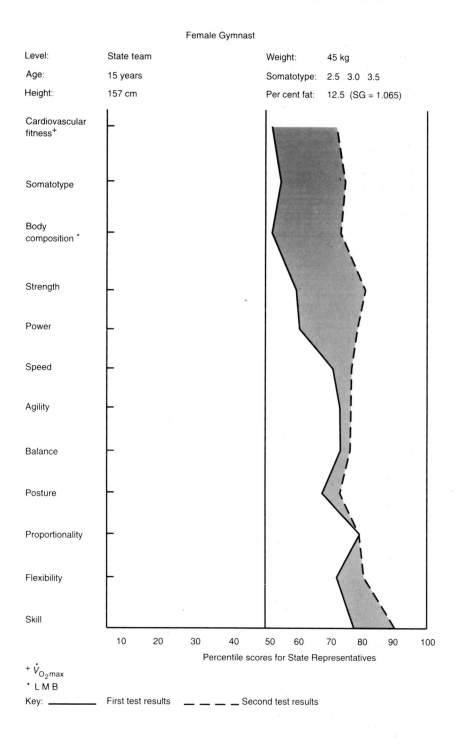

Fig. 11.2 The profiles of a female state-level gymnast recorded before and after a 20 month intervention programme (Bloomfield 1979).

shows data from an international level male oarsman under *score* and his profile graph under *percentile scores*. Further, the profile should be drawn simply so that athletes can easily understand it, because they should take part in the discussion with the coach and the relevant sports scientist. The following evaluations of several profiles will enable the reader to understand the procedure better.

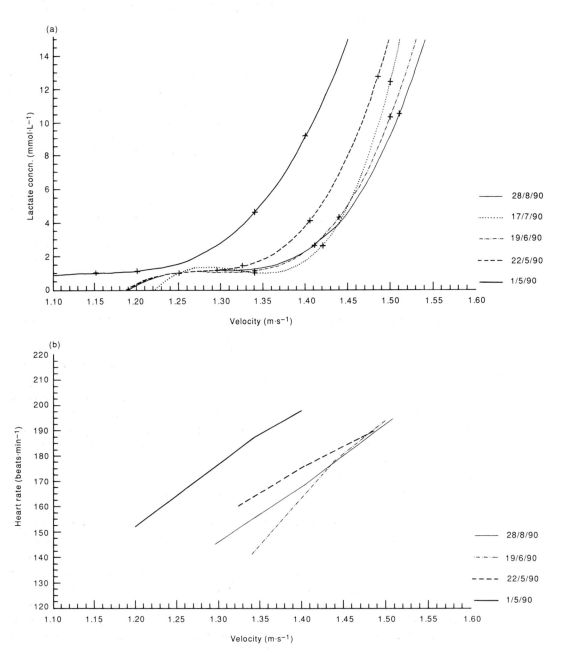

Fig. 11.3 A serial profile of an elite-level swimmer showing: (a) lactate and (b) heart rate curves over a 4 month training period (S. R. Lawrence personal communication).

Fig. 11.4 The psychological profile of a state-level junior tennis player (Ackland 1989).

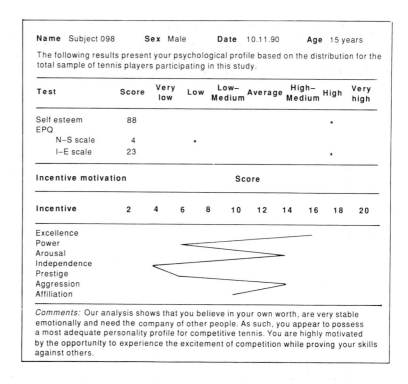

| Name Subject 098 | Sex Male | Date 10.11.90 | Age 15 years |

The following results present your psychological profile based on the distribution for the total sample of tennis players participating in this study.

Test	Score	Very low	Low	Low–Medium	Average	High–Medium	High	Very high
Self esteem	88						*	
EPQ								
N–S scale	4		*					
I–E scale	23						*	

| Incentive motivation | | Score | | | | | | | |

Incentive	2	4	6	8	10	12	14	16	18	20
Excellence										
Power										
Arousal										
Independence										
Prestige										
Aggression										
Affiliation										

Comments: Our analysis shows that you believe in your own worth, are very stable emotionally and need the company of other people. As such, you appear to possess a most adequate personality profile for competitive tennis. You are highly motivated by the opportunity to experience the excitement of competition while proving your skills against others.

Anatomical and Physiological Profiles

To date, the bulk of sports profiling has been done in this area because international norms have been more available. It should be stated, however, that profiling is a very personal thing and to be really effective, it should be repeated at various intervals. Figure 11.2 illustrates a profile in which the athlete was first tested to generally profile them, then at a later time was re-tested to see whether the intervention programme on which they had been placed had improved their physical and physiological status (Bloomfield 1979).

The athlete in Fig. 11.2 is a female gymnast of linear build with low levels of strength and power, but high levels of skill. She had a somatotype which rated 2.5–3.0–3.5 with a percentage fat level of 12.5. She was given a general strength training programme over and above her normal training three times a week for 20 months. During this time her somatotype changed to a 2.0–4.0–3.0 and her percentage body fat was reduced to 9.6. The dotted line on the right-hand side of the original graph shows the other changes which were made during this time.

With individuals preparing for international events, serial profiles are often carried out on a limited range of physiological variables during the heavy training period. This is done in order to monitor the athlete's adaptation to the stress of heavy training and is shown in a graphical form and compared with times performed in trials or races (Fig. 11.3).

Psychological Profiles

This type of profile is a little less objective than the anatomical and physiological type. It is nevertheless a valuable tool for the coach and sports scientist. Normally, only one profile is constructed on the athlete's behavioural variables and this acts as a baseline for coaches to understand their athletes better. Figure 11.4 illustrates a profile of a state-level junior tennis player, while Fig. 11.5 portrays a TAIS profile of a young tennis player who has recently gone on to become an outstanding inter-

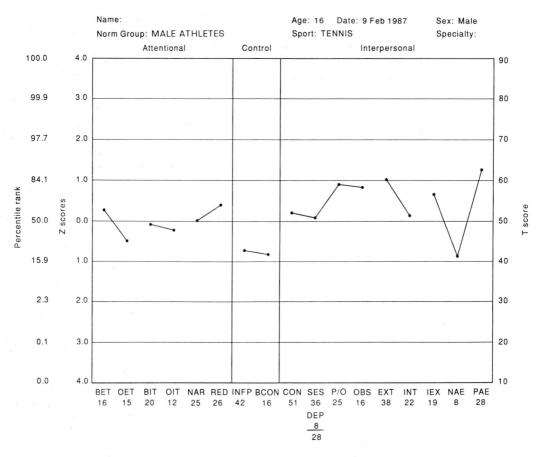

Name: Age: 16   Date: 9 Feb 1987   Sex: Male
Norm Group: MALE ATHLETES   Sport: TENNIS   Specialty:

Fig. 11.5 A TAIS profile of an international level junior tennis player (J. Bond, pers. comm., 1990).

national professional tennis player. Another elite tennis player's POMS profile sheet is shown in Fig. 8.6 in Chapter 8.

In conclusion, J. Bond (personal communication) feels that psychological profiles are a valuable tool in identifying talent, but he warns that they must only be used as a guide and are best done in conjunction with other sports science tests.

PROGRAMME DEVELOPMENT

After the profile has been evaluated, the decision should be made as to whether the individual needs an intervention programme. Whether one is needed or not, the coach and athlete should confer at this stage, as the status of each team member in comparison with other athletes of a similar level, or the ranking on each variable within the team or squad, should also be known by the individual. In some cases athletes can even take part in the development of their own programme, especially if they are mature individuals.

It is important at this point that a formal intervention programme be devised which is in a printed form. Targets or goals should be realistic and the competitor should be clear as to what these are and how they can be achieved. The coach should also set the time of the next test battery, whether it be 3 or 6 months hence, or at the beginning of the next season. This gives the athlete a target date to be aimed for, rather than a nebulous period over which the programme should be carried out.

CONCLUSION

Until recently profiling has been done only randomly in various institutes and centres of excellence throughout the world. Now that more international sports science literature is available with which to make comparisons between athletes, and more test protocols are becoming internationally standardized, profiling is becoming an important feature of the elite athlete's development.

REFERENCES

Ackland T. R. & Bloomfield J. (1993) Stability of proportions through adolescent growth. *Proceedings of the Annual Meeting of the Australian Sports Medicine Federation*, Melbourne 1993.

Ackland T. R., Elliott B. C., Blanksby B. A., Hood K. P. & Bloomfield J. (1989) Profiling junior tennis players, Part 2: The practical application of normative data. *Australian Journal of Science and Medicine in Sport* 21, 22–24.

Alabin V., Nischt G. & Jefimov W. (1980) Talent selection. *Modern Athlete and Coach* 18, 36–37.

Bayer L. & Bayley N. (1959) *Growth Diagnosis*. University of Chicago Press, Chicago, IL.

Bloomfield J. (1979) Modifying human physical capacities and technique to improve performance. *Sports Coach* 3, 19–25.

Bloomfield J., Ackland T. A. & Elliott B. C. (1994) *Applied Anatomy and Biomechanics in Sport*, pp. 267–281. Blackwell Scientific Publications, Melbourne.

Coopersmith S. (1967) *The Antecedents of Self-Esteem*. Freeman, San Francisco, CA.

Elliott B. C., Ackland T. R., Blanksby B. A., Hood K. P. & Bloomfield J. (1989) Profiling junior tennis players, Part 1: Morphological, physiological and psychological normative data. *Australian Journal of Science and Medicine in Sport* 21, 14–21.

Eysenck W. (1968) *Manual for the Eysenck Personality Inventory (Junior)*. CA: Educational and Industrial Testing Service, San Diego, CA.

Greulich W. & Pyle, S. (1959) *Radiographic Atlas of Skeletal Development of the Hand and Wrist*. Stanford University Press, Stanford, CA.

Hahn A. (1990) Identification and selection of talent in Australian rowing. *Excel* 6, 5–11.

Komadel L. (1988) The identification of performance potential. In Dirix A., Knuttgen H. & Tittel K. (eds) *The Olympic Book of Sports Medicine I*, pp. 275–285. Blackwell Scientific Publications, Oxford.

Lowery G. (1978) *Growth and Development of Children*, 7th edn, pp. 96–97. Year Book Medical Publishers, Chicago, IL.

Malina R. & Bouchard C. (1991) *Growth, Maturation and Physical Activity*, pp. 60–64, 83–84, 96–100, 202–203, 445–458. Human Kinetics Publishers, Champaign, IL.

McNair D. M., Lorr M. & Droppleman L. F. (1971) *EDITS Manual for POMS*. CA: Educational and Industrial Testing Service, San Diego, CA.

Martens R. (1977) *Sport Composition Anxiety Test*. Human Kinetics Publishers, Champaign, IL.

Morgan W. P. (1980) Test of champions: The iceberg profile. *Psychology Today* 19, 92–93, 97–99, 102, 108.

Nideffer R. M. (1976) Test of attentional and interpersonal style. *Journal of Personality and Social Psychology* 34, 394–404.

Sloane K. (1985) Home influences on talent development. In Bloom B. S. (ed.) *Developing Talent in Young People*, pp. 440–444. Ballantine Books, New York.

Tanner J. (1989) *Foetus into Man*, pp. 65–70, 178–221. Castlemead Publications, Ware.

Widmeyer W. N., Brawley L. R. & Carron A. V. (1985) *The Measurement of Cohesion in Sport Teams: The Group Environment Questionnaire*. Sport Dynamics, London.

Wilmore J. H. & Costill D. L. (1994) *Physiology of Sport and Exercise*, p. 109. Human Kinetics Publishers, Champaign, IL.

SECTION 4

SPORTS MEDICINE

CLASSIFICATION OF INJURIES AND MECHANISMS OF INJURY, REPAIR, HEALING AND SOFT TISSUE REMODELLING

B. W. Oakes

In musculoskeletal practice it is important to develop clinical skills and to establish an accurate diagnosis with anatomical precision to manage a patient optimally. Management regimens are based on both the previous practical experience of the clinician and of other researchers working on animal or human subjects. This chapter briefly reviews recent basic science information in relation to mechanisms of injury to muscle, bone, articular cartilage and ligament/tendon and their repair response, and relates this to practical clinical patient management.

CLASSIFICATION OF INJURIES

Sports injuries can be classified by their cause (Corrigan 1968; Williams & Sperryn 1976) or by the tissue which is injured. However, an understanding of both is needed if the sports physician is to give the patient optimal care during the recovery period.

MECHANISMS OF INJURY

These can be divided into primary and secondary injury. Three major types of primary injury are recognized.

Primary Injury

DIRECT OR EXTRINSIC INJURY

This type of injury may result from external causes such as a collision with another athlete or being struck by a piece of equipment used by an opposing player or team-mate, such as a cricket ball or a hockey stick. This may lead to head injury, joint injury, skin abrasions or muscle contusion. The forces involved in this type of injury are often great because of the momentum involved with both the player(s) and the implement; hence severe injuries occur such as fractures, joint dislocations and Grade 2 and 3 ligament injuries to both the ankle and the knee joints.

INDIRECT OR INTRINSIC INJURY

These injuries are caused by the individual athlete and are commonly seen as, for example, muscle tears following inadequate 'preseason' and 'inseason' stretching, where muscle length is not adequate to perform a particular skilled manoeuvre. The muscle–tendon unit is overloaded, often under eccentric loading conditions, with the inevitable consequences of a partial tear or even a complete rupture of that muscle–tendon unit.

OVERUSE INJURY

Acute repetitive friction

This may occur if continually apposed structures are in constant contact, such as in the iliotibial band syndrome or semimembranosus bursitis in relation to the tendon of the semimembranosus and the medial head of the gastrocnemius tendon. Tenosynovitis and tenovaginitis are further examples of injuries which result from continuous frictional wear between the tendon and its associated synovial sheath.

Chronic repetitive micro-fatigue

This failure can result in such injuries as Achilles tendinitis or Osgood-Schlatter's disease at the tibial tuberosity epiphysis in adolescent boys. Inadequate footwear without medial arch support in distance runners may lead to 'medial arch strain' especially if the inverter muscle group is weak or fatigued. Stress fractures are another example of repetitive micro-fatigue.

Secondary Injury

SHORT TERM

This injury often follows one which has been previously mismanaged. It is common with muscle–tendon unit tears when the pain of the acute inflammatory phase has settled down in the second or third week of treatment. At this time the athlete believes that an adequate load-bearing scar has formed and commences the rehabilitation exercise at full power or speed, which may cause a 're-tear' at the previously injured site. A similar situation can occur with unrecognized stress fractures, especially of the tibia or the metatarsals, where the athlete may rest for a short period (perhaps 2 weeks) until the pain of the acute injury subsides and then on commencement of exercise the pain returns as the microfractures 'open' again on loading.

LONG TERM

This occurs in situations where a long-term injury can lead to other degenerative problems. An example of this is seen in degenerative knee osteoarthritis as a result of cruciate ligament rupture or meniscal damage.

TISSUE-BASED CLASSIFICATION OF INJURY

For the practising clinician this classification is useful and is as follows:

Soft Tissue Injuries

Skin and deep fascia

- Muscle–tendon unit and tendoperiosteal attachments to the skeleton
- Muscle compartments, for example, the anterior compartment of the leg
- Joints and their associated structures including dislocation, subluxation and fracture dislocation with ligamentous and ligament–bone junction injuries, fibrocartilage or meniscal damage, capsular and synovial tearing, bursitis, tenosynovitis and tenovaginitis
- Intervertebral disc annulus fibrosis disruptions

Hard Tissue Injuries

- Acute bone fractures including osteochondral fractures and avulsion fractures
- Periostitis, for example, 'shin' soreness and posteromedial tibial syndrome
- 'Stress' fractures due to repetitive cyclical loading on normal bone
- Hyaline articular and epiphyseal cartilage injuries

Special Tissues or Organ Injuries

- Brain and peripheral nerves
- Eye, nose, sinuses, larynx, teeth
- Thoracic, abdominal and pelvic organs

GENERAL PATHOLOGY OF THE REPAIR PROCESS

Alvarez et al. (1987) describe three phases of the repair response which can be applied to tissues in general. Following this, the specifics of repair in ligament/tendon, articular cartilage and fibrocartilage are discussed in more detail (Fig. 12.1).

The Acute Inflammatory Response (Approximately 0–72 h After Injury)

Immediately after the tissue is injured there is cell necrosis and then a remarkably uniform vascular response to injury occurs. Small capillary rupture leads to immediate haemorrhage and these capillaries

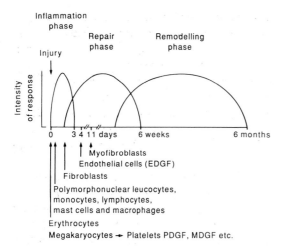

Fig. 12.1 The three phases of healing and the cells involved.

then undergo vasoconstriction within about 5–10 min. This phase is then followed by vasodilation. Coincident with this vasodilation is the leakage of plasma from the postcapillary venules, which is due to the separation of endothelial cells, and the capillary basement membrane is exposed directly to the luminal plasma. Local lymphatic capillaries can also be ruptured as they are more fragile than blood-vascular capillaries and this causes more fluid leakage into the damaged area. Fibrin from the vascular compartment and other components of the blood-clotting system quickly plug the damaged capillaries as well as the lymphatics and hence this latter blockage effectively stops any drainage from the injured area.

The local vasodilation, leakage of fluid from the ruptured capillaries and cessation of lymphatic drainage from the injured area lead to the classical signs of inflammation: redness, swelling and heat. Pain may be due to the local tissue pressures and to the release of local chemical mediators such as histamine from mast cells, as well as serotonin and heparin. It appears that the action of these amines is not on the capillaries but on the postcapillary venules, which are only 20–30 μm in size. Kinins and prostaglandins (PGE_1 and PGE_2) are also released and the latter appear to have strong vaso-active, permeability increasing and lymph flow promoting properties. It appears that the pros-

taglandins are terminal mediators of the acute inflammatory response and the use of aspirin and indomethacin, which are potent inhibitors of pros-taglandin synthesis, is thus indicated as anti-inflammatory agents in sports injuries. Prostaglan-dins may also have a significant effect on connective tissue remodelling. Growth factors such as platelet-derived growth factor (PDGF) and others from monocytes are also present in this early stage and these are important in directing fibroblast prolifer-ation for the next stage of repair.

Chemotactants such as PDGF attract a rapid accumulation of polymorphonuclear neutrophilic leucocytes, lymphocytes and macrophages into the injured area. Macrophages appear to be essential for the progression of the repair process. This is because they are long-lived cells and apart from their well known phagocytic properties, they release further angiogenic and fibroblast growth factors, which are essential to the next repair phase. The use of systemic hydrocortisone results in a mono-cytopenia, and antimacrophage serum used locally reduces the number of macrophages and wound debridement and the synthetic activity of fibroblasts is significantly delayed.

Matrix and Cellular Proliferation Phase (Approximately 72 h to 6 weeks +)

This phase is characterized by the proliferation of capillaries and fibroblasts which synthesize a collagen/proteoglycan matrix and together form the 'granulation' tissue classically seen in open wounds. Neovascularization during this repair phase is derived from the existing capillary network by a budding process, which eventually fills in the damaged area and is probably under the control of growth factors, such as transforming growth factor-β (TGF-β) as well as endothelial cell derived growth factor (ECDGF). Fibroblasts initially lay down small diameter Type III collagen, which may then be partially converted to larger diameter Type I collagen in the next phase of wound remodelling. It is during this phase that fibroblasts start to commence traction on the collagen fibrils deposited, causing wound contraction. This is the forerunner for the next phase of collagen remodelling. Fibro-nectin is a high molecular weight glycoprotein found on the surface of cells, which mediates the adhesion of fibroblasts to the fibrin network and facilitates their migration in this phase. It also acts as an anchoring compound between the newly synthesized collagen fibrils and the fibroblasts. It appears that during this phase of collagen deposition, the large diameter collagen fibrils present in normal non-injured ligaments and tendons are never re-formed and that the mechanism of repair in adult tissues in any site in the body is by the deposition of a large amount of smaller diameter collagen fibrils, which may be an admixture of Types I and III collagen. This 'scar tissue' leads to a change in the material properties of the tissue, especially in ligaments and tendons where large collagen fibrils determine the tensile strength of these special tissues and where the collagen is oriented in parallel bundles with a classic collagen 'crimp'.

Remodelling and Maturation Phase of Healing (Approximately 6 Weeks to Several Months)

It is during this phase that special cells called myofibroblasts, which contain the contractile actin proteins, interact with the newly laid down collagen fibrils and continue contraction of the collagen fibril framework established during the repair phase. They also reorientate the collagen fibrils in the direction of loading, especially during ligament repair. Collagen maturation also continues and generally cell numbers decrease within the tissue. Early motion of ligaments as opposed to immobilization appears to translate mechanical signals to the fibroblasts at this stage to assist in the remodelling process of removal of early poorly oriented collagen fibrils and deposition of new collagen fibres in the direction of loading. Similarly, early motion and cyclical loading of bone appear to speed up this remodelling phase during bone fracture repair.

BASIC BIOMECHANICS OF TISSUE INJURY

Muscle–Tendon–Bone Injury

The basic causes of intrinsic muscle injury are still not entirely clear, but have been attributed to inadequate muscle length and strength, for example, 'tight' hamstrings, especially in adolescent boys, muscle fatigue and inadequate kinesthetic skills. It is also clear that the majority of muscle injuries occur in the lower limb and most involve the 'two-joint muscles', the hamstrings and the rectus femoris, probably because of the complex reflexes involved in simultaneous co-contraction and co-relaxation involved with these two muscle groups (Oakes 1984).

Both concentric and eccentric muscle–tendon unit loading can cause muscle–tendon–bone junction injury. The use of eccentric muscle loading to cause increased muscle hypertrophy, as against the use of more conventional concentric loading, has led to the phenomenon of eccentric muscle soreness, which is now known to be due in part to muscle sarcomere disruption at the Z lines (Fridén et al. 1983). Eccentric muscle–tendon–bone load can generate more force than concentric contractions and may be the mechanism by which the patellar tendon and its attachments lead to tendo-periosteal partial disruptions at both the superior and inferior poles of the patella. Recent studies by Chun et al. (1989) demonstrated that the infero-medial collagen fibre bundles of the human patellar tendon, when subjected to mechanical stress, fail at loads which are much less than the lateral fibre bundles. The biological reasons for this are not clear at present, but it helps to explain the prevalence of inferomedial tenderness which is such a common cause of anteromedial knee pain or 'jumper's knee'.

Muscle–Tendon Junction

Failure at this junctional region is commonly seen in the clinical situation. There is an increased membrane 'infolding' of the terminal end of the last muscle sarcomere, which has important mechanical implications for reducing the stress at this critical junctional region. It has been determined that a typical vertebrate fast twitch cell can generate about 0.33 MPa of stress across the cell. The stress placed on the cell's junctional complex at the muscle–tendon junction by the complex folding of the terminal sarcomeres experiences a maximal stress of 1.5×10^4 Pa which is much less than 33×10^4 Pa and this difference may determine whether mechanical failure occurs at this junctional region. With muscle injury at this site, it is probable that this complex sarcomere muscle membrane infolding (which increases the surface area and hence decreases substantially the stress at the muscle–tendon junction) is probably not reproduced following repair. This may be an explanation for the occurrence of 're-tears' at this junction in athletes with previous injury and repair to this region.

Tendon Injury

Tendon injury is not uncommon in sport because of the heavy loads applied. Komi (1987) has measured the high forces generated in the human Achilles tendon with the surgical introduction of a calibrated buckle transducer for short periods of time. Forces of up to 4000 N were recorded in the Achilles tendon with toe running; thus it is not surprising that with repetitive loadings of these magnitudes, micro-fatigue failure could occur with long-distance running, especially in an Achilles tendon with a small cross-sectional area (Engstrom et al. 1985).

Spontaneous Tendon Rupture

This is uncommon in the young athlete and usually occurs in the older sportsperson, where it is mostly associated with the degenerative pathology of the collagen fibrils.

LIGAMENTS AND TENDONS

Structure and Biomechanics of Ligaments and Tendons

The mature adult ligament and tendon are composed of large diameter Type I collagen fibrils (>1500 Å diameter) tightly packed together with a small amount of Type III collagen dispersed in an aqueous gel which contains small amounts of proteoglycan and elastic fibres. The outstanding feature of both these unique load-bearing tissues is the collagen 'crimp', which is a planar wave pattern found extending in phase across the width of all tendons and ligaments. This collagen 'crimp' appears to be built into the tertiary structure of the collagen molecule and is probably maintained *in vivo* by inter- and intramolecular collagen cross-links as well as a strategically placed elastic fibre network. The 'crimp' may help to attenuate muscle loading forces at the tendoperiosteal junction as well as the musculotendinous junction.

Ligament and tendon injury can be closely correlated with the load–deformation curve (Butler et al. 1979; Oakes 1981). The load–strain curve can be divided into three regions (Fig. 12.2):

- The 'toe' region or initial concave region represents the normal physiological range of ligament/tendon strain up to about 3–4% of initial length and is due to the flattening of the collagen 'crimp'. Repeated cycling within this 'toe' region or 'physiological strain range' of 3–4% can normally occur without irreversible macroscopic or molecular damage to the tissue. This may perhaps be up to 10% in cruciate ligaments due to the intrinsic macrospiral of collagen cruciate fibre bundles

- The second part of the load–deformation curve is the linear region, where pathological irreversible ligament/tendon elongation occurs due to partial rupture of intermolecular cross-links. As the load is increased further, intra- and intermolecular cross-links are disrupted until macroscopic failure is evident clinically. The early part of the linear region corresponds to mild ligament tears or Grade 1, 0–50% fibre disruption and the latter part to Grade 2, and 50–80% fibre disruption, where there is obvious clinical laxity on stress testing. Grade 1 and 2 injuries always have some pain after the initial trauma and usually with a Grade 2 injury the athlete cannot continue activity, which is a 'rough' guide to the clinical severity of the injury

- In the third region, if continued loading occurs, the linear part of the curve flattens and then the 'yield' or failure point is reached at 10–20% strain, dependent upon ligament/tendon fibre bundle macro-organization. In this region complete ligament or tendon rupture occurs at 'maximal breaking load' and this is the dangerous Grade 3 ligament rupture on clinical testing. It is 'dangerous' because the athlete has severe momentary pain when the trauma is applied and then little pain after, and the athlete and often inexperienced examiners believe the injury is trivial and treat it as such with disastrous consequences (Fig. 12.2).

There has been a considerable amount of work done on the biomechanical properties of the human knee ligaments, with the anterior cruciate ligament (ACL) dominating research because of its key role in anteroposterior stability of the knee. Rotational injury to the knee with the foot fixed, as well as hyperextension of the knee, appear to be the two key mechanisms involved in ACL disruption. Forces of the order of 2000 N are required to disrupt the

ACL and are even higher for the posterior cruciate ligament (PCL). Direct falls on to the tibia or collisions with opponents, such that there is a posterior displacement force of the tibia on the femur, appear to be a common mechanism for PCL injury. Collateral ligament injury involves excessive varus, valgus or rotational forces. The ligament–bone junction, with its special fibrocartilage transition zone, is a common region of clinical failure. Recent experimental animal work indicates that ligament mid-substance strain is much lower than at the insertion sites and this appears to be due to a differing collagen fibre crimp amplitude and angle. This higher strain at the insertion sites, together with ligament insertion geometry, could be an explanation of preferential failure at some of the sites.

Correlation of Collagen Fibril Size with Mechanical Properties of Tissues

Parry *et al.* (1978) have completed detailed quantitative morphometric ultrastructural analyses of collagen fibrils from a large number of collagen-containing tissues in various species. They concluded that:

- Type 1 oriented tissues such as ligament and tendon have a bimodal distribution of collagen fibril diameters at maturity
- The ultimate tensile strength and mechanical properties of connective tissues are positively correlated with the 'mass average diameter' of collagen fibrils. In the context of response of ligaments to exercise, they also concluded that the collagen fibril diameter distribution is closely correlated with the magnitude and duration of loading of tissues

COLLAGEN FIBRIL DIAMETER QUANTIFICATION WITH AGE AND CORRELATION WITH ACL TENSILE STRENGTH

Oakes (1988) measured collagen fibrils at various ages of the rat, from 14 days fetal to 2 year old senile adult rats. The mean diameter and the range of fibrils from the largest to the smallest for each time interval were plotted against age and are shown in Fig. 12.3. The mean fibril diameter begins

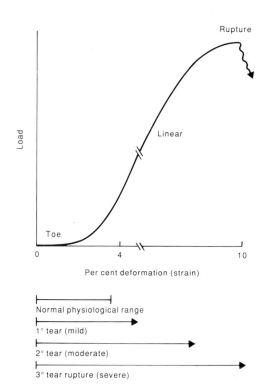

Fig. 12.2 The load–deformation (strain) curve for ligament/tendon and the clinical correlation with the grading of the injury. Note the 'toe' region of the curve is entirely within the normal physiological range and that greater than approximately 4% strain causes tissue damage.

to plateau at about 7 weeks postnatal. Also plotted on this figure is the separation force required to rupture the ACL as a function of age. Special grips were used in this study to obviate epiphyseal separation and 70% of the failures occurred within the ACL. It can be seen that the two curves closely coincide, indicating a close correlation between the size of the collagen fibrils and the ultimate tensile strength of the ACL, as has been suggested by Parry *et al.* (1978). This rapid increase in collagen fibril size over 6 weeks in the growing rat is not seen during normal ligament/tissue repair.

Work by Shadwick (1986) has also elegantly demonstrated a clear correlation between collagen fibril diameter and the tensile strength of tendons. He determined that the tensile strength of pig flexor tendons was greater than that of extensor tendons and that this greater flexor tendon tensile strength was correlated with a population of larger diameter collagen fibrils not present in the weaker extensor tendons.

EFFECTS OF IMMOBILIZATION ON LIGAMENTS AND SYNOVIAL JOINTS

There is articular cartilage atrophy with proteoglycan loss and an associated fibrofatty connective tissue that is synovial-derived, which adheres to the articular cartilage. Ligament insertion sites are weakened and the ligament itself has increased compliance with reduced load to failure. This is due to loss of collagen mass which may occur with only 8–12 weeks immobilization and may take up to 1 year to recover after mobilization. Capsular changes include loss of water due to loss of glycosaminoglycans (GAG), including hyaluronic acid, which leads to joint stiffness (Akeson *et al.* 1987). Joint immobilization is to be avoided if possible to prevent the above changes from occurring as they may take many months to recover (Fig. 12.4).

BONE

Acute fractures of long bones and their individual biomechanical considerations cannot be covered in detail in this chapter except to mention that large bending, torsional and compressive forces are involved. Fortunately, they are not common in sport but do occur occasionally with player collisions.

More common are avulsion fractures associated with excessive loading of tendons and ligaments. A typical avulsion fracture is to the dorsal bone of the base of the distal phalanx or 'mallet finger' injury, when the extended finger is forced into flexion if

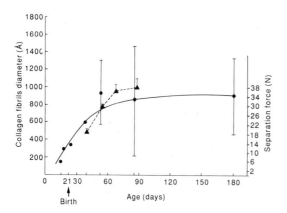

Fig. 12.3 A comparison of growth in the mean diameter of collagen fibrils (solid circle) (bar represents the largest and smallest fibrils) and tensile strength (solid triangle) with age in the growing rat anterior cruciate ligament. Note both curves plateau at about 90 days after conception or about 70 days after birth.

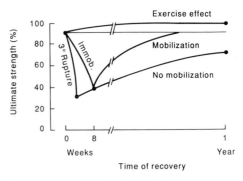

Fig. 12.4 The effects of immobilization, mobilization and exercise on ligament ultimate tensile strength (UTS) recovery. After a relatively short period of immobilization of about 8 weeks, ligament tensile strength takes many months to recover — with no mobilization it may take up to 1 year! Note that the effect of exercise on the ligament UTS is small. (Modified from Woo *et al.* 1987.)

hit by a ball. A similar injury is the 'rugger-jersey' finger when the volar aspect of the base of the distal phalanx is avulsed due to acute overload during finger flexion, as the player grasps the jersey of his opponent during tackling.

Perhaps less commonly understood are the mechanisms involved in the development of stress fractures.

Bone fatigue failure is currently topical because of the large numbers of individuals involved in distance running or jogging who sustain stress fractures. Also of particular interest is the onset of osteoporosis in long-term amenorrhoeic marathon runners (Drinkwater *et al.* 1984). Of clinical interest is the relationship of the quality of the bone matrix and especially bone mineral density (BMD) and the formation of stress fractures, particularly in running athletes. Carbon *et al.* (1990) found no such relationship in a study on stress fracture formation in elite female athletes. Bennell *et al.* (1994) have shown a correlation between spine BMD and stress fracture formation, but they did not show any correlation for leg BMD. However, it must be remembered that bone strength is related to bone mass: the lower the bone mass, the higher the prevalence of fractures (Riggs & Melton 1986).

The 'threshold level' of physical activity or mechanical loading at which bone remodels positively or accumulates microdamage has not been defined. In fact the concept of microdamage is poorly defined, except in terms of the status or integrity of the bone prior to a 'clearly' diagnosable problem such as a stress fracture. Carter *et al.* (1981) have demonstrated that repetitive cyclical physiological loading *in vitro* can cause a progressive gradual loss of stiffness and ultimate strength due to microcracks. Bone was shown to have extremely poor fatigue resistance and fully reversed cyclic loading to one-half of the yield strain caused fatigue fracture in 1000 cycles. Carter *et al.* (1981) compared their strain ranges (0.005–0.010) and fatigue results and extrapolated these data to that which may occur in bone *in vivo* with the clinical experience of fatigue fractures among military recruits and athletes. They concluded that military recruits would within 6 weeks (the earliest appearance of stress fractures) accumu-

late a loading history equivalent to 100–1000 miles of very rigorous exercise, which they calculated as equivalent to 100 000–1 000 000 loading cycles. From their data extrapolation they predicted cyclic strain ranges of 0.0029 and 0.0019, respectively, for fatigue fractures in these recruits (Fig. 12.5).

Carter *et al.* (1981) further determined that tensile fatigue caused failure at the cement lines, which resulted in debonding of the osteons from surrounding interstitial bone, whereas compressive fatigue resulted in the formation of 'diffuse shear microcracks throughout bone which are oblique to the loading direction'. They also estimated the fatigue strength of bone as being about 7 MPa at 10^7 cycles and suggested that this extremely low value for fatigue strength of human cortical bone would require that our bones are constantly accumulating fatigue damage during daily activities and that the processes of normal bone remodelling and repair are necessary for long-term structural integrity of bone. The use of plasma hydroxyproline levels, which is a measure of bone resorption, may be a useful clinical marker for predicting the onset of stress fractures of bone in those who are vigorously exercising (Marguia *et al.* 1988). (For further de-

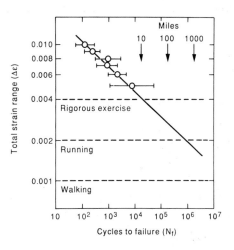

Fig. 12.5 The *in vitro* strain-related fatigue behaviour of cortical bone compared with the levels of cyclical strain range that are expected during various *in vivo* activities. Note that prolonged rigorous exercise may lead to cortical fatigue or 'stress' failure as may prolonged running. (Carter *et al.* 1981. With permission.)

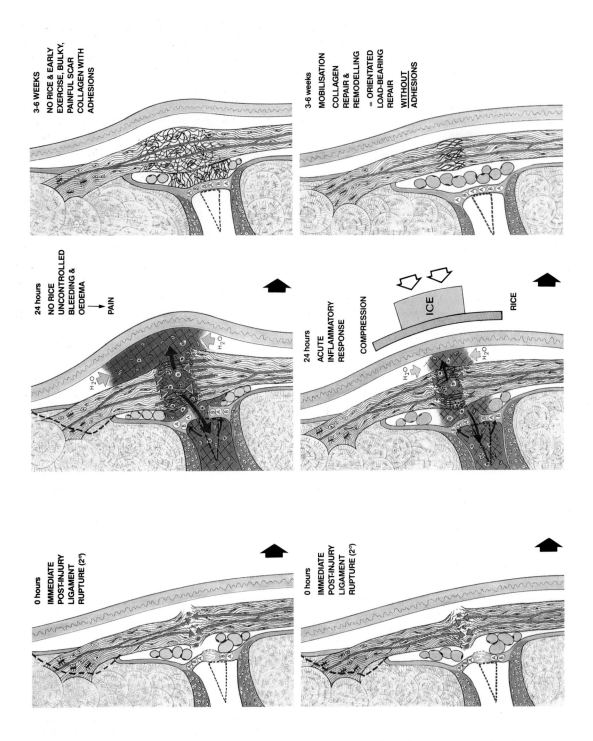

Figs 12.6 & 12.7 Ligament repair with and without 'RICE' (rest, ice, compress, elevate) management and early mobilization.

tailed reading on the mechanical adaptation of bone, see Martin & Burr 1989 and Burr & Martin 1992.)

In another study Rubin *et al.* (1987) measured the velocity of ultrasound across the patella and tibia in 98 volunteers before and after running the Boston Marathon. In summary, they found that absolute sound velocities were 2.9% higher in those runners finishing in less than 3 h compared with those finishing after 3 h. Tibial velocities in males were 8.8% higher than in female runners. The mean velocity across the patella of three wheelchair racers was 28% lower than the mean combined patellar velocity measures in all runners. They suggested that 'faster' velocities were associated with bone that was more suited to greater functional demands. Also it was shown that there was a 1.6% increase in ultrasonic velocity across the tibia, and a 3.5% increase across the patella between pre- and post-race velocities, indicating that change had occurred within the bone during the race. The nature of this change is speculative at present, but it may well be due to fatigue fracture damage as has been postulated by Carter *et al.* (1981). However, with fatigue fractures one would expect a marked decrease in sound velocity. They suggested that the increase in sound transmission observed post-race may be due to other organic mechanisms such as proteoglycan orientation. Unfortunately, individual biomechanical profiles which may have identified structural abnormalities likely to promote a damaging overload situation were not reported.

PATHOLOGY IN SPECIFIC TISSUES

Ligament and Tendon Repair (Figs 12.6 and 12.7)

Although the above tissues are different in their cell types they are included together in this section of the chapter. ACL injuries, which are in a category of their own, are dealt with later in the section.

ACUTE INFLAMMATORY PHASE (UP TO 72 H)

The gap in the ligament/tendon is filled immediately with erythrocytes and inflammatory cells, especially polymorphonuclear leucocytes. Within 24 h monocytes and macrophages are the predominant cells

which actively engage in phagocytosis of debris and necrotic cells. These are gradually replaced by fibroblasts from either intrinsic or extrinsic sources and these commence the initial deposition of the Type III collagen scar. At this stage collagen concentration may be normal or slightly decreased, but the total mass of ligament collagen scar is increased. Glycosaminoglycan content, water, fibronectin and DNA content are increased (Fig. 12.8).

PROLIFERATION (4– 6 WEEKS +)

During proliferation fibroblasts predominate, water content remains increased and collagen content increases and peaks during this phase (3–6 weeks). Type I collagen now begins to predominate and GAG concentration remains high. The increasing amount of scar collagen and reducible cross-link profile have been correlated with the increasing tensile strength of the ligament matrix. Recent quantitative collagen fibril orientation studies indicate that early mobilization of a ligament at this stage (within the first 3 weeks) may be detrimental to collagen orientation. After this time there is experimental evidence that mobilization increases the tensile strength of the repair and probably enhances this phase and the next phase of remodelling and maturation (Vailas *et al.* 1981; Hart & Danhers 1987; Woo *et al.* 1987).

With this basic biological knowledge there is now a rationale for the use of 'early controlled mobilization' of patients with ligament trauma. The use of a limited motion cast with an adjustable double action hinge for the knee joint is now

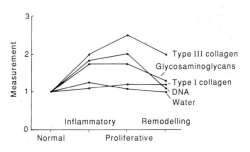

Fig. 12.8 Ligament repair during the phases of healing and the 'normalized' content of Type I and III collagen, water, DNA and glycosaminoglycans. (Woo & Buckwalter 1988. With permission.)

accepted and encourages more rapid repair and remodelling, as well as preserving quadriceps muscle bulk. Patients are now usually mobilized in a limited motion cast at 3 weeks rather than the previously empirical time of 6 weeks.

REMODELLING AND MATURATION (6 WEEKS TO 12 MONTHS)

There is a decreasing cell number and hence decreased collagen and GAG synthesis. Water content returns to normal and collagen concentration returns to just below normal, but total collagen content remains slightly increased. With further remodelling there is a trend for scar parameters to return to normal, but the matrix in the ligament scar region continues to mature slowly over months and even years. Collagen fibril alignment in the longitudinal axis of the ligament occurs even though they are small diameter collagen fibrils (Fig. 12.9).

Occasionally, calcium apatite crystals are deposited in the damaged tissues and the classic site for this to occur is in the rotator cuff supraspinatus tendoperiosteal attachment to the greater tubercle of the humerus.

Achilles tendon injuries, especially partial tears, present a dilemma for the clinician in that they are often difficult to manage, although Stanish *et al.* (1986) claim good clinical results from graded eccentric loading regimens. The authors have examined Achilles tendon biopsies of patients with chronic localized tears and more generalized thickened tender chronic Achilles tendons. The feature which characterized the pathology ultrastructurally was the persistence of small diameter collagen fibrils.

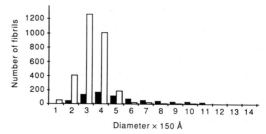

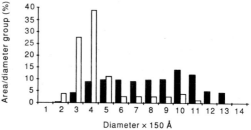

Fig. 12.10 A comparison of the number of fibrils versus fibril diameter in patients with normal tendon Achilles (solid square) and chronic Achilles tendinitis (open square) and also expressed as per cent area occupied for each diameter group versus diameter. Note the preponderance of small diameter fibrils in 'repairing' chronic Achilles tendinitis. The large normal fibrils are not replaced.

The large fibrils of the original tendon do not appear to be replaced in either a repairing tendon or ligament (Fig. 12.10).

Clinical and Ultrastructural Observations on Achilles Tendon Injuries

This section relates the three phases of healing of soft tissues with those seen in Achilles tendon injuries. Achilles tendon injuries can be classified as described above for ligament injury, that is, Grades 1–3 with Grade 3 being complete rupture. Several patient histories are used to illustrate these three phases of healing and attempted repair.

GRADE 3, COMPLETE RUPTURE

Patient profile: Footballer aged 26, accelerating to avoid an opponent. The clinical signs were a palpable defect of the tendo-Achilles as well as a positive Thompson's sign. A biopsy was taken during surgical repair.

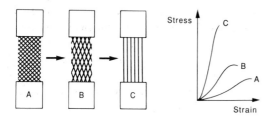

Fig. 12.9 The effect of collagen repair with identical fibrils but different geometry and their corresponding load–strain response to tensile testing. (Modified from Viidik 1980. With permission.)

With this disastrous injury there is both collagen bundle failure and vascular disruption and hence bleeding, which is a feature of these injuries. This trauma to the tendon initiates the acute inflammatory phase and microscopically there is massive red cell extravasation and fibrin clot formation as well as collagen fibril disruption. The damaged tendon becomes oedematous and polymorphonuclear monocytes migrate into this area and release their lysosomal contents, actively phagocytosing cellular and other debris. Macrophages also move into the rupture site and commence phagocytosis of damaged cells and tissue. This phase lasts 0–72 h or more and is followed by the repair phase.

GRADE 2, TEAR

Patient profile: Footballer with a 6 month old painful and thickened tendo-Achilles. Operation: Excision of the paratenon and a tendon incision to remove damaged, haemorrhagic and necrotic regions. A biopsy was also taken.

Light microscopy demonstrated a thickened paratenon and an oedematous and thickened tendon. Ultrastructurally, many fibroblasts had dilated rough endoplasmic reticulum and prominent nucleoli, indicative of increased collagen synthesis. Apart from the many free red blood cells the other feature was the prevalence of many small diameter collagen fibrils not aligned or closely packed (180–200 Å diameter) in among the older larger pre-existing fibrils ranging from 800 to 1500 Å diameter. Polymorphonuclear monocytes and macrophages were not common at this stage and this may reflect the slowness of repair in this unique tissue.

This biopsy demonstrated the features of the repair phase which follows the acute inflammatory phase and lasts from after the first 72 h to 4–6 weeks, but in this patient the repair phase was prolonged because of continued activity by the athlete. This is a common problem with this type of athlete because when they run the Achilles tendon pain usually subsides and then returns on 'cool-down', often being acute. In other patients where there is less florid tendinitis and the tendon is clinically painful but not obviously enlarged, discrete areas of increased cellularity can be seen in the tendon in the form of free red blood cells, cell debris and viable fibroblasts surrounded by both large and many small diameter collagen fibres. These areas are almost 'walled-off' from the densely packed collagen of the rest of the tendon by a fibrin precipitate. These discrete areas are probably due to collagen fibre ruptures or 'micro-tears' corresponding to the early part of region 2 of the load–deformation curve. There is as yet no evidence that the use of massage or 'deep friction' enhances this repair phase.

GRADE 1, INJURY

Patient profile: Runner, aged 25, with a painful tender lump in the Achilles tendon for 18 months. A biopsy was obtained at open operation.

The lump at operation was firmer than the rest of the tendon and was slightly darker in colour. Light microscopy of the biopsy taken from the nodule showed that the changes in the collagen bundles were very subtle. There was less regular 'crimping' of the collagen bundles and they were not as tightly packed. However, ultrastructurally the cause of this less regular collagen crimp was obvious: in between the large diameter fibrils were many small diameter fibrils less well oriented longitudinally. These tendons were interpreted as being in the remodelling phase as there were no increased fibroblast numbers in the nodules and no inflammatory cells were observed.

The mechanism of acute complete rupture in young athletes during acceleration in sprinting indicates that the gastrocnemius–soleus complex can generate sufficient force to rupture the tendon. However, tendon strength usually exceeds that of its muscle by a factor of 2 and hence rupture is unusual. The mechanisms involved in partial Grade 1 and 2 tears in the Achilles tendon are less clear. Viidik (1973) has shown that rat tendons *in vitro* undergo increasing deformation or 'plasticity' if cycled to loads less than one-tenth of their failure load. The strain or deformation is well before region 2 or the linear part of the load–strain curve begins. Similar observations have been made both *in vivo* and *in vitro* for rat knee joint ligaments by Weisman *et al.* (1980). It is possible that in distance runners a similar fatigue plasticity and elongation occurs in the tendon and this causes the micro-ruptures and repair nodules already described.

The notion that some running athletes may not have an Achilles tendon of sufficient cross-sectional area to sustain the repetitive tendon loading of distance without injury has been investigated by Engstrom et al. (1985). In an elegant study they used ultrasound to measure the cross-sectional area of the human Achilles tendon in vivo and validated this technique as a reliable method by using cadaver Achilles tendons. Two groups of distance athletes with and without Grade 1 Achilles tendinitis who were age-, weight- and distance-matched had their Achilles tendon cross-sectional area measured using the ultrasound technique. The athletes with Grade 1 type Achilles tendinitis had an approximately 30% decrease in the cross-sectional area of their Achilles tendons ($P<0.05$). This indicates that a major mechanism in this common type of injury may simply be fatigue creep failure of Achilles tendon collagen. Komi (1987) has recently developed an in vivo buckle transducer which was placed around the Achilles tendon in a number of subjects. Direct force measurements were made on several subjects who were involved in slow walking, sprinting, jumping and hopping after calibration of the transducer. During running and jumping, forces close to the previous estimated ultimate tensile strength of the tendon were recorded. This indicates that fatigue creep in a small cross-sectional tendon is a possible mechanism of injury, without the need to invoke other lower limb biomechanical pathology as has been suggested by Williams (1986). For an excellent review of the surgical management of Achilles tendon overuse injuries, see Schepsis et al. (1994).

ACL injuries appear to be unique in that the chondrocyte-like cells in this special ligament apparently have a limited capacity to proliferate and synthesize a new collagen matrix and hence repair appears to be limited. Collagenase release may also influence the effectiveness of the repair process.

Collagen Remodelling and Fibril Size in ACL Grafts

In order to gain some biological insight into collagen remodelling mechanisms within human cruciate ligament grafts, biopsies were obtained from auto-enous ACL grafts of patients subsequently requiring arthroscopic intervention because of stiffness, meniscal and/or articular cartilage problems or removal of prominent staples used for fixation. Most of the ACL grafts were from the central one-third of the patellar tendon as a free graft (Oakes 1988).

The results (Fig. 12.11) from the collagen fibril diameter morphometric analysis in all the ACL grafts clearly indicated a predominance of small diameter collagen fibrils. Absence of a 'regular crimping' of collagen fibrils was observed by both light and electron microscopy, as was a less ordered parallel arrangement of fibrils. In most biopsies capillaries were present and most fibroblasts appeared viable.

Quantitatively, the following occurred (Fig. 12.11, insets):

- Large diameter collagen fibres (>1000 Å diameter) form a large proportion (approximately 45%) of the percentage cross-sectional area in the normal human patellar tendon
- Collagen fibrils (<1000 Å diameter) form a large proportion (approximately 85%) of the percentage cross-sectional area in the normal human ACL
- In all the ACL grafts, collagen fibrils (<1000 Å diameter, majority 250–750 Å diameter) are the major contributor to the collagen fibril cross-sectional area, be they 'young' (9 months) or 'old' grafts (6 years).

The conclusion from this study is that the predominance of the small diameter collagen fibrils (<750 Å) and their poor packing and alignment in all the ACL grafts irrespective of the type of graft, their age and the surgeon, may explain the clinical and experimental evidence of a decreased tensile strength in such grafts compared with the normal ACL. It appears that in the adult, the 'replacement fibroblasts' in the remodelled ACL graft cannot re-form the large diameter, regularly crimped and tightly packed fibrils seen in the normal ACL even after 6 years, which was the oldest graft analysed.

Fig. 12.11 The transverse sections through collagen fibrils of: (a) the normal young adult patellar tendon (mean of six biopsies); (b) normal young adult ACL (mean of six biopsies); (c) Jones' free grafts (mean of nine biopsies) — all ×34 100. Insets: shown on the left are the number of fibrils versus diameter; on the right the per cent area occupied/diameter group. Note the preponderance of small diameter fibrils in the graft (c), and the large fibrils in the patellar tendon (a) not seen in the 'normal' anterior cruciate ligament (b).

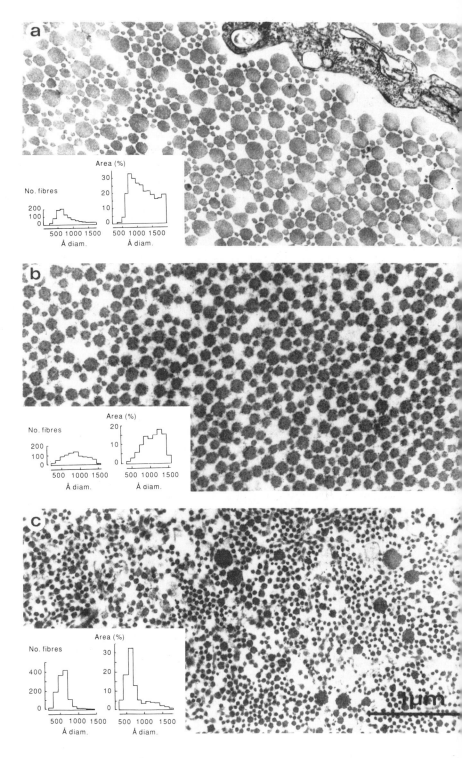

HUMAN ACL HAMSTRING AND ILIOTIBIAL BAND ACL AUTOGRAFTS

Since Oakes (1988), the author has taken more ACL autograft biopsies from patients who have had a strip of iliotibial tract used as an ACL replacement or who have had medial hamstring grafts. Fifteen iliotibial ACL autografts (graft age, 10 months to 6 years) and nine hamstring grafts (graft age 10 months to 6 years) have been quantitated for collagen fibril size. Eighteen ACL graft biopsies have been obtained from other surgeons (national and international). The mean percentage area/diameter fibril groups for the normally used graft tissues, that is, normal patellar tendon, normal iliotibial tract and normal semitendinosus, were compared with the normal ACL and the mean percentage area/diameter groups for 39 Jones' free grafts, nine hamstring grafts and 15 iliotibial tract grafts. With all these autogenous grafts, small fibrils (<100 nm) predominate when compared with the normal ACL collagen fibril profile and some large fibrils are present in the hamstring grafts. These large fibrils are probably remnants of the original large fibrils in the normal hamstring tendons, rather than being formed from pre-existing medium-sized fibrils. This persistence of a small number of large fibrils in the hamstring grafts is not seen with the iliotibial band or the patellar tendon autografts.

The observations in these studies suggest that loadings on the normal iliotibial band and ACL may be similar because of the remarkable similarity in their fibril profiles. Higher 'normal' loadings are postulated for the patellar and hamstring tendons because of their distinct bimodal profiles, with a greater proportion of their cross-sectional area found in the larger fibril populations.

The unimodal profile of small diameter fibrils was observed in most of the ACL autografts whether they were patellar, hamstring tendon or iliotibial in origin. This was a constant observation indicating that collagen remodelling occurs with all these tissues within 3–4 months post-surgery and is independent of the surgeon. This predominance of small collagen fibrils within the ACL grafts is the probable explanation of the less than optimal results obtained in some patients and accounts for the macroscopic diminished quality of these grafts

especially if directly viewed within 1 year of surgery. Large fibrils were observed in a few biopsies obtained from autografts older than 12 months but these were the exception. In human ACL allografts paradoxically more of the larger fibrils survived 12 months compared with the autografts (Oakes 1993; Shino et al. 1995).

The persistence of the small collagen fibril population within these ACL autografts suggests that these fibrils are derived from synovial/vascular stem cells and this notion correlates with the large amount of small proteoglycan and hyaluronate found within ACL autografts in a recent goat study (Oakes 1993, 1994; Ng et al. 1995).

A similar long-term (8 years post-grafting) ultrastructural study of collagen remodelling in human ACL allografts has been completed in collaboration with K. Shino (Oakes 1993; Shino et al. 1995).

The origin of the 'replacement' fibroblasts which remodel the ACL grafts is not known at present. It is the author's view that they do not come from the graft itself, although some of these cells may survive due to diffusion. The bulk of the stem cells involved in the remodelling process is probably derived from the surrounding synovium and its vasculature.

ARTICULAR CARTILAGE

Our understanding of the repair processes in articular cartilage is still very rudimentary. The complex three-dimensional array of Type II collagen fibrils embedded in a rich cartilage specific–proteoglycan matrix seen with normal articular cartilage is difficult to repair and/or replace in the adult (Mankin 1982; Woo & Buckwalter 1988).

Response of Articular Cartilage to Superficial Lacerative Injury

If a simple wedge-shaped laceration is made down to the calcified zone of articular cartilage, the acute inflammatory phase does not occur because articular cartilage is avascular. Chondrocyte death adjacent to the defect occurs and those chondrocytes that survive close to the defect undergo a short-lived proliferative response over a period of approximately 1 week. However, chondrocytes are not mobile cells and they do not migrate into the defect and any matrix which they do synthesize and deposit is within their own vicinity. Probably because this process is avascular there is no fibrin deposited in the defect and hence there is no structural framework and no growth factor stimulus for the proliferation and normal influx of inflammatory cells as described above for ligament repair. Hence fibroblasts do not migrate into the defect and no collagen repair occurs. These lesions remain essentially unchanged over several years and they do not appear to progress to osteoarthritis (Fig. 12.12).

Recently, Hunziker and Rosenberg (1994) have used both 'free' and 'bound' TGF-β incorporated into liposomes which were in turn incorporated into a fibrin clot used to fill partial thickness articular cartilage defects in adult rabbits and mini-pigs. They demonstrated remarkably good short-term repair with chondrocytes and a cartilage-like matrix up to 12 months post-surgery. They demonstrated that the cells which filled these partial articular cartilage defects were derived from the synovium and that the TGF-β caused the transformation of these synovial cells to chondrocytes.

This work is very exciting in that for the first time a biological mechanism has been demonstrated to repair these partial defects and this approach could easily be applied clinically.

FULL THICKNESS ARTICULAR CARTILAGE DEFECTS WHICH BROACH THE SUBCHONDRAL BONE

In this situation as distinct from the above, an acute inflammatory response can occur and the defect fills with fibrin and a vascular repair response rapidly occurs. A new subchondral bone plate forms and the articular cartilage defect above becomes filled with a new tissue which is not the normal combination of Type II collagen and the large specific proteoglycan of articular cartilage. This new tissue is composed of a combination of Type I and II collagen and a 'cartilage type of proteoglycan'. Even 1 year after injury there is still 20% Type I collagen. This new matrix is inferior mechanically to normal articular cartilage and eventually it breaks down and undergoes fibrillation and degeneration and can lead to the development of osteoarthritis (Fig. 12.13).

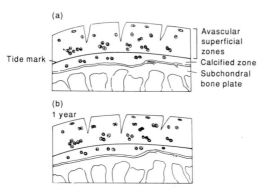

SUPERFICIAL INJURY RESPONSE (vertical or tangential):

- Vigorous repair response for 2 weeks
- Fibrocartilaginous repair
- No repair at 1–2 years and hence
- Poor matrix at >1 year but,
- No OA evident

Fig. 12.12 The response of hyaline articular cartilage to superficial injury of the avascular superficial zone (a). At 1 year there is little repair evident after an initial fibrocartilaginous repair (b). This type of injury does not proceed to osteoarthritic cartilage damage.

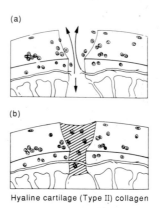

DEEP INJURY (through subchondral bone):

- Vigorous repair response for 2 weeks
- Clot and deposition of a more Type I matrix
- Modulation of fibrous repair
- Mixture of hyaline and fibrocartilage at 12 months with Type I and some Type II

Fig. 12.13 The repair response of hyaline articular cartilage to deep injury through the subchondral bone plate (a). At 12 months the repair tissue is a mixture of hyaline and fibrocartilage with Type I and some Type II collagen (b). There is some proliferation of chondrocytes adjacent to the cut surface.

Blunt Trauma

Blunt trauma to articular cartilage (below the level to cause fracture) such as a direct fall on to the patella, can also cause chondrocyte changes and altered matrix in terms of collagen–proteoglycan relationships, with a loss of proteoglycan in the deeper layers and alterations in the calcified zone. This type of cartilage injury may lead to chondromalacia patellae independent of patellar maltracking problems.

Salter (1989) has demonstrated the possibility of using uncommitted stem cells found in the 'cambium' layer of the periosteum to repair full thickness defects in articular cartilage. Loading and joint motion appear to be important determinants in chondrogenic stem cell differentiation toward a chondrocyte, which synthesize a 'neoarticular cartilage matrix'. The nature of the signals at the molecular level which determine these events needs to be further established.

At the macro-level of real patients some important studies have emerged in relation to long-distance running. It has always been intuitively felt that long-distance running or even simple jogging could lead to excessive joint wear, especially in the lower limb joints such as the hip, knee and ankle joints and that this could lead to the premature onset of degenerative osteoarthrosis. There have been few studies reported on the relationship between running and osteoarthritic change in the major lower limb joints. However, Puranen et al. (1975) examined the hip joints in 74 former champion runners and concluded that running did not contribute to osteoarthritic development of the hip joint. Panush et al. (1986) also came to the same conclusion when they compared clinical and radiological indices of joint degeneration in 17 male marathon runners with a mean age of 56 years, who ran an average of 44.8 km·week^{-1} for 12 years, with 18 similar non-runners who were matched for age, height and weight. Lane et al. (1986) in a similar study compared 41 long-distance runners aged 50–72 years with 41 matched community controls. Radiological analyses of hands, lateral lumbar spine and knees were performed without knowledge of running status and a computerized tomography scan of the first lumbar vertebrae quantitated bone mineral content. Both male and female runners had 40% more bone mineral than matched controls. No differences were observed in joint space narrowing, crepitation, joint stability or symptomatic arthritis between the two groups.

These studies are at variance with animal models of arthritis, where it has been postulated that repetitive impact loading leads to fatigue fractures of the subchondral bone, which then stiffens the loading response of the articular cartilage and after 12–30 months leads to histological and biochemical manifestations of cartilage degeneration (Radin 1987).

Recent work by Vingard et al. (1993) indicates that men who have long-term exposure to sports of all kinds, especially track and field and racquet sports, had a relative risk of developing osteoarthritis of the hip of 4.5 compared to those with low exposure. Men who, in addition, were exposed to high physical loads both from their occupation and sports had a relative risk of 8.5 of developing osteoarthrosis of the hip compared with those with low physical activity in both activities. A recent comprehensive review of the effects of exercise on articular cartilage as a cause of osteoarthritis has just been completed (Buckwalter et al. 1994).

FIBROCARTILAGE MENISCI OF THE KNEE JOINT

These C-shaped special load-bearing and sharing structures between each femoral and tibial condyle are prone to tearing under the large compressive, torsional and shearing loads applied to them. The location of the tear dictates the response to the injury. If the injury occurs in the periphery of the meniscus where there is ready blood supply (peripheral 25–30%), a reparative response can occur with fibrovascular scar repair occurring. If the injury occurs in the avascular inner region, the repair response is minimal and the lesion usually fails to heal. A partial meniscectomy is then necessary.

MUSCLE

Muscle contusions are common sporting injuries and are usually caused by contact with opponents or equipment. Muscle repair after injury follows the three phases already outlined. The phenomenon specific to muscle is the ability of skeletal muscle fibres to regenerate in phases II and III of the repair process (Garrett 1988; Lieber 1992; Crisco *et al.* 1994).

Experimental blunt lesions have been investigated in the rat gastrocnemius. Soon after injury there is an intense inflammatory reaction and haematoma formation. Later dense scar formation and varying degrees of muscle regeneration occur together with capillary ingrowth. If the muscle is mobilized there is a more intense inflammatory reaction which settles more rapidly, but with more scar formation than in immobilized muscle. Biomechanical testing shows faster recovery of tensile muscle strength in the mobilized muscle. Collagen synthesis is maximal between 5 and 21 days after injury. There are two

competing processes occurring during muscle healing: first, the regeneration of the disrupted muscle fibres; and second, the production of connective tissue collagen. This collagen can act as a barrier to muscle fibre regeneration, as well as acting as an adhesive 'glue' between muscle fibres, causing muscle stiffness and lack of extensibility.

Treatment by immobilization after injury limits the size of the connective tissue zone at the site of injury and penetration of regenerating muscle fibres through this connective tissue is more prominent; but the orientation of the muscle fibres is complex and not parallel with the uninjured muscle fibres. However, immobilization for more than 1 week is followed by marked muscle atrophy.

Treatment by mobilization, when combined with a sufficient period of immobilization following injury (approximately 5 days for the rat) is followed by good penetration of regenerating muscle fibres through this connective tissue is more prominent; but the orientation of the muscle fibres is complex and not parallel with the uninjured muscle fibres.

Fig. 12.14 The repair of a muscle tear at the musculotendinous junction with and without the 'RICE' (rest, ice, compress, elevate) regimen and early mobilization and stretching.

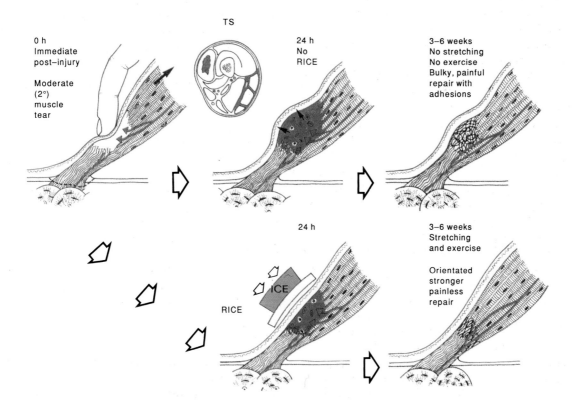

Summary of the Trends in the Experimental Animal Results

Immobilization following injury is required to allow granulation tissue to form in the injured area with sufficient tensile strength that it will not rupture during 'early' muscle fibre contraction. The length of the immobilization time is dependent on the grade of the injury; hence the more severe the injury, the more time is required for adequate granulation tissue deposition and mechanical strength. Mobilization is required for the original tensile strength of the muscle to be restored and to allow regenerating muscle fibres to penetrate and orientate through the resorbing connective tissue scar.

Intrinsic Muscle Contraction-induced Injury

Eccentric exercise in both humans and animals has demonstrated that injuries can be sustained using this system to train skeletal muscle. At the light microscopic level only about 5% of the fibres show evidence of injury, whereas at the ultrastructural level some 50% of the fibres show evidence of disruption, which is probably the basis of the 'delayed muscle soreness' that occurs after intense exercise.

Muscle Strain Injury

Although the muscle–tendon unit may undergo injury along any part of its length, it is a common clinical observation that failure often occurs at junctional sites such as the bone–tendon junction or the myotendinous junction (Taylor *et al.* 1993; Fig. 12.14).

In recent experiments with a rabbit, the muscle tendon units were stretched to breaking point. For all muscles tested the failure occurred consistently near the myotendinous junction and the rate of stretch did not appear to be important. This failure at or near the terminal sarcomeres may be due to the increased stiffness of these sarcomeres compared with those in the middle of a fibre. The reasons for this terminal sarcomere stiffness are not clear, but

may be related to the increased infolding of the cell membrane and increased basement membrane collagen in this zone.

Incomplete tears also occur at the myotendinous junction and are followed by three phases of repair. Even with severe tears/strain injury induced experimentally, immediate post-injury peak tensile loads are 63% of controls and strain to complete rupture is about 80% of controls, indicating that severely injured muscle retains enough structural strength to allow early limited functional rehabilitation. This is designed to maintain muscle tone and ranges of motion and confirms the earlier clinical work done in Australia (Corrigan 1965). However, the injured muscle is placed at a significant risk for complete rupture if the muscle is subjected to high tensile forces such as in premature early athletic competition. Recent experimental work by the same group (Obremski *et al.* 1994) indicates that the use of piroxicam (Feldene) immediately following a severe strain injury does not interfere with contractile and tensile strength recovery of injured muscle over a 1 week post-injury period. They concluded that non-steroidal anti-inflammatory drugs (NSAID) may be beneficial in the early post-injury period, but this must be weighed against the potential for NSAID to delay the inflammatory and muscle regenerative processes associated with injury.

With prolonged muscle elongation achieved by immobilization coupled with stretching, new sarcomeres are added at this junctional region or they are deleted if the muscle is immobilized in a shortened position. Intramuscular connective tissue (collagen) also changes and with muscle immobilized in a shortened position, there is an increase in the intramuscular collagen. This is responsible for the increased passive stiffness in the muscle which can be reversed by electrical stimulation of the muscle, indicating that lack of muscle activity is the important factor in determining the increased collagen in the immobilized shortened muscle. Recent work also indicates that short periods of passive stretching of immobilized muscle (30 min daily) is sufficient to prevent this increase of interstitial collagen in immobilized muscle.

Muscles that are stretched and innervated not

only have an increased number of sarcomeres but also have less intramuscular connective tissue, with the result that they are more compliant with passive elongation. This important biology of muscle has direct relevance to muscle stretching in the athlete and the prevention of muscle tears.

Therefore a warm-up period is always recommended for athletes to prevent muscle injury. Recent animal experimental work has confirmed that one maximal muscle stimulation lasting only 10–15 s causes the stimulated muscles to develop more force and to be able to stretch further before failure than non-stimulated muscles. This also has very important clinical applications.

CONCLUSIONS

As a general rule it appears that ligaments (with the exception of the ACL) and tendons heal well with adequate collagen formation. Also, early 'controlled' mobilization appears to be beneficial in minimizing joint stiffness and increasing the tensile strength of the repair collagen.

Muscle injury also responds well to careful early mobilization, depending upon the grade of the injury. Successful early contraction depends upon the time required for the granulation repair tissue (collagen and capillaries) to withstand the loading of early muscle contraction, which in turn facilitates myotube regeneration and penetration of the collagen in the repair zone. With the advent of growth factors being available in usable quantities articular cartilage repair may be a future clinical possibility.

Acute bone fractures and stress fractures require immobilization for adequate repair. Occasional undiagnosed chronic stress fractures in the navicular or scaphoid bones may require grafting.

REFERENCES

Akeson W. H., Amiel D., Abel M. F., Garfin S. R. & Woo S. L-Y. (1987) Effects of immobilization on joints. *Clinical Orthopedics Related Research* **219**, 28–37.

Alvarez O. M., Uitto J. & Perejda A. J. (eds) (1987) Pharmacological and environmental modulation of wound healing. In *Connective Tissue Disease, Molecular Pathology of the Extracellular Matrix*, Vol. 12, *The Biochemistry of Disease*, pp. 367–383. Marcel Dekker, New York.

Bennell K., Malcolm S., Thomas S., McCrory P., Ebeling P., Brukner P. & Wark J. (1994) A prospective study investigating risk factors for stress fractures in female track and field athletes. Abstract. *Proceedings of the International Conference of Science and Medicine in Sport, October*, Brisbane.

Buckwalter J. A., Lane N. E. & Gordon S. L. (1994) Exercise as a cause of arthritis. In Kuettner K. & Goldberg V. (eds) *New Horizons in Osteoarthritis*. American Academy of Orthopaedic Surgeons, Port Ridge, IL.

Burr D. B. & Martin R. B. (1992) Mechanisms of bone adaptation to the mechanical environment. *Triangle* **31**, 59–76.

Butler D. L., Grood E. S., Noyes F. R. & Zernicke R. F. (1979) Biomechanics of ligaments and tendons. In Hutton R. S. (ed.) *Exercise and Sports Sciences Reviews*, **6**, 125–181. Franklin Institute Press, PA.

Carbon R., Sambrook P. N., Deakin V., Fricker P., Eisman J. A., Kelly P., Maguire K. & Yeates M. G. (1990) Bone density of elite female athletes with stress fractures. *Medical Journal of Australia* **153**, 373–376.

Carter D. R., Caler W. E., Spengler D. M. & Frankel V. H. (1981) Fatigue behaviour of adult cortical bone: The influence of mean strain and strain range. *Acta Orthopedica Scandinavica* **52**, 481–490.

Chun K. J., Butler D. B., Bukavec M. J., Gibbons M. J. & Stouffer D. C. (1989) Spatial variation in material properties in fascicle–bone units from human patellar tendon. *ORS Transactions* **14**, 214.

Corrigan A. B. (1965) The immediate treatment of muscle injuries in sportsmen: A trial involving direct contusion injuries. *Medical Journal of Australia* **25**, 926–928.

Corrigan A. B. (1968) Sports injuries. *Hospital Medicine* **2**, 1328–1334.

Crisco J. J., Jokl J., Heinen G. T., Connell M. D. & Panjabi M. M. (1994) A muscle contusion injury model. Biomechanics, physiology and histology. *American Journal of Sports Medicine* **22**, 702–710.

Drinkwater B. L., Nilson K., Chesnut C. H., Bremmer W. J., Shainholtz M. S. & Southworth M. B. (1984) Bone mineral content of amenorrheic and eumenorrheic athletes. *New England Journal of Medicine* **311**, 277–281.

Engstrom C. M., Hampson B. A., Williams J. & Parker A. W. (1985) Muscle–tendon relations in runners. *Abstract of the Proceedings of the Australian Sports Medicine Federation*, p. 56.

Fridén J., Sjöström M. & Ekblom B. (1983) Myofibrillar damage following intense eccentric exercise in man. *International Journal of Sports Medicine* **4**, 170–176.

Garrett W. E. (1988) Injuries to the muscle–tendon unit. In Bassett F. H. III (ed.) *Instructional Course Lectures*, Vol. 37, 275–282. American Academy of Orthopedic Surgeons, Park Ridge, IL.

Hart D. P. & Danhers L. E. (1987) Healing of the medial collateral ligament in rats. *Journal of Bone and Joint Surgery* **69A**, 1194–1199.

Hunziker E. B. & Rosenberg L. (1994) Induction of repair in partial thickness articular cartilage lesions by timed release of TGF-β. *Transactions of Orthopaedic Research Society* **19**, 236.

Komi P. V. (1987) Neuromuscular factors related to physical performance. In Russo P. & Balnave R. (eds) *Muscle and Nerve, Factors affecting Performance* (Proceedings of the 6th Biennial Conference), pp. 114–132. Sports Sciences & Research Centre, Cumberland College of Health Sciences.

Lane N. E., Bloch D. A., Jones H. H., Marshall W. H., Wood P. D. & Fries J. F. (1986) Long-distance running, bone density, and osteoarthritis. *Journal of the American Medical Association* **255**, 1147–1151.

Lieber R. L. (1992) *Skeletal Muscle Structure and Function. Implications for Rehabilitation and Sports Medicine*, Chapter 6. Williams and Wilkins, Baltimore, MD.

Mankin H. J. (1982) Current concepts review: The response of articular cartilage to mechanical injury. *Journal of Bone and Joint Surgery* **64A**, 460–465.

Marguia M. J., Vailas A., Mandelbaum B., Norton J., Hodgdon J., Goforth H. & Riedy M. (1988) Elevated plasma hydroxyproline: A possible risk factor associated with connective tissue injuries during overuse. *American Journal of Sports Medicine* **16**, 660–664.

Martin R. B. & Burr D. B. (eds) (1989) Mechanical adaptation. In Martin R. B. & Burr D. B. (eds) *Structure, Function and Adaptation of Compact Bone*, pp. 143–185. Raven Press, New York.

Ng G. Y., Oakes B. W., Deacon O. W., McLean I. D. & Lampard D. (1995) A three year study of the biomechanics of patellar tendon autograft for anterior cruciate ligament reconstrruction in the goat. *Journal of Orthopedic Research* (in press).

Oakes B. W. (1981) Acute soft tissue injuries — Nature and management. *Australian Family Physician* **10** (Suppl.), 1–16.

Oakes B. W. (1984) Hamstring injuries. *Australian Family Physician* **13**, 587–591.

Oakes B. W. (1988) Ultrastructural studies on knee joint ligaments: Quantitation of collagen fibre populations in exercised and control rat cruciate ligaments and in human anterior cruciate ligament grafts. In Woo S. L-Y. & Buckwalter J. (eds) *Injury and Repair of the Musculoskeletal Tissues*, Section 2, pp. 66–82. American Academy of Orthopedic Surgeons, Park Ridge, IL.

Oakes B. W. (1993) Collagen ultrastructure in the normal ACL and in ACL graft. In Jackson D. *et al.* (eds) *The Anterior Cruciate Ligament: Current and Future Concepts*, pp. 209–217. Raven Press, New York.

Oakes B. W. (1994) Tendon–ligament basic science. In Harries M., Micheli L. J., Stanish W. D. & Williams C. (eds) *The Oxford Textbook of Sports Medicine*, pp. 493–511. Oxford University Press, Oxford.

Obremski W. T., Seaber A. V., Ribbeck B. M. & Garrett W. E. (1994) Biomechanical and histologic assessment of a controlled muscle strain injury treated with Piroxicam. *American Journal of Sports Medicine* **22**, 558–561.

Panush R. S., Schmidt C., Caldwell J. R. *et al.* (1986) Is running associated with degenerative joint disease? *Journal of the American Medical Association* **255**, 1152–1154.

Parry D. A. D., Barnes G. R. G. & Craig A. S. (1978) A comparison of the size distribution of collagen fibrils in connective tissues as a function of age and a possible relation between fibril size and distribution and mechanical properties. *Proceedings of the Royal Society London B*, **203**, 305–321.

Puranen J., Ala Ketola L., Peltokallio P. & Saarela J. (1975) Running and primary arthritis of the hip. *British Medical Journal* **2**, 424–425.

Radin E. L. (1987) Osteoarthrosis. What is known about prevention? *Clinical Orthopedics Related Research* **222**, 60–65.

Riggs B. L. & Melton L. J. (1986) Involutional osteoporosis. *New England Journal of Medicine* **314**, 1676–1686.

Rubin C. T., Pratt G. W., Porter A. L., Lanyon L. E. & Poss R. (1987) The use of ultrasound *in vivo* to determine acute change in the mechanical properties of bone following intense physical activity. *Journal of Biomechanics* **20**, 723–727.

Salter R. B. (1989) The biologic concept of continuous passive motion of synovial joints: The first 18 years of basic research and its clinical application. *Clinical Orthopedics Related Research* **242**, 12–25.

Schepsis A. A., Wagner C. & Leach R. E. (1994) Surgical management of Achilles tendon overuse injuries. *American Journal of Sports Medicine* **22**, 611–619.

Shadwick R. E. (1986) The role of collagen crosslinks in the age related changes in mechanical properties of digital tendons. *Proceedings of the North American Congress of Biomechanics* **1**, 137–138.

Shino K., Oakes B. W., Inoue M., Horibe S., Nakata K., Maeda M. & Ono K. (1995) Human ACL allografts —an electronmicroscopic analysis of collagen fibril populations. *American Journal of Sports Medicine* (in press).

Stanish W., Rubinovich R. M. & Curwin S. (1986) Eccentric exercise in chronic tendinitis. *Clinical Orthopedics Related Research* **208**, 65–68.

Taylor D. C., Dalton J. D., Seaber A. V. & Garrett W. E. (1993) Experimental strain injury. Early functional and structural deficits and the increased risk of injury. *American Journal of Sports Medicine* **21**, 190–194.

Vailas A. C., Tipton C. M., Matthes R. D. & Gart M. (1981) Physical activity and its influence on the repair process of medial collateral ligaments. *Connective Tissue Research* **9**, 25–31.

Viidik A. (1973) Functional properties of connective tissues. *International Review of Connective Tissue Research* 6, 127–215.

Viidik A. (1980) Interdependence between structure and function in collagenous tissues. In Viidik A. & Vuust J. (eds) *Biology of Collagen*, pp. 257–280. Academic Press, New York.

Vingard E., Alfresson L., Goldie I. & Hogstedt C. (1993) Sports and osteoarthrosis of the hip. An epidemiologic study. *American Journal of Sports Medicine* 21, 195–205.

Weisman G., Pope M. H., Johnson R. J. (1980) Cyclical loading in knee ligament injuries. *American Journal of Sports Medicine* 8, 24–30.

Williams J. G. P. (1986) Achilles tendon lesions in sport. *Sports Medicine* 3, 114–135.

Williams J. G. P. & Sperryn P. N. (1976) (eds) *Sports Medicine*, 2nd edn, p. 244. Arnold, London.

Woo S. L-Y. & Buckwalter J. A. (eds) (1988) *Injury and Repair of the Musculoskeletal Soft Tissues*, pp. 465–482. American Academy of Orthopedic Surgeons, Park Ridge, IL.

Woo S. L-Y., Inoue M., McGurk-Burleson M. & Gomez M. A. (1987) Treatment of the medial collateral ligament injury. II: Structure and function of canine knees in response to differing treatment regimens. *American Journal of Sports Medicine* 15, 22–29.

CHAPTER 13

PRINCIPLES OF TREATMENT AND REHABILITATION

C. R. Purdam, P. A. Fricker and B. Cooper

With an understanding of the processes of inflammation and healing as outlined in Chapter 12, this chapter considers the effects of injury on an athlete and the processes necessary to enable him or her to resume training and competition as quickly and as safely as possible. The evaluation of injuries to different tissues of the body is discussed in addition to the various methods of treatment, including the electrotherapy modalities, manual therapy techniques, pharmaceuticals and acupuncture. The chapter also reviews the objectives of treatment and rehabilitation and provides a framework for assessment of an athlete prior to resumption of competition.

THE GRADING OF INJURY

To assist in the assessment and management of an injury, it is valuable to have a frame of reference which indicates the degree of injury and associated disability. The terms 'partial' and 'complete', and 'mild' and 'severe' add little to understanding the inherent changes in those tissues that are injured.

Blazina (1973) has devised a grading of injury, which is applicable to overuse soft tissue injuries in particular, and runs from 0 to 4, with Grade 4 being the most severe. The Sports Medicine Unit at the Australian Institute of Sport has modified this to a grading scale from 1 to 3. Such a scale may be used in both acute and chronic injuries, and enables the coach, the athlete, and the therapist to relate the

nature of injury to associated disability and impairment of performance.

Table 13.1 outlines a system of grading for acute soft tissue injury and refers to Chapter 12 for the histopathological findings associated with each grade of injury. Table 13.2 provides a summary of grades of overuse injury.

Treatment and recovery from any injury should progress through the grades (from 3 to 1) with improved functional ability evident at each grade.

The grading system as outlined is only a guide as there are specific changes which may be associated with particular structures: for example, calcification is more likely in some tendons (the Achilles and supraspinatus, for example) and the medial ligament of the knee (Pellegrini-Stieda's disease), while other tendons and ligaments rarely calcify despite chronic inflammation. Nevertheless, the grading system describes the ability to perform and can be used to assess recovery from the injury, whatever the diagnosis.

With respect to bone and joint problems, these tend to present differently and be more an 'all or nothing' phenomenon. Stress fractures may present with severe disability (Grade 3) after a short period of pain — for example, femoral neck and tarsal navicular fracture — and during recovery may 'regress' through the grades. Similarly, joint injuries such as osteochondritis dissecans can present quite suddenly after a vague prodrome of diffuse joint discomfort.

Table 13.1 Grading of traumatic soft tissue injuries

Grade	Symptoms	Signs	Histopathology
1	Mild to moderate pain	Minimal to mild swelling, tenderness Can weight bear or tolerate loading stress	Up to 50% fibre disruption with local inflammatory changes Some local haemorrhage
2	Moderate pain	Moderate swelling, tenderness, perhaps bruising Pain on weight bearing or stress testing Evidence of ligament laxity but 'end point' noted	50–80% fibre disruption Inflammatory changes, plus haemorrhage
3	Moderate to severe pain	Severe or marked swelling and tenderness with bruising Unable to weight bear and function severely affected No 'end point' to stress testing; joint laxity	Complete disruption of structure Pronounced bleeding and inflammatory changes

Table 13.2 Grading of overuse soft tissue injuries

Grade	Symptoms	Signs	Histopathology
1	Ache after activity	May be mild local tenderness	Local inflammatory or adaptive changes
2	Ache or pain at onset of activity but disappears with warm-up. Reappears after activity	Local tenderness Some limitation of range or movement, weakness and painful to test	Inflammation of injured tissue with involvement of contiguous structures. (e.g. bursitis) May be adhesions
3	Constant ache or pain exaggerated by any activity. Eventually necessitates cessation of activity	Local tenderness, loss of movement, weakness and perhaps muscle wasting	Extensive inflammatory changes scar formation, adhesions May be calcification or degenerative change

FIRST AID IN SPORT

It is now well established that 'first aid' for injury in sport is summarized by the acronym RICE*, which stands for rest, ice, compression and elevation, and forms the basic protocol for treatment of acute injuries over the first 72 h. In many cases it is also useful for the treatment of chronic injuries or acute presentations of chronic injuries. Table 13.3 outlines the RICE* treatment programme.

It is recommended that such first aid should be adhered to for 2–3 days after injury and supported, if appropriate, by the use of non-steroidal anti-inflammatory medication. The various physiotherapy modalities, exercise programmes and manual therapy are generally instituted on day 3, after the initial phase of inflammation has subsided.

THE OBJECTIVES OF TREATMENT AND REHABILITATION

Table 13.4 provides a schema for treatment and rehabilitation of injury. The initial aims of treatment are to assist healing, to regain length and strength of damaged tissues (undergoing fibrosis) and to regain function, in that order.

The final functional result of treatment must include cardiovascular fitness, endurance, speed and psychomotor skills. All these components of performance necessitate attention to the specific timing

Table 13.3 The RICE* programme for immediate treatment of acute (soft tissue) injury

Rest:	Rest the injured tissue.
	Modify activity to maintain fitness, strength and skill as much as possible.
Ice:	Apply ice to the area of injury for 10–15 min every 45–60 min. This minimizes oedema, bleeding, pain and associated muscle spasm, and decreases the metabolic rate of the underlying tissue.
Compress:	Compression bandages (not tourniquets) are used to minimize the bleeding and oedema and must be comfortably tight. A crepe or elastic bandage is recommended.
Elevate:	Elevation of the injured tissue minimizes the effect of gravity on accumulating blood and oedema at the site of the injury.

Note: This programme is administered for the first 72 h after injury and is supported by appropriate diagnosis and management by qualified medical practitioners.
*Recent usage has added P and D to RICE where P stands for 'protection' (from further injury) and D stands for 'diagnosis' (which must be obtained from appropriately qualified practitioner(s)): thus PRICED.

Table 13.4 A schema for treatment and rehabilitation of injury

Process	Phase	Management
Injury	Acute phase	RICE programme
Inflammation	Phases of fibroplasia,	Anti-inflammatory medication
Adhesions	vascularization	Physiotherapy modalities
		Stretching
		Massage (unless risk of myositis ossificans exists)
Scarring	Phase of cicatrization	Modified activity
Contracture		Hydrotherapy
		Massage
		Stretching
Muscle wasting		Strength training (concentric, eccentric)
Weakness		Activity
Loss of proprioception		Balance-board ('wobble-board') exercises
		Mini-trampoline, skipping
		Light activity
Loss of skill		Skill training, e.g. running/swerving (cutting),
Inability to perform		throwing/catching, skipping/hopping
		More intense activity

of rehabilitative exercises such as hydrotherapy, and drills such as running, swerving (cutting), hopping, jumping and skipping, together with counselling which relates to the re-development of self-confidence, achievement of performance goals and overcoming the fear of re-injury.

As a rule of thumb, time required for initial healing and recovery of different tissue types is as follows:

- Muscles — 6 weeks
- Tendons and ligaments — 12 weeks
- Bone and joints — 6–12 weeks (Woo & Buckwalter 1987)

It must be emphasized that certain structures such as substitution repairs of the anterior cruciate ligament (ACL) take up to 12 months to regain functional strength after injury. Similarly, longer periods may be necessary if any aspect of first aid, treatment and rehabilitation of injury has been neglected.

THE PHYSICAL MODALITIES

A range of physical modalities is available for the management of sports injuries. These can be divided into electrotherapeutic modalities, manual techniques and exercise therapy.

Electrotherapy

INTERMITTENT PRESSURE THERAPY

Many athletic injuries, particularly those occurring distally in a limb, produce significant soft tissue (extra-articular) oedema. Intermittent compression devices are valuable in the acute and subacute phases of injury, to assist in the removal of this exudate, reducing the likelihood of organization of this oedema with resultant secondary fibrosis. These pumps are less effective in dealing with intra-articular fluid, especially since an irritated or damaged synovium continues to produce exudate.

Intermittent pressure therapy may be used on a daily basis in conjunction with ice application and stimulation currents with pad electrodes or with magnetic field therapy.

ULTRASOUND

Ultrasound units supply a mechanical wave, which is transmitted from the sound head to the tissues through a coupling medium such as aqueous gel. Most machines operate at about 1 MHz, although some machines can provide varying frequencies from 0.75 to 3.0 MHz. The higher frequency has a greater absorption in superficial tissues. The lower frequency is more suited to deeper structures such as muscle (Gieck & Saliba 1990). The higher frequencies do not penetrate as deeply as the lower frequencies.

Ultrasound is also selectively absorbed at the periosteum and it should be noted that higher doses may irritate this tissue. For this reason, ultrasound has been used as a diagnostic device for detecting stress fractures (Lowdon 1986).

Ultrasound is used in both continuous and pulsed or intermittent modes, the latter allowing utilization of the mechanical but not the heating effect of ultrasound.

The non-thermal effects of ultrasound are primarily those of an increase in the diffusion of fluids or ions across membranes, notably calcium. The response to changes in intracellular calcium ions can be synthesis (of collagen), secretion (of chemotactic agents and wound factors) or motility changes of pericytes, fibroblasts and endothelial cells) (Dyson 1987).

The thermal effects of continuous ultrasound produce a temporary increase in the extensibility of tissues with a high collagen content such as tendons, joint capsules and ligaments. Continuous ultrasound has been shown to increase the rate of healing of punctured rat tendon compared with untreated controls in terms of tensile strength and collagen deposition (Jackson *et al.* 1991).

Ultrasound may be used together with various water or gel-based pharmaceutical preparations, a technique known as phonophoresis. The ultrasound drives the active substance into affected tissues to provide a deep, yet well localized, deposition of this substance. Such drugs include 1 or 10% hydrocortisone cream and heparin/hyaluronidase preparations, which are available for treatment of soft tissue contusions.

Depending on the lesion ultrasound may be given on a twice daily basis for 5–8 min at a time. Low dose ($0.5 \ W \cdot cm^{-1}$) may be used initially and then increased after the acute phase of injury. Ultrasound should not be administered over an area of active bleeding nor over infected areas, prosthetic devices, screws and plates. Caution should be exercised when treating near the heart, endocrine and special sense organs and open epiphyses.

SHORT WAVE DIATHERMY

Short wave diathermy units generate radio-frequency waves (27.12 MHz) of sufficient intensity to induce a deep heating effect in the tissues. This is greatest in skin and fat when applied through an electrostatic condenser field (with pads or plates) or in blood and muscle if an electromagnetic inductor field (or coil) is used. The induction coil also provides a greater magnetic field response.

Currently, short wave diathermy is most frequently employed in the pulsed mode permitting much higher intensities. These give a greater penetration, without the effects of raising tissue temperature to a dangerous level (Wilson 1972). Indeed many pulsed short wave units are used in a primarily athermic mode, where no warmth is perceived by the patient at all.

The literature to date suggests pulsed short wave diathermy increases the rate of healing in acute soft tissue lesions, particularly so in the skin and nervous system. Chronic injuries fare less well (Goats 1989).

Pulsed short wave diathermy is reportedly useful in the treatment of ankle sprains, hand injuries, arthritis and in the resolution of haematomas (in rats; Goats 1989).

PULSED MAGNETIC THERAPY

Pulsed magnetic field units consist of a low-frequency generator driving a coil applicator. The applicator is placed in either a coplanar fashion over the lesion or, alternatively as a drum encircling the region. Drums may be relatively large to accommodate the trunk or smaller to encircle the limbs.

Magnetic field units commonly generate frequencies of between 2 and 100 Hz at nominal strengths of between 50 and 100 G ($5-10 \times 10^{-3}$ T). In the authors' experience pulsed magnetic therapy at lower frequencies appears to have a positive effect on periosteal and tenoperiosteal lesions and may provide symptomatic improvement for tendon and bony lesions through the frequency.

In general, lower doses are utilized initially for acute lesions. There is much to be learned regarding doses and frequencies; however, it appears that many lesions receive benefit from relatively long treatment times, that is between 1 and 12 h. Current practice with this form of therapy prescribes up to 12 h daily for the management of stress fractures of the tibia, fibula and tarsal navicular in particular and in the management of delayed union in fractures of the scaphoid.

LASER THERAPY

The use of lasers in medicine has expanded during the last 10 years. While high-powered lasers are restricted to surgical use, the lower powered 'soft' lasers have been shown to be effective in stimulating wound healing (Kokino et al. 1985) and also in pain reduction (England et al. 1985).

The 'soft' laser makes use of either helium–neon or gallium arsenide diodes, which have different characteristics as a result of their emission wavelengths. The helium–neon units have a wavelength of 632.8 nm, which is primarily absorbed in the skin to a depth of 3 mm. These units are most effective for skin lesions or the stimulation of auricular acupuncture points.

The gallium arsenide units commonly emit coherent light at a wavelength of 904 nm (infra-red) and have a penetration of up to 4 cm, which allows effective treatment of both superficial and deep lesions and acupuncture points. Some units offer a mix of both diodes.

Laser units have been shown to be effective in reducing pain and inflammation in acute and chronic injuries as well as stimulating wound healing in superficial and deep lesions. Treatment techniques vary, but are generally divided into acupuncture or trigger point stimulation, or that of laser therapy, where a hand-held or operated beam scans the lesion. Treatment times and intensities vary according to the technique used and the area of the lesion (Molenaar 1988).

Laser therapy is contra-indicated in the presence of acute infections, pregnancy, pelvic and abdominal lesions, malignancy, retinal damage and with concurrent use of photosensitive medication. It should be used with caution near pacemakers, on patients with poor calcium assimilation (due to laser effect on the sodium–calcium pump), on pain of unknown cause and on patients with coronary or peripheral vascular conditions (Jackson et al. 1990).

ELECTRICAL STIMULATORS

Transcutaneous electrical nerve stimulators (TENS) offer a very portable form of electrotherapy with battery powered units typically no larger than two matchboxes, and generally produce square and/or spiked waveforms at low frequencies (0–200 Hz). Pulse width may be varied between 50 and 250 ms with narrower pulse widths offering deeper penetration. The longer pulse widths, in conjunction with high currents, are used where muscle contraction is desired.

TENS machines are valuable for control of pain and/or muscle spasm and are typically used with long application times. They are reported to be useful in the treatment of reflex sympathetic dystrophy (Ladd et al. 1989), spinal lesions, postoperative pain in the early phase, and peripheral periarticular, articular and musculotendinous unit injuries.

Normal function is encouraged by reducing the pain of the lesion. However, it is imperative that an accurate diagnosis is reached prior to treatment, because TENS may mask pain and permit activity which then results in the development of a more serious lesion, such as a stress fracture.

INTERFERENTIAL STIMULATION

Interferential therapy induces a low-frequency current in tissues by intersecting two medium frequency currents to produce a lower beat frequency at the site of interference. The medium frequency currents are commonly of the order of 4000 Hz, with a difference in currents of between 1 and 200 Hz. Most machines are 'two-dimensional' using pad electrodes in combination with suction. Also available is a 'three-dimensional' unit (Siemens 'Electrodynator') which, it is claimed, allows the current to be biased to either electrode, facilitating more localized treatment of superficial or deep injuries.

Interferential stimulation units are useful in managing pain, muscle spasm, oedema or circulatory disorders. Common therapeutic applications include joint dysfunction, subacute or chronic muscle injuries, compartment syndromes and thoracic or lumbar spinal injuries. Interferential stimulation has also been reported to be of benefit in cases of delayed bony union (Ganne 1988).

Interferential therapy should not be used in infected areas, on patients with deep venous thrombosis, tumours, pacemakers, over the area of a pregnant uterus or where there is risk of exacerbating haemorrhage.

HIGH-VOLTAGE GALVANIC ('d.c.') STIMULATORS

These stimulators generate a biphasic pulse of very high amplitude (up to 500 V), but by virtue of a very short pulse width have a relatively low average current density. This means that charge buildup under the electrodes is minimized, reducing the problem of electrical burns, even with very small electrodes. The stimulators use a large indifferent electrode in combination with one or two active electrodes, which range in surface area from 20–30 cm^2 down to probes of 2 cm^2 or less. Treatment frequencies may vary from 1 to 100 Hz and electrode polarity is reversible. Treatment applications commonly include reduction of pain, muscle spasm and

oedema, although the mechanism for this remains unclear (Mohr et al. 1987; Reed 1988). High-voltage stimulators may also be used for muscle stimulation. The probe electrodes are a very effective, non-invasive method of desensitizing chronic irritable scar tissue and may also be used over acupuncture or trigger points. It is important to use caution with this technique.

ELECTRICAL MUSCLE STIMULATORS

These stimulators are used either to assist in the rehabilitative processes of improving strength in atrophied muscle or to assist strength gains in the normal athlete. The latter has yet to be fully substantiated; however, strength gains are believed to occur by enhancing the output of the motor neurons, leading to adaptive changes in the contractile elements of the muscle. Increases in muscle girth and strength and decreases in subcutaneous fat are claimed following long-term protocols on athletic subjects (Kots 1977).

Electrical muscle stimulators are commonly square or sinusoidal wave generators of variable pulse width and frequency (50–2500 Hz). Electrodes may be arranged in bipolar fashion along the muscle, or more usually in a unipolar fashion, with one electrode over the origin of the spinal nerve root and the other over the motor nerve. Kots' protocol recommends a 10–15 s stimulation followed by 50 s of rest for 10 repetitions, 5 days a week (Kots 1977).

It is recommended that contractions are maximal to gain most benefit, ideally being greater than maximal volitional contraction. To facilitate this, it is helpful to position the patient so that the muscle group being stimulated works against a resistance and is close to its optimal length.

Manual Techniques

These include therapeutic massage, joint mobilizing and manipulative techniques, and therapeutic stretching of musculotendinous units and other soft tissues.

THERAPEUTIC MASSAGE

Massage probably originated from a primary instinct

to rub any sore part of the body and can be defined as 'the controlled and specific manipulation of the soft tissues of the body for a therapeutic purpose'. Massage treatment can vary depending on the desired result of treatment and the physical and mental state of the patient.

Massage techniques

At the commencement of a massage, oil is applied to the hands and then, by stroking and light effleurage movements, it is applied over the area to be massaged. The following techniques are used:

- *Effleurage*. This consists of rhythmic, flowing, stroking actions over the area being massaged. The purposes of effleurage are to spread the oil, warm and prepare the area being massaged, soothe the patient, encourage local blood and lymph flow, and allow the masseur to detect any areas of tightness that require further work
- *Frictions*. These are short 'back and forth' massage strokes, used over areas of tight muscle or tendon soreness, either with or across the grain of the muscle or tendon. They are performed using thumb or fingertips with substantial pressure and are used to break up muscular 'tight spots' and adhesions and to produce a 'counter irritation' effect. Frictions can be very effective in the treatment of lateral epicondylitis and chronic hamstring origin tendinitis. Frictions, however, must not be used on acute muscle tears or contusions because of the risk of further haemorrhage or the development of myositis ossificans
- *Pressure point techniques*. These have their origins in oriental massage, but are now a major part of mainstream sports massage. The basis of these techniques is to locate and to gradually apply thumb or finger pressure to an area of muscle spasm, to hold the pressure for a few seconds until the tightness is felt to release, then to relax the pressure (Fig. 13.1). Small frictions may be used while the pressure is being applied. A line or lines of such points may be used on a tight muscle. Empirical evidence suggests that this form of massage for muscle tightness produces far less residual soreness

than the deep friction method, perhaps due to a lesser disturbance of muscle tissue.

Techniques such as 'Shifting' and 'Dynamic massage' incorporate the passive movement of the affected muscle while point pressure is being applied. Pressure techniques may also be used on trigger points as described by Travell and Simons (1983) and on suitable traditional acupuncture or shiatsu points.

- *Kneading*. This is the rhythmic lifting and squeezing of muscle tissue, alternating left and right hands in opposing directions. The technique is used over the whole of the muscular area being treated, to loosen muscle and to encourage local blood and lymph flow
- *Petrissage*. This is aimed primarily at increasing peripheral circulation and general soft tissue

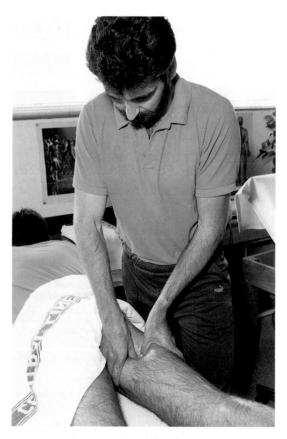

Fig. 13.1 Localized pressure techniques may be used to assist the release of muscle spasm.

stimulation. Petrissage involves kneading, grasping and compressing, and rolling and squeezing muscle tissue. This technique breaks up adhesions between skin and deeper layers and is used to loosen fibrous or scarred tissue

- *Tapotement.* This includes light striking or percussive movements, performed with cupped hands, pummelling with the side of fisted hands or chopping with the ulnar borders of the hands. The chief aim of tapotement is stimulation of the area
- *Vibrations.* These are performed by the masseur, tensing the hand and arm and pressing on the area to be treated with light pressure, inducing vibration with the fingertips

Other techniques

The masseur may also employ passive stretching during treatment or use additional equipment, such as an electric vibratory massager, Chinese spoons, Chinese vacuum cups, or other devices to enhance treatment.

Types of massage

In the field of sports medicine, massage can be divided into four main categories: relaxation, maintenance and recovery, pre-event and specific treatment. Table 13.5 outlines these various types.

Table 13.5   Massage for athletes

Relaxation	Light massage Deep massage 60–90 min Effleurage, kneading, stroking
Maintenance and recovery	Directed at tissues used in training and competition or employed after hard training sessions or post-competition Effleurage, deep effleurage, kneading, petrissage, tapotement
Pre-event	Used as 'warm-up' Brisk effleurage, kneading, friction, petrissage, tapotement, stroking and rolling
Specific treatment	Variable but typically involves friction, deep effleurage and pressure point techniques

Table 13.6   Contra-indications to massage for athletes

Bleeding, contusions
Coagulation disorders (e.g. haemophilia)
Skin infections
Myositis ossificans
Burns
Skin rashes
Insect bites, snake bites, etc.
Fracture
Varicose veins
Local tumours
Skin fragility (e.g. aged, corticosteroid induced)

Contra-indications to massage

In some situations massage should not be used and Table 13.6 lists the contra-indications to massage.

JOINT MOBILIZATION AND MANIPULATION

In the ongoing management of sports patients a frequent complaint is back and neck pain. Many of these presentations do not involve major pathology but are associated with the loss of the normal range of joint motion. Peripheral joint conditions which are accompanied by reduced joint movement are also common. Thus, passive movement procedures to restore the range of joint movement have an important role in sports physiotherapy. Mobilization is the use of graded oscillatory techniques, whereas manipulation requires the use of high-velocity localized thrust procedures. Both techniques are used in a wide variety of sports injuries involving vertebral and peripheral joints.

Vertebral joints

Zygoapophyseal and disc injuries occur in many sports, with the former being more common. These injuries are caused in several ways, namely by hyperextension, hyperextension and rotation, or forced movements of lateral flexion which may damage the zygoapophyseal joints and associated soft tissue structures. Movements of flexion combined with rotation are more likely to damage the disc. Direct trauma which occurs in body contact sports may result in injury to the soft tissue supporting the vertebral column and result in more serious disruption to the zygoapophyseal and costovertebral joints. Occasionally, severe trauma may result in fractures particularly of transverse and spinous processes.

Early differential diagnosis between zygoapophyseal joint and intervertebral disc injuries is often very difficult. Damage to either structure may present with very similar signs and symptoms in the early stage, for example, acute local pain and marked restriction of movement. In these acute situations a careful history must be obtained to identify the movement which caused the injury in the first phase. This is followed by an accurate vertebral column examination. There is a tendency for apophyseal joint dysfunction to present with restricted extension and lateral flexion towards the side of the pain or a combination of these movements. Occasionally, flexion is involved in the acute stage; however, this is more common with disc injury and movements appear more irregular with disc disruption.

Dural tension tests may appear to be positive in zygoapophyseal injuries in the early stages and can cause a degree of confusion.

Apophyseal and disc injuries may require the use of mobilization and manipulation procedures, the former syndrome usually responding quickly, while the latter is more difficult. If the disc is prolapsed, then passive movement procedures usually have minimal beneficial results and may aggravate the injury.

The use of X-rays in the early stage of acute traumatic injury is important to evaluate damage. Common bony injuries in the vertebral column include a fractured transverse process in the lumbar spine, fractured ribs in the thoracic spine and fractured spinous processes, as in the cervical spine. More serious vertebral body or laminar fractures are less common. Careful examination of movement and resulting signs and symptoms may alert the examining physician to such conditions.

The diagnosis of early pars interarticular defects or stress fractures is often difficult. Repeated hyperextension of the lumbar spine, especially if associated with rotation, is the major factor in its onset. The history and physical examination require careful interpretation, and X-ray examination often coupled with reversed gantry computerized axial tomography views are required to confirm the diagnosis.

The use of the computerized tomography (CT) scan is also often necessary to highlight disc involvement in pain or vertebral column origin. Care must be taken, however, in the interpretation of the CT scan results and careful correlation with clinical signs is essential (see Chapter 17 for further details).

Peripheral joints

Ligamentous and capsular contraction, which may be late manifestations of trauma, often require mobilization and manipulation to restore full range. Restriction of movement following injury is most common in the ankle region, particularly the subtalar joint (Fig. 13.2). However, inferior tibiofibular, talocrural, intertarsal and metatarsophalangeal joints often remain restricted in movement following ligamentous injury. The relatively uncommon 'dropped cuboid' syndrome only responds adequately to localized thrust and manipulative procedures.

The restoration of full peripheral joint range is essential following soft tissue injury and trauma and it is in this area that the use of mobilization techniques are especially important.

On occasions, mechanical dysfunction in the vertebral column and sacro-iliac joints can refer symptoms into the thorax and the upper and lower limbs, mimicking peripheral soft tissue injuries.

Unresponsive 'rotator cuff' symptoms and 'tennis elbow' may have their origins in the joints of the lower cervical spine. Similarly, groin or hip pain and chronic or recurrent 'hamstring' tears may reflect pain referred from lumbar or sacro-iliac joints.

Careful vertebral column and peripheral joint examination is required in these cases and the use of mobilization or manipulation of the appropriate vertebral joints may produce very dramatic improvement in what appears to be unresponsive soft tissue injuries.

ASSESSMENT

In the treatment of both vertebral and peripheral joint conditions by mobilization and manipulation, careful and accurate assessment is essential if acceptable results are to be achieved (see Table 13.7). This assessment is carried out primarily in relation to range of movement, pain response and 'end feel'

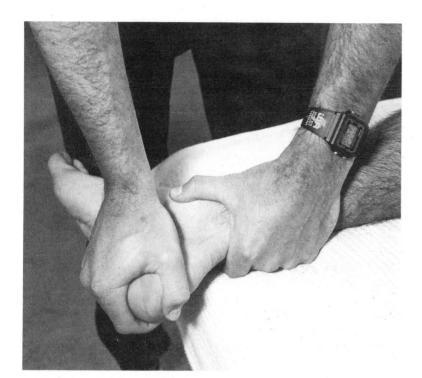

Fig. 13.2 Subtalar joint mobilization is often indicated following ankle joint injury.

of the joint, the latter usually in relation to muscle spasm. Changes in one or all three have to be carefully interpreted in order to assess the efficacy of the treatment.

The assessment of the unstable joint, more easily diagnosed in the case of peripheral than vertebral column joints, requires different management. Often the use of mobilization or manipulative procedures are used to excess on unresponsive joint symptoms, resulting in aggravation of symptoms or occasionally causing a joint to become symptomatically hyper-mobile.

The latter is more commonly seen with excessive manipulative treatment being given to vertebral column joint dysfunctions resulting in constant recurrence, despite apparent initial improvement in signs and symptoms. Stabilizing and strengthening exercises are therefore essential in hypermobility problems of the vertebral column or peripheral joints mentioned previously.

For detailed discussion of this wide area, the reader is referred to the work of Cyriax (1975), Kaltenborn (1976), Grieve (1981), McKenzie (1981), Maitland (1986, 1990) and Bourdillon (1987).

THERAPEUTIC STRETCHING

Stretching of the musculotendinous unit or other soft tissues is frequently used as a therapeutic technique. Stretching reduces increased tone or

Table 13.7 Contra-indications to mobilization and manipulation

Absolute
Malignancy
Spinal cord involvement, e.g. cauda equina, neurological disorders
More than one spinal nerve involved
Fracture
Acute inflammatory arthritis, e.g. rheumatoid arthritis
Septic arthritis, ankylosing spondylitis, gout
Vascular anomalies, e.g. vertebral artery involvement
Anticoagulant medication
Worsening neurological signs
Hypermobility (generalized and specific)
Osteoporosis
Relative
Neurological signs
Spondylolisthesis
Pregnancy
Gross protective muscle spasm

tightness in an affected muscle and may be used in the treatment of painful trigger areas (Travell & Simons 1983). One of the most commonly used stretching techniques is that of proprioceptive neuromuscular facilitation (PNF) stretching (Knott & Voss 1968). PNF may be used both in treatment and as part of an athlete's warm-up (see Chapter 1) and utilizes the phenomenon whereby maximal muscle relaxation follows maximal contraction. The therapist isometrically resists a maximal contraction of muscle at its mid-range or outer range for a period of 6–10 s and then follows this with a passive stretch of the muscle to the point of discomfort for 15–20 s. This is then repeated several times and is most effective where muscle spasm provides the limitation to the muscle length. In terms of short-term gains in flexibility, the most effective method is reported to be the CRAC method (contract–relax followed by antagonist contraction, Moore & Hutton 1980). For example, with the hamstring group, the athlete performs a maximal contraction followed by relaxation and active contraction of the hip flexors/quadriceps. This method produces the largest gains in hip flexion compared with static and contract–relax methods, despite the latter being associated with the highest electromyographic (EMG) activity. The effects of these forms of stretching may be enhanced by the use of the deeper forms of massage mentioned previously. It is unrealistic to expect short periods of stretching to affect the overall resting length of normal (uninjured) musculotendinous units, but such stretching may lengthen those units affected by pain or spasm. Athletes wishing to increase the overall length of a muscle group need to embark on a long-term programme of sustained stretching on a regular basis. The best examples of this are the stretching programmes used by gymnasts, where one muscle group, for example the hamstrings, may be stretched for 30 min or more at a session.

Janda (1983) has investigated the response of different muscle groups to dysfunction in the musculoskeletal unit. He states that phasic muscles, that is, those composed predominantly of fast twitch Type II fibres used in more explosive activities, atrophy and weaken, whereas the postural muscle groups, those comprising relatively more slow-twitch Type I fibres, tend to be tight. This leads to predictable patterns of tightness and weakness in the muscles around an affected joint. Recognition of these patterns allows the therapist to be more specific in tailoring the stretching and strengthening components of a rehabilitation programme.

Exercise Therapy

CRYOKINETICS

Cryokinetics combines the use of ice and exercise in the management of acute, subacute or chronic joint and musculotendinous unit injuries, or where the rehabilitation process is inhibited by the presence of muscle spasm. Ice is used for its anaesthetic effect (by slowing nerve conduction) and for its ability to decrease metabolic demands of injured tissue.

The technique involves prolonged cooling of the affected area(s) by icing, using either an ice bath or ice packs. This is then followed by brief alternating periods of 2–3 min of stretching or range of movement exercises and further icing under close supervision. The athlete is thus able to accelerate the exercise component of rehabilitation with a reduced risk of exacerbation.

Exercise is a powerful method of decreasing inflammatory stasis and removing inflammatory exudate via lymphatic drainage and increased circulatory flow; therefore the use of cold and exercise may provide outstanding results in the management of acute soft tissue injuries (Knight 1985).

Contra-indications to cryokinetic therapy include Raynaud's disease, insufficient vascular supply to the area being treated and regions where superficial nerves such as the common peroneal may be injured by excessive cooling

CONTINUOUS PASSIVE MOTION

Continuous passive motion (CPM) has been used predominantly in the post-surgical phase of orthopaedic management of sports injuries. The benefits to the patient include a reduction in postoperative joint stiffness, less soft tissue adhesions, improved nourishment of the articular cartilage in the potentially hazardous postoperative period and a better preservation of the enzyme systems of the involved muscle groups. CPM is widely used following surgery for ACL reconstruction, post-manipulation, following repair of intra-articular and extra-articular fractures of the tibia or femur and following peri-articular trauma or procedures involving the extensor mechanism of the knee (McCarthy *et al.* 1992).

At the Australian Institute of Sport CPM has been used in the management of muscle tears, with good results (Stanton 1988). This may be commenced as early as 1 h after injury together with ice therapy. We have found an earlier return to function using this method presumably by the inhibition of the formation of a painful or irritable scar.

RANGE OF MOVEMENT EXERCISES

These exercises are prescribed as a follow-up to joint mobilization techniques. Their purpose is to retain or restore range of movement to affected joints. The exercises may be performed in a number of ways, using sustained holds, rhythmic motion or 'hold–relax' techniques.

PROPRIOCEPTIVE EXERCISES

On many occasions following traumatic injury or prolonged periods of disuse, static or dynamic joint position sense may be reduced. This may result from damage to the proprioceptive mechanism (stretch receptors in the joint capsule, or the muscle spindles or Golgi tendon organs within the musculotendinous units). It may also result from compensatory change in normal motor control. Proprioceptive re-education is particularly important in athletes where ligamentous integrity of the joint is lost, increasing the demands on those stabilizing muscles acting over the affected joint.

Proprioceptive exercises involve either reducing the various cues to position sense from systems outside of the joint *per se*, such as sight, touch and pressure, or by increasing the difficulty of the joint exercises by adding distractions. These are of primary importance in the rehabilitation of all joints, in particular the knee, ankle and spine. Examples of proprioceptive exercises of the lower limb include wobble-board balancing exercises while bouncing a ball, mini-trampoline drills and exercises which include skipping, hopping, throwing and catching.

MOTOR CONTROL EXERCISES

Chronic injuries in particular may produce or result from ineffective or inappropriate motor function. Failure of a muscle group to provide adequate tension when required through a range of movement during activity, produces postural or dynamic imbalance which increases biomechanical stresses on portions of the musculoskeletal system during athletic activity.

Biofeedback with EMG devices is a useful tool in assisting the re-education process and is generally used in the clinical setting; although where this is not available the therapist may use palpation and vocal feedback (Fig. 13.3).

As the patient develops a greater appreciation of the motor pattern required, specific exercises may be added to the home exercise regimen. These exercises are directed at muscles performing a stabilizing function, for example, the deep calf flexor in controlling pronation at the ankle, the hamstrings in limiting anterior tibial excursion of the ACL deficient knee, the hip abductors/external rotators in controlling the pelvis during the stance phase of gait, or the scapular stabilizers or rotator cuff in controlling shoulder function.

Sahrmann (1993) suggests a method of assessment and re-education of the stabilizing function of individual muscles or muscle groups in terms of their optimum length–tension relationship.

ISOMETRIC EXERCISE

This static system of exercise is used in the early stages of rehabilitation of the musculotendinous unit, to assist in the maintenance of muscle strength and tone when the patient is not able to move the joint or has limited movement. In the latter situation where some movement is possible, contractions performed at various joint angles may also be carried out (see Chapter 1 for further details).

CONCENTRIC EXERCISE (ISOTONIC)

This includes any exercise where shortening of the exercised muscle occurs. Isotonic exercise requires resistance to a movement and should replicate the normal action of the muscle group. Resistance may be applied using a wide range of devices including

Fig. 13.3 Biofeedback devices are a useful adjunct in motor re-education.

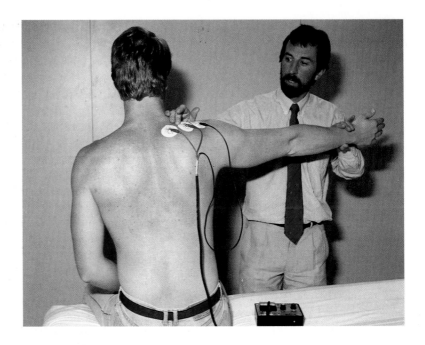

bodyweight, free weights, springs, pulleys, rubber bands, and a variety of exercise machines, which are comprehensively covered in Chapter 1.

ECCENTRIC EXERCISE

When considering the exercise prescription, one should bear in mind that in most athletic activities muscles perform in a stretch–shortening cycle (Komi 1984). In this fashion, elastic energy is stored in the muscle group during an eccentric contraction and this is then utilized in part in the subsequent concentric contraction, greatly increasing mechanical efficiency. In rehabilitating lesions of the tendon, musculotendinous junction or tenoperiosteal junction, exercises emphasizing eccentric contraction have been shown to be beneficial (Curwin and Stanish 1984). To achieve good clinical results the region should be relatively asymptomatic prior to commencement of such exercise. Eccentric and concentric exercises are discussed in full in Chapters 1 and 2.

PHARMACOLOGICAL THERAPY

The processes of inflammation relate to the metabolism of phospholipids and their arachidonic acid metabolites. The various pharmaceutical agents employed to control inflammation act at different points in the metabolic pathways by inhibiting the various enzymes involved (Fig. 13.4).

The initial step in arachidonic acid metabolism involves cleavage of arachidonic acid from the phospholipid in the cell's plasma membrane. Further metabolites are formed via the cyclo-oxygenase and lipoxygenase pathways (Fig. 13.4) and all cells have the capacity to metabolize arachidonic acid.

Although the prostaglandins (PG) have not been fully evaluated as yet, it is known that PGE is released by polymorphonuclear cells during phagocytosis and is chemotactic for leucocytes — enhancing inflammation. The leukotrienes act to increase permeability of blood vessels and induce bronchospasm, mimicking the effect of histamine.

Corticosteroids act early in the arachidonic acid pathway by inhibiting the formation of arachidonic acid from phospholipid (Fig. 13.4). As such, corticosteroids are the most potent of the anti-inflammatory medications used in the treatment of injury in sport. Non-steroidal anti-inflammatory agents act later in the arachidonic pathway to inhibit the production of prostaglandins and leukotrienes.

Non-Steroidal Anti-inflammatory Drugs

Table 13.8 lists commonly used non-steroidal anti-inflammatory drugs (NSAID) by their trade and generic names. Recommended doses are provided as a guide only.

NSAID should be prescribed as soon as possible after injury, as inhibition and not reversal of inflammation, is the principle of treatment. Current practice dictates that 3–5 days of full dosage of NSAID may achieve much in minimizing the time taken to recover from soft tissue injury.

Long-term use of NSAID depends on the clinical signs and symptoms of inflammation, such as oedema, tenderness, erythema, pain and the period of 'morning stiffness', or the time required to 'warm up' and move the affected tissue more comfortably. One should be alert for possible side-effects, although most of these tend to present within the first days or weeks of treatment.

The principal side-effects of NSAID involve the gastrointestinal tract, inducing nausea, gastric erosions, erosive gastritis or peptic ulceration. The combination of enteric-coated NSAID and cyto-protective agents such as H_2-receptor blockers can reduce the incidence of such gastrointestinal side-effects. Aggravation of asthma may also occur and agranulocytosis and significant fluid retention are encountered rarely. Practitioners should become familiar with the use of one or two NSAID, as side-effects and efficacy for various conditions differ.

Corticosteroids

Injections of corticosteroids are commonly used in the treatment of athletic injuries (Table 13.9). The indications for use are those of local treatment of inflammatory conditions of soft tissues: tendons, ligaments and muscles. Acute and chronic conditions may respond to injection, especially when supported by 'active rest' of the injury, physiotherapy and judicious rehabilitation exercises. Particular conditions which respond well to corticosteroid injection include supraspinatus tendinitis, subacromial bursitis, iliotibial band friction syndrome and trochanteric bursitis. It is important for long-term

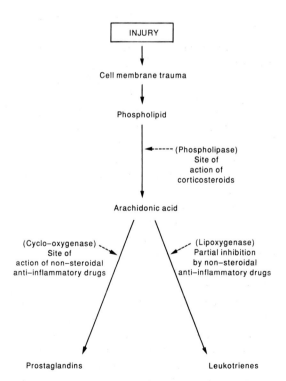

Fig. 13.4 Schema of arachidonic acid metabolism (adapted from Petersdorf *et al.* 1983).

Table 13.8 NSAIDs commonly used in the treatment of injury

Generic name	Dosage (mg·day^{-1})
Propionic acid derivatives	
Flurbiprofen	100–300
Ibuprofen	800–320
Ketoprofen	100–200
Naproxen sodium	825–1100
Tiaprofenic acid	600
Indole derivatives	
Indomethacin	75–150
Sulindac	200–400
Diclofenac	150–200
Others	
Tenoxicam	10–20
Piroxicam	10–20
Phenylbutazone	400–600
Salicylic acid	1800–2400
Diflunisal	500–1000
Aspirin-enteric coated	1950–5200

results to address the underlying biomechanical contributing factors. Caution must be exercised when repeated injections are given to the same site, as there is always the risk of rupture of the structure which has been injected, and a 10 day rest is advised after an injection for this reason. It is also important never to inject corticosteroids into a tendon or ligament and one should also be aware that repeated injections of corticosteroids into joints may induce a crystal arthropathy.

Corticosteroid injections are not advised for bone injuries, particularly stress fractures, or epiphyseal/ growth plate conditions such as Osgood-Schlatter's disease and Sever's disease, because they have a catabolic effect on bone.

The use of corticosteroid injections is deemed a notifiable practice under International Olympic Committee (IOC) rules and further information on this can be obtained in Chapter 26.

Analgesics

It is important that analgesics be considered as a form of therapy distinct from anti-inflammatory agents.

Because analgesics inhibit the perception of pain (nociception) the concept of analgesics 'masking pain' is a familiar one to sports physicians, and due consideration of this action of analgesics must be made when prescribing for athletes who may injure themselves through activity while on treatment.

Analgesics may be considered in two forms: oral and injectable. Injected lignocaine has a limited place in the treatment of injury (sutures etc.) and in the diagnosis of painful conditions such as acromio-clavicular joint disruptions and interdigital neuromas. Care must be taken to use those anal-

gesics permitted by the IOC. Particular note should be taken of morphine and pethidine, which are banned under Olympic rules.

Aspirin (acetylsalicylic acid) is the most widely used analgesic in Western society. Its remarkable efficacy lies in its actions as an analgesic, antipyretic (reducing a fever), anti-inflammatory and uricosuric (promoting the excretion of uric acid by the kidneys) agent. In addition, it is readily absorbed from the stomach and intestine and excreted by the kidney.

As aspirin reduces platelet stickiness it must not be given to those who bleed readily, for example haemophiliacs. Similarly, aspirin may produce peptic ulceration, gastric erosions and bleeding and care should be taken to avoid using aspirin in people suffering dyspepsia or ulcers. Furthermore, it should be noted that asthmatics exhibit notable sensitivity to aspirin and fatal reactions have been reported.

Overdose with aspirin produces tinnitus (ringing in the ears), dizziness, sweating, nausea, vomiting and mental confusion. Lethal doses are reported in the region of 25–30 g and it should be noted that aspirin is not recommended for children under 12 years of age.

Paracetamol acts as an analgesic and antipyretic and is a very suitable alternative for people with dyspepsia or ulcers, or who are sensitive or allergic to aspirin. It should be used carefully in those with liver or kidney problems, as paracetamol is metabolized by these organs.

Overdosage produces vomiting, bleeding from the stomach or intestine, liver damage, cerebral oedema and kidney damage and may be fatal. Paracetamol does cross the placenta and is excreted in breast milk; however, there are no reports of fetal damage with a normal dose of paracetamol.

TOPICAL AGENTS: RUBEFACIENTS AND ANTI-INFLAMMATORIES

Table 13.10 lists topical agents in common use by athletes and trainers in particular. There is debate about the nature of any therapeutic effect of such agents, particularly as the depth of penetration of such preparations in therapeutic quantities appears to be questionable. However, the act of massage may contribute to the beneficial effects which have been reported.

Table 13.9 Injectable corticosteroid preparations commonly used in the treatment of injury

Generic name	Dosage (mg·mL⁻¹)
Betamethasone	5.7
Methylprednisolone acetate	40
Triamcinolone acetate	10

Table 13.10 Topical agents — rubefacients and anti-inflammatories — in common use

Generic name	Dosage
Indomethacin 1% solution	4 times daily
Phenylbutazone	3 times daily
Methyl salicylate compounds	3–4 times daily
Benzydamine	3–4 times daily
Nonylvanillamide butoxyethyl nicotinate	1–2 times daily
Adrenal extracts	2–3 times daily

Note: Agents such as 'Hirudoid', 'Lasonil', etc. are heparin based and used for bruising and contusions.

ACUPUNCTURE

Acupuncture has recently achieved a place in modern sports medicine and is often used when conventional therapies fail.

The earliest acupuncture records date back to 2000 BC, during the reign of the Yellow Emperor of China. It was during the Han Dynasty (206 BC–AD 25) that the *Nei Ching*, otherwise known as the *Yellow Emperor's Classic of Internal Medicine*, first appeared in the Imperial Court Annals. Political events after 1949 encouraged the resurgence of the use of acupuncture and from then on acupuncture research has greatly increased.

The Mechanisms of Acupuncture

Modern neurophysiological research in pain control has thrown considerable light on the mechanisms of acupuncture. It is now known that stimulation of a large diameter afferent nerve causes the release of opioid-like polypeptides in the spinal cord and brain. This in turn either inhibits incoming nociceptive impulses or helps to modulate the perception of pain in the higher centres. The exact mechanisms of the action of acupuncture may not only be by one particular mode of action, but possibly by two or three occurring concurrently.

The first action is one of segmental inhibition. Stimulation of a paravertebral segment causes the release of endorphins in the spinal cord. This has the effect of inhibiting the incoming nociceptive sensations at the spinal marginal neurons in Lamina I and the wide dynamic range neurons in Lamina IV–VI.

The second mode of action, and the most important in acupuncture analgesia, is that of diffuse noxious inhibitory control. In this action, stimulation of a painful area such as the trigger point, causes a nociceptive impulse to be relayed to the mid-brain, where stimulation of the nucleus raphe magnus causes the activation of the descending modulatory pathway to release serotonin and also possibly noradrenaline in the spinal cord segment. This has the effect of inhibiting the incoming nociceptive impulses caused by the injury. Acupuncture and TENS are considered to act principally via this modality and thus relate to the gate control theory of pain (Melzack & Wall 1965).

A third and better known mode of action is a humoral one, whereby low frequency stimulation of an acupuncture point causes release of [β-endorphins from the hypothalamus and pituitary glands into the cerebrospinal fluid and bloodstream. This is responsible for the euphoria that is sometimes seen during or after treatment.

Treatment of Sports Injuries

The treatment of soft tissue injuries with acupuncture differs from the use of acupuncture for other problems in a fundamental way:

- For most medical disorders a diagnosis is made with reference to the Chinese philosophy regarding the relevant channels thought to pervade the body, following which appropriate points are chosen in order to normalize the disorder
- In using acupuncture for the treatment of soft tissue problems, the primary points for treatment are the centres of soreness or trigger points which the Chinese call 'Ah shi' points. Traditional channel points are used as secondary support points in this type of treatment
- The major form of modern acupuncture is still the use of filiform needles, often disposable for convenience, sometimes with the addition of electrical needle stimulation via a type of low-frequency TENS machine made for that specific purpose
- Laser acupuncture is also used, especially for children or patients opposed to the use of

needles, but suffers from the need to treat one point at a time and is less potent except on the more superficial points. Low-powered 'soft' lasers are used

- Other forms of point stimulation, such as TENS and other electronic stimulators, or acupressure are also viable means of treatment in the absence of, or in addition to, the use of needles. The burning of Moxa (a herbal stick made mostly of mugwort) over points is also still used for some conditions and provides localized heat and infra-red radiation to the area

In general, acupuncture is used in the treatment of a wide range of acute and chronic soft tissue injuries and in support of conventional treatment for many other conditions.

CONCLUSIONS

After an athlete has been injured, it is necessary for the physician and therapist to ensure that recovery includes all aspects of performance. These include strength, speed, endurance, power, skill, flexibility and, above all, confidence.

Before providing the athlete/patient with the 'all clear' to resume normal sport activity, a check-list of the factors mentioned previously should be addressed and the correction of any deficiencies attended to promptly. A sports psychologist can contribute to full recovery using techniques previously discussed in Chapter 10. The coach is very important in this situation, as it is his or her judgement which usually provides the best assessment of recovery and the coach often understands the athlete better than the other professionals who help to service him or her.

In the event of any disability arising from injury, it is the therapist's duty to ensure that resumption of sport does not further endanger the athlete. Some attention may also have to be paid to the use of protective devices, protective taping or strapping, and orthotics to allow continued participation at minimal risk. Education of the athlete is also important because the athlete may be unaware of the mechanism of his or her injury, or of the rationale behind the rehabilitation programme which has been instituted.

Resumption of sporting activity should imply a full understanding by the athlete and coach of the processes involved in the production of the injury and the measures necessary to prevent recurrence.

REFERENCES

Blazina M. (1973) Jumper's knee. *Orthopaedic Clinics of North America* **4**, pp. 665–678. W. B. Saunders, Philadelphia.

Bourdillon J. F. (1987) *Spinal Manipulation*, 4th edn. Heinemann Medical Books, Norwalk, CT.

Curwin S. & Stanish W. (1984) *Tendinitis: Its Etiology and Treatment*, pp. 157–165. The Collamore Press, D.C. Heath & Company, Lexington, MA.

Cyriax J. (1975) *Textbook of Orthopaedic Medicine*, Vols I and II. Baillière Tindall, London.

Dyson M. (1987) Mechanisms involved in therapeutic ultrasound. *Physiotherapy* **73**, 116–120.

England J. M., Coppock J. S., Struthers G. R. & Bacon P. A. (1985) An observer blind trial of IR ceb mid laser therapy in bicipital tendonitis and supraspinatus tendonitis. *Proceedings from International Congress on Laser in Medicine & Surgery*, Monduzzi Editore Sp.A, Bologna, Italy, June, pp. 413–414.

Ganne J. M. (1988) Stimulation of bone healing with interferential therapy. *Australian Journal of Physiotherapy* **34**, 9–20.

Gieck J. H. & Saliba E. (1990) Therapeutic ultrasound: Influence on inflammation and healing. In Leadbetter W. B., Buckwalter J. A. & Gordon S. L. (eds) *Sports Induced Inflammation*, pp. 479–492. American Academy of Orthopedic Surgeons, Park Ridge, IL.

Goats C. F. (1989) Pulsed electromagnetic (short-wave) energy therapy. *British Journal of Sports Medicine* **23**, 213–216.

Grieve G. (1981) *Common Vertebral Joint Problems*. Churchill Livingstone, Edinburgh.

Jackson B. A., Schwane J. A. & Starcher B. C. (1991) Effect of ultrasound therapy on the repair of Achilles tendon injuries in rats. *Medicine and Science in Sports and Exercise* **23**, 171–176.

Jackson R., Fitch K. & O'Brien M. (eds) (1990) *Sport Medicine Manual*, pp. 372–374. IOC Medical Commission, Lausanne.

Janda V. (1983) *Muscle Function Testing*, pp. 224–227. Butterworths, London.

Kaltenborn F. (1976) *Manual Therapy for the Extremity Joints*. Olaf Norlis Bokhandel, Oslo.

Knight K. (1985) *Cryotherapy: Theory, Technique and Physiology*, pp. 55–90. Chattanooga Corporation, Chattanooga, TN.

Knott M. & Voss D. (1968) *Proprioceptive Neuromuscular Facilitation. Patterns and Techniques*, 2nd edn, pp. 98–100. Harper & Row, New York.

Kokino M., Temilli Y., Tozun R., Alati M., Altug T. & Beckman M. (1985) Effect of laser radiation on tendon healing. *Proceedings from International Congress on Laser in Medicine and Surgery*, Monduzzi Editore Sp.A, Bologna, Italy, June pp. 405–411.

Komi P. (1984) Physiological and biomechanical correlates of muscle function: Effects of muscle structure and stretch shortening cycle on force and speed. *Exercise and Sports Sciences Reviews*, **12**, pp. 81–121. Lexington, MA.

Kots Y. M. (1977) Notes from lectures and laboratory periods. *Canadian Soviet Exchange Symposium on Electrostimulation of Skeletal Muscle*, p. 4. Concordia University, Montreal, Canada.

Ladd A. L., DeHaven K. E., Thanik J., Patt R. B. & Feuerstein M. (1989) Reflex sympathetic imbalance. *American Journal of Sports Medicine* **17**, 660–668.

Lowdon A. (1986) Application of ultrasound to assess stress fractures. *Physiotherapy* **72**, 160–161.

Maitland G. D. (1986) *Vertebral Manipulation*, 5th edn. Butterworths, London.

Maitland G. D. (1990) *Peripheral Manipulation*, 3rd edn. Butterworths, London.

McCarthy M. R., O'Donoghue P. C., Yates C. K. & Yates-McCarthy J. L. (1992) The clinical use of continuous passive motion in physical therapy. *Journal of Orthopaedic and Sports Physical Therapy* **15**, 132–139.

McKenzie R. (1981) *The Lumbar Spine — Mechanical Diagnosis and Therapy*. Spinal Publications, Waikane, New Zealand.

Melzack R. & Wall P. D. (1965) Pain mechanisms. *Science* **150**, 971.

Sahrmann S. A. (1993) Muscle imbalances in the athletic female. In Pearl A. J. (ed.) *The Athletic Female*, pp. 209–217. Human Kinetics Publishers, Champaign, IL.

Stanton P. (1988) CPM for muscle injuries. In Torode M. (ed.) *The Athlete Maximizing Participation and Minimizing Risk*, pp. 95–102. Cumberland College of Health Sciences, Sydney.

Travell J. G. & Simons D. G. (1983) *Myofascial Pain and Dysfunction*, pp. 5–21, 86–87 Williams and Wilkins, Baltimore, MA.

Wilson D. H. (1972) Treatment of soft tissue injuries with pulsed electrical energy. *British Medical Journal* **2**, 269–270.

Woo S. L-Y. & Buckwalter J. A. (eds) (1987) *Injury and Repair of the Musculoskeletal Soft Tissues*. American Academy of Orthopaedic Surgeons, Park Ridge, IL.

CHAPTER 14

IMAGING IN SPORTS MEDICINE

I. F. Anderson and J. A. Booth

Athletes, whether elite or recreational, spend a great deal of time and effort in training and competing in their chosen sports. Consequently, when an injury occurs, it concerns them greatly because it interferes with their performance. A high level of expertise is then demanded of the sports medicine doctor whom they will expect to diagnose and treat their problems effectively and quickly. The provision of this service is only possible if the doctor receives dependable and accurate support from the imaging specialties.

REQUIREMENTS FOR A HIGH STANDARD OF IMAGING SUPPORT

The musculoskeletal system of the modern athlete is placed under previously unseen stress and as a consequence, the field of sports medicine is rapidly changing, having to diagnose and treat an increasing number of injuries, the majority of which are specific to athletes and often specific to a particular sport. In addition, the old and the young are also in regular training for sport, ensuring a continuing variation in the type of injury seen.

For a radiologist and nuclear medicine physician to play a valuable part in this changing scene, they should:

- Be interested in sports medicine and have a

good working relationship with the sports physician
- Have an understanding of the specific injuries encountered in various sports, and the specialized views needed to demonstrate these conditions
- Have a willingness to keep up with the latest developments in imaging technology and its application to sports medicine
- Have access to specific imaging modalities

Most sports-related injuries are due to overuse and are often difficult to diagnose. It is important therefore that a team approach is taken by the medical personnel involved, to prevent wasted time and expense by following the correct diagnostic protocols.

Each imaging modality used in the diagnosis of sports injuries has a specific role. However, they all have their limitations and this should be appreciated by the sports clinician. The following modalities are currently available: plain film radiography; conventional tomography; nuclear medicine; diagnostic ultrasound; arthrography; computerized tomography (CT); magnetic resonance imaging (MRI); and other less common modalities, such as digitized imaging, infra-red medical thermography, magnification radiology, image intensification and xerography.

PLAIN FILM RADIOGRAPHY

Plain film radiography remains the cheapest and most efficient way of imaging. Almost all sporting injuries require a high quality series of radiographs as the initial and often the only imaging investigation. Their production requires the use of modern machinery, employing an X-ray tube with a fine focal spot and modern film screen combinations. Probably the most important factor in producing a high quality radiograph is the technical skill of the radiographer, which enables precise positioning and correct exposure factors to be used (Clark 1979).

The radiologist and radiographer should plan a series of films which include a basic series, with the occasional addition of specific projections to help with the diagnosis. In all plain film radiography for sports injuries, an attempt must be made to image both the bone and the surrounding soft tissue, as considerable information can be lost with high contrast films of bones and joints. It is possible with correct film screen combinations, a fine focal spot X-ray tube and careful selection of developer temperature, to show definition of both the trabecular pattern and cortex of bone together with adjacent soft tissue structures. Single-coated, orthochromatic high-speed film has been developed basically for mammography, but it produces excellent detail for extremity imaging.

The following discussion on radiographic technique and projections is restricted to sports-oriented injuries in these areas where difficult diagnostic problems are often encountered.

Hand and Wrist

Plain films play the major role in the investigation of hand and wrist injury. Radiography of the hand is usually relatively easy, due to its mobility. The wrist is anatomically complex and superimposition occurs in each view of a routine series of radiographs. Therefore, even after obtaining a high-quality series of plain films, changes can be difficult to interpret and extra views can be of assistance. Bone scans, CT and MRI are also used to unravel the anatomy and image subtle bone changes, with ultrasound and MRI helpful in demonstrating changes in tendons, ligaments and other soft tissues.

The Hand

Routine views

Two views are normally obtained:

- A posteroanterior view is taken with the hand lying flat on the cassette. The hand is in a 'neutral' position with the shoulder, elbow and wrist at the same level and the elbow flexed at 90°. The X-ray beam is centred over the head of the third metacarpal
- A posteroanterior oblique view is obtained with elevation of the radial side of the hand. The fingers are separated to reduce superimposition

In the majority of cases these views provide all the information that is required but occasionally an area is not well demonstrated by these views and, depending on the clinical picture, further positions are helpful.

Additional views: Lateral views of the finger

Use in tendon injury

Extensor tendon Injury to the extensor mechanism produces a number of finger deformities seen best in a true lateral view of the finger.

A 'mallet finger' deformity is produced by an injury to the extensor tendon insertion at the base of the distal phalanx. This is common in sport and is particularly prevalent in ball handling sports. With stretching or rupture of the tendon, a flexion deformity is the only change seen in the lateral view of the finger and an ultrasound scan can be used to make this diagnosis. The other types of 'mallet finger' deformity can be defined on plain films. Commonly, a small avulsed fragment is seen separated from the base. Less commonly, a large fragment is separated and volar subluxation of the distal phalanx may occur. In the immature skeleton, separation of the epiphysis at the base of the distal phalanx may be evident.

The early diagnosis of 'boutonnière deformity' is important. This occurs with an injury to the extensor tendon at its insertion at the base of the middle phalanx and is usually due to blunt trauma or acute flexion. Delay in diagnosis often means that the deformity becomes irreversible. It is rare to see a fragment avulsed from the base of the middle phalanx with this injury and a flexion deformity at the proximal interphalangeal joint may be the only radiological sign available in the lateral view. The complete 'boutonnière deformity' with hyper-extension of the metacarpophalangeal joint, flexion of the proximal interphalangeal joint and extension of the distal interphalangeal joint, is not seen until late in untreated cases (Fig. 14.1). 'Pseudobouton-nière deformity' results from a hyperextension injury causing damage to the volar plate at the proximal interphalangeal joint. Fibrosis and, occasionally, calcification occurs producing a flexion contracture of the proximal interphalangeal joint. When calcification is present, this requires a lateral view for demonstration.

Injury to the extensor mechanism at the meta-carpophalangeal joint does not produce specific changes on plain films. Caused usually by a direct blow, fibres holding the extensor tendon are damaged centrally and the tendon subluxes, usually to the ulnar side. A flexion deformity may be observed at this joint on a plain film.

Flexor digitorum profundus Injury to the flexor digitorum profundus classically occurs in football when a player grasps the jersey or sweater of an opposition player and, if the grasp is broken, the finger may be forcibly extended. This causes an avulsion of the flexor digitorum profundus from its insertion at the base of the distal phalanx. This injury is known as 'jersey finger' and the ring finger is most commonly affected. Three degrees of deformity are described and these can be assessed on plain film if a bony fragment has been separated. More often, ultrasound and MRI are necessary to show how far the tendon has retracted after rupture. *Type 1* deformity is when a large fragment is separated from the volar tip of the distal phalanx with the volar plate attached. The attachment of the plate prevents retraction and there is only slight displacement. *Type 2* deformity occurs when avulsion of the tendon itself has occurred, allowing retraction. This retraction usually extends back to the level of the hiatus of the flexor digitorum sublimis near the proximal interphalangeal joint. A *Type 3* deformity is where a complete avulsion of the flexor mechanism has occurred, allowing re-traction of the flexor digitorum into the palm of the hand.

Use in the diagnosis of fractures

A true lateral view is important in assessing whether a fracture is present, identifying involvement of an articular surface and assessing displacement of fragments. Where a fracture involves more than 40% of an articular surface, open reduction is usually necessary (Fig. 14.2). Consequently, appropriate views must be obtained to allow this assessment to be made and to detect evidence of instability with subluxation. Good quality radio-graphs are particularly necessary in those fractures which are traditionally difficult to treat. They include a fracture of the metaphysis at the base of the proximal phalanx, a condylar and a bicondylar fracture.

Additional views: Reversed oblique view

The reversed oblique view is obtained in the posteroanterior position with elevation of the medial side of the hand. This view is particularly useful for demonstrating a fracture at the base of the fifth metacarpal. The view is used both for the diagnosis of the fracture and assessment of displacement which commonly occurs. The metacarpal shaft becomes both displaced and angulated dorsally.

Additional views: Special views of the thumb

The thumb lies in a different axis from the other digits and requires specific views. A true antero-posterior and lateral view of the thumb allows careful assessment of the first carpometacarpal joint. The presence of a Bennett's fracture or a Rolando's fracture can be diagnosed and the displacement of the fragments assessed. Accurate assessment of the proximal interphalangeal joint and metacarpophal-angeal joint of the thumb are only possible with these views, together with examination of the sesamoid bones. These bones occasionally fracture following direct trauma in ball sports and these fractures are particularly seen in cricketers.

Additional views: Lateral and lateral oblique views of the hand

With metacarpal fractures, a lateral view is necessary in assessing the angulation and shortening, which is present at the fracture site. Often, in a true lateral, definition is obscured by overlying metacarpals and a 30° lateral view is often helpful in overcoming this problem. A common metacarpal fracture involves the neck of the fifth metacarpal with anterior tilting of the metacarpal head. Although this is attributed to sporting activity, it occurs more commonly in street fighters.

The Wrist Joint

The wrist is a complex joint and injuries are usually subtle with occult fractures, fracture dislocations, carpal malalignments and instabilities often difficult to diagnose.

Routine views

Posteroanterior view For this view to be precise and reproducible, the film is taken with the palm flat on the cassette and the elbow resting on the table at the same height as the shoulder. The view highlights the following:

- The alignment of the carpal rows describing smooth arcs at the radiocarpal and intercarpal joints. These arcs are disrupted by carpal subluxations and fractures (Fig. 14.3)

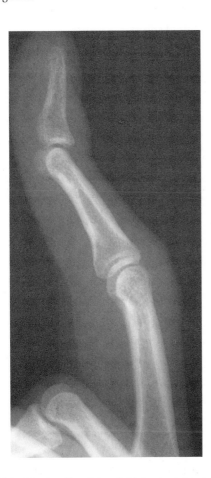

Fig. 14.1 'Boutonnière deformity' following injury to the extensor tendon and its insertion at the base of the middle phalanx. It is recognized by extension of the distal interphalangeal joint and flexion of the proximal interphalangeal joint.

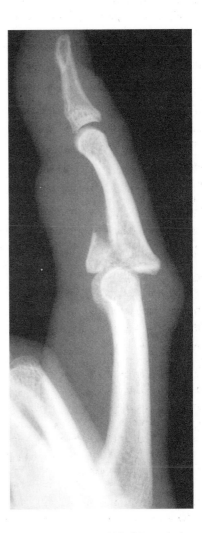

Fig. 14.2 Where more than 40° of the articular surface is separated by a fracture, subluxation usually occurs, requiring surgical reduction.

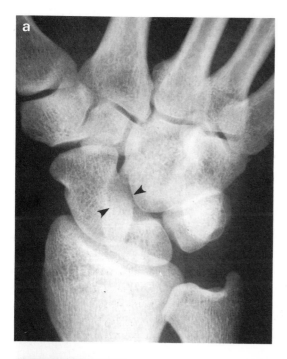

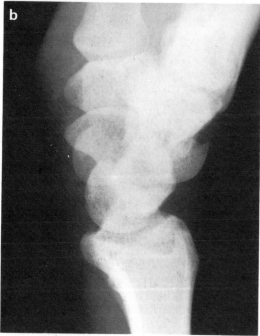

Fig. 14.3 (a) There is an abnormal widening of the joint space between the scaphoid and the capitate. All the intercarpal joint spaces should be equal. (b) A lateral view of the same patient shows a fracture of the capitate with dorsal displacement of the proximal fragment.

- The scapholunate joint space, which is normally the same width as the other intercarpal joints (1–2 mm). A widening of this joint is due to a rupture of the scapholunate ligament and is the commonest cause of carpal instability (Gilula & Weeks 1978)
- A correct exposure on a high detail film screen combination should demonstrate soft tissues as well as bony detail. Tendons on both the medial and lateral aspects of the wrist joint and the scaphoid fat pad are important to examine in this view

Oblique view — Posteroanterior A postero-anterior position with 45° obliquity (thumb elevated), displays the scaphotrapeziotrapezoid joints and the mid-carpal joints particularly well.

Lateral view The importance of an accurate lateral position must be stressed, as considerable information is present in a carefully positioned film. As with a posteroanterior view, the shoulder and elbow must be at the same height as the wrist, with the elbow flexed at 90° and the dorsal surfaces of both the metacarpals and the radius in a straight line. The relationship between the two rows of carpal bones and their relationship to the distal radial articular surface are assessed in this neutral position.

Additional views: Specific carpal views

The shape of the carpal bones makes imaging with plain films difficult and sometimes impossible. By changing the obliquity of the wrist and the X-ray tube, the great majority of carpal fractures can, with care, be demonstrated, although CT may often be a more efficient way of achieving a diagnosis.

Scaphoid series Most fractures of the carpal bones (70–80%) involve the scaphoid bone. This is a common injury in sport, resulting from a fall on the outstretched hand. Stress fractures are uncommon but can occur in gymnasts following repeated compression and dorsiflexion loads. In addition to the three routine views, a specific view of the scaphoid is also taken. This is obtained with the wrist in ulnar deviation and the tube tilted proximally. This tends to elongate the scaphoid and demonstrates the waist of the scaphoid particularly well. Magnification views are also occasionally used for imaging the scaphoid. In practice, if a small focal spot X-ray tube and a fine detail film and screen combination are used, magnification views provide little additional information.

Hook of hamate views A fracture of the hook of hamate is occasionally seen as the result of a sporting injury due to direct trauma. This occurs in racquet sports, golf and in baseball where the tip of the hook impacts against the grip at impact, either with a mishit or a checked shot.

An easy profile view of the hook of hamate can be obtained and to achieve this the wrist is placed in the lateral position with radial deviation. A pad is placed under the head of the fifth metacarpal to help maintain this position and the wrist is then supinated slightly. With the thumb abducted, the

tube is then centred over the base of the fifth metacarpal. Figure 14.4 shows a fracture of the hamate using this method of imaging.

A further view of the hamate can be obtained using a carpal tunnel view. The wrist is dorsiflexed and the X-ray beam angled to profile the carpal tunnel.

Triquetrum and pisiform view The wrist is placed in an anteroposterior oblique position with an obliquity of approximately 60° with the thumb elevated. This position demonstrates the articulation between the pisiform and triquetrum and profiles the pisiform.

Trapezium view An oblique posteroanterior view of the wrist, taken with ulnar deviation, helps to demonstrate the margins of the trapezium. The anterior margin of the trapezium can be well demonstrated in a lateral projection and is particularly well profiled in a carpal tunnel view.

Additional views: Instability series

Normal wrist function requires both movement and stability often while subjected to considerable static and dynamic loading. This function is particularly important in the athlete whose wrist is used to position the hand precisely and to transmit force from the forearm to the hand as in throwing, golf or racquet sports. In sports such as gymnastics and swimming, force is transmitted from the hand to the forearm.

Stability of the wrist is provided by the shape of the carpal bones and ligaments, both interosseous and intracapsular. When collapse occurs under a compressive force, injury to an interosseous ligament has usually occurred. Initially, the collapse occurs intermittently and becomes a dynamic instability occurring in certain positions accompanied by certain movement speeds. With repetitive loading, the stability may become static.

An attempt is made to image a largely dynamic problem by taking a series of films stressing each interosseous group of ligaments in turn.

- A posteroanterior view may show evidence of a static instability. The usual change which is seen is a widening of the scapholunate joint

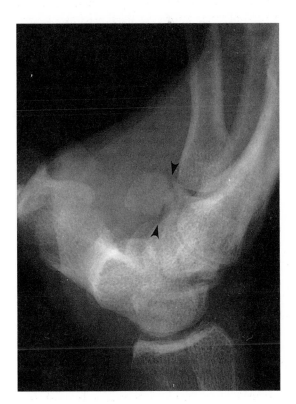

Fig. 14.4 A fracture of the hook of hamate can be easily demonstrated as described in the text

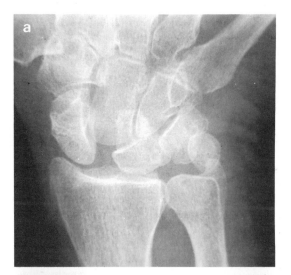

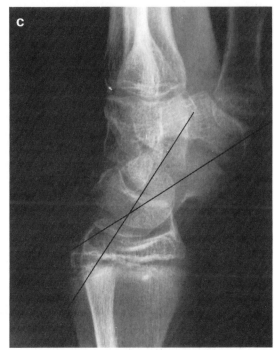

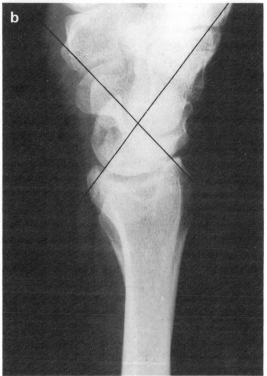

Fig. 14.5 (a) A scapholunate ligament rupture is present producing widening of the scapholunate joint space. (b) A rupture of the scapholunate ligament (DISI) produces an increase in the scapholunate angle in the lateral view due to dorsal rotation of the lunate. (c) A rupture of the lunotriquetral ligament (VISI) causes a decrease in the scapholunate angle, with palmar rotation of the lunate.

space (Fig. 14.5a). Occasionally, widening of the lunotriquetral space can be suspected, but usually the instability produced by lunotriquetral ligament rupture and mid-carpal instability is dynamic, requiring stress views for the diagnosis to be made

- A posteroanterior view with ulnar deviation stresses the radial side and demonstrates scapholunate ligament rupture. This manoeuvre may also produce a mid-carpal instability. A posteroanterior view with radial deviation tests the integrity of the lunotriquetral ligament
- An anteroposterior view with a clenched fist forces the capitate back into the proximal row of carpal bones stressing both the scapholunate and lunotriquetral ligaments, producing joint space widening if ligament damage is present
- A lateral view in the neutral position often holds the key to the diagnosis of carpal instability. Rupture of the scapholunate ligament is the most common cause of carpal instability and produces a dorsal intercalated segment instability (DISI). Following rupture of this

ligament, the lunate and triquetrum rotate independently of the scaphoid and the lunate is seen in the lateral view to rotate dorsally. This is demonstrated in Fig. 14.5b. With rupture of the lunotriquetral ligament, the lunate and scaphoid rotate independently of the triquetrum and the lunate rotates anteriorly. This is a volar intercalated segment instability (VISI) and is demonstrated in Fig. 14.5c. The lunotriquetral angle has also been described as a sensitive assessment of lunotriquetral ligament rupture. The relationship between the capitate and lunate should also be assessed in this view. The axis of the lunate and long axis of the capitate should be almost in a straight line. A 10% variation is accepted as normal and mid-carpal instability should be suspected if this angle lies outside 10°

- A lateral view with flexion and extension demonstrates abnormal movement in both the lunocapitate joint and the lunoradial joint. The total normal arc described between full flexion and extension should be approximately 120°. About a third of this movement occurs at the lunoradial articulation with the majority of movement occurring at the lunocapitate joint. Abnormal movement can be detected by careful examination of these views, and studied further by using image intensification

- Mid-carpal stress views. The relationship between the proximal and distal rows of the carpals is best assessed in the lateral view by examining the lunocapitate joint. When mid-carpal instability is present, dorsal or volar force causes abnormal movement with subluxation of the capitate from the lunate fossa and manual traction is needed during this manoeuvre. On release of the stress in the abnormal patient, the distal row of carpal bones snaps back into normal alignment. Palmar mid-carpal instability may also be produced occasionally by ulnar deviation.

Because of the dynamic nature of this condition, fluoroscopy and video are an obvious method of demonstrating the presence of carpal instability and this is discussed later in the chapter.

Distal radio-ulnar joint

Plain films can help in the diagnosis of instability of the distal radio-ulnar joint and assessment of ulnar variance.

Instability of the distal radio-ulnar joint requires a careful lateral view in the neutral position to detect displacement of the head of the ulna. Films of the distal radio-ulnar joint are then taken in supination and pronation and any widening of the joint space is abnormal. If widening occurs with supination, a volar subluxation is present and if subluxation occurs following pronation, a dorsal subluxation can be diagnosed. Sometimes stress pronation and supination are necessary to demonstrate instability of the joint. Following abnormal plain films, CT is the examination of choice for demonstrating subluxation of the head of the ulna from the sigmoid notch. Assessment can be made of the shape of the sigmoid notch which together with the pronator quadratus, the triangular fibrocartilage and the extensor retinaculum contributes to the stability of the distal radio-ulnar joint.

The extensor carpi ulnaris is also a stabilizer of the distal radio-ulnar joint and tenosynovitis or subluxation of this tendon may be associated with instability. Swelling along the line of the tendon or possible associated calcification can be seen on plain films and, if present, careful inspection of the distal radio-ulnar joint is advisable.

Ulnar variance has important associations and ulnar minus variance (a short ulna) has been associated with avascular necrosis of the lunate and tears in the triangular fibrocartilage before 30 years of age. A relatively long ulna, ulnar plus variance, is associated with ulnolunate abutment, chondromalacia of the lunate and perforation of the triangular fibrocartilage. Ulnar plus variance is occasionally seen in gymnasts where premature closure of the distal radial epiphyseal plate is caused by an injury to it.

Stress reaction in the distal radial epiphyseal plate is also seen in gymnasts with widening of the epiphyseal plate (Fig. 14.6).

Carpal tunnel view

This view is obtained with the wrist in dorsiflexion

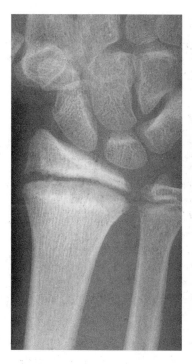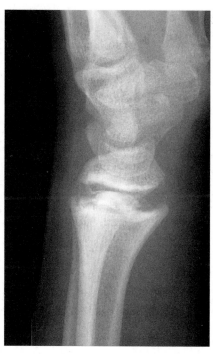

Fig. 14.6 A stress reaction with widening of the distal radial epiphyseal plate occurs in gymnasts.

and the X-ray beam angled through the carpal tunnel. This view is useful in demonstrating the hook of hamate, the pisiform bone and the volar aspect of the trapezium.

Radiocarpal joint

The articular surfaces of the radiocarpal joint can be easily demonstrated with the palm of the hand lying on a 20° wedge, elevating the fingers. A tube angled slightly towards the elbow is also used.

Soft tissue changes

Changes in the soft tissue around the wrist provide valuable clues to underlying changes in tendons and bones.

In the lateral view, two important fat planes should be examined. The pronator quadratus fat plane lies between the pronator quadratus muscle and the volar tendon sheaths. This is seen on the anterior aspect of the distal radius. With trauma to the distal radius, this fat plane becomes obliterated or bowed anteriorly (Fig. 14.7). This is a very sensitive indicator of the presence of injury to the distal radial epiphyseal plate in children and may be

the only sign present. The dorsal fat plain at the wrist becomes deformed in almost all scaphoid fractures and deserves careful examination.

In the posteroanterior view of the wrist, the scaphoid fat pad should be identified and examined. This lies between the radial collateral ligament and the abductor pollicis brevis tendon. This becomes obliterated or deformed by oedema when a scaphoid fracture is present.

When tenosynovitis of the abductor pollicis longus and the extensor pollicis brevis tendons is present, soft tissue thickening can be observed over the lateral margin of the radial styloid. With a fine detail film, the margins of the tendon can normally be identified and, when inflammatory changes are present, the margins become difficult to define. Similarly, swelling along the medial aspect of the wrist is produced by tendinitis of the flexor carpi ulnaris.

Progress films

If a scaphoid fracture is present, a progress examination is important to assess union. Also if the initial examination appears normal and clinical

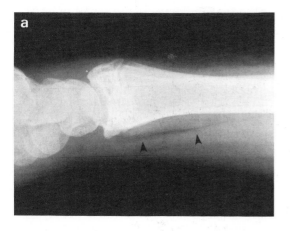
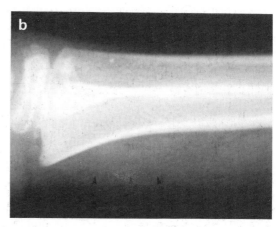

Fig. 14.7 (a) This is a normal pronator quadratus fat plane (arrows). (b) With a fracture of the distal radial epiphyseal plate there is partial obliteration, displacement and bowing of the pronator quadratus fat plane.

suspicion persists or if there are changes in the adjacent fat planes, re-examination of the wrist in 10–14 days will help identify subtle fractures. Bony resorption makes a fracture line more easily identified. The diagnosis may still be in doubt even after a second examination and a further progress examination or bone scan should then be considered.

The Elbow Joint

The indications for plain film radiography of the elbow joint following sporting injuries result from either acute trauma or overuse.

ACUTE TRAUMA

The fractures most commonly encountered in athletes are as follows:

- A fracture of the radial head or neck
- A supracondylar fracture of the humerus — this is the second most common fracture in the immature skeleton
- Avulsion fractures and traction apophysitis, particularly involving the medial epicondyle and the apophysis of the olecranon

Routine views following trauma

An anteroposterior view This is performed with the elbow extended, the hand supine and with the shoulder, elbow and wrist at the same level.

The lateral view The lateral view is positioned with the elbow flexed at 90°, the hand lateral and, again, the shoulder, elbow and wrist are at the same level. This view demonstrates the margins of the trochlear notch, the radial head, the olecranon process and the supracondylar region of the distal humerus. The soft tissue changes produced by trauma are seen in this view.

Oblique view with 45° external rotation This profiles the anterior and anterolateral margins of the radial head and neck and the articular surface of the capitellum.

Deep fat planes at the elbow Anterior and posterior fat pads are an important indicator of trauma, being extrasynovial but intracapsular, and are displaced with a joint effusion. When an effusion is present, a careful examination for a subtle fracture is important and if a fracture cannot be identified, a progress examination in 10–14 days is usually advisable. The supinator fat plane is a lucent line seen in the lateral view 4–5 cm in length, running parallel to and about 1 cm anterior to the proximal radius. This is displaced or obliterated with fractures of the radial head and neck.

Additional views

Tangential view of the olecranon With the shoulder and humerus at the same level, the elbow is fully flexed and the palm of the hand rests on the shoulder, with the tube slightly angled towards the shoulder. This view demonstrates the olecranon process and also details of the posterior joint compartment.

Oblique view with 45° internal rotation This view profiles the tip of the coronoid process and the margin of the trochlea.

Additional radial head views With care, the entire circumference of the radial head can be visualized by various supinated and pronated flexion views. The elbow and shoulder are at the same level with 60° elbow flexion. The radial head is rotated by supinating and pronating the hand, displaying particularly the posterior half of the radial head, an area which is difficult to see on other views.

OVERUSE INJURIES

Joint injuries

Throwing injuries, in particular, create an instability in the elbow joint by damaging and stretching the ulnar collateral ligament. Its anterior oblique band, the prime stabilizer of the elbow, is largely affected. This instability in the medial side of the elbow produces a number of changes which are as follows:

- An impingement of the radial head on the capitellum occurs and this may result in osteochondritis dissecans of the capitellum in the young athlete or degenerative change in the more mature athlete
- Traction produces bony spurs from the medial aspect of both the coronoid process and the medial epicondyle with areas of ossification occasionally occurring within the ulnar collateral ligament (Fig. 14.8)
- Instability allows impingement on the margins of the olecranon fossa and cartilaginous damage which leads to degenerative change is common. Localized changes of osteochondritis dissecans may appear, eventually producing loose bodies (Fig. 14.8)

Tendon injuries

Throwing produces inflammatory changes in the flexor–pronator group medially and in the triceps posteriorly, while racquet sports often produce a lateral epicondylitis.

Routine overuse series

Anteroposterior view This view demonstrates the presence of spurs, bony erosion or soft tissue calcification indicative of epicondylitis and the early changes of osteochondritis dissecans in the capitellum.

Lateral view The identification of the fat lines in this view demonstrates the presence of a joint effusion.

Oblique view With 45° external rotation, the radiocapitellar articulation is well demonstrated.

The tangential view of the olecranon This demonstrates changes resulting from impingement (Fig. 14.8).

Additional views

The following views assist in the more difficult diagnoses:

- An oblique view with 45° internal rotation demonstrates the ligamentous attachments to the lateral epicondyle and may show the presence of calcification or bony erosion of the epicondyle
- A view of the elbow joint with valgus stress (Rijke *et al.* 1994) establishes instability due to damage to the ulnar collateral ligament and is performed with the elbow flexed between 30° and 40° (Fig. 14.8)
- The proximal radioulnar joint is shown in an anteroposterior view with 15° of external rotation separating the radius and the ulna

The Shoulder Joint

The shoulder joint is commonly injured and is difficult to image. To do this well requires particular precision and attention to detail. Imaging of the shoulder is difficult because the anatomy is complex and changes seen in overuse injuries occur in the places most difficult to access. Further, some of the significant changes occur within tendon substance itself.

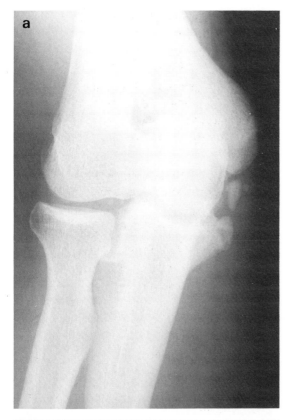

ACUTE TRAUMA

Routine views

Anteroposterior view: Internal and external rotation This view is obtained with the patient standing with the scapula flat against the bucky with the primary beam angled at 15°–20° to the feet to demonstrate better the space between the acromion and the humeral head. In this position, films are taken with external and internal rotation. External rotation often demonstrates an avulsion fracture of the greater tuberosity and the internal rotation view may demonstrate the presence of a defect in the posterolateral aspect of the humeral head (Hill-Sachs' lesion) produced by a previous glenohumeral dislocation.

Fig. 14.8 (a) Changes resulting from baseball pitching ('thrower's elbow') are present with ossification in the line of the ulnar collateral ligament, spur formation on the medial aspect of the coronoid process and loose bodies on the medial aspect of the radiocapitellar articulation are demonstrated. (b) A tangential view of the olecranon demonstrates fragmentation of the lateral margin of the trochlea due to repeated impingement by the olecranon. This abnormal laxity is made possible by an injury to the ulnar collateral ligament. (c) A valgus stress view demonstrates instability produced by an injury to the ulnar collateral ligament.

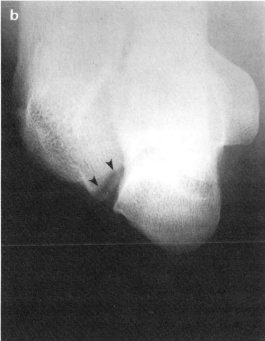

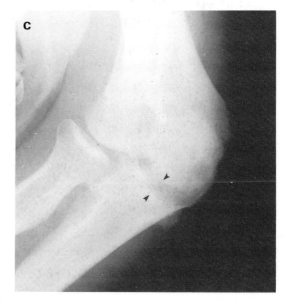

Glenohumeral joint view An anteroposterior view, with the primary beam passing along the plane of the articular surface of the glenoid fossa, requires the patient to be further inclined to approximately 40°. This view allows the joint space to be assessed.

Lateral view Following trauma, a lateral view is essential to assess whether a dislocation is present, by evaluating the relationship between the glenoid and the humeral head.

Axial view There are two methods to obtain this view, and both may be difficult when the patient has had a fracture or dislocation around the shoulder joint. The first is to have the patient supine, with the arm abducted to 90° with the cassette resting above the shoulder. The tube is then angled towards the head. The second is obtained with the patient sitting with the arm abducted at 90° and with the cassette placed beneath the axilla. This view demonstrates the relationship between the humeral head and the glenoid, but has the further advantages of imaging the anterior and posterior glenoid margins.

CHRONIC TRAUMA

Chronic trauma to the shoulder is common, usually as a result of overuse with repetitive microtrauma, commonly to the rotator cuff tendons.

The two major clinical groups are the impingement/rotator cuff group and the instability group and these provide most of the diagnostic problems presenting to a sports medicine clinic.

Shoulder instability group An instability series includes an *anteroposterior* view as well as *internal and external rotation*. These are performed as with acute trauma. The internal rotation view is valuable for the demonstration of an osteochondral fracture on the posterolateral aspect of the humeral neck (a Hill-Sachs' lesion). An *axial view* is performed as previously described. In this view, a fragment can occasionally be seen separated from the posterior aspect of the glenoid rim, produced by posterior dislocation.

West Point view A West Point view is performed with the patient in the prone position, with the arm abducted at 90° and with the forearm and hand

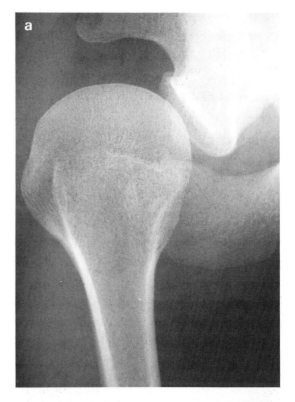

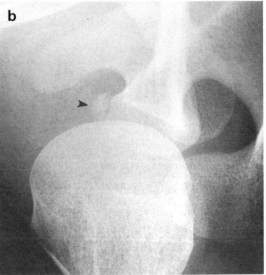

Fig. 14.9 (a) Normal axial view fails to demonstrate the separated fragment. (b) A West Point projection profiles the antero-inferior corner of the glenoid rim and is a most useful projection for demonstrating separated fragments.

hanging over the side of the table. The tube is angled at 25° to the head and 25° medially. This view has been found to be helpful in identifying small fragments separated from the anterior and antero-inferior aspects of the rim of the glenoid (Fig. 14.9). The West Point and axial views are also useful in combination to demonstrate displacement of the apophyses of the coracoid and the acromion.

Additional views

Notch view (Stryker's view; Hall *et al.* 1959) This is performed with the patient supine, the hand flat on top of the head and the shaft of the humerus parallel to the patient's body. The shoulder is flexed slightly beyond 90° with minor internal rotation. There is a 10° tilt of the tube to the head. About 75% of recurrent shoulder dislocations have a defect on the posterolateral aspect of the humeral neck (a Hill-Sachs' lesion) produced by impaction of the humerus against the interior rim of the glenoid, which often occurs in collision sports (Fig. 14.10).

Impingement — rotator cuff group Problems can arise in the supraspinatus tendon as it passes through the rigid tunnel produced by the acromion, acromioclavicular joint, the neck of the scapula and the acromioclavicular ligament anteriorly. This canal can become reduced in size due to bony spurs or the tendon may increase in size due to oedema. These views are used to help demonstrate a reason for a bony impingement or provide plain X-ray evidence of tendinitis. They include the following:

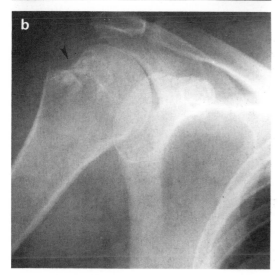

Fig. 14.10 The mechanism of production of a Hills-Sach lesion is well demonstrated. (a) With glenohumeral dislocation, the humeral head impacts against the glenoid rim. (b) On reduction of the dislocation, a large posterolateral defect persists.

- *Anteroposterior View: Internal and external rotation.* With external rotation the greater tuberosity is clearly profiled and demonstrates any supraspinatus calcification which may be present. Internal rotation shows infraspinatus and teres minor calcification with subscapularis calcification located adjacent to the lesser tuberosity in the region of the glenohumeral joint. Caudal angulation also helps to assess the distance between the humeral head and the acromion process which, if reduced, indicates rotator cuff degeneration
- *Anteroposterior joint view.* This joint view is essential in assessing the width of the glenohumeral joint and in determining whether degenerative changes are present
- *Lateral view (tunnel view).* The bony tunnel through which the supraspinatus passes can be examined with a carefully taken lateral view. A 20–25° caudal tube tilt enables the primary

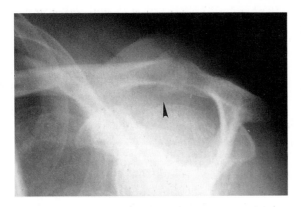 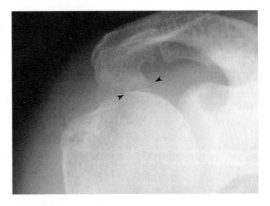

Fig. 14.11 (a) A lateral view with caudal tube tilt demonstrates the pathway of the supraspinatus and may demonstrate bony causes for impingement. A bony spur is shown at the anterior margin of the acromion. (b) A 30° caudal tube angulation in an anteroposterior projection will profile a bony spur at the anterior margin of the acromion.

beam to pass along the line of the supraspinatus. The arc described by the acromion and acromio-clavicular joint is then examined for bony irregularities which cause impingement (Fig. 14.11)

- *Axial view.* The axial view is taken as previously described. With impingement, the anterior margin of the acromion can be examined and an os acromiale excluded

Additional views

30° Caudal angulation   An additional view, which is helpful in demonstrating bony spur formation, is an anteroposterior view of the shoulder with a 30° caudal angulation of the X-ray tube (Kilcoyne *et al.* 1989). This demonstrates the anterior margin of the acromion (Fig. 14.11b).

Bicipital groove view   The long head of the biceps may become inflamed as it passes beneath the transverse humeral ligament and this injury is often seen in throwers, gymnasts and swimmers. This

view may show encroachment on the groove by a spur. Tendon calcification, however, is rarely present. The simplest way to produce this view is for the patient to sit with the elbow resting on the X-ray table and the humerus slightly extended. A film is placed under the humeral head, and the bicipital groove is profiled.

Hip and Groin Region

The most commonly encountered sporting injuries of the hip and groin requiring radiology are stress fractures of the pubic rami, 'groin strains', avulsion fractures and stress fractures of the femoral neck.

STRESS FRACTURES OF THE PUBIC RAMI

These fractures involve the inferior pubic ramus and are most commonly seen in female joggers and long-distance runners. As with all stress fractures the radiological signs of callus formation and resorption along the margins of the fracture may be delayed.

Routine views

The following views can be helpful when diagnosing stress fractures of the pubic rami:

- An anteroposterior view of the pelvis
- The obturator foramen view. The margins of the obturator foramen are displayed with the patient prone, the opposite side of the body elevated to about 15° and the X-ray tube angled slightly towards the feet

'GROIN STRAIN' AND OSTEITIS PUBIS

Groin strain is a relatively common sporting injury and is produced by several different causes. Most 'groin strains' appear to be due to lesions at the origin of the adductor longus, adductor brevis or gracilis. Other injuries in this region occur to the pubic tubercle, superior pubic ligament or conjoint tendon. Osteitis pubis is commonly seen on plain films, affecting one or both sides of the symphysis, usually with sclerosis and erosion of the margin(s) of the joint (see Chapter 20).

Routine views

The following views may be helpful in the diagnosis of 'groin strain':

- An anteroposterior view of the pelvis
- A coned view of the pubic bones with the patient in a supine position and the tube angled to the head

Additional views

Craniocaudal view This view of the symphysis pubis can be obtained with the patient sitting on the table leaning backwards, supported by the arms. A straight tube is used and this view shows both the anterior and posterior margins of the symphysis pubis.

Instability views of the symphysis This examination is performed using a posteroanterior projection, centred on the symphysis pubis, initially with weight evenly taken on both feet. Films are then taken with weight being borne alternately on

each foot 'flamingo views'. This demonstrates instability of the symphysis pubis, with abnormal movement (>2 mm of vertical shift) occurring at this joint.

AVULSION INJURIES

Excessive muscular stress can produce characteristic avulsion fractures with separation of their tendinous attachments. In the adolescent, inflammatory changes at the apophyses or avulsion of the apophyses also occur. Several avulsion injuries in the pelvis, particularly in young athletes, have the following radiographic features:

- Avulsion of the apophysis of the ischial tuberosity occurs with violent contraction of the hamstrings. In the acute injury the curvilinear apophysis may be separated, whereas in the more chronic injury demineralization and fragmentation of the apophysis will be seen. This injury is characteristically found in hurdlers, sprinters and long jumpers (Fig. 14.12)
- Avulsion of the anterior superior iliac spine is the second most commonly encountered pelvic injury (Fig. 14.13)
- Avulsion of the anterior superior iliac spine is associated with stress at the origin of the tensor fasciae femoris and the sartorius muscle. This injury can be seen in sprinters (Fig. 14.14)

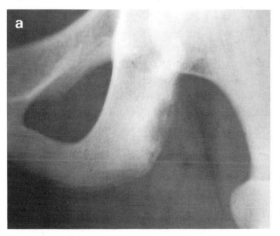
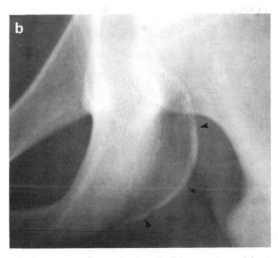

Fig. 14.12 Stress to the hamstring attachment may produce: (a) a bony resorption and sclerosis; (b) an acute avulsion with displacement of the apophysis, in this case, produced by hurdling.

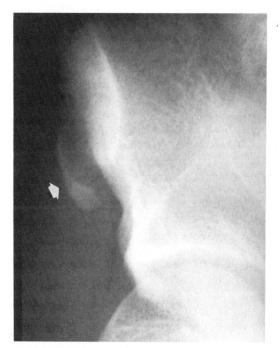

Fig. 14.13 A separation of the anterior inferior iliac spine is present (arrow). This is produced by a contraction of the rectus femoris.

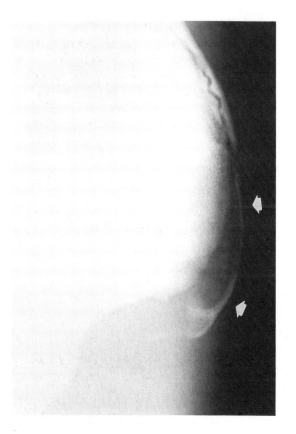

Fig. 14.14 The anterior superior iliac spine has been avulsed and is best displayed by elevating the unaffected side and using a soft tissue technique.

- Avulsion of the apophysis of the iliac crest may occur in the adolescent with violent contraction of the abdominal muscles. This injury is seen in runners and weight-lifters
- Avulsion of the greater trochanter can be produced by gluteal muscle contraction
- Avulsion of the apophysis of the lesser trochanter results from traction by the psoas major during strenuous hip flexion

Routine views

An anteroposterior view The ischial tuberosity, the anterior iliac spines and iliac crest can all be seen on an anteroposterior view of the pelvis. This, combined with the lateral view of the hip joint will adequately demonstrate an avulsion of either trochanter.

Additional views

Ischial tuberosity Elevation of the affected side to approximately 20° obliquity better demonstrates the ischial tuberosity.

Iliac crest and anterior iliac spines The iliac crest and the anterior iliac spines are often not well shown on a routine anteroposterior view. To better demonstrate both the anterior superior and anterior inferior iliac spines, a soft tissue film is helpful. It should be centred on the particular spine, with elevation of the unaffected side (Fig. 14.14). Often a soft tissue film is also required to demonstrate the apophysis of the iliac crest. Slight displacement of the apophysis is often only evident after comparison with the normal side.

FEMORAL NECK FRACTURES

Stress fractures of the femoral neck may be seen in runners and can occur at several sites on the femoral neck and upper femoral shaft. The commonest site is at the inferior aspect of the base of the femoral neck (Fig. 14.15), with the second most common at the superolateral aspect of the neck. The third site of a stress reaction in this region is subtrochanteric at the medial aspect of the upper femoral shaft where a periosteal reaction occurs at the insertion of the adductor brevis.

Routine views

The following views are taken for these injuries:

- Anteroposterior view of the pelvis
- Anteroposterior view of the hip
- Lateral view of the hip

The Knee Joint

The knee is a complicated joint which is subjected

to varied stresses in sport. The following major problems arise: fractures; extensor mechanism injury; degenerative changes; osteochondritis dissecans; patellofemoral problems; and soft tissue changes.

FRACTURES

Sports injuries tend to be of three major types and are as follows:

Stress fractures   The commonest site of a stress fracture is the medial tibial condyle. This is seen as a sclerotic band with or without an associated periosteal reaction. Stress fractures are also seen involving the neck of the fibula and the patella, but are not as common at these sites.

Avulsion fractures   The following avulsion fractures occur in the knee joint:

- The tibial attachment of both the anterior (ACL) and posterior cruciate ligaments (PCL) may be avulsed (Fig. 14.16)
- A small bone fragment is occasionally avulsed

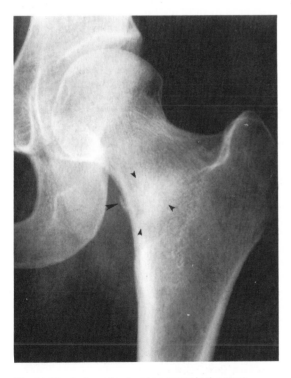

Fig. 14.15   A stress fracture is present in the most commonly encountered site, at the base of the femoral neck on its inferior aspect. There is characteristic sclerosis (small arrows) and cortical irregularity (large arrow) present.

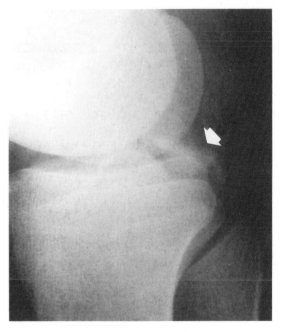

Fig. 14.16   There is a separation of the tibial attachment of the PCL which has a characteristic appearance in this lateral view of the knee.

from the femoral attachment of the ACL on the lateral wall of the intercondylar notch

- A sliver of bone may become avulsed from the lateral aspect of the lateral tibial condyle, by the inferior meniscal capsular ligament. This fracture (Segond fracture; Goldman *et al.* 1988) almost always indicates the presence of an ACL rupture and meniscal injury (Fig. 14.17)
- A patellar fragment is quite commonly avulsed from the medial margin of the patella by the medial retinaculum, following patellar dislocation

Osteochondral fractures   These are seen following impingement by either the patella on a femoral condyle after direct trauma to the patella, or by a femoral condyle on the neighbouring tibial plateau following either a forced valgus or varus stress. When there is an osteochondral fracture of the femoral condyle secondary to patella trauma, an area of demineralization may be the only radiological sign on plain film.

Routine views

Anteroposterior view   This view should routinely be taken with the patient standing erect, although occasionally weight-bearing is difficult after trauma.

Lateral view   The lateral view is performed with 20°–30° of knee flexion.

Intercondylar view   This may not be possible after severe knee trauma, as it requires the knee to be flexed at 45°.

Patellofemoral view   Following trauma a view without distortion (such as Merchant's view) is preferred.

Additional views

Cross-table lateral views   Following trauma a fluid level can sometimes be demonstrated in the suprapatellar extension when a haemarthrosis is present. The fluid level represents a fat–fluid level indicating the presence of a fracture with escape of marrow fat into the joint space (Fig. 14.18).

Oblique view   This view of the knee is helpful in imaging the patella in a patient who cannot flex the knee.

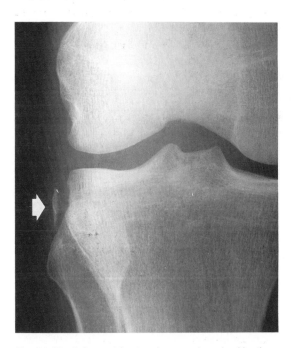

Fig. 14.17   A Segond fracture is present, avulsed by the inferior meniscal capsular ligament. The presence of this fracture almost always indicates an ACL rupture and meniscal injury.

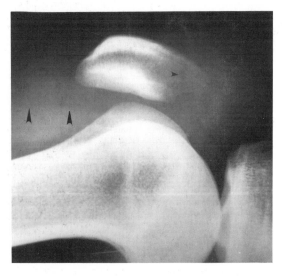

Fig. 14.18   A fat-fluid level is well demonstrated in a cross-table lateral view (arrows). Marrow fat has escaped into the joint from a patellar fracture.

EXTENSOR MECHANISM INJURIES

Repetitive stress to the extensor mechanism of the knee produces a number of conditions, seen most frequently in the adolescent athlete. Following repetitive jumping, an injury to the quadriceps tendon and its patellar attachment may occur. Radiologically, ossicles can be seen in the quadriceps tendon, or there may be fragmentation or a spur formation at the superior pole of the patella. Stress to the extensor mechanisms of the knee joint may also produce a stress fracture of the patella, which is usually transverse. Changes at the inferior pole of the patella are also seen and are characteristically associated with jumping sports. These changes (Sinding-Larsen-Johansson disease), produce fragmentation associated with some thickening of the upper end of the patellar tendon. Osgood-Schlatter's disease is by far the most common change resulting from extensor mechanism stress injury. The aetiology is considered to be chronic stress on the tibial tubercle apophysis and in the initial stages tissue swelling over the tubercle and loss of definition of the margins of the adjacent patellar tendon may be the only signs. Fragmentation of the apophysis often occurs with some displacement of the fragments (Fig. 14.19).

Routine views

The routine knee series is the same as for trauma.

Additional views

Soft tissue lateral view This view is helpful when Osgood-Schlatter's disease or Sinding-Larsen-Johansson disease are suspected as soft tissue swelling may be the only sign. A similar view of the other knee is also valuable as the condition may be bilateral (Fig. 14.19).

Additional patellar views These views are necessary when a stress fracture of the patella is suspected. In this situation an oblique view is valuable. The definition of the patella is improved by imaging the knee in a posteroanterior rather than an anteroposterior direction.

DEGENERATIVE DISEASE

Routine views

In addition to the routine views required for the trauma, an additional weight-bearing posteroanterior view of the knee is also performed. To do this, the knee is flexed at 45° with the patella resting against the cassette and the tube is angled at 10° towards the feet. This view is thought to be more sensitive to early narrowing of articular cartilage and a discrepancy of more than 2 mm in the width of the medial and lateral compartments indicates significant cartilage thinning. The routine anteroposterior view with weight-bearing cannot be replaced by this view, as it is important for the assessment of tibiofemoral alignment.

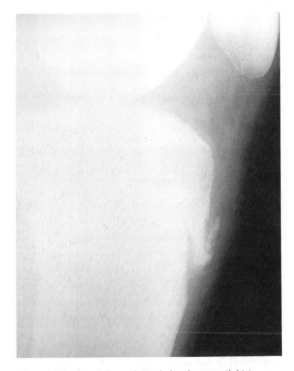

Fig. 14.19 A soft tissue lateral view is essential to demonstrate the changes of osteochondritis of the tibial tuberosity (Osgood-Schlatter's disease). It is important to demonstrate the presence of the soft tissue swelling as this is an indicator of activity.

Additional views

A long weight-bearing anteroposterior view of both legs is helpful in assessing tibiofemoral alignment and should be routine preceding a tibial osteotomy.

In addition, anteroposterior views in abductor and adductor stress may also be helpful prior to a tibial osteotomy, to demonstrate abnormal joint laxity.

OSTEOCHONDRITIS DISSECANS

The commonest location of osteochondritis dissecans in the knee joint is the lateral aspect of the medial femoral condyle. The process is also seen in the lateral compartment and on the articular surface of the patella (Fig. 14.20). Quality radiographs are essential as early changes may be quite subtle and a small area of demineralization may be the only radiological sign.

Fig. 14.20   (a) Osteochondritis dissecans of the articular surface of the patella is relatively uncommon. (b) In this case there is displacement of a fragment producing a loose body.

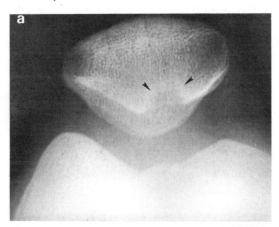

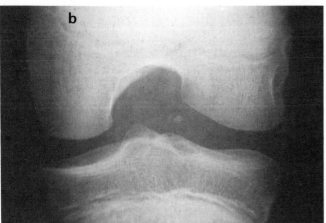

Routine series

The series required is the same as for degenerative disease with a posteroanterior 45° weight-bearing film included routinely.

PATELLOFEMORAL DISORDERS

Radiologically, these disorders fall into groups A and B. The former includes patellofemoral instability, tracking problems and chondromalacia patellae, while the latter comprises degenerative disease, osteochondritis dissecans, avulsion fractures and osteochondral fracture of the femoral condyles.

GROUP A

There are several factors which influence patellofemoral abnormalities. These are dynamic in nature and it is often not possible for plain radiography to contribute significantly to their diagnosis. Associated conditions such as patellofemoral dysplasia and tibiofemoral malalignment may be imaged and occasionally definite evidence of instability can be seen. More often than not, particularly with chondromalacia, no radiological signs are available, as the associated factors such as increased loading, or pressure on the articular cartilage cannot be appreciated radiologically. The patella may appear well centred on a static film, but may not be stabilized.

Radiology of the patellofemoral articulation

The majority of instabilities are thought to occur at about 20° of knee flexion and certainly before 30°, when the patella enters the sulcus and begins seating. Unfortunately, a patellofemoral view under 30° usually has the tibial tuberosity projected over the joint, thus obscuring detail. At about 60° flexion, good contact between the articular surfaces occurs and towards 90° contact abnormalities such as osteoarthritis are best demonstrated. An easy, routine method of visualizing the patellofemoral articulation is the Hughston view, in which the patient is prone with the knee flexed between 50° and 60° and the tube is angled at 30° to the femur. This view is good for assessing the sulcus as the lateral condyle profile is at its greatest height at 55° (the normal sulcus angle is 118° for this method). The best method of imaging the patellofemoral joint is the Merchant's view (Merchant *et al.* 1974). This method requires the patient to sit on the table with the leg over the table end, resting on a fixed angle frame. The knee is flexed at 45° with the ankle fixed by straps. The film is held by a cassette holder anterior to the shin, enabling the film to be taken at 90° to the X-ray beam with the tube angled at 30° to the femur. As there is no distortion, this is the preferred method for excluding osteoarthritis, a patellar fracture, an osteochondral fracture of the femur condyle or osteochondritis dissecans. The only disadvantage of this method is, as with other static methods, that it may not show evidence of subluxation or instability, which may occur in the first 30° of flexion.

Additional views

An attempt can be made to appreciate the dynamic nature of patellofemoral disorders by taking a series of films at 30°, 60° and 90° of flexion (Newberg & Seligson 1980). These views can sometimes provide information about the character of the articular cartilage of the patellofemoral joint.

All the above methods are performed with relaxation of the quadriceps; however, films taken with the quadriceps contracted may add a further dynamic dimension. Turner and Burns (1982) have described an axial technique with the patient standing with the knee flexed at 40°.

Teige (1988) has developed a technique to demonstrate lateral and medial instability. The knees are placed on a Merchant frame and stress is applied to both the medial and lateral margins of the patella in turn, both with and without quadriceps contraction.

Routine views

Anteroposterior view: Erect The anteroposterior view is helpful in assessing tibiofemoral alignment, height of the patella and position of the tibial tuberosity.

Lateral view The position of the patella is assessed in the lateral view.

Patellofemoral view A Merchant's view is the preferred imaging technique, but if a Merchant's frame is unavailable, a Hughston's view will suffice.

GROUP B

This group requires undistorted, precise imaging; therefore the same routine series is used as with group A, and the use of a Merchant's frame is important.

SOFT TISSUE CHANGES

In the lateral view of the knee with 20°–30° flexion, the collapsed suprapatellar extension of the knee joint creates a sharply defined vertical line between the anterior suprapatellar fat and the prefemoral fat pad. This line is usually between 5 and 10 mm in width and thickening of this line indicates an effusion.

Soft tissue thickening along the line of the medial collateral ligament may be the only radiological indication of injury to this ligament and the presence of soft tissue calcification (Pellegrini-Stieda calcification) medial to the medial femoral condyle indicates previous damage. Soft tissue definition behind the knee joint may demonstrate the presence of a Baker's cyst and ossicles are occasionally seen within the cyst.

The Ankle

Sporting injuries which occur in this region of the body are normally the result of either acute trauma or overuse.

ACUTE TRAUMA

An inversion injury to the ankle joint occurs regularly in agility sports. Ankle fractures are usually obvious when the malleoli are involved, but occasionally the changes are quite subtle and careful radiography with the use of additional views may be necessary to show a fracture. Three fractures in particular are subtle and are commonly overlooked. They are as follows:

- An osteochondral fracture of the talar dome
- A fracture of the anterior process of the calcaneum
- A fracture of the posterior process of the talus

The base of the fifth metatarsal is also often included in an ankle series and if so should be examined for an avulsion fracture.

Routine views

The anteroposterior view is taken with 15°–20° of internal rotation of the foot to demonstrate better the medial articular space.

The lateral view requires slight internal rotation of the foot and a small sponge is placed under the lateral aspect of the forefoot. Both malleoli should be superimposed in the correctly positioned film.

An oblique view with 45° internal rotation demonstrates the lateral joint space and the lateral corner of the dome of the talus. To prevent the calcaneum overlying the tip of the lateral malleolus, the foot is dorsiflexed.

Additional views

With 45° of external rotation a further view of the talar dome is obtained when there is a clinical suspicion of an osteochondral fracture. This is known as the opposite oblique view.

In the plantar flexion view of the talar dome, a fracture may be seen on this projection which cannot be seen with other views (Fig. 14.21).

Anteroposterior radiographs to obtain stress views with both varus and valgus stress and lateral radiographs with anterior and posterior stress may be used to assess ligamentous damage in the ankle.

The identification of an effusion depends on retaining the soft tissue detail. This can be seen in the lateral soft tissue view.

OVERUSE

In the region of the ankle joint, stress fractures often occur in the distal shaft of the fibula and the distal tibial metaphysis. With more chronic overuse, impingements may occur with plantar and dorsiflexion of the ankle joint. Anterior impingements are usually due to an anterior tibial spur, with a further contribution being made by a bony spur arising from the dorsal aspect of the neck of the talus (produced by stress at the insertion of the anterior capsular ligament). A posterior impingement is most often due to a posterior tibial spur impinging on a prominent posterior process of the talus or an os trigonum. In ballet dancers the presence of an os trigonum alone may produce an impingement.

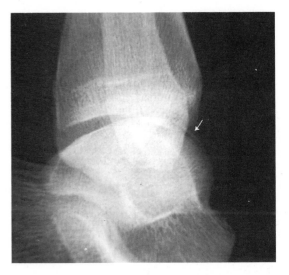

Fig. 14.21 With dorsiflexion of the ankle, an osteochondral fragment has been separated from the talar dome. The fragment would not have been detected on a neutral lateral view due to superimposition of the malleoli over the talar dome.

Routine views

These views are identical to those taken for trauma.

Additional views

As with stress fractures elsewhere, a progress examination after 10–14 days will help with the diagnosis (Fig. 14.22).

Plantar and dorsiflexion lateral views are useful in demonstrating the presence of anterior and posterior impingements.

Occasionally, calcification indicative of calcific tendinitis can also be identified in a soft tissue lateral view.

Heel and Tarsal Region

Sporting injuries in this region may include the following:

- Stress fractures may involve the talus adjacent to the subtalar joint and are also seen in the calcaneum, the navicular and the cuboid
- Degenerative joint changes
- Haglund's syndrome (Pavlov *et al.* 1982)

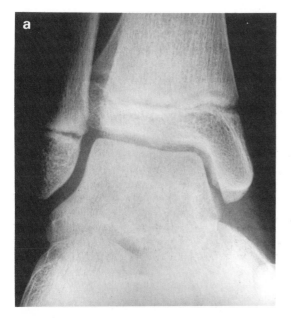

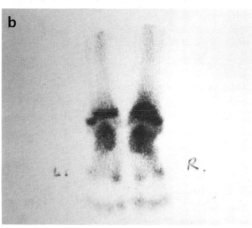

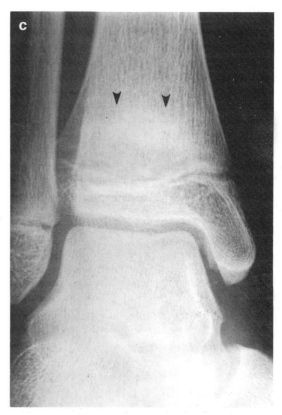

Fig. 14.22 A schoolboy cross-country runner developed a painful ankle. (a) The initial examination is normal. (b) A bone scan, however, was abnormal, with increased uptake of isotope in the distal tibial metaphysis. (c) A progress film in 10 days shows the classic appearance of a stress fracture (arrows).

- Plantar fasciitis
- Osteochondral fracture of the navicular

Routine views

Subtalar joint The internal oblique view of this joint is similar to an internal oblique view of the ankle joint, except that the X-ray beam is angled at 15° towards the head and the beam is centred 3 cm below the lateral malleolus. Forty degrees of angulation shows the posterior articulation of the subtalar joint and 20°–30° demonstrates the middle articulation. Fifteen degrees, however, produces a good overall view of the three articular surfaces.

In the external oblique view the beam is angled at 15° to the head and is centred 2.5 cm below the medial malleolus.

The axial Harris-Beath view is similar to a penetrated axial view of the calcaneum with slight internal rotation of the foot defining the posterior subtalar articulation, the middle articulation and the anterior articulation between the talus and calcaneum adjacent to the talocalcaneonavicular joint.

Stress fractures of the talus adjacent to the sub-talar joint may be difficult to identify as bony compression occurs and instead of the articular surfaces being parallel, some concavity of the talar articular surface results (Fig. 14.23).

Calcaneum Routine views of the calcaneum are taken in both the lateral and axial positions. Stress

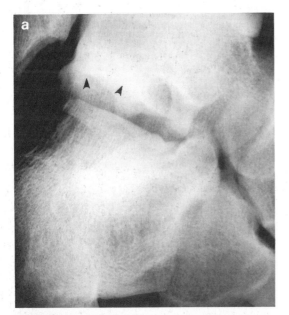

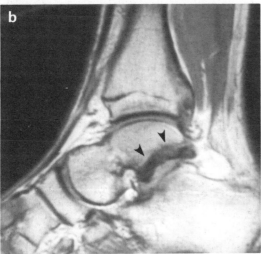

Fig. 14.23 (a) A cricketer with chronic ankle pain has bowing of the articular surface of the talus, shown in this view of the subtalar joint. (b) MRI confirms the presence of a stress fracture with some compression.

fractures of the calcaneum are characteristically identified as bands of sclerosis oriented parallel to the posterior margin of the calcaneum.

Mid-tarsal region A routine series includes the anteroposterior, oblique and lateral views. The anteroposterior view may demonstrate small fragments which have separated from the lateral aspect of both the calcaneum and cuboid bones characteristically occurring adjacent to the calcaneocuboid articulation. The oblique view of the foot is the best single view in assessing the mid-tarsal joints and is also helpful in profiling the anterior process of the calcaneum, which is a commonly overlooked site of fracture. Small fragments separated from the dorsal aspect of the head of the talus and navicular usually require a lateral view.

Additional views

Navicular views An anteroposterior view with elevation of the forefoot profiles the articular surfaces of both the talonavicular and naviculo-cuneiform articulations. Slight external rotation of the foot allows better demonstration of the tubercle of the navicular. The diagnosis of stress fractures of the navicular is often delayed, due to its often vague presentation and difficulty in seeing the fracture on a plain film (Kahn et al. 1992). Bone scans and CT play an important role in this diagnosis.

Soft tissue lateral view A lateral view of the heel is helpful in demonstrating Haglund's syndrome (Fig. 14.24).

A soft tissue lateral view demonstrates the presence of plantar fasciitis. In the acute stage there is localized soft tissue swelling with resultant loss or displacement of normal tissue planes. More chronic changes are characterized by the presence of a plantar (calcaneal) spur and possibly calcification within the plantar fascia.

The margins of the Achilles tendon are well defined in a soft tissue lateral view and acute rupture results in widening of the tendon, loss of the normal sharp delineation between the tendon and adjacent fat and the pre-Achilles fat pad is partially obliterated.

Achilles tendinitis can be diagnosed by calcifi-

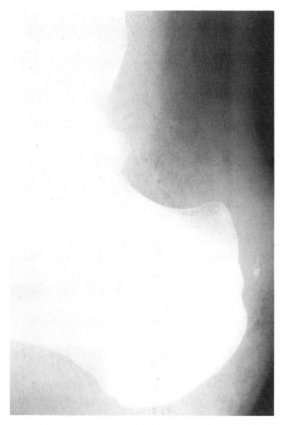

Fig. 14.24 The changes of Haglund's syndrome are present with: (a) Achilles tendinitis manifest by thickening of the tendon and calcification within the tendon. (b) Obliteration of the angle between the Achilles tendon and the calcaneum produced by retrocalcaneal bursitis. (c) A prominent bursal projection. (d) Swelling over the Achilles insertion produced by tendo-Achilles bursitis.

cation within the Achilles tendon or possibly by localized expansion of the tendon. This change is better defined by MRI or ultrasound scan.

The Forefoot

Sport may produce stress fractures of the metatarsals, changes in the sesamoid bones or an avulsion fracture of the base of the fifth metatarsal.

Routine views

These are taken in the anteroposterior and oblique projections.

Additional views

Sesamoid views The sesamoid bones can be profiled either by the patient lying prone with the toes dorsiflexed or in the supine position with the great toe held in dorsiflexion. The X-ray beam is directed tangentially, clearly demonstrating both sesamoids and their articulations with the head of the first metatarsal. Acute fracture of a sesamoid may be seen after acute trauma, but the most common change follows overuse with avascular necrosis, compression and fragmentation affecting the sesamoid (Fig. 14.25).

Progress views Metatarsal stress fractures are relatively common in athletes and with continuing pain, progress films are useful. Often a fracture line cannot be detected and a localized periosteal

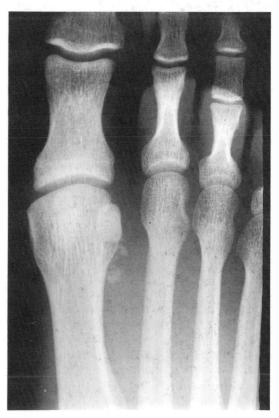

Fig. 14.25 A painful foot in a young cricketer shows fragmentation and distraction of the proximal pole of the lateral sesamoid. This has occurred as the result of stress.

reaction may be the only finding. In ballet dancers a diffuse thickening of the cortex of the second, and often third, metatarsals usually develops in response to stress. In this group, stress fractures of the base of the second metatarsal characteristically occur and may only be seen on MRI (Harrington *et al.* 1993).

Of particular interest is the fracture of the proximal shaft of the fifth metatarsal (to be distinguished from the avulsion fracture at the base of the fifth metatarsal). This fracture of the shaft, known as a Jones' fracture, may be either a stress fracture or follow an acute injury. Because it heals slowly, progress films of a Jones' fracture are important to assess union, as non-union is a common complication of this fracture.

Lateral view A lateral view may be useful in assessing the alignment of a metatarsal fracture and soft tissue changes on both the plantar and dorsal aspects of the metatarsals.

CONVENTIONAL TOMOGRAPHY

Complicated tomographic procedures have now been effectively replaced by CT and MRI. However, where anatomy is complicated by overlapping bones, conventional tomography can be a quick, cheap and efficient method of demonstrating the anatomy and defining pathological changes.

Complex joints such as the temporomandibular, sternoclavicular, atlanto-axial and apophyseal joints can be very easily defined. If a spinous process of a thoracic vertebra or a sternal fracture is to be demonstrated, a tomogram in the lateral position can quickly supply the required definition. Clinicians tend to think only of the high technology modalities of CT and MRI when often simple tomography can provide the answer.

NUCLEAR MEDICINE

In nuclear medicine the patient is given a radioactive isotope attached to a pharmaceutical, which is designed to localize in a specific tissue or enter a particular metabolic pathway in the body. It is then tracked, using a detector called a gamma camera. Compared with X-rays, the nuclear medicine procedure is less a representation of anatomy and much more an indicator of physiological and biochemical processes.

Equipment

The nuclear medicine department should be able to perform both planar and tomographic imaging. For planar imaging the gamma camera can operate either in stationary mode for spot views of one region at a time, or in sweep mode to survey the whole skeleton quickly but with slightly less resolution. The tomographic capability is known as single photon emission computerized tomography (SPECT). In this method the gamma camera rotates around the patient detecting the gamma ray emissions. A computer subsequently reconstructs the data to map the distribution of the isotope in slices, usually in three orthogonal planes (transverse, coronal and sagittal). The method is the emission equivalent of X-ray CT.

The Technetium Bone Scan

The radioactive isotope technetium-99m is complexed with methylene diphosphonate (MDP) for bone scanning. Following an intravenous injection, it is tracked through the perfusion or dynamic phase and after several minutes of equilibration, a blood pool image may be obtained (Fig. 14.26a). After 2 or 3 h, delayed images show activity in the skeleton. This is often referred to as a 'three-phase bone scan'. The first phase is the radionuclide angiogram; the second is the blood pool image; the delayed image represents the third phase.

Radiation Dosimetry

The wide distribution of the radiopharmaceutical results in radiation exposure to various organs (Weber *et al.* 1989). This is compared with the exposure from standard X-rays in Table 14.1. Drinking additional water and frequent bladder emptying reduces radiation to the bladder and nearby structures such as the gonads, bone marrow and fetus. Bone scans are usually avoided on pregnant patients. The calculated dose to the fetus is

Fig. 14.26 Stress fractures.
(a) A blood pool image with hyperaemia in the mid-shaft of both tibiae. (b) A delayed anterior image with bilateral tibial stress fractures and a stress fracture of the shaft of the second left metatarsal. (c) A lateral view of a left tibial stress fracture, Grade II. (d) A lateral view of the right tibial stress fracture, Grade I.

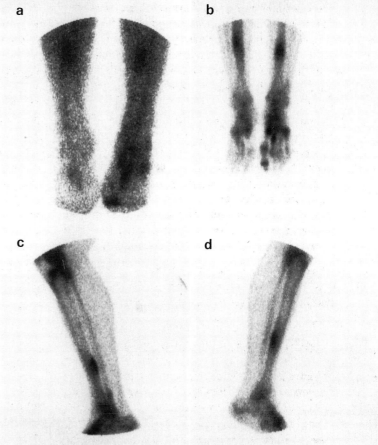

acceptably low, however, should this occur (Hendrick *et al.* 1988).

Nursing mothers having bone scans with technetium-99m–MDP have been advised to discard milk produced during the first 4 h after tracer administration and then to resume breast feeding (Romney *et al.* 1986).

Normal and Pathological Bone Scan

The bone agent is deposited predominantly in association with the calcium phosphate complex. The degree of uptake is related to the local blood supply and activity of the local osteoblastic process. Sites of bone stress will therefore show increased

Table 14.1 A comparison of radiation doses from a standard bone scan and X-rays of the spine and pelvis (mGy)

	Bone scan dose from 15 mCi (570 MBq) technetium ^{99}m	X-ray dose lumbosacral spine, pelvis (anteroposterior and lateral)	
Bone surfaces	34.5		
Bladder wall	19.5		
Red bone marrow	5.0		
Ovary	1.8	2.61	0.75
Testis	1.2	0.04	0.86

Zwas *et al.* (1987).

uptake due to increased remodelling. The bone scan is thus able to distinguish metabolically active from inactive pathology, to separate older injuries from more recent ones, and to monitor the response to therapy.

The bone scan is extremely sensitive in reflecting early pathological changes. In contrast, X-rays demonstrate pathology in terms of relative increase or decrease of bone mineral, a process which may take weeks or months to develop a recognizable pattern of disturbance such as the X-ray appearance of a stress fracture. They often, however, give a much more specific diagnosis, and correlation of the scan with corresponding X-rays is often necessary.

Because of the shared local blood supply, synovitis for example causes increased uptake in periarticular bone. Not uncommonly, the area of increased uptake on the bone scan may be more extensive than the precise limits of the pathology, a feature attributed to local hyperaemia. The kidneys and bladder are seen normally and urine contamination may cause artefacts. Extraosseous activity may also be seen in the breasts, calcified areas (cartilage, myositis ossificans) and rhabdomyolysis.

Clinical Implications of Bone Scan Sensitivity to Accelerated Remodelling

The following implications should be noted:

- The bone scan provides an objective assessment regarding the presence of bone pathology in patients with symptoms difficult to evaluate and may often be the only positive objective finding
- It is so sensitive that a negative study strongly suggests that soft tissue is the more likely cause of symptoms
- The early recognition of bone stress should allow therapeutic intervention before the development of more serious injury, resulting in less disruption to training
- When the isotope uptake pattern is non-specific, it is important to consider carefully the scan in its clinical context and to correlate it with X-rays when necessary

- Areas of increased uptake gradually become less intense over a period of months. This helps distinguish old from recent events and may predict a risk of recurrence of symptoms if full activity is resumed
- X-ray positive and bone scan negative findings usually indicate old changes unlikely to be the cause of present symptoms
- Understanding the underlying physiological basis of bone scan isotope uptake helps explain areas of increased cortical uptake in asymptomatic but very active individuals
- In general a normal X-ray should be followed by a bone scan for patients with persisting symptoms. Not uncommonly patients have distressing symptoms which persist for weeks or months undiagnosed, because investigation ceased after an initial X-ray

Bone Stress

Roub et al. (1979; Fig. 14.27) developed a concept of bone reaction to stress by a process of remodelling as a continuum, beginning with mild changes in an asymptomatic individual. They saw this continuing through to the point of clinical fracture and incorporated into it the spectra of changes seen on bone scan and X-rays. They suggested that a stress fracture was a part of this continuum, rather than an isolated event and so included the stage of focal uptake on the bone scan in a symptomatic patient, usually weeks before the X-ray became positive. Scintigraphic uptake at non-painful sites in athletes is also part of this continuum (Matheson et al. 1987).

Stress Fractures

Radionuclide bone scanning is the imaging method of choice for demonstrating stress fractures (Daffner & Pavlov 1992). It is rarely negative early in the course of a stress injury and while the appearance is not specific, when taken in the clinical context, other causes rarely confuse.

A system of grading stress fractures has been prepared by Zwas et al. (1987), as is shown in Table 14.2. This assessment requires two orthogonal views

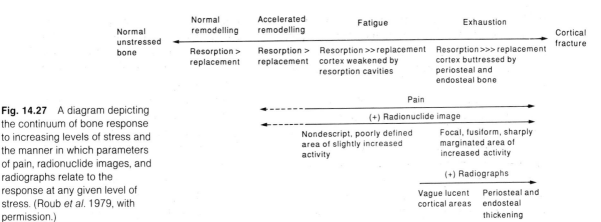

Normal unstressed bone	Normal remodelling	Accelerated remodelling	Fatigue	Exhaustion	Cortical fracture
	Resorption > replacement	Resorption > replacement	Resorption >> replacement cortex weakened by resorption cavities	Resorption >>> replacement cortex buttressed by periosteal and endosteal bone	

Fig. 14.27 A diagram depicting the continuum of bone response to increasing levels of stress and the manner in which parameters of pain, radionuclide images, and radiographs relate to the response at any given level of stress. (Roub *et al.* 1979, with permission.)

Pain

(+) Radionuclide image

Nondescript, poorly defined area of slightly increased activity

Focal, fusiform, sharply marginated area of increased activity

(+) Radiographs

Vague lucent cortical areas

Periosteal and endosteal thickening

on the delayed images (Fig. 14.26). Hyperaemia on the dynamic and blood pool phase is not necessary for the diagnosis of stress fractures but it is an increasing feature of the more severe grades of injury. The more advanced grades require much stricter and longer curtailment of activity. Grade 1 and 2 abnormalities usually return to normal on the bone scan by 2–3 months, while Grade 4 abnormalities may take 6 months or more (Matin 1979).

'Shin Splints' (Medial Tibial Stress Syndrome; Mubarak *et al.* 1982)

In this condition, delayed phase images show linear increase in cortical uptake of the isotope, often of varying intensity and corresponding to the posteromedial portion of the tibia in its distal two-thirds, that is at the attachment of the soleus muscle (Fig. 14.28). The dynamic and blood pool phases are

Table 14.2 Grades of stress fracture (bone scan appearance)

Grade	Description
1	Small, ill-defined lesion with mildly increased activity in the cortical region
2	Larger than Grade 1, well-defined, elongated with moderately increased activity in the cortical region
3	Wide fusiform lesion with highly increased activity in the corticomedullary region
4	Wide extensive lesion with intensely increased activity in the transcorticomedullary region

normal. A similar traction periosteal reaction may be seen anteriorly (tibialis anterior) and in the medial fibula (tibialis posterior or flexor hallucis longus). The differentiation of stress fractures from 'shin splints' is a major contribution of the bone scan; however, this is occasionally difficult and the two may coexist.

Low Back Pain

Among the many causes of low back pain the main contributions of the bone scan are as follows:

- The diagnosis of recent stress fractures of the pars interarticularis, when the X-ray is frequently negative (Fig. 14.29)
- The further evaluation of pars defects seen on plain X-rays, where a negative scan usually indicates an old injury which is not responsible for the patient's symptoms

SPECT imaging greatly improves the sensitivity and accuracy of the procedure (Bellah *et al.* 1991) by improving the inherent contrast between the abnormality and the normal bone, as well as providing more accurate localization. Early detection is obviously important for management and a progress study may also be helpful in planning return to competition (Jackson *et al.* 1981). The scan sometimes shows an abnormality in the pars opposite to the one with a stress fracture. It is usually less intense and is due to secondary strain

Fig. 14.28 A medial tibial stress syndrome (bilateral 'shin splints'). BP = blood pool image, which is normal. All other views are delayed and show in different views the pattern of extended patchy uptake along the posteromedial cortex.

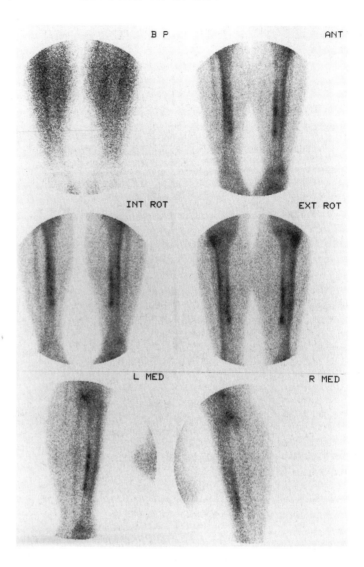

consequent upon the primary lesions. For the same reason scan uptake is sometimes seen on the opposite side to that of a well established spondylolysis (Elliott *et al.* 1988).

Occasionally, the scan detects other causes of back pain not discovered on X-rays, such as sacroiliitis, subtle fractures of the vertebral end plates and spinous or transverse process, osteomyelitis, osteoid osteoma, osteoblastoma or even malignant tumours. Figure 14.29e shows a lesion in the lamina of a vertebra localized on a scan which was not seen on plain X-ray and subsequently proven to be an osteoid osteoma at surgery.

Enthesopathy

The insertions of tendons and ligaments into bone may also produce increased remodelling which is secondary to traction trauma. Sports enthesopathies therefore usually demonstrate increased uptake at these sites, which may be useful in differential diagnosis (Fig. 14.30).

Fractures

The bone scan can be very valuable in occult fractures. The best examples are the scaphoid bone,

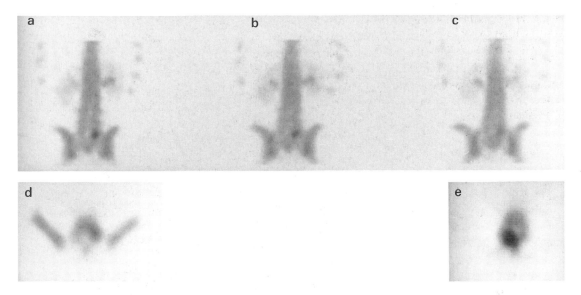

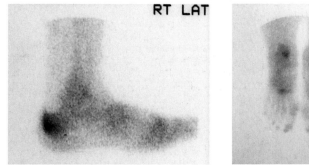

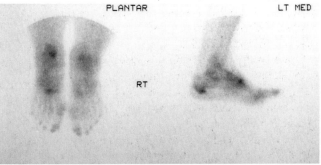

Fig. 14.29 A pars interarticularis stress fracture and osteoid osteoma of the lamina (a–c) Coronal reconstructions of a SPECT study of a lumbosacral spine of a patient with a stress fracture of the pars interarticularis of the left side of L5 A focal area of increased uptake is seen on those slices near to the vertebral body (d) A transverse reconstruction through stress fracture of the same patient as in a–c (e) A transverse reconstruction of a SPECT study in a patient with an osteoid osteoma Note that the focus is centred on the lamina, an unusual site for a stress fracture

the neck of the femur, ribs and osteochondral fractures of the talar dome and around the knee. Bone scintigraphy has been shown to be a good screening procedure which can exclude a talar dome fracture (Urman *et al.* 1991; Fig. 14.31). In a blinded prospective study of patients who sustained an acute internal derangement of the knee Marks *et al.* (1992) found bone scintigraphy detected all the subchondral fractures demonstrated on MRI as well as avulsions of ligaments and more subtle MRI — silent bone injuries.

It has been demonstrated that the bone scan is positive within 24 h in 95% of patients under 64 years of age and is very rarely negative in anyone with a fracture which is at least 3 days old (Matin 1979). Different bones behave differently with fractures in the vicinity of joints showing early uptake and rapidly becoming intense in a few days whereas fractures of the axial skeleton and shafts of long bones take significantly longer (Spitz *et al.* 1993). Peak activity is reached 2–5 weeks after

Fig. 14.30 (a) An Achilles insertion tendinopathy (b) A plantar fasciitis

trauma. Persistence of scan abnormalities depends also on the presence of fixation devices and any malalignment. Rib fractures normalize most quickly, with 80% of them normal by 1 year. Long bones and vertebrae often take more than a year and in unfavourable circumstances may take many years to become normal.

Joint Injuries and Joint Disease

The bone scan is very sensitive to synovitis and to the early changes of degenerative disease, which has a characteristic appearance. It has been shown to be useful in identifying acute ligamentous injuries and subchondral plate fractures. In the evaluation of knee pain a high sensitivity for both chondromalacia (Kohn *et al.* 1988) and meniscal lesions (Marymont *et al.* 1983; Mooar *et al.* 1987) has been demonstrated.

Muscle Injuries

Bone scan agents have been known for years to localize in recent myocardial infarctions and have been used to assist with this diagnosis. Whatever the mechanism, and there are many theories, the bone agents localize in injured skeletal muscle as well as in the smooth muscle of the heart.

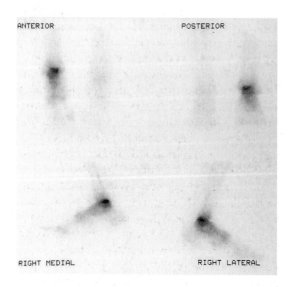

Fig. 14.31 A talar dome fracture

Reflex Sympathetic Dystrophy

The typical appearance of a positive three phase bone scan in reflex sympathetic dystrophy is as follows:

- An increased blood pool on the radionuclide angiogram
- Increased activity on the blood pool image
- Diffuse periarticular increase in activity on the delayed images (Holder *et al.* 1992; Fig. 14.32)

The appearances on the radionuclide angiogram and blood pool images have been variable and an atypical pattern where both have been reduced has been described by Heck (1987).

DIAGNOSTIC ULTRASOUND

Diagnostic ultrasound initially found wide application in obstetrics, especially after the development of grey scale imaging in the early 1970s. It has since found innumerable applications throughout the body, especially in the abdomen and the pelvis. Muscle and tendon ultrasound is a more recent application, which has been facilitated by the development of high frequency transducers with a

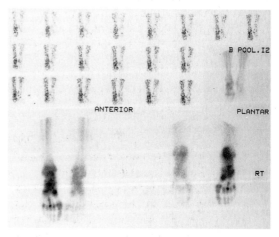

Fig. 14.32 Reflex sympathetic dystrophy. Note the increased activity in the affected right limb on the angiogram and blood pool images. The delayed images show increased periarticular uptake throughout the right foot. Note also the stress fracture in the third right metatarsal.

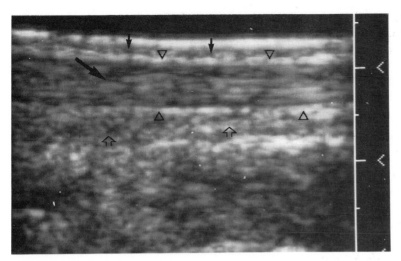

Fig. 14.33 A normal Achilles tendon. Peritendon (arrowheads); tendon (large arrow); retro-Achilles fat (small open arrows); subcutaneous fat (small closed arrows).

much improved near field resolution and real time capability. There is no doubt that this increasing use is attributable to its safety and the profound technological improvements.

The fundamental principle of diagnostic ultrasound is to interrogate the tissues with pulses of high frequency sound, usually in the range of 2–10 MHz and to use the time between pulses to record the echoes returning from tissue interfaces. The echoes are processed in terms of their location of origin and their amplitude and from this information a grey scale image is obtained of a cross-section of tissue examined by the sound beam.

Technical Factors

There are several technical factors of which the reader should be aware. They are as follows:

- As most muscles and tendons of clinical relevance are superficial, high frequency transducers can be used to give very detailed images
- The region of the image adjacent to the transducer is prone to artefacts and inferior resolution and when imaging very superficial structures, such as the Achilles tendon, it is necessary to interpose a thick coupling layer of material between the transducer and the skin surface. This is usually a water bag or pliable gel
- When scanning muscles and especially tendons, it is important to keep the ultrasound beam

perpendicular to the direction of the muscle or tendon fibres. Echoes are returned from the fibres only when the sound beam strikes them at 90° or close to it. This is possible only with linear array transducers and sector scanners are not suitable. Sports medicine clinicians should ensure that this equipment is available before requesting these investigations

Normal Appearances

The normal tendon has a wavy linear pattern on longitudinal scans (Fig. 14.33). Provided the ultrasound beam is perpendicular, it is considerably more echogenic than muscle and usually a little less echogenic than subcutaneous fat. The peritendon appears as a thin echogenic line on both sides of the tendon on central longitudinal scans. Muscles are quite hypoechoic and longitudinal scans show oblique echogenic bands corresponding to the supporting connective tissue. The sound does not penetrate through bones and the tissues behind the bone lie in an acoustic shadow (Fig. 14.34).

Most muscles, tendons, bursae, fascial planes, vessels and even the larger nerves are now accessible to high resolution imaging with ultrasound, both at rest and during movement. As ultrasonologists become increasingly familiar with the anatomy and the range of normal and pathological appearances, many more valuable uses will be found for its use in sports medicine.

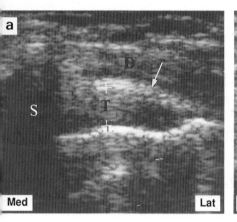

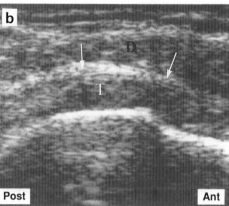

Fig. 14.34 A normal rotator cuff. (a) A longitudinal echogram of the normal rotator cuff. (b) A transverse echogram of the normal rotator cuff. D = deltoid muscle. T = rotator cuff tendon. S = acoustic shadow behind the acromion. Arrows indicate the plane of the subdeltoid bursa.

Pathological Appearances

Ultrasound enables identification of the pathological state of tendons and surrounding soft tissues and of both inflammatory and degenerative changes in nature.

The early changes of tendinitis do not cause recognizable changes on ultrasound. Swelling, which can be difficult to assess, may be the only sign.

Reduced echogenicity and loss of the normal longitudinally organized wavy texture are signs of more severe tendinitis (Figs 14.35 and 14.36). Calcific changes are generally easily appreciated, as is shown in Fig. 14.37.

Increased echogenicity of Kager's triangle has been described as a sign of peritendinitis of the Achilles tendon and thickening of the peritendon is

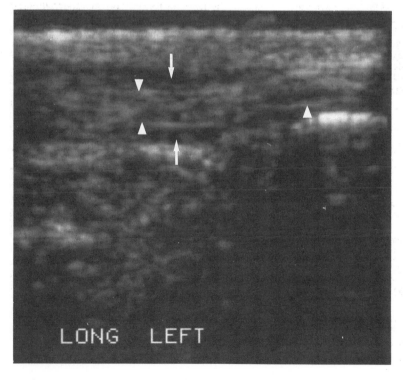

Fig. 14.35 A diffuse tendinitis and peritendinitis of the Achilles tendon. Boundaries of abnormal tendon (arrowheads); hypoechoic thickening of the peritendon (arrows).

readily appreciated, albeit sometimes with indistinct boundaries between the tendon itself and its surrounding tissues.

Acute tears, as in the Achilles tendon, result in markedly hypoechoic areas representing haematomas between the torn ends (Fig. 14.38). These areas are usually arranged transversely but are sometimes longitudinal. A similar appearance, but not quite as hypoechoic, is seen in patellar tendinitis (jumper's knee) in the tendon immediately below the lower pole of the patella (Fig. 14.39).

Chronic tears, as in the rotator cuff, result in localized thinning of, or a defect in, the tendon (Fig. 14.40).

Cystic lesions may be recognized as in the Achilles and patellar tendons and bursitis is recognized as a layer of fluid in the plane of the bursa (Fig. 14.41).

Compressive muscle injuries (contusions) when imaged acutely (Fig. 14.42a) are echogenic and may be ill-defined becoming hypoechoic and better defined over the next few days (Fig. 14.42b). Echogenicity returns as healing progresses. Haematomas are initially hypoechoic and may show posterior acoustic enhancement like other fluid collections. With time they gradually resorb and are replaced by more echogenic reparative tissue.

Painful foci in tendons (Fig. 14.43) and some muscle haematomas may be very small; therefore, when scanning these patients it is most important to pay careful attention to the precise area of tenderness if many abnormalities are not to be overlooked.

Specific Examples of the Use of Ultrasound in Sports Medicine

ACHILLES TENDON

Ultrasound can diagnose partial (Fig. 14.38) and complete tears in this tendon. The gap between the frayed ends of the torn tendon can be measured to help decide whether surgery is necessary.

Ultrasound can probably provide objective evidence of the degree of damage to the tendon in cases of chronic tendinitis (Figs 14. 35 and 14.36) and may thereby help in deciding whether to persist with conservative measures or whether to recom-

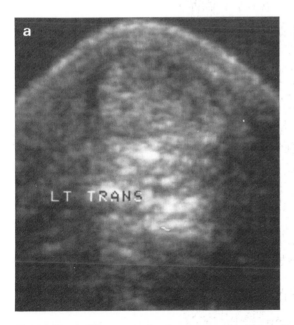 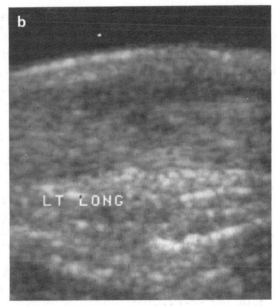

Fig. 14.36 A diffuse severe tendon degeneration The peritendon is involved but is more difficult to differentiate from the tendon than in the case illustrated in Fig. 14.35. (a) Transverse echogram. Multiple tiny hypoechoic foci (?cystic) are seen throughout the tendon. (b) Longitudinal echogram. Note the marked thickening of the tendon with gross disruption of the normal wavy linear appearance of the tendon.

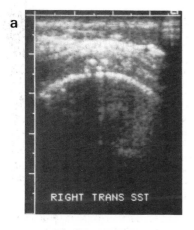

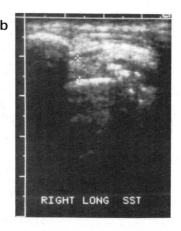

Fig. 14.37 A calcific tendinitis of the supraspinatus tendon. (a) A transverse echogram of the right rotator cuff. (b) Longitudinal echogram of the right supraspinatus tendon (SST). Cursors mark the superficial and deep limits of the tendon. Note the cluster of highly echogenic foci of calcification.

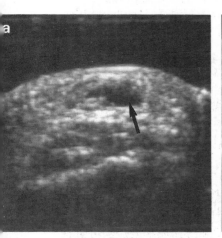

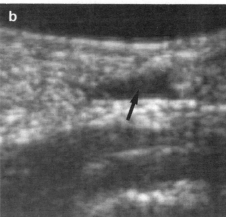

Fig. 14.38 An Achilles tendon tear. (a) A transverse echogram. The arrow points to an irregular hypoechoic region medially representing the area of disruption. (b) A longitudinal echogram. The arrow points to the tear.

mend surgery. According to Mathieson *et al.* (1988) a normal ultrasound in a symptomatic patient may reliably predict a successful response to conservative therapy; however, the place of ultrasound imaging of the Achilles tendon is still being evaluated.

KNEE LESIONS

Tears of the patellar tendon, tendinitis, bursitis involving any of the many bursae around the knee, cartilaginous and bony loose bodies, Baker's cysts and their rupture are all readily recognized.

Patellar tendinitis (jumper's knee) is characterized by an irregular hypoechoic area situated centrally in the tendon, just below the inferior pole of the patella. This usually extends along the tendon for 1 or 2 cm with associated local swelling (Fig. 14.39). Occasionally, tendinitis extends the whole length

of the tendon with thickening and abnormal echo appearance.

ROTATOR CUFF

The evaluation of the rotator cuff is one of the most difficult in diagnostic ultrasound and consequently the most operator dependent. Many imaging modalities have been applied to the problem of subacromial pain syndrome and Stiles and Otte (1993) have recently provided an excellent review of their strengths and limitations. Some authors have reported a high rate of successful identification of complete tears with ultrasound. Figure 14.34 depicts the appearance of the normal rotator cuff. When the cuff tears the deltoid muscle and subdeltoid bursa and fat fall into the space created and in so doing move closer to the humeral head, thereby

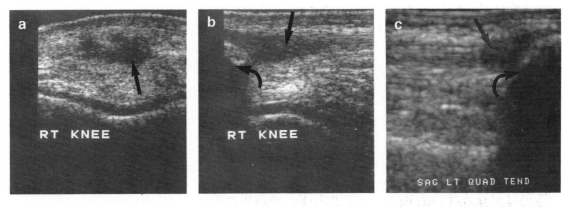

Fig. 14.39 A patellar tendinitis. (a) A transverse echogram. Note the irregular hypoechoic region expanding the central portion of the patellar tendon. (b) A longitudinal echogram. Note the focal hypoechoic area within the tendon extending inferiorly from the lower pole of the patella. (c) A quadriceps tendinitis. Note the similar appearance to a patellar tendinitis occurring in the quadriceps tendon immediately above the patella. Area of tendinitis (straight arrows); inferior and superior poles of the patella (curved arrows).

Fig. 14.40 A complete tear of the rotator cuff. (a) A normal tendon on the left side. Cursors indicate the superficial and deep limits of the tendon. (b) A complete tear on the right side. Arrows indicate plane of defect due to rupture.

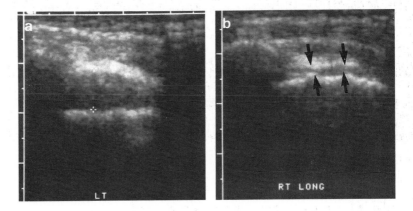

causing a contour abnormality of the deep surface of the deltoid. With complete avulsion of the cuff from the greater tuberosity it retracts under the acromion and is no longer visualized (Fig. 14.40). With small or partial tears the contour abnormality and focal thinning may be subtle. Fluid is commonly seen in the subdeltoid bursa. Details of the technique, diagnostic criteria and pitfalls are well described by Middleton (1992). The biceps tendon is easily examined with ultrasound and is a routine part of the shoulder examination. Abnormalities frequently exist with rotator cuff pathology.

CALF PAIN

Ultrasound is extremely valuable in the diagnosis of acute calf pain. Muscle tears are readily recognized. Blood is often seen between the soleus and gastrocnemius muscles thought to be due to a tear at the muscle–aponeurosis boundary.

The differential diagnosis may include superficial or deep venous thrombosis and ultrasound has largely replaced X-ray venography as the modality of choice for diagnosing or excluding venous thrombosis. The secret of gaining an accurate diagnosis of the cause of calf pain using ultrasound, is

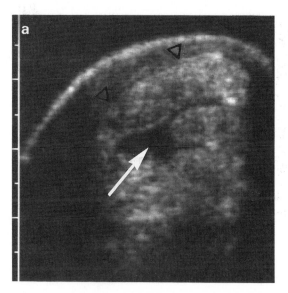 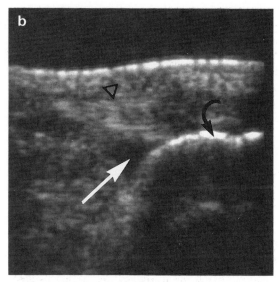

Fig. 14.41 A retro-Achilles bursitis. (a) A transverse echogram of the right Achilles tendon. Note the anechoic layer of fluid deep to the tendon and pooling also deep to the medial side. (b) A longitudinal echogram. Posterior surface of the Achilles tendon (arrowheads); fluid in the bursa (white arrow); posterior surface of the os calcis (curved arrow).

to pay particular attention to the precise area(s) of pain and tenderness indicated by the patient and not be confined to a protocol where only the veins are examined.

ARTHROGRAPHY

Valuable information about joints, tendon sheaths and bursae can be obtained by the introduction of a contrast medium and then imaging by routine radiography, conventional tomography or CT.

Since the introduction of these techniques, the development of arthroscopy and arthroscopic surgery have caused modification of the indications and methods of arthrography. Now with the introduction of MRI, further inroads have been made into the place of arthrography and it is conceivable that all arthrography will eventually be replaced by non-invasive imaging techniques. At the present time, arthrography is useful in the wrist and shoulder joints with a possible application in the elbow, hip, knee and ankle also.

Wrist Joint

Following sporting injuries, arthrography of the wrist may be used to diagnose injuries to the triangular fibrocartilage or interosseous ligaments. The wrist joint is divided into four separate compartments which are as follows:

- The first carpometacarpal compartment
- The carpometacarpal cavity extending between the distal row of carpal bones and the bases of the second, third, fourth and fifth metacarpals
- A mid-carpal cavity, extending between the proximal and distal carpal rows
- The radiocarpal cavity which is separated from the inferior radio-ulnar cavity by the triangular fibrocartilage

Following trauma, if communication can be demonstrated between these cavities, injury to interosseous ligaments or the triangular fibrocartilage has occurred (Fig. 14.44).

Opacification of tendon sheaths and bursae has limited clinical application in the hand and wrist;

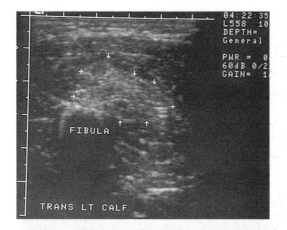

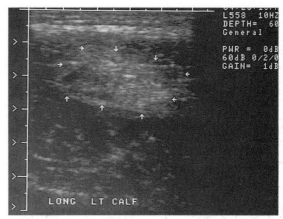

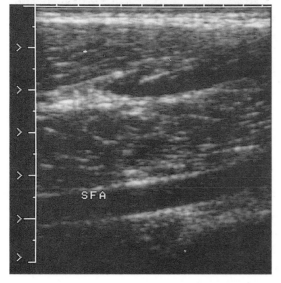

Fig. 14.42 (a) Area of increased echogenicity 1 day after muscle injury. (b) Haematoma in muscle several weeks old showing small fluid area and torn muscle, which on real-time imaging could be seen to move in the fluid area with transducer pressure (bell-clapper sign). SFA = superficial femoral artery.

however, these soft tissue structures, particularly in the carpal tunnel, can be well demonstrated by MRI.

Shoulder Joint

Following sporting injury, there are two indications for shoulder arthrography, namely:

- Rotator cuff tears
- The identification of glenoid rim fractures

ROTATOR CUFF TEARS (BURK *ET AL.* 1989)

Following a complete tear, abnormal communication can be demonstrated between the glenohumeral joint cavity and the subacromial bursa. With the use of double contrast arthrography, the width of the tear can be identified and the adjacent rotator cuff tendons assessed.

With incomplete tears, either the deep or superficial surface of the rotator cuff may be involved. After a glenohumeral joint injection the partial tear on the inferior aspect of the tendon may be demonstrated with contrast medium entering the tear within the tendon. Tears on the superior surface of the tendon cannot be demonstrated on glenohumeral arthrography and can be difficult to demonstrate with subacromial bursography.

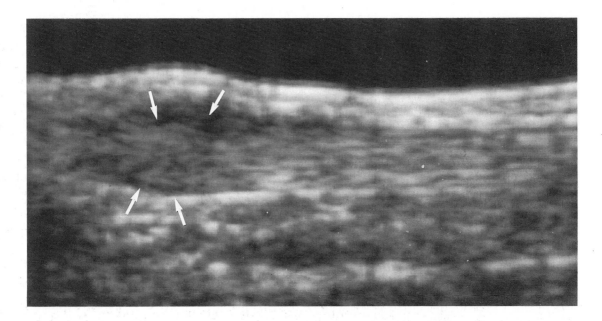

Fig. 14.43 A focal area of tendinitis and peritendinitis in the Achilles tendon, felt as a tender nodule. Note the slight swelling and decreased echogenicity of the tendon and the marked hypoechoic thickening of the peritendinous tissues (arrows).

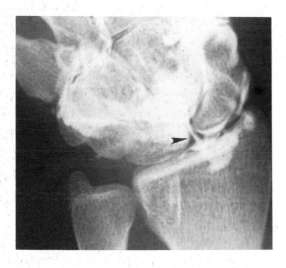

Fig. 14.44 Wrist arthrography demonstrates a rupture of the scapholunate ligament. The interpretation of this finding is difficult as this appearance is often seen in a 'normal' wrist after adolescence.

GLENOID RIM FRACTURES

Following a glenohumeral dislocation, the glenoid labrum can become completely detached. In this injury the osseous Bankart lesion can usually be seen with plain radiography, particularly employing a West Point view, but labral fragments or separated osteochondral fragments may require CT after double contrast arthrography for identification.

Other Joints

The role of arthrography in examination of the elbow, hip, knee and ankle has diminished with the availability of arthroscopy, CT and MRI. There may still be a place for double contrast arthrography in the elbow, hip and ankle to identify suspected intra-articular osteochondral loose bodies which cannot be detected by other means. It is sometimes difficult using other modalities to determine whether ossicles are loose bodies or if they lie outside the joint space, related to the capsule or the synovium.

The wide use of arthroscopy and availability of MRI have almost completely eliminated the indications for knee arthrography and when MRI becomes easily accessible, it is doubtful whether knee arthrography will continue to be performed.

COMPUTERIZED TOMOGRAPHY

The use of CT for musculoskeletal imaging has changed with the introduction of MRI and its place in diagnostic protocols will change further with increasing availability and development of MRI. Nevertheless, CT has a unique ability to display precise bone detail and even in centres where MRI is available, CT is usually the preferred method of imaging bone trauma. CT also has the advantages of being easily available and is currently a relatively low-cost method of imaging compared with MRI.

CT is particularly useful in those areas where plain film radiography is difficult. One such region is the spine and CT is indispensable when significant spinal injury has occurred. Adequate plain films are often difficult to acquire in the traumatized patient and CT can be used to establish the presence of a fracture or subluxation, and in particular to demonstrate displacement of fragments.

CT is playing a strong supporting role to plain film radiography as a means of diagnosing the presence of a fracture and delineating its extent, in anatomically complex regions. Following a sporting injury its major application is in the identification of small bony fragments and osteochondral bodies within joints. An example of its use is shown after hip trauma or dislocation, where CT provides considerable benefit in the imaging of the acetabulum and the femoral head. Bony superimposition and the curves of both the acetabulum and femoral head make identification of small fractures difficult on routine radiography (Fig. 14.45).

After glenohumeral dislocation, bony fragments separated from the glenoid rim may be identified by CT and if the separated fragment is largely cartilaginous, a CT examination after the introduction of air into the shoulder joint readily defines the fragment (Singson et al. 1987). Other occult fractures such as an osteochondral fracture of the dome of the talus (Fig. 14.46), a fracture of the hook of the hamate and osteochondral fractures around the knee joint are often best displayed by CT. With a high-resolution bone algorithm and appropriate window settings for bone detail, precise imaging can be achieved.

MRI has taken over the majority of the soft tissue imaging previously performed by CT. The major continuing contribution which is made by CT in defining soft tissues changes has been in the diagnosis of low back pain, demonstrating intervertebral disc herniations and the relationship of the herniation to the neighbouring nerve root. There is also an excellent demonstration of the epiphyseal joints.

CT remains the imaging method of choice for spinal injuries and low back pain, with much to offer in defining occult fractures and intra-articular osteochondral fragments. At the present time CT occupies a valuable position in many diagnostic protocols.

MAGNETIC RESONANCE IMAGING

MRI is a new technology which produces images of both bone and soft tissue. MRI offers considerable

Fig. 14.45 Small fractures around the hip joint are well shown by a CT scan. This case shows a fracture of the posterior margin of the acetabulum and a fragment of bone separated from the femoral head, lying within the joint.

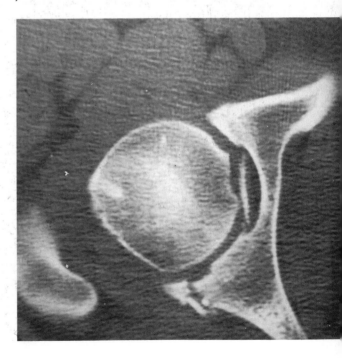

benefits in the diagnosis of sporting injuries with a non-invasive method of imaging injuries, some of which cannot be diagnosed by any other modality. An exhaustive discussion on the physics of MRI is beyond the purpose of this chapter; however, a knowledge of the general principles involved is useful in interpreting the images (Vaughan 1989). When the patient is placed in a strong magnetic field, the body's protons, previously oriented in a random manner, are aligned in the direction of the magnetic field. (The hydrogen proton is the basis of MRI because of its wide distribution in tissues.) These protons do not align perfectly with the axis of the field, but rotate around the axis. This is called precession. Each hydrogen proton precesses around the axis of the magnetic field (Z-axis) at a

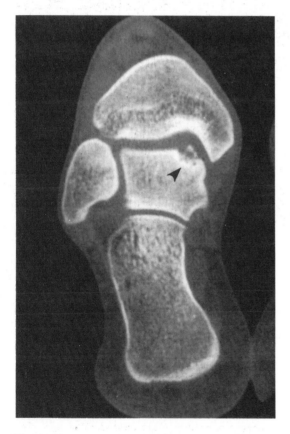

Fig. 14.46 Fragmentation of the medial corner of the talar dome is well demonstrated in this view. Sclerosis of the fracture bed indicates that the fracture is of long standing.

common frequency. With radiofrequency pulses, a further magnetic field is applied at 90° to the Z-axis at a resonant frequency of the hydrogen proton (in both X and Y axes). A pulse of sufficient strength is used to rotate the net magnetization vector into the transverse plane (90° pulse) or around into the opposite direction (180° pulse). When the radiofrequency pulse ceases, the protons return to their initial state of equilibrium in the Z-axis, at a rate dependent on the type of tissue. The return to equilibrium is called relaxation and is characterized by two time constraints, T_1 and T_2. T_1 is the time in which the strength of the magnetic field on the Z-axis has recovered 63% of its original value. Hydrogen protons in different tissues recover at different rates (T_1 ranges from 200 to 2000 ms). When the radiofrequency pulse ceases, the protons rotate in a random fashion causing loss of energy. There is a decay of the XY magnetism, losing 63% of its initial value in a time T_2 (most tissues have a T_2 between 20 and 300 ms). The movement of protons during this recovery produces a signal which differs for different tissues.

Fortunately, for most sports injuries, surface coils can be used to receive the MR signal, improving spatial resolution of the signal by reducing signal-to-noise ratio. This means that the part examined lies in the centre of the magnet to produce proton alignment in the Z-axis and the part is placed within a small coil that acts as a signal receiver. The resulting emitted radiofrequency signals of different frequency are computer reconstructed into an image, each point of which relates to the intensity of the MR signal obtained from a volume of tissue (voxel).

As with all modalities a differentiation between tissues and tissue planes is the basis of imaging and with MRI, image contrast results from a variety of factors including signal intensity, the pulse sequence used and the tissue's proton behaviour. The contrast in musculoskeletal MRI is largely dependent on fat, in fat pads, between tissue planes and within the bone marrow. Contrast between tissues can be increased by changing parameters and techniques. On T_1-weighted images a high signal is obtained from subcutaneous and marrow fat, while a lower signal is obtained from articular cartilage, with only a moderate signal from muscle and fluid. Ligaments, tendons and cortical bone have no signal intensity; therefore this spectrum lends itself extraordinarily well to musculoskeletal imaging. The major disadvantage of T_1-weighted imaging is differentiation between fluid, muscle and articular cartilage, which all have similar signals. This differentiation can be achieved by producing a T_2 weighted image, which displays fluid with a bright signal which is even more intense than fat, making the presence of a collection of fluid such as an effusion easy to identify (Fig. 14.47). Inflammatory reactions seen in sporting injuries have considerable fluid associated with the process and conditions such as tenosynovitis can be confidently diagnosed.

More recently developed techniques have markedly improved the display of subtle changes in the medulla, by suppressing the signal from normal fat. Bone bruising, stress fractures and subchondral bony changes are very well demonstrated (Fig. 14.48). Other sequences have enabled improved visualization of both synovium and articular cartilage (Peterfy *et al.* 1994). Gadolinium-containing compounds have helped to produce the MR arthrogram and, when administered intravenously, increase the signal intensity of the inflamed synovium.

Apart from the clear demonstration of anatomy, MRI provides other advantages. Unlike CT, any imaging plane can be selected that will display a particular anatomy. A further obvious advantage is the use of an electromagnetic field rather than ionizing irradiation and the method appears to be free of biological side-effects.

At the moment the high cost of MRI tends to act as a deterrent to its use. However, there has been some decrease not only in the initial cost of the equipment but also in its running costs. Nevertheless, even at its present level of cost, its ability to make definitive diagnoses makes the modality cost-effective, as a number of previously employed diagnostic steps can be omitted. This is particularly the case if the patient is a professional sportsperson or an elite athlete, when a delayed or incorrect diagnosis can affect his or her future. Currently, MRI should be included in the diagnostic protocol for a number of musculoskeletal conditions and it is certain that its use will greatly increase.

Bone Imaging

MRI is very sensitive to changes in bone marrow. On a T_1-weighted image these changes reduce the

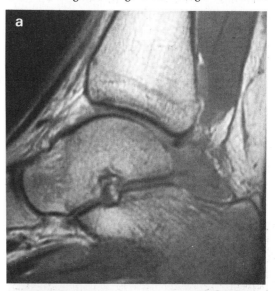

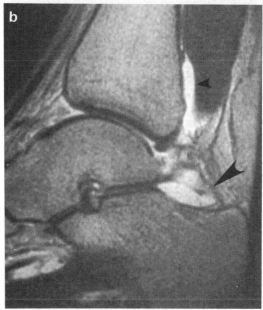

Fig. 14.47 (a) A ballerina who complained of a posterior impingement is shown to have an abnormal mass of tissue behind the ankle joint on a sagittal T_1-weighted image. (b) On a T_2-weighted image this mass becomes bright and is fluid in a bursa. Fluid is also seen to track up the flexor hallucis longus.

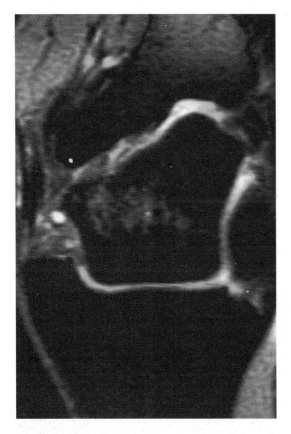

Fig. 14.48 Using a fat suppression technique, the inflammatory reaction associated with bone stress can be well demonstrated.

normal signal and the involved area is well contrasted with a surrounding normal bright signal of marrow fat. Following acute trauma, reactive changes in the neighbouring marrow cause a decreased signal on a T_1-weighted image and the area affected is often remarkably extensive. This reaction makes the identification of a minimal fracture possible (Fig. 14.49). This is most useful for minor osteochondral fractures of the femoral condyles or of the talar dome. In particular, with osteochondral fractures, trabecular compression may be the only change present. This has previously been difficult to diagnose, as all tests apart from a bone scan are negative, but can now be easily demonstrated on MRI. It is important to recognize this change and to anticipate the tendency of these areas to become avascular and fragment-producing as in the case of

an osteochondritis dissecans or a subchondral cyst (Anderson *et al.* 1989).

In the more chronic injury, the medullary changes are generally more organized. With osteochondral fractures, abnormal areas can be seen, sharply demarcated from the surrounding normal marrow. Occasionally, as shown in Fig. 14.50, quite extensive marrow changes in the cancellous bone may be present with the overlying articular cartilage being normal at arthroscopy.

Soft Tissue Imaging

Normal ligaments and tendons have few mobile protons and have a very low signal intensity on both T_1- and T_2-weighted images. Images along the long axis of these structures are obtained together with axial images. Most attention has been paid to the knee joint where imaging of the patellar tendon, the collateral ligaments, the menisci and both the ACL and PCL are easily obtained. Patellar tendinitis, which is seen in jumping sports, can be recognized as an area of high signal within the tendon material (Fig. 14.51) while tears and partial tears in the cruciate ligaments can also be imaged. Early indications are that the accuracy of diagnosing

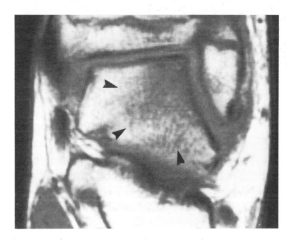

Fig. 14.49 A minimal osteochondral fracture of the lateral aspect of the talar dome is difficult to define but the marked reaction in the surrounding medulla makes its identification simple. The reaction is produced by oedema in the acute stage and later by an inflammatory infiltrate and fibrocartilage.

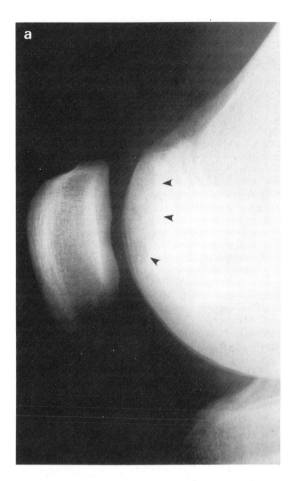

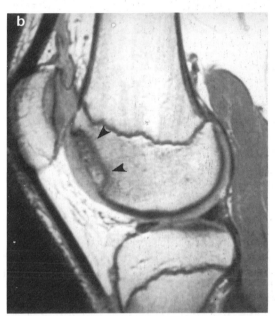

Fig. 14.50 (a) Following direct trauma to the patella, a well-defined area of demineralization is seen in the lateral femoral condyle, behind the patella. (b) An MRI shows an abnormal area in the subchondral medulla, with a mixed signal and a well defined margin. The appearances are almost certainly avascular following trauma and are similar to those associated with osteochondritis dissecans. The overlying articular cartilage was normal and no abnormality could be detected during arthroscopy.

meniscal tears is comparable with that obtained by arthroscopy (Crues *et al.* 1987; Fig. 14.52). Tendon injury in the foot and around the ankle can also be clearly demonstrated and in the heel, the presence of retrocalcaneal bursitis, Achilles tendinitis or injury to the Achilles tendon can be shown.

Initial experience with rotator cuff degeneration and tears has been disappointing but the development of a specific surface coil for the shoulder will improve the quality of these images. Supraspinatus impingements, however, are now well demonstrated (Fig. 14.53).

At the wrist joint, MRI has been helpful in imaging soft tissues including tenosynovitis, structures within the carpal tunnel and the triangular cartilage.

The future of MRI in sports medicine is exciting and the development of lower cost machines, improved software and surface coils, will place the technology within the reach of all athletes in the near future.

Selection of Patients for MRI

Plain film radiography should be always performed as the initial examination. If this is normal a progress examination in 10–14 days is appropriate to help identify subtle fractures. If the second examination is also normal and clinical suspicion of bone injury persists, a bone scan should be used to assess whether osteoblastic activity is occurring. Those patients with a positive bone scan may then benefit from an MRI. It is also particularly helpful in diagnosing avascular necrosis, its sensitivity being at least equivalent to the sensitivity of bone scanning in determining the presence of avascular changes.

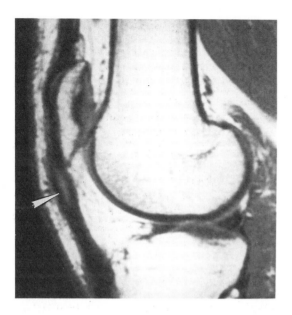

Fig. 14.51 Patellar tendinitis can be diagnosed by demonstrating an area of high-intensity signal within the tendon substance. This is an area of cystic degeneration.

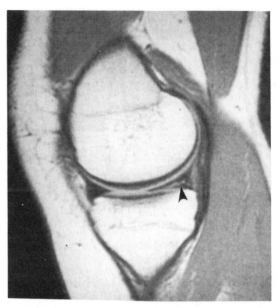

Fig. 14.52 Most menisci contain an area of degeneration shown by a high-intensity signal. When this change extends to an articular surface of the meniscus, a tear is present. In this case, the tear is located inferiorly.

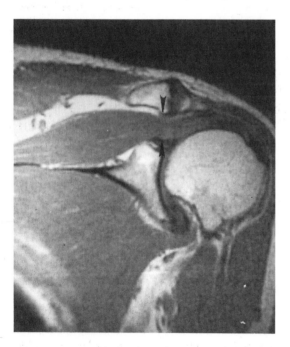

Fig. 14.53 Hypertrophic changes in the acromioclavicular joint, produced in this case by psoriatic arthritis, cause impingement on the supraspinatus muscle belly as it passes beneath the joint.

MRI also has the additional advantage of demonstrating the margin of the avascular area which is of importance if surgical intervention is planned.

DIGITIZED IMAGING

The early digital film processing systems appeared to offer a method of significantly improving the quality of diagnosis in musculoskeletal radiology. By manipulating the image, the abnormality could be made more conspicuous by improving visual perception (Sartoris & Sommer 1984). It is unquestionably far easier to evaluate an image which is digitized using zoom and contrast manipulation rather than having to view a radiograph with a bright light or magnifying glass. However, the initial promise of an increased diagnostic ability of this imaging technique has not been realized. The clarity of bone and soft tissue lesions can be improved using edge enhancement and optimal contrast resolution, but there is no difference in the ability to detect a lesion. For musculoskeletal work, a fine detail film–screen combination is used and the spatial resolution obtained, particularly with radiographic magnification, cannot be achieved by digital systems. Digitizing a radiographic image therefore cannot improve the inherent resolution and consequently no further information can be provided. Most digital systems have been developed for chest radiography where the spatial resolution required is about one-third that needed for bone detail. Consequently, these systems are not suitable for musculoskeletal imaging if an increased diagnostic ability is required.

There are, however, other advantages offered by digital technology. Image retrieval and storage is easier, there are no film costs, there is elimination of lost records and the images can be transmitted by teleradiography to be more available to clinicians. Further developments in digitization will be interesting to follow and may eventually offer a real diagnostic benefit in musculoskeletal imaging for sporting injuries.

INFRA-RED MEDICAL THERMOGRAPHY

The place of infra-red thermography in the diagnosis of musculoskeletal conditions is currently being examined. It is possible that thermography will play a small, but interesting, role and for this reason a discussion of this modality is included especially in the diagnosis of selected musculoskeletal conditions.

Thermography measures the infra-red energy emitted by the skin, expressed as thermal images. Normally, the temperature of opposite limbs and opposite sides of the trunk differ by as little as 0.3°C, or less (with the exception of the forearms). Studies suggest that a variation of 0.5°–0.7°C is indicative of dysfunction and there is a correlation between the existence of painful conditions and an abnormal thermographic pattern. Physiologically, changes in the skin temperature are produced by the alteration of cutaneous blood flow under the control of the autonomic nervous system, so that abnormal thermograms occur in the presence of vasomotor dysfunction. This is a change which cannot be demonstrated by conventional radiographic modalities.

Use in Sporting Injuries

Thermal asymmetry is almost always present in patients with nerve root compression with a decreased temperature in the involved segment. Thermography therefore can play a part in the evaluation and progress of peripheral nerve injury, such as ulnar nerve entrapment and carpal tunnel syndrome. It also appears to have a part in evaluating the presence of reflex sympathetic dystrophy. In the early stages, thermography may demonstrate temperature changes indicating vasomotor instability. The affected extremity initially is warmer, but after 4–5 months a reduction in temperature due to vasoconstriction is recorded.

MAGNIFICATION RADIOGRAPHY

Magnification of a bony trabecular pattern or a cortical margin may enable the identification or confirmation of a subtle fracture.

There are two ways of obtaining magnification using plain film radiography, which are as follows:

- Optical magnification is achieved using a high detail film. The resultant image is viewed using a hand lens or may be projected on to a screen. All musculoskeletal radiography should be of a high enough quality to allow optical magnification
- Radiographic magnification. Geometric enlargement is produced by using a fine focal spot X-ray tube and separating the object and film to achieve the required magnification

A suspected scaphoid fracture is the classic situation where magnification techniques can occasionally be definitive. Usually, there is suspicion of a fracture on the normal scaphoid series using optic magnification, and a radiographic magnification film may confirm the findings. The most convenient method of producing a high class magnification radiograph is to use a mammographic unit with magnification capabilities. A modern unit has an X-ray tube with 100 μm focal spot enabling fine detail to be obtained at a $\times 2$ magnification.

More often than not, when a cortical break is seen on a magnified radiograph, other than with a scaphoid, a progress examination or possibly a bone scan is required for confirmation of the findings.

IMAGE INTENSIFICATION

Modern screening units have excellent detail resolution producing good bone and soft tissue images on the monitor and fluoroscopic monitoring has many applications.

Often dynamic problems are impossible to appreciate on routine radiography but may be observed on screening. Such problems as carpal instability, flexion and extension problems of the spine and possibly patellofemoral instabilities can be examined. Many units also have video and cineradiography available and this can be extremely useful in recording instabilities that occur only on certain degrees of movement.

Stress can be easily applied to joints under direct vision and conditions such as subluxation of the acromioclavicular joint or instability of the ankle can be easily observed.

When there is an impingement affecting the normal range of joint movement, screening may identify the offending bony spur or confirm that the impingement is soft tissue, possibly requiring an MRI for further evaluation.

Where the anatomy is difficult to display, image intensification can offer valuable help. For example, positioning the wrist to profile the hook of hamate is normally difficult; however, if the wrist is first positioned under image intensification control and then a high detail film taken, a potentially difficult task is made easy. Other uses include the screening during arthrography and monitoring needle placements.

Although image intensification has much to offer in evaluating sports injuries, it is often overlooked. This is a low cost and freely available modality and may often be the only method of imaging dynamic abnormalities of joints.

XEROGRAPHY

This technique was basically developed for mammography, but has been found to be useful in musculoskeletal imaging. The xerographic image has the following advantages over routine radiography:

- Edge enhancement enables imaging of soft tissue structures, which may not have significant different radiographic densities but have well defined edges. Individual muscles can be defined and soft tissue masses such as a haematoma, popliteal cyst, etc. can be clearly identified. CT has far better density resolution and must be preferred to xerography as a method of soft tissue imaging
- Xerography enables all radiographic densities to be displayed on the one image. Detail from the skin surface to the trabecular pattern of bone can be demonstrated

Xerography has never been widely used, as there are only a limited number of systems available and the method also uses a relatively high dose of irradiation. Nevertheless, xerography has a small following in musculoskeletal imaging, and the modality is employed particularly for imaging metallic prostheses, to confirm that solid bony consolidation has occurred around the prosthesis and to detect early resorption.

CONCLUSIONS

All modalities have their strengths and weaknesses and the limitations of plain film radiography have already been considered. If it is not possible to locate the problem using a plain film technique then further examination is necessary. Although this will depend on the site and type of injury, nuclear medicine is often the easiest method of selecting patients who will benefit from a further examination using such techniques as a CT scan or MRI. It should not be forgotten, however, that there are several other modalities discussed in this chapter which may also be of considerable benefit.

REFERENCES

Anderson I. F., Crichton K. J., Grattan-Smith T., Cooper R. A. & Brazier D. (1989) Osteochondral fractures of the dome of the talus. *Journal of Bone and Joint Surgery* 71, 1143–1152.
Bellah R. D., Summerville D. A., Treves S. D. & Micheli

L. J. (1991) Low back pain in adolescent athletes: Detection of stress injury to the pars interarticularis with SPECT. *Radiology* **180**, 509–512.

Burk D. L., Karasick D., Kurtz A. B. *et al.* (1989) Prospective comparison of MR imaging with arthrography, sonography and surgery. *American Journal of Roentgenology* **153**, 87–92.

Clark K. C. (1979) *Positioning in Radiology*, 10th edn, pp. 1–125. William Heinemann Medical Books, London.

Crues J. V., Mink J., Levy T. L., Lotysch M. & Stoller D. W. (1987) Meniscal tears of the knee: Accuracy of MR imaging. *Radiology* **164**, 445–448.

Daffner R. H. & Pavlov H. (1992) Stress fractures: Current concepts. *American Journal of Roentgenology* **159**, 245–252.

Elliott S., Hutson M. A. & Wastie M. L. (1988) Bone scintigraphy in the assessment of spondylolysis in patients attending a sports injury clinic. *Clinical Radiology* **39**, 269–272.

Gilula L. A. & Weeks P. M. (1978) Post-traumatic ligamentous instabilities of the wrist. *Radiology* **129**, 641–651.

Goldman A. B., Pavlov H. & Rubenstein D. (1988) The Segond fracture of the proximal tibia. *American Journal of Roentgenology* **151**, 1163–1167.

Hall R. H., Isaac F. & Booth C. R. (1959) Dislocations of the shoulder with special reference to accompanying small fractures. *Journal of Bone and Joint Surgery* **41**, 489–494.

Harrington T., Crichton K. J. & Anderson I. F. (1993) Stress fractures at the base of the second metatarsal in ballet dancers. *American Journal of Sports Medicine* **21**, 591–598.

Heck L. L. (1987) Recognition of atypical reflex sympathetic dystrophy. *Clinical Nuclear Medicine* **12**, 925–928.

Hendrick W. R., DiSimone R. N., Wolf B. H. & Langer A. (1988) Absorbed dose to the fetus during bone scintigraphy. *Radiology* **168**, 245–248.

Holder L. E., Cole L. A. & Myerson M. S. (1992) Reflex sympathetic dystrophy in the foot: Clinical and scintigraphic criteria. *Radiology* **184**, 521–535.

Jackson D. W., Wiltse L. L., Dingeman R. D. & Hayes M. (1981) Stress reactions involving the pars interarticularis in young athletes. *American Journal of Sports Medicine* **9**, 304–312.

Khan K. M., Fuller P. J., Brukner P. D., Kearney C. & Burry H. C. (1992) Outcome of conservative and surgical management of navicular stress fracture in athletes — Eighty six cases proven with computerized tomography. *American Journal of Sports Medicine* **20**, 657–666.

Kilcoyne R. F., Reddy P. K., Lyons F. & Rockwood C. A. (1989) Optimal plain film imaging of the shoulder impingement syndrome. *American Journal of Roentgenology* **153**, 795–797.

Kohn H. S., Guten G. N., Collier B. D., Veluvolu P. & Whalen J. P. (1988) Chondromalacia of the patella: Bone imaging correlated with arthroscopic findings. *Clinical Nuclear Medicine* **13**, 96–98.

Marks P. H., Goldenberg J. A., Vezina W. C., Chamberlain M. J., Vellet A. D. & Fowler P. J. (1992) Subchondral bone infractions in acute ligamentous knee injuries demonstrated on bone scintigraphy and magnetic resonance imaging. *Journal of Nuclear Medicine* **33**, 516–520.

Marymont J. V., Lynch M. A. & Henning C. E. (1983) Evaluation of meniscus tears of the knee by radionuclide imaging. *American Journal of Sports Medicine* **11**, 432–435.

Matheson G. O., Clement D. B., McKenzie D. C., Taunton J. E., Lloyd-Smith D. R. & Macintyre J. G. (1987) Scintigraphic uptake of Tc-99m at non-painful sites in athletes with stress fractures: The concept of bone strain. *Sports Medicine* **4**, 65–75.

Mathieson J. R., Connell D. G., Cooperberg P. L. & Lloyd-Smith D. R. (1988) Sonography of the Achilles tendon and adjacent bursae. *American Journal of Roentgenology* **151**, 127–131.

Matin P. (1979) The appearance of bone scans following fractures, including immediate and long-term studies. *Journal of Nuclear Medicine* **20**, 1227–1231.

Merchant A. C., Mercer R. L., Jacobsen R. H. & Cool C. R. (1974) Patellofemoral congruence. *Journal of Bone and Joint Surgery* **56**, 1391–1396.

Middleton W. D. (1992) Ultrasonography of the shoulder. *Radiologic Clinics of North America* **30**, 927–940.

Mooar P., Gregg J. & Jacobstein J. (1987) Radionuclide imaging in internal derangements of the knee. *American Journal of Sports Medicine* **15**, 132–137.

Mubarak S. J., Gould R. N., Lee Y. F., Schmidt D. A. & Hargens A. R. (1982) The medial tibial stress syndrome: A cause of shin splints. *American Journal of Sports Medicine* **10**, 201–205.

Newberg A. H. & Seligson D. (1980) The patellofemoral joint: 30°, 60° and 90° views. *Diagnostic Radiology* **137**, 56–61.

Pavlov H., Henaghan M. A., Herch A., Goldman A. B. & Vigorita V. (1982) The Haglund syndrome: Initial and differential diagnosis. *Diagnostic Radiology* **144**, 83–88.

Peterfy C. G., Majumdar S., Lang P., van Dijke C. F., Sack K. & Genant H. K. (1994) MR imaging of the arthritic knee; improved discrimination of cartilage, synovium and effusion with pulse saturation transfer and fat-suppressed T_1-weighted sequences. *Radiology* **191**, 413–419.

Rijke A. M., Goitz H. T., McCue F. C., Andrews J. R. & Berr S. S. (1994) Stress radiography of the medial elbow ligaments. *Radiology* **191**, 213–216.

Romney B. M., Nickoloff E. L., Esser P. D. & Alderson P. O. (1986) Radionuclide administration to nursing mothers: Mathematically derived guidelines. *Radiology* **160**, 549–554.

Roub L. W., Gumerman L. W., Hanley E. N., Williams Clark M., Goodman M. & Herbert D. (1979) Bone stress: A radionuclide imaging perspective. *Radiology* **132**, 431–438.

Sartoris D. J. & Sommer F. G. (1984) Distal film processing: Applications to the musculoskeletal system. *Skeletal Radiology* **11**, 274–281.

Singson R. D., Feldman F. & Bigliani L. (1987) CT arthrography patterns in recurrent glenohumeral instability. *American Journal of Roentgenology* **149**, 749–753.

Spitz J., Laver I., Tittel K. & Weigand H. (1993) Scintimetric evaluation of remodelling after bone fractures in man. *Journal of Nuclear Medicine* **34**, 1403–1409.

Stiles R. G. & Otte M. T. (1993) Imaging of the shoulder. *Radiology* **188**, 603–613.

Teige R. A. (1988) Stress X-rays for patellofemoral instability. Monograph accompanying exhibit at the 3rd European Congress of Knee Surgery. Amsterdam, 1988.

Turner G. W. & Burns C. B. (1982) Erect position tangential projection of the patella. *Radiology Technology* **54**, 11–14.

Urman M., Ammann W., Sisler J., Lentle B. C., Lloyd-Smith R., Loomer R. & Fisher C. (1991) The role of bone scintigraphy in the evaluation of talar dome fractures. *Journal of Nuclear Medicine* **32**, 2241–2244.

Vaughan B. (1989) Magnetic resonance imaging physics and technical aspect. *Australian Radiology* **13**, 34–39.

Weber D. A., Todd Makler P. Jr, Watson E. E. & Coffey J. L. (1989) MIRD dose estimate report no. 13. radiation absorbed dose from Technetium-99m-labelled bone imaging agents. *Journal of Nuclear Medicine* **30**, 1117–1122.

Zwas S. T., Elkanovitch R. & Frank G. (1987) Interpretation and classification of bone scintigraphic findings in stress fractures. *Journal of Nuclear Medicine* **28**, 452–457.

CHAPTER 15

INJURIES TO THE HEAD, EYE AND EAR

A. P. Garnham

HEAD INJURY

Head injury implies injury to the skull, the meningeal membranes and associated blood vessels surrounding the brain and the substance of the brain itself.

In contact sports injury may result from a collision between players or from contact with the ground or playing field structures. A blow need not be directly to the head itself to produce a brain injury. In non-contact sports, playing implements are the most likely causes of direct injury, although accidental collision between players and the ground or structures are also of importance.

Boxing is unique in that the intention is to land repeated blows to the head which can cause a significant brain injury, that is, a knock-out.

Head injuries in sport are divided into three categories:

- Skull fractures which occur with or without brain injury; the fracture itself is of less concern than damage to the structures within
- Localized trauma to the head which may induce focal internal head injury, such as contusion of the cerebral cortex, extradural haematoma, subdural haematoma and intracerebral haemorrhage. These injuries produce two-thirds of the deaths from head injuries
- Diffuse injuries which involve widespread disruption of neurological structures without obvious localized damage. They are the major cause of long-term neurological disability

Mechanisms of Injury

Force to the head can be static or dynamic. Static loading implies the gradual application of a force and is unlikely to occur in sport. Dynamic loading is the rapid application of force and can be either of the impact type, when force is applied directly, or impulsive loading where the load is set in motion and accelerated or decelerated by a blow to the body which does not strike the head. Impulsive injuries are common in sport, where players' bodies collide, but there is no impact to the head. A blow to a helmet causes impulsive, rather than impact loading, as the head may be accelerated or decelerated, but is not struck directly.

Acceleration (or deceleration) results in either a linear translational or a rotational movement:

- Linear translational acceleration results in a focal structural injury, but does not cause concussion. Local trauma, such as fracture occurs, possibly accompanied by damage to immediate underlying structures. The brain is protected well by the skull and cerebrospinal fluid from such forces. Helmets are designed to diffuse linear acceleration forces
- Rotational acceleration may result from impact or impulsive loading and has now been clearly

implicated as the major mechanism of intra-cranial injury (Genarelli 1991). Experimental evidence has shown that rotational forces can reproduce the entire spectrum of intracranial injuries. Shearing, tension and compression forces are produced within the skull, with shearing forces being the most likely to cause neuronal injury. Distant to the site of impact, contusion, diffuse injury and subdural haema-toma may result. The brain tolerates rotational forces poorly, there being no innate protective mechanism. Protective devices are relatively ineffective at controlling the rotational acceler-ation of the head, greatly lessening their effec-tiveness in this situation

Management

Whenever an impact to the head has occurred or unconsciousness has resulted from any cause, the full spectrum of head and spinal injury must be considered. If a player is unconscious, management must centre on adequate protection of the cervical spine while ensuring general supportive measures such as securing clear airways. In this situation play must be stopped if the rules permit and the player must be removed from the playing area immediately. In the case of the conscious player, the possibility of severe cervical spine injury must be excluded before removal from the playing area is undertaken. Assessment of head injury should not be done on the field but performed carefully on the sideline or in the dressing room.

Once the player has been removed from the field, frequent neurological observations (every 15 min) should be commenced including the following:

- Conscious state. Any change, whether sudden or gradual, demands assessment in hospital
- Headache. The location, nature and severity of any headache must be noted and regularly checked. Worsening headache may indicate cerebral oedema and/or haematoma
- Pupils. Any change in pupil size or abnormal reaction to light indicates the need for hos-pitalization
- Eye movement. The player should be asked whether double vision is present and full eye

movements must be tested. The sixth cranial (abducens) nerve is usually the first to be affected in intracranial injury and results in a loss of lateral gaze
- Nausea and vomiting. These symptoms are indicative of rising intracranial pressure
- Orientation and intellectual function. The examiner should check the patient's knowledge of the immediate environment, people, place, current score, etc.
- Pulse rate. A slowing of the pulse rate is associ-ated with increasing intracranial pressure
- Blood pressure. A rise in blood pressure is indicative of rising intracranial pressure

Conscious state is the single most important sign and must be monitored closely. Changes in pulse rate and blood pressure are late signs indicative of catastrophic injury.

Hospital admission must be arranged if there is persistence or deterioration of any of the above signs. It is reasonable to relieve discomfort resulting from head or other injuries; however, the effects of analgesic administration must be considered when assessing the neurological state. Narcotic analgesics are not advised as they may affect both pupil size and conscious state. Hence they should not be used in the presence of abnormal neurological signs.

Concussion

A definition of concussion proposed by the Com-mittee on Head Injury Nomenclature of the Con-gress of Neurological Surgeons USA (1966) is a 'clinical syndrome characterized by immediate and transient post-traumatic impairment of neural function, such as alteration of consciousness, distur-bance of vision and equilibrium due to brain stem involvement'. From this definition it is important to note that loss of consciousness (LOC) need not occur. A wide variety of neurological symptoms may be experienced, but none are permanent. Many classifications of concussion have been proposed based on immediate and residual effects. A clinically useful classification is as follows:

- Grade 1 (mild) — no LOC and post-traumatic amnesia (PTA) of less than 30 min

- Grade 2 (moderate) — LOC less than 5 min or PTA greater than 30 min
- Grade 3 (severe) — LOC greater than 5 min or PTA greater than 24 h (Cantu 1986)

PTA is the period of loss of memory of the concussive event and subsequent events until full recall of recent events is regained, not including those events during the period of amnesia.

Using this classification, the management of concussion proceeds as outlined in Table 15.1. It

Table 15.1 Management of concussion

Grade 1	As consciousness has not been lost, Grade 1 injury may be difficult to recognize unless mistakes in play are being made. For example, there is impairment of intellectual function and memory with the interpretation and assimilation of new information most likely to be affected. As soon as a Grade 1 concussion is recognized the player should leave the field and neurological observations commence. In addition to the observations outlined above, tests of mental and physical dexterity must be undertaken if return to play is being considered. The player must be able to run and perform game skills, comment on the ongoing play and perform rapid mental arithmetic. If headache or dizziness exist or concentration is impaired, there must not be a return to play. Occasionally, a heavy blow to the face or upper abdomen may result in vagus nerve excitation and vasovagal syncope (fainting). This can be distinguished from unconsciousness caused by head injury by the site of the blow, the delay between the blow and LOC and the characteristic slow bounding pulse of a vasovagal episode.
Grade 2	Initial management is as above; however, recovery of consciousness within the 5 min period alters further management. The player must be removed from the game and neurological observations commenced. If consciousness has not been lost, but the player is in PTA, return to play is forbidden.
Grade 3	The head and neck must be immobilized and immediate transfer and admission to hospital must be arranged. Cervical spine and significant intracranial injury must be presumed until actively excluded.

Adapted from Cantu (1986).

must be emphasized to the player that any concussion involves a degree of brain injury and the affected brain must be allowed to recover. The player should take time off from work and training and have plenty of sleep. Family, work-mates and team-mates should be informed that any persistent headache, dizziness, irritability, emotional or personality change and impairment of concentration or memory, imply incomplete recovery and further evaluation must be performed. Often the player is unaware of, or even denies, the presence of such symptoms and in this situation comprehensive neuropsychological assessment should be undertaken, particularly if other investigations detect no abnormality.

Return to play on the same day as head injury can only *ever* be considered in the case of mild concussion and only then after a complete and careful assessment by a medical practitioner. In all other cases, once the acute phase has passed, further detailed assessment must be performed before permitting return to training and competition.

Worsening or persistence of any head injury symptoms, including headache beyond 24 h requires further full evaluation. Radiological investigation of the head and neck should be considered in every case and performed in the majority of them (see below). Investigation should exclude any significant intracranial injury. It must be remembered that shearing forces can tear blood vessels causing intracerebral or extracerebral bleeding without LOC.

Recovery from concussion is variable and no firm guide-lines can be used to estimate the duration of absence from competition. Mandatory periods of exclusion from competition have been legislated in a number of contact sports. However, such mandatory recovery periods take no account of the wide individual variation of recovery. After any concussive episode the player must be cleared by a medical practitioner before returning to training. This clearance should include a full neurological assessment and assessment of mental and physical skills, including reaction time. Simple neuropsychological and reaction time tests have been developed which can objectively and reliably measure return to a baseline level of cognitive function, and have been shown to correlate well with clinical recovery

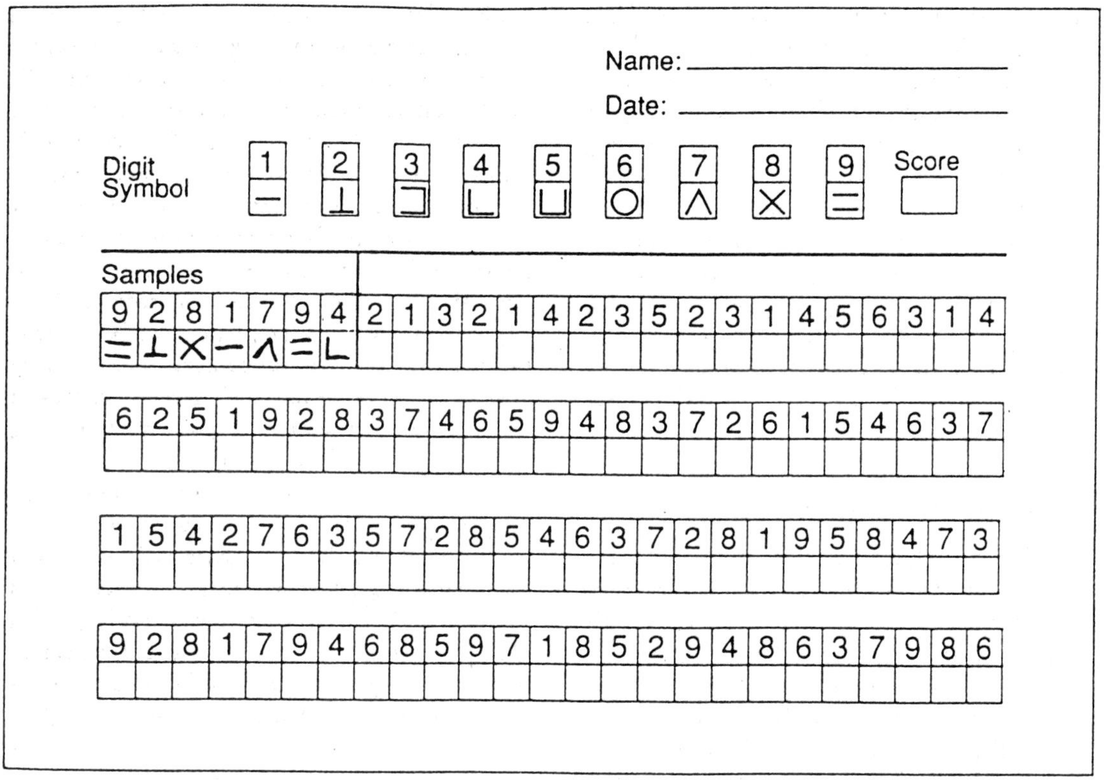

Fig. 15.1 Digit Symbol Substitution Test. As many boxes as possible are completed in 90 s (Dicker 1991).

(Fig. 15.1). These tests are best administered pre-season to the entire team in order to determine baseline function. However, repeated tests commenced only after injury will indicate progression of recovery. Testing is only useful as an objective measure of recovery and is not a diagnostic test for concussion. At the professional level a player may be assessed several times weekly. On return to training the player should complete several training sessions free of symptoms before being declared fit for competition. The co-operation of the coach is invaluable in assessing recovery of playing skills. Any recurrent symptoms demand further rest and reassessment (Alves 1991; McCrory et al. 1994).

Criteria for management of repeated concussion have been proposed by several authorities. However, these criteria are again dependent upon the imposition of mandatory periods of exclusion from competition. Each episode of head injury must stand alone in its assessment. The guide-lines above should be applied in every instance of concussion. There is no evidence that previous concussions have any influence on recovery from subsequent concussion. Where findings suggest long-term neurological impairment, it is likely that previous, more severe brain injury has been misdiagnosed as concussion and thorough investigation must be carried out.

Any persistent abnormality on computerized tomography (CT) or magnetic resonance imaging (MRI) scan, or the need for intracranial surgery, implies a major risk with any return to contact sport and the player should be counselled against this. The so-called post-concussive syndrome is a form of long-term brain injury usually resulting from high-velocity trauma rather than forces commonly encountered in sport. Again lengthy, if not permanent, absence from contact sport is advised. In the situation where a player returns to competition after concussion on the same day or soon after, the second impact syndrome has been described. This involves not only the increased risk of the concussed player suffering a second injury but also the pathological effects of a second injury, which are magnified in the presence of any existing damage. Fatal brain swelling has been recorded following two apparently mild concussions in one game of contact sport. In these cases the player was not fully medically assessed prior to return to play and a potentially catastrophic injury, or ongoing impairment of function had not been excluded. Medico-legal consequences of incomplete assessment of the concussed player are likely to be severe (McCrory et al. 1994)

Imaging of Head Injuries

Careful consideration should be given to the choice of imaging modality when investigating head injury. Plain X-ray is readily available and relatively cheap, but is useful only in the demonstration of linear skull fractures, where it is the modality of choice. Plain films have almost no place in determining intracranial pathology. Angiography offers information about vascular injury and the displacement of normal vascular structures, but has been surpassed by non-invasive techniques.

CT scanning is now widely available and is the most commonly used modality. It is the investigation of choice for all bony injuries, other than linear skull fractures, when the plane of the fracture may coincide with the axis of the scanner, rendering the fracture line invisible. Clinically significant subdural and epidural haematomas are well demonstrated on CT scans. Diffuse neuronal injury is generally seen only when relatively severe. However, when soft tissue injury is associated with bony injury, as in depressed skull fracture, CT remains the preferred modality. CT can be performed rapidly, and there are no contra-indications to its use. Intravenous contrast media are rarely necessary in head trauma investigation.

MRI is the best modality for demonstrating diffuse intracranial soft tissue injury, both acute and chronic. MRI is able to detect changes of diffuse axonal damage resulting from the shearing forces arising in sporting injury. These changes will not be visible in an acute injury of mild to moderate severity, but will be seen in acute severe or chronic injuries. Axonal damage cannot be seen on CT. Small subdural haematomas, which do not require surgery can also be detected on MRI, but not CT. However, MRI is a slow procedure, taking approximately 30 min for a complete examination. It cannot be performed on uncooperative or claustrophobic patients. MRI is difficult to perform on critically ill or ventilated patients, because of the physical constraints of the scanner and the fact that there must be no metal present within the extremely powerful magnetic field. MRI is relatively expensive and currently confined to major centres, making accessibility a significant barrier to its use.

The choice between the superior soft tissue imaging of MRI and the relative ease of performing CT sometimes makes the choice of investigation difficult. In emergency situations it is often best to organize early CT scanning, following up with MRI if indicated. Discussing the circumstances with a radiologist is often useful in making an appropriate decision (Jahre et al. 1991).

Skull Fracture

Fractures are most likely to occur from high velocity impact often with a relatively small object such as a bat or ball, or from a fall on to a hard playing surface (such as ice or asphalt). In the case of a large scalp haematoma or area of localized pain or tenderness, one must suspect an underlying fracture. There may be diffuse swelling over the fracture site rather than the usual lump (haematoma) and management of any suspected skull fracture consists of immediate X-ray and referral to a specialist.

A non-depressed, linear fracture heals within a few weeks without special treatment. Brain injury, however, is implied in any depressed fracture and hospital treatment is essential.

The site of the fracture is important. For example, a fracture in the temporoparietal area may damage the underlying middle meningeal vessels, resulting in extradural haemorrhage (Fig. 15.2a). Fracture of the frontal bone is likely to involve the frontal sinus and prophylactic antibiotics should be commenced immediately to prevent meningitis,

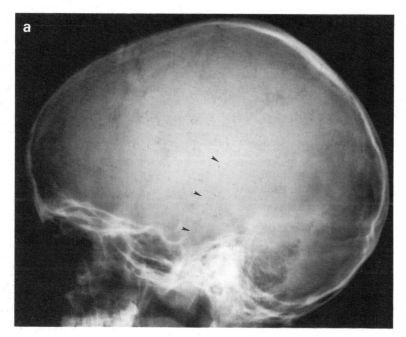

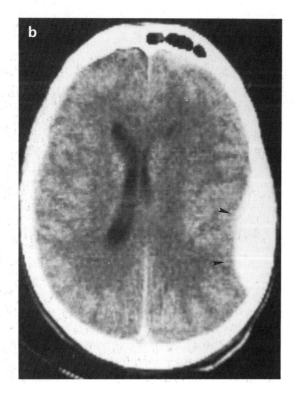

Fig. 15.2 (a) There is a linear fracture (arrows) extending from the parietal eminence into the temporal fossa. This fracture will cross branches of the middle meningeal vessels. (b) A CT scan shows a resultant extradural haematoma (arrows) due to bleeding from the meningeal vessels. Note the compression and shift of the ventricular system to the right.

followed by referral to a neurosurgeon for further management. Skull base fractures, often with cerebrospinal fluid leaks (otorrhoea or rhinorrhoea), also require antibiotics and specialist referral. Cerebrospinal fluid leakage can be confirmed by the use of glucose test strips, which yield a positive result. Whenever a fracture passes through a foramen of the skull there is likely to be damage to the structures within that foramen.

Intracranial Haemorrhage

Intracranial haemorrhage is the most likely cause of death from head injury. Rapid accurate assessment and appropriate specialist referral are essential if fatalities are to be avoided. Four types of intracranial haemorrhage occur and all are dangerous.

EXTRADURAL HAEMATOMA (FIG. 15.2b)

The meningeal blood vessels supply the dura mater and many small vascular branches supply the skull. A shearing force from a rotational injury or a direct blow causing a fracture (most commonly of the temporal bone) tears the meningeal blood vessels and produces bleeding between the skull and the dura mater, which may rapidly form a large haematoma, compressing the brain and inducing a decrease in conscious state. After an LOC from the initial injury, the player may recover and appear well for several hours before lapsing into unconsciousness, possibly after experiencing a headache which steadily increases in intensity. There are also changes in pupil size and the other neurological observations discussed previously. Transport by ambulance to a hospital with neurosurgical facilities must be arranged immediately. The lucid interval which may occur with this injury emphasizes the importance of careful observation of all who suffer a head injury.

SUBDURAL HAEMATOMA

This is the most common form of sports-related intracranial haemorrhage. Tearing of a vein over the brain surface results in 'low-pressure' bleeding between the brain and the dura mater and there may be associated damage to small arteries and to the brain substance. Subdural haemorrhage can result from any severe blow. As early symptoms are usually the result of primary brain damage, immediate CT or MRI scanning and hospital treatment is required. Late presentation of chronic subdural haematoma is seen less often in sport than in the general population, as the associated loss of skills and performance caused by the cortical atrophy usually results in early presentation by athletes. However, the possibility of a subdural haematoma must be checked by CT or MRI scan when even mild symptoms and signs persist for weeks after a head injury.

INTRACEREBRAL HAEMORRHAGE

Injury to the brain substance can tear vessels within it. In such cases the primary brain injury is severe and consciousness is not regained or there is a rapid progression into unconsciousness. Immediate hospital management is therefore necessary.

SUBARACHNOID HAEMORRHAGE

Any head injury can result in bleeding from the small surface vessels of the brain, commonly from a cerebral aneurysm or arteriovenous malformation.

This bleeding is normally of 'low pressure' resulting in a headache (which is usually severe) and abnormal neurological signs often develop. Lumbar puncture is the most sensitive diagnostic test. Hospital treatment is required.

Management of Intracranial Haemorrhage

In each of the four types of haemorrhage the importance of immediate hospital treatment, including CT or MRI scanning, cannot be over-emphasized.

The player must be transported in the 'coma position' with the airways secured. Any resuscitation equipment available should be used to achieve maximum oxygen saturation of the blood by hyperventilation. If progressive neurological signs are present with worsening unconsciousness, a 70 kg adult can be given 100 mg dexamethasone or 1 g methylprednisolone sodium succinate intravenously as a statim dose (Bruno *et al.* 1987).

Headache

Any complaint of a headache with a history of head trauma must be regarded as being due to that trauma and treated accordingly.

If trauma has been excluded, a history must be taken to ascertain whether the headache is of cervical origin, caused by exertion, or by factors not directly related to sport or exercise, such as migraine or anxiety. Appropriate investigations should then be undertaken in each case (Cacayorin *et al.* 1987).

Exertional headaches are most often associated with strength training, as maximal weight-lifting efforts can produce systolic blood pressures of up to 400 mmHg, with leg exercise generally producing higher pressures than arm exercise. The Valsalva manoeuvre, which is the compression of blood vessels by muscular tension and the constriction of other blood vessels, contributes to this rise in pressure. Intracranial haemorrhage can be caused by such high blood pressure and persistent or severe headache must be investigated. Treatment entails moderation and modification of the training regimen (McCarthy 1988).

Runners, swimmers and other athletes may also suffer exertional headache. The onset of headache is often quite rapid and severe, followed by a lingering dull ache. Exertional headaches may be related to elevated blood pressure or the result of unknown mechanisms. Dehydration is a frequent associated factor and the athlete should be advised to maintain adequate fluid intake during and after exercise. Treatment requires moderation and modification of training and a degree of patience. The combination of these usually ensures a return to full competition within a short period of time. Standard analgesics may also be used once any pathology has been excluded.

Migraine may be triggered by exertion, hypoglycaemia, glare and stress, exhibiting typical features and responding to standard treatment. Trauma to the head may also produce what the player describes as a typical migraine headache. As late migraine symptoms are very similar to concussion, caution should be exercised in these cases.

Dysautonomic cephalgia is the result of direct trauma to sympathetic nerve fibres accompanying the carotid arteries in the anterior triangle of the neck. This condition is characterized by a unilateral headache, associated with Horner's syndrome and excessive sweating. Treatment with Propranolol is often effective, but it must be remembered that this agent is banned in competition in some sports under International Olympic Committee regulations (Brukner & Khan 1993; see Chapter 26).

Chronic Brain Injury

Players involved in any contact sport who suffer repeated cerebral injury may exhibit features of chronic impairment of brain function. This is seen most commonly in boxing and is referred to as 'punch drunkenness', or chronic traumatic encephalopathy of the boxer. It is characterized by features of extrapyramidal neurological disturbances and cerebellar signs, such as abnormal gait and coordination, tremor of the hands and body and slurred speech. The condition is progressive and the likelihood of suffering from it is proportional to the number of blows sustained to the head. Four stages of the condition are recognized by neurolo-

gists, the final stage being a persistent Parkinsonian state with florid psychiatric signs. The first two stages are reversible, if no further head trauma is sustained.

Clinical examination, electroencephalography, neuropsychological evaluation, CT scanning and MRI-based studies have demonstrated neurological damage in a high percentage of the boxers tested. However, epidemiological studies making use of well matched controls and allowing for the degree of exposure to head trauma are difficult to perform. Hence, both the absolute risk of chronic traumatic encephalopathy and the relative risk when compared with other contact sports are unknown (Jordan 1992). Steps have been taken in amateur boxing to lessen the risk of acute and chronic brain injury. Changes include the use of head guards, more heavily padded and better designed gloves and the shortening of contests. However, none of these measures has yet been scientifically shown to decrease risk.

Prevention of Head Injury

Every sporting body must critically examine the incidence and severity of head injuries in their respective sports in order to legislate for safe conduct. Practices such as spear tackling in gridiron and tunnelling in basketball are rightly banned because of the high risk of head and cervical spine injury. Endorsement of safe practice by elite players and firm disciplinary action by administrators in response to unsafe play, can effectively reduce the incidence of injury. The vigilance of sports medicine personnel has led to many beneficial rule changes. This is an area where there is always room for improvement and good communication between practitioners and administrators should lead to progressively safer sport.

Sport-specific protective headwear has been developed for a wide variety of sports, and ideally all such equipment should satisfy the following criteria:

- Provide adequate protection from injuries
- Be affordable
- Be comfortable to wear
- Be light in weight

- Should allow adequate adjustment to achieve perfect fit
- Should not impair central or peripheral vision
- Should not impair hearing
- Should not impair reaction time
- Must be securely fastened but easily removed
- Damage to the helmet must not produce dangerous fragments
- Must not increase the risk of cervical spine injury
- Must not provide a target for opponents
- Must not be useful as an offensive weapon
- Should clearly indicate use for single or multiple impacts
- Must not impair thermal regulation
- Should carry approval of the appropriate National Standards Association and the relevant sporting body for which it is in use

From the participant's point of view, the major criteria are cost, comfort, acceptance and use by peers and availability in team colours.

Helmets have been demonstrated to be effective in reducing head injury in high-velocity sports such as cycling, in sports where there is a risk of missile injury such as baseball and cricket and where there is a risk of falls on to hard surfaces such as gridiron and ice hockey (Hodgson 1991).

In cycling, where helmet usage is mandatory both in competition and for recreational use in many Australian states, two points are very important. First, most cycling helmets are designed to withstand a single impact only, and after such an event the helmet must be destroyed to prevent further use and a new one obtained. This must be clearly indicated by labelling (Ellis *et al.* 1994). Second, cycling helmets in particular have often

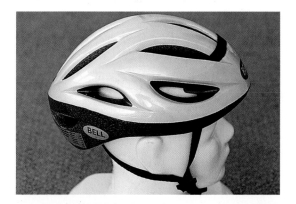
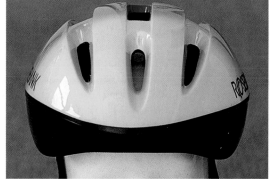
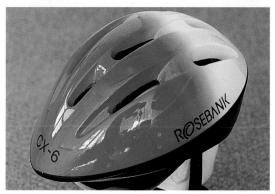
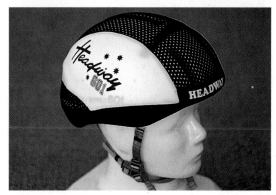

Fig. 15.3 Examples of cycling helmets. (a–c) Thin shell helmets, lightweight but protective. Note the air vents and streamlining. (d) Cloth-covered soft shell. The use of this type is not recommended.

been described as 'too hot', and this objection has been raised to avoid their use. Modern helmets with better design do not impair heat loss (Gisolfi *et al.* 1988; Fig. 15.3a–c).

Helmets must not increase the risk of head or other injuries, to the player or others. In rugby football a major objection to hard helmets is their use as an intentionally offensive weapon. The helmet may also encourage a false sense of security and the player may indulge in dangerous play. In Australian football, as the incidence of significant unintended head injury is quite low, the use of helmets in this sport has been critically examined with respect to its benefits. Any helmet which may effectively protect against concussion, with present technology, makes the player's head a larger target in a collision. A larger and heavier target is likely to suffer a greater rotational acceleration force, thereby increasing the risk of intracranial injury (McCrory *et al.* 1994). Cloth-covered cycling helmets have been implicated in an increased incidence of cervical spine injuries. The cloth covering may grip the ground, slowing movement of the head while inertia carries the body forward, increasing forces on the neck (Ellis *et al.* 1994; Fig. 15.3d).

The mouthguard remains the single most useful protective device available for those sports which do not or cannot make use of helmets. A well fitted mouthguard stabilizes the mandible relative to the cranium, thereby diminishing concussive forces as well as affording facial and dental protection (Greenberg & Springer 1991). Chapter 16 deals with this valuable protective device in more detail.

Strengthening of the neck musculature is believed to decrease the incidence and severity of head and cervical spine injuries in rugby and gridiron, by assisting to brace the head and neck against rotational forces.

THE INJURED EYE

Adequate visual acuity is essential both for effective performance and for prevention of eye injuries. Testing of visual acuity should be routine in any general medical examination.

Athletes with the following conditions should be counselled to avoid contact sports altogether, and to make use of protective eyewear whenever playing other sports which present a risk of eye injury:

- The presence of only one good eye
- Severe amblyopia (lazy eye)
- Myopia (short sightedness) of greater than 6 dioptres, as the elongated globe increases the risk of retinal injury
- A history of retinal detachment, or a pre-retinal detachment condition
- Diabetic retinopathy
- Marfan's syndrome
- Recent eye surgery (Vinger & Knuttgen 1988)

The anatomy of the eye is demonstrated in Fig. 15.4.

Eye Injury

Table 15.2 lists signs and symptoms indicative of serious eye injury. In such cases removal of the player to a suitable area for examination and possible referral to specialist medical facilities are required.

If the eyelids are swollen and shut and cannot be opened voluntarily, no attempt should be made to open them.

In order to proceed with an eye examination one requires a clean location away from the competition area with adequate lighting, preferably a torch. The following equipment should be available:

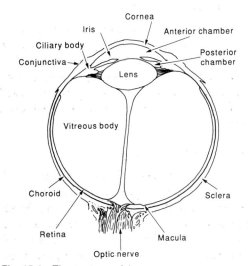

Fig. 15.4 The anatomy of the eye.

Table 15.2 Signs and symptoms of serious eye injury

Persistent blurring of vision not cleared by blinking
'Double' vision
Loss of part or all of the visual field in one or both eyes
Photophobia
Stabbing, piercing or throbbing eye pain
Acuity of less than 6/9 (where acuity is normally 6/6)

- Sterile single use containers of fluorescein stain, mydriatic drops and topical anaesthetic drops
- Equipment for removing foreign bodies, including cotton buds, sterile needle, dental burr and saline solution
- An ophthalmoscope

A brief history must be taken, noting factors such as a foreign body, possible penetration of the eye by a sharp implement, or rupture resulting from a blunt instrument or projectile.

The pupils must be carefully examined for light and accommodation reflexes, and comparative size and shape. Patients should be asked if they have pre-existing irregular or unequal pupils. The swinging flashlight test indicates damage to the optic nerve or retina. When a light is swung from the normal to the injured eye, pupillary dilation in the injured eye indicates a positive test (Levy 1986).

The lids should be everted to look for foreign bodies or signs of trauma. Lacerations and bruising around the eye should be examined, particularly with regard to the lacrimal apparatus. Visual fields should be assessed with care, with any defect being rechecked and recorded. Eye movements must be tested fully.

Fundal examination should be carried out, and if available, slit-lamp examination should also be undertaken. The visual acuity must be tested and recorded. A makeshift test can be used, such as reading various type sizes on a newspaper or reading nearby signs.

Specific Injuries of the Eye

ANTERIOR CHAMBER

Conjunctival foreign body

A foreign body in the conjunctiva is painful and usually obvious. It may result from dirt or mud being thrown or thrust into the eye, usually in the course of contact sports involving tackling and contact with the ground. Irrigation with sterile saline solution or the use of a cotton bud to remove a loose body is generally adequate, but referral to an ophthalmologist is recommended if the body is not readily removed. The upper and lower lids should be everted to ensure no other foreign material is present.

Corneal foreign body

Foreign bodies in the cornea arise from the same mechanism outlined earlier and local anaesthetic drops are useful for examination and treatment. Saline irrigation or light brushing with a cotton bud mostly suffices; however, if the foreign material is embedded, a sterile dental burr or sterile needle held at a tangent to the cornea can be used to scrape the material out. This should be done by an ophthalmologist if available, as a shallow layer of cornea may be removed and great care must be taken, particularly over the pupil. Fluorescein dye should be instilled to delineate the resultant abrasion and highlight any other superficial injury. Chloramphenicol ointment should then be applied and the eye padded. With an anaesthetized eye the player must not take part in further activity in order to avoid the risk of further eye injury.

Chemical burns

These may result from swimming pool chemicals or from lime used in line marking on playing fields. The eyes must be copiously irrigated with water for up to 20 min with the lids held open. Full examination with fluorescein dye may reveal generalized superficial corneal injury, which may require hospital treatment.

Corneal abrasion

Corneal abrasion may occur from a fingernail scratch or similar injury and is painful, usually producing tears. It is normally accompanied by photophobia. Fluorescein dye delineates the injury and all such abrasions must be fully assessed to exclude deep laceration. Contact lenses are frequently associated with corneal abrasions and should not be worn until the injury has healed. It should also be noted that a 'lost' contact lens may sometimes be found beneath the upper or lower eyelid. A firmly applied eye-pad helps relieve pain, while chloramphenicol eye drops or eye ointment is used 4-hourly to prevent infection. The injury should be reviewed daily until the wound has healed.

Tetanus prophylaxis must be considered for all corneal injuries. Local anaesthetic drops must never be used as a long-term analgesic as they damage the corneal surface.

Corneal laceration

Corneal laceration is an extension of the above and must always be treated with great care, hospital treatment being mandatory. It must be assumed that the injury is penetrating and steps must be taken to ensure that there is no increase in intra-ocular pressure. Squeezing the eyes closed, physical activity and pressure on the globe of the eye all increase intraocular pressure and risk loss of the eye. An intraocular foreign body may be present and this possibility should be excluded by radiographic examination. The eye should be lightly padded, and transfer to hospital arranged. If this is to be by air transport, air pressure must be maintained so as not to induce herniation of ocular contents. A herniated iris can appear as a corneal foreign body and similarly a subconjunctival lump

may be the result of prolapse through a scleral tear (Vinger 1986). No topical preparations should be used if there is any possibility of perforation.

Subconjunctival haemorrhage

This common injury may arise from a blow to the eye, or from intravascular pressure changes during weight-lifting or SCUBA diving. No treatment is required as the haemorrhage resolves spontaneously within 1–3 weeks; however, if the patient has hypertension it should be further investigated. If no posterior limit to a traumatic subconjunctival haemorrhage can be seen, the bleeding may have tracked forward from an orbital or cranial injury and this must be actively excluded by careful examination and radiological investigation.

Hyphaema

A hyphaema is a haemorrhage into the anterior chamber of the eye, with the bleeding coming from small vessels of the iris. This is usually the result of a blunt trauma, particularly after being struck in the eye by a ball. The injury causes immediate blurring of vision and pain in the eye, with photophobia and redness following within minutes. Examination reveals fresh bleeding, which settles within hours to form a fluid level in front of the iris. There may also be a corneal abrasion. Hyphaema is by far the most common sports-

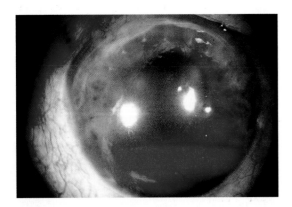 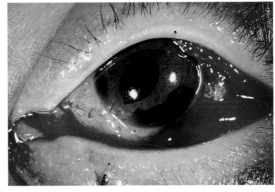

Fig. 15.5 (a) Hyphaema. (b) Hyphaema with iris trauma and subconjunctival haemorrhage. (Courtesy of Medical Illustration, Royal Victorian Eye and Ear Hospital.)

related eye injury requiring hospital admission. Squash and badminton are the sports most often involved (Fong 1994; Fig. 15.5a,b).

Associated injuries involving the orbit, ciliary body and retina are common and the eye must be examined by a specialist. The patient often feels drowsy, which may be the result of a concussive injury, or from the hyphaema itself. Once the hyphaema is recognized, the eye should be padded, the patient rested and hospital treatment arranged. The haemorrhage usually clears in 3–5 days, but in about 20% of injuries, secondary haemorrhaging occurs. The patient must rest in bed and aspirin should be avoided. The major complications are ocular hypertension and delayed development of chronic glaucoma leading to visual impairment. Hence, long-term specialist follow-up is necessary and further trauma must be avoided (Brucker *et al.* 1991)

Traumatic iritis

Less severe blunt trauma can cause an inflammatory iridocyclitis. The eye becomes red, the pupil may be constricted (miosis) or dilated (mydriasis) and blurring of vision and photophobia are common. In traumatic mydriasis, the pupil may be minimally reactive to light and irregular in shape.

Other injuries should be excluded and early specialist treatment must be arranged.

Injury to the lens

Blunt trauma can result in the development of 'rosette-like' traumatic cataract over a period of months. Dislocation or subluxation of the lens results in iridodonesis, a trembling of the iris with quick visual movements, and vitreous humour may appear in the anterior chamber of the eye. Immediate hospital treatment is required.

Injury to the lacrimal system

Trauma to the eye and lacerations may result in damage to the tear ducts. Such damage may be obscured by local swelling and any injury to the medial margins of the eyelids, particularly associated with absent or excessive tear production should be referred for specialist management.

Injury to the eyelids

Laceration of the eyelids can result from any type of direct trauma and since the lids often tend to hold themselves closed, the full extent of injury may not be recognized. The laceration must be explored, the lid fully everted and coexistent injuries to the eye and bony orbit excluded. If fat is seen in an eyelid wound this signals orbital septum penetration. Blunt trauma may cause minor laceration, but this can be associated with extensive rupture of the tarsal plate of the upper eyelid which is detected only by eversion of the lid. Specialist surgical treatment is essential in order to prevent functional and cosmetic deformity in any situation where the tarsal plate is at risk.

Retinal injury

Injury to the retina may occur in the absence of damage to the anterior segment of the eye. Once suspected, any retinal injury requires immediate ophthalmological assessment.

Retinal haemorrhage and oedema usually involve the macular area, resulting in blurred vision, and a whitish appearance is seen on examination as distinct from the usual red-orange of a healthy retina. Peripheral oedema of the retina may be asymptomatic and usually resolves over weeks with no permanent sequelae.

Retinal detachment

This injury is usually the result of a blow to the eye caused by, for example, a squash ball during a match. It may not, however, become symptomatic for weeks after the injury. The patient may complain of seeing flashes of light, 'floaters', or a 'curtain' across the field of vision. On examination, the area not yet separated is red, well demarcated and most commonly in the temporal quadrant of the retina. After detachment, the area appears grey and the retinal blood vessels almost black. Surgery is necessary for the repair of retinal detachment and is now usually done by laser.

Choroid rupture

This may also result from a blow to the eye as above, and is often associated with retinal

Fig. 15.6 There is a 'blow-out' fracture of the floor of the left orbit. The bone fragment (white arrow) forms a trapdoor and early herniation of intraorbital fat through the opening is shown (open arrow). There is considerable displacement and deformity of the inferior rectus muscle (black arrow).

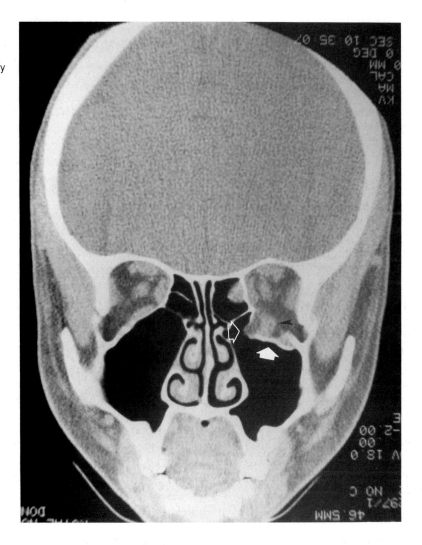

haemorrhage. On examination whitish circumscribed areas concentric with the disc margin are seen and prolonged rest is necessary for resolution.

Optic nerve injury

Severe blunt injury to the head, eye or orbit as in motor vehicle accidents may injure the optic nerve and produce permanent blindness. There may be abnormal pupillary responses to light and on ophthalmoscopy the nerve appears pale and swollen. Urgent referral to a medical specialist is required.

Orbital injury

Fracture of the orbital floor, or 'blow-out' fracture, may result from squash when the ball strikes the eye, or in punching or kicking sports. The blunt trauma causes a sudden increase in intraorbital pressure. Usually the orbital margins remain intact, but the very thin orbital floor offers least resistance and consequently fractures. Herniation of orbital contents may occur through the bony defect (Fig. 15.6).

Clinical features of a 'blow-out' fracture include

double vision (diplopia), restriction of eye movement, protruding eye and downward displacement of the eye, together with anaesthesia or hyperaesthesia in the distribution of the intraorbital nerve on the cheek below the injured eye. The inferior rectus muscle is most often affected, and causes diplopia on upward gaze. Initial findings of restricted eye movement, diplopia and sensory change over the cheek and upper gums may be the result of soft tissue swelling alone. Other clinical signs may not appear until later. The possibility of fracture must be assessed by a radiological examination. The fracture itself is often not visible; however, there may be clouding of the maxillary sinus. A more certain diagnosis is made by the finding of tissue herniated into the maxillary sinus. Where there is any doubt, CT scans offer the most accurate imaging of the area and show the fracture site and herniation (Levy 1986).

On diagnosis, antibiotics must be commenced to prevent orbital cellulitis and specialist consultation is required to determine further treatment. Many fractures can be treated conservatively with full resolution of symptoms, others require immediate repair, or delayed repair should diplopia persist.

Medial orbital wall fracture

This fracture occurs less often, but in similar circumstances to a 'blow-out' fracture. A communication with the ethmoid sinus results and subcutaneous emphysema (collection of air) about the nose and eyelids, accentuated by blowing the nose, is usually found. Radiographs may show air in the orbit and CT scans may be necessary if this is not demonstrated. Treatment with antibiotics is advised and surgery is only required if there is entrapment of the medial rectus muscle.

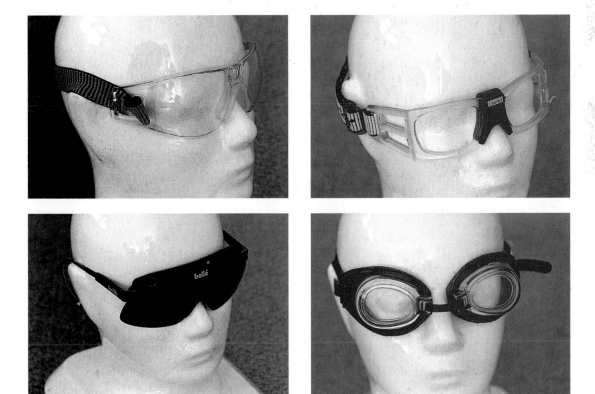

Fig. 15.7 Examples of polycarbonate eyewear. (a) Protective glasses for squash. (b) Protective glasses with corrective lenses. (c) Sports sunglasses with corrective lenses. (d) Swimming goggles with corrective lenses.

Prevention of Eye Injuries

Severe eye injuries are often associated with the sports of squash and badminton. The ball or shuttlecock is usually the cause of injury, as it can penetrate the orbit and strike the eye directly, at velocities of up to 230 k.p.h. in both sports (Vinger 1991; Fong 1994). Protective goggles which have passed vigorous testing standards are available for squash, and as they do not impair the visual field, should be considered mandatory. Numerous studies have shown that experienced elite squash players tend to suffer more eye injuries because of their style of play and further studies have demonstrated that eye injuries become virtually non-existent with the routine use of approved protective eyewear (Easterbrook 1987, 1988; Fig. 15.7a). Lensless eye guards for squash have been widely promoted. The ball is able to penetrate these guards, increasing the risk of serious eye injury. They should never be used.

In sports where a larger ball is used the risk of the ball penetrating the orbit is much less. Most eye injuries in football and basketball are the result of accidental contact with another player rather than the ball (Vinger 1991). In these sports eye protection for players with normal vision is not essential.

Spectacles or goggles, whether for correction of vision or eye protection, must be adequate for the sport concerned. A wide variety of spectacles specifically designed for sporting use are available. Glass lenses should never be used, regardless of whether they are described as 'safety' or 'toughened'. CR39 is the most widely used lens material in prescription spectacles. It is quite strong, but does not withstand the impact of a squash ball. Polycarbonate is the best material for protective lenses; however, it may not be available for some prescription lenses. Polycarbonate is many times stronger than CR39 and can withstand the impact of gunshot (Vinger 1991). Frames must also be strong and suitably designed and not allow the lens to pop out on impact (Easterbrook 1987). Contact lenses may be more suitable for correcting acuity for many sports because they do not interfere with the field of vision and do not fog. However, they are not protective in any circumstances and should be combined with suitable eye protection for all high-risk activities, such as squash. Hard lenses are dangerous if there is any risk of trauma to the eye.

In cricket the batsman facing a fast rising ball, or the close-in fielder, runs a significant risk of sustaining a 'blow-out' fracture of the orbit and protective helmets must include adequate eye and facial protection. The same applies to other sports such as ice-hockey and lacrosse (Jones & Tullo 1986).

The damaging effect on the eye of prolonged exposure to ultraviolet light is now widely recognized. Ultraviolet light levels are high throughout summer, particularly during the middle part of the day. Snow reflects approximately 10 times as much ultraviolet light as other surfaces and is particularly dangerous to the eye. Lens damage leading to cataract formation is the major concern. Damage to the cornea, choroid and retina also occurs. Many purpose designed sports sunglasses are now available, which almost totally eliminate ultraviolet penetration. Good design allows an unrestricted field of vision and excellent clarity, so there should be no impairment of visual performance. As lenses are generally constructed of polycarbonate they also protect against trauma. Their use is strongly recommended for sports where there is a high level of ultraviolet exposure, particularly cricket, tennis, golf, skiing and cycling. Modified sports sunglasses are available for those who require corrective lenses (Carson & Taylor 1994; Fig. 15.7b–d).

INJURY TO THE FACE AND NOSE

Soft Tissue Lacerations

Lacerations are commonly encountered in contact sports such as boxing, football and field hockey and a number of factors must be borne in mind with respect to the repair of these lacerations. They are as follows:

- Infection often results from contamination through the mouth and nose or from playing surfaces. Prophylactic antibiotics and a tetanus toxoid injection should be administered in the majority of cases
- The cosmetic repair of a laceration is important

and the player must always be made aware of the possible outcomes if returning to activity before the wound has healed. Complications which can occur are wound breakdown, infection and an excessive scar

- Underlying structures in the soft tissues, such as muscles, nerves and the parotid gland, must be considered in the repair of what may seem to be a minor superficial laceration
- Deeper structures may be damaged but disguised by local oedema or haematoma. Fractures of the frontal sinuses are particularly important in this regard and radiological examination is strongly recommended

Acute Management of the Bleeding Wound

Bleeding wounds of the head or face are one of the most common injuries encountered in team sports, whether contact be intended or accidental. Concerns about the risk of transmission of HIV, hepatitis B and other infectious diseases have led to many sporting bodies formulating policy to deal with this situation. Most require removal of the bleeding player until all bleeding has ceased and the wound is adequately covered. In competition, rapid and effective treatment is essential.

Rapid haemostasis can be achieved by the use of firm pressure to the wound. If the wound continues to bleed, calcium alginate dressings are very effective, releasing calcium ions into the wound and forming a sodium alginate gel over the wound. This gel can then be washed off and the wound repaired with no impairment of healing. Gauze soaked in adrenaline 1:1000 and applied to the wound is also effective. Petroleum jelly and other preparations used as haemostatics impair wound healing unless carefully washed out of the wound before repair.

Disinfection of the area and removal of any dirt or other debris should then be undertaken. Alcoholic iodine is the most effective skin bactericide, but allergic reactions are common. Alcoholic chlorhexidine and Povidone-iodine are nearly as effective. These preparations should be allowed to dry on the area to achieve full effect. Local stinging is transient, and wound healing when closure is immediate is not impaired. Any dirt etc. in the wound must be

meticulously removed to prevent infection and to prevent subsequent tattooing of the skin.

Wound closure can be achieved with sutures, tissue adhesive or adhesive dressings. On the face sutures should be non-absorbable monofilament of 5/0 or 6/0 thickness to minimize scarring, and should be inserted with suitable local anaesthetic cover. Cyano-acrylate tissue adhesives produce the best cosmetic result on small, clean, dry wounds. The wound should be stretched, adhesive applied along its length and then held for 1 min. Adhesive strips also provide effective rapid closure of small, superficial wounds, as long as the skin is dry. Tincture of benzoin applied to unbroken skin improves adhesion. On the very sweaty player, obtaining a dry surface can be very difficult and so a temporary closure may have to be made and dressings applied liberally until formal repair can be undertaken after the game. Skin staplers should never be used on the face. Staples are cosmetically unacceptable, being equivalent to 2/0 suture material, and present a risk of further tissue damage on return to play. Staplers do not offer more rapid repair than the above methods.

Once the wound has been repaired, it must be effectively dressed to allow continued play without further bleeding. On dry wounds, adhesive polyurethane dressings are ideal as they are waterproof, allow inspection of the wound and permit gaseous exchange, thus not delaying healing. If the wound is still oozing, hydrocolloid dressings are most effective, being flexible, resilient and absorptive. If the wound is very moist, polyurethane foam offers greater absorptive capacity. The wound should then be liberally bandaged or taped to ensure dressings remain in place. Cohesive bandages, or elastic adhesive tapes applied circumferentially are most effective (D. MacLellan, Wound Foundation of Australia, personal communication).

The Scalp

The scalp is frequently lacerated and may bleed profusely because of its copious blood supply. Repair by suturing can be undertaken rapidly. If bleeding is not controlled by direct pressure, ligation of the bleeding vessel may be necessary.

The loose plane between the galea aponeurotica

and the skin is a potentially large tissue 'space' after wound closure. The floor of a wound must be explored to exclude skull fracture, then irrigated and pressure applied to prevent haematoma formation in this 'space'.

The Forehead and Eyebrows

Significant structures in this area include the frontalis muscle, the facial nerve and the frontal sinus. The frontalis muscle can be repaired with the use of deep sutures. The temporal branch of the facial nerve runs approximately 1 cm lateral to the eyebrow, innervating the frontalis muscle. Should there be asymmetry on raising the eyebrows or on wrinkling the forehead, the patient with a laceration in this area should be referred immediately for formal exploration by a surgeon.

Frontal sinus fracture may produce a palpable depression and long-term deformity. More importantly, a communication with the cerebrospinal fluid can result in an associated risk of meningitis. Appropriate radiological evaluation and referral to a neurosurgeon should be undertaken.

The eyebrows, when interrupted by a laceration must be meticulously repaired, as a 'stepped' eyebrow is cosmetically undesirable. Eyebrows should never be shaved, as correct realignment by suturing becomes extremely difficult.

The Face

The anatomical position of the parotid duct must be located and injury excluded by careful exploration with a fine probe.

The facial nerve may be at risk, particularly at its marginal mandibular branch which runs over the margin of the jaw and the platysma. If injury to this nerve has occurred the ability to lower the corner of the mouth will be lost and an asymmetrical smile results. Lacerations involving the orbicularis oris muscle must be carefully repaired by suture to avoid asymmetry about the mouth (White et al. 1989).

In general, wounds heal well when they occur parallel to the lines of facial expression, while 'perpendicular' lacerations often result in disfiguring scars. Careful debridement of these wounds improves the result. Tissue adhesive or adhesive strips are ideal for smaller wounds. Sutures should be used for the repair of gaping or deep facial lacerations and sutures should be removed after 5 days. The wound should then be protected by adhesive strips for a further week and kept dry during the first 2 weeks to minimize scarring. Subsequently, sunlight should be avoided to achieve optimal fading of the scar.

Solar Injury

Sports played outdoors during the summer months expose the face to high doses of ultraviolet light. The major causative role of ultraviolet light in all types of skin cancer, particularly malignant melanoma, is now well recognized. The use of hats and ultraviolet shielding creams is strongly recommended for all participants.

The Mouth and Lips

These highly vascular areas bleed profusely but heal quickly. Lacerations often result from compressive forces such as a punch or push against the lips and teeth in contact sports. Every external laceration in this area should be explored to be sure it does not extend through to the mucosal surface of the mouth. Absorbable sutures should be used to close the mucosal surface and a deep layer may be necessary to approximate the orbicularis oris muscle. If the muscle is not closed, an unsightly local depression may result.

The vermilion border of the lip must be precisely realigned when this region of the face is torn. When a laceration of the lip does not involve the vermilion border, does not gape and bleeding has ceased, suturing may be unnecessary as rapid healing occurs.

Fracture of the Zygoma

The fractured zygoma (or cheekbone) is the result of a direct blow, usually sustained during participation in contact sports, or an injury by a hard ball, equipment, fist or boot. The two most common types of fractures are the depressed fracture of the zygomatic arch and the trimalar fracture. The latter is where the zygoma fractures at its attachment to the temporal, frontal and maxillary bones. In either case, associated orbital injury is frequent and must be actively excluded by careful examination and X-ray.

The player typically complains of an inability to open the jaw when zygomatic arch fragments are depressed. In the trimalar fracture, the associated intraorbital nerve injury causes sensory loss of the cheek. Inspection of the face reveals bruising and swelling, but bony deformity may not be apparent. Viewing the face from above and carefully comparing the contours of the cheeks is a good method of detecting the deformity. Careful palpation and comparison with the normal side reveals a depression or step in the bone structure if local swelling and tenderness are not too severe (Cannell 1986).

Radiological investigation should be undertaken, requesting specific views of areas of suspected injury. Fractures should be evident and the maxillary sinus may be opacified by blood, indicating damage to the orbital floor and perhaps herniation of the orbital contents.

Antibiotics must be administered immediately, but surgical repair may be delayed on specialist advice to allow swelling to settle. Trimalar fractures require reduction and wiring or packing and elevation if the fracture is depressed. Sport should be avoided for at least 3 weeks after surgical repair.

Sinus Fractures

Fractures of the walls of the maxillary, ethmoid and frontal sinuses can occur in isolation as a result of a direct blow. However, damage to orbital and intracranial structures usually accompanies the sinus injury and management of these two problems is the first priority. Fracture of the sinus produces soft tissue crepitus directly overlying the sinus and fracture of the ethmoid produces crepitus on the medial wall of the orbit. X-rays reveal opacification of the affected sinus or an air–fluid level and air may be seen in the adjacent soft tissues. For isolated maxillary or ethmoid sinus fracture, sport should be avoided for a week and management is by use of antibiotics and strict avoidance of nose-blowing. In the case of the frontal sinus, cosmetic deformity may result, or with a posterior wall fracture, cerebrospinal fluid leakage is likely. Antibiotic therapy should be started immediately and specialist treatment sought. Repair of the sinus is usually necessary and one should also be aware of the complications of chronic sinusitis and osteomyelitis (Handler 1991).

Fractures of the Maxilla and Mandible

These injuries are discussed in Chapter 16.

Injuries of the Nose

There are four common results of injury to the nose, which may coexist. These are as follows:

- Fracture of the nasal bones
- Fracture or dislocation of the nasal septum
- Septal haematoma
- Epistaxis (nose-bleed)

FRACTURE OF THE NASAL BONES

Nasal fracture is a common result of a direct blow to the nose, for example in boxing. A lateral force produces a depressed fracture of one side of the nose, while a 'front-on' blow splays the bridge of the nose and often fractures both nasal bones. Immediate reduction is possible but this should only be undertaken by a specialist medical practitioner as there is a significant risk of a sharp bony fragment tearing nasal arteries and producing severe epistaxis.

Swelling of the nose occurs rapidly with a fracture and diffuse swelling may mask a severe future deformity, while unilateral swelling may suggest an apparent bone deformity where none exists. Ice packs are useful to limit swelling and, once other injuries to the nasal structures have been excluded, the athlete should be reviewed in 5–7 days to assess deformity and possible obstruction of nasal passages. Immediate referral to a surgeon for reduction should occur if such a problem is apparent. X-rays are generally of little value as the diagnosis is clinical and X-rays need only be taken when other bony injuries are suspected.

Once reduction of the nasal fracture has been performed, a plaster splint may be worn for approximately a week if the reduction is unstable. Return to contact sports should be delayed for at least 3 weeks after reduction as the risk of redisplacement is high. If early reduction of a fracture is not undertaken and a marked deformity of the nose persists, rhinoplasty (nasal surgery) can be undertaken at the end of the competitive season. In contact sports it may be preferable to delay such surgery until the end of the player's career if the surgeon's 'good work' is not to be undone by further trauma.

Major complications with nasal fracture include associated injuries to the orbit, fractures of the ethmoid labyrinth, loss of the sense of smell (anosmia) by trauma to the olfactory nerve and severe epistaxis if the anterior ethmoidal artery is torn.

Orbital examination must be a routine part of the examination of a nasal injury and radiological examination should be undertaken if there are suspicious signs. Leakage of clear fluid from the nose (rhinorrhoea) suggests cerebrospinal fluid leak and a communication of air with the ethmoid labyrinth, requiring immediate surgical repair. Prophylactic antibiotics must be commenced immediately to prevent meningitis and if there is any discharge from the nose test strips to detect the presence of glucose in the fluid can confirm the presence of cerebrospinal fluid.

Occasionally the lamina papyracea is fractured, resulting in a communication between the nose and the orbit. Blowing the nose in this situation causes periorbital swelling and surgical emphysema in the form of air collecting underneath the skin. However, if nose blowing is avoided the injury heals spontaneously within a week. Prophylactic antibiotics and referral to a surgeon are strongly recommended (Brookes & McKelvie 1986).

FRACTURE OF THE NASAL SEPTUM

This can occur with or without nasal fracture and symptoms are those of a unilateral sensation of 'a blocked nose' and sometimes pain of the forehead and/or cheek. Direct examination of the septum with the patient's head tilted back and the nostrils well lit makes the diagnosis easier. A formal septoplasty is often necessary. This procedure may be performed at the end of a player's career, as the nasal structure is weakened by the initial injury and is susceptible to repeated injury.

SEPTAL HAEMATOMA

This injury results from direct trauma and is commonly associated with fracture, but it may occur in isolation. Bleeding within the nasal septum produces a swelling which looks like a cherry within the nose on examination. There is often a complete obstruction of one or both nostrils. This is tested by occluding one nostril and asking the patient to blow through the nose. Immediate treatment is necessary to prevent local infection which can result in cavernous sinus thrombosis (a blood clot close to the brain). On recognition of the haematoma the patient should be immediately referred to a surgeon for incision, drainage and packing of the area and prophylactic antibiotics should be commenced. If the injury is neglected, 'death' of the septal cartilage results and produces an ugly 'saddle-nose' deformity which may require extensive plastic surgery.

EPISTAXIS

Most often bleeding from the nose is not severe and arises from Little's area of mucosa on the anterior nasal septum. Bleeding may be spontaneous or result from trauma. Immediate management consists of firmly pinching the soft tissues of the nose between the finger and thumb for at least 5 min. Ice applied to the bridge of the nose will promote local vasoconstriction and the head should be tilted forward in order to prevent swallowing or inhaling blood.

If bleeding is severe, blood loss should be estimated and regular measurements of pulse and blood pressure undertaken to detect the effects of blood loss (shock). Immediate control of bleeding is best achieved by nasal packing with ribbon gauze impregnated with a vasoconstrictive agent, but this is only effective if the medical practitioner has experience in the correct nasal packing technique. An alternative is the use of an inflatable device such as a balloon catheter. Where these measures are not available, a cotton ball or tampon impregnated with adrenaline 1:1000 may be used to stem the blood loss. If the bleeding point can be identified, it may be cauterized at a suitable medical facility, or surgical treatment may be necessary.

INJURIES TO THE EAR

Injuries to the external ear are relatively common in the various contact football codes and in wrestling, boxing and the martial arts. They basically fall into two categories: lacerations and auricular haematomas. Middle ear injuries usually result from direct trauma. Damage to the inner ear may be caused by excessive noise, or be associated with intracranial trauma.

External ear injury may be prevented by any form of helmet that covers the ear, while permitting effective hearing. Closely fitted soft shell helmets are available for this purpose in those sports where hard shell helmets are not permitted. Rugby players make use of elastic headbands or adhesive tape to prevent ear trauma. Rigid ear protectors are used in water polo to minimize middle ear damage.

Lacerations

The external ear has a well developed blood supply and there is a high potential for ragged wounds to heal well with competent early management. The damaged area must be meticulously cleaned, the cartilage of the ear should be identified and approximated, but not closed. The perichondrium should be closed with absorbable sutures and the skin layer should be finally repaired separately with non-absorbable material. Sutures should not pass through cartilage as they produce an irritative perichondritis; however, suturing may be necessary after avulsion injuries (Brookes & McKelvie 1986). Broad-spectrum antibiotics should be prescribed for all lacerations of the ear. Avulsed portions of the ear can be successfully reattached with immediate repair, producing better results than delayed repair.

Auricular Haematoma

Shearing forces to the ear can produce bleeding between the perichondrium and cartilage, causing local swelling (and loss of the ear's contours), or what is generally termed a 'cauliflower ear'. If treatment is delayed organization of the haematoma results in a permanent 'cauliflower ear', which is then very difficult or impossible to restore. The haematoma must be aspirated as soon as possible and then firmly dressed to prevent reaccumulation of blood.

To dress the ear a liberal quantity of cotton wool should be dampened with mineral oil or collodion, and then packed firmly and evenly to restore every contour of the ear on both surfaces. A firm crepe bandage should then be wrapped around the ear and the head and left in place for 1 week.

With any injury to the external ear, hearing must be tested and the middle ear examined to exclude associated injury such as rupture of the tympanic membrane which is discussed in the next section.

Lacerations of the ear canal may heal with subsequent canal stenosis (narrowing) and may require surgery at a later time.

The Middle Ear

A slap, punch or other trauma to the ear, particularly when the canal is filled with water in aquatic sports, such as water polo or water skiing, may result in a rupture of the tympanic membrane (ear drum). Such an injury with a sudden sharp pain and often tinnitus (ringing in the ears) can usually be diagnosed by history alone, particularly as the canal may be filled with blood, which hides the perforation. The ear should be kept dry and it is wise to administer prophylactic antibiotics. Small perforations of the ear drum will heal within a few weeks and mild conductive deafness, if present, should also resolve. If the perforation is large, or not healing within 4 weeks, specialist medical referral is essential. Grafting of the tympanic membrane gives good results.

Barotrauma to the ear is discussed in detail in Chapter 25.

The Inner Ear

Sensorineural deafness is not uncommon among sporting shooters and participants in sports involving motorized vehicles, where sound-limiting devices such as mufflers are deficient or non-existent. Competitors should be warned of the risk to their hearing and appropriate ear protectors employed.

Closed head injuries can permanently damage the vestibulocochlear structures of the inner ear by a number of means. Fractures of the petrous temporal bone may directly damage structures of the inner ear, resulting in permanent deafness and a blow to the fixed head can cause labyrinthine concussion. Rapid acceleration or deceleration forces to the head can tear the auditory nerve and these injuries may produce vertigo and deafness. In each case, the immediate management of head injury should be instituted as recommended in the early part of this chapter. Bleeding from the ear, haemorrhage through the tympanic membrane and cerebrospinal fluid discharge from the ear are all signs of intracranial injury and must be checked.

CONCLUSIONS

In contact sports the player runs a definite risk of injury to the head, eye or ear. Where contact is not allowed, accidental collisions with other players or their equipment, and sometimes even the facility in which they are competing, can badly injure them. It is by the modification of rules and the use of carefully designed protective equipment that many injuries to the head can be minimized and it should be the goal of all those persons connected with the safe conduct of the sport to see that this occurs.

REFERENCES

Alves W. M. (1991) Football-induced mild head injury. In Torg J. S. (ed.) *Athletic Injuries to the Head, Neck, and Face,* 2nd edn, pp. 283–304. Mosby Year Book, St Louis, MO.

Brookes G. B. & McKelvie P. (1986) Otorhinolaryngology. In Helal B., King J. & Grange W. (eds) *Sports Injuries and Their Treatment,* pp. 101–119. Chapman & Hall, London.

Brucker A. J., Kozart D. M., Nichols C. W. & Raber I. M. (1991) Diagnosis and management of injuries to the eye and orbit. In Torg J. S. (ed.) *Athletic Injuries to the Head, Neck, and Face,* 2nd edn, pp. 650–670. Mosby Year Book, St Louis, MO.

Brukner P. & Khan K. (1993) Headache. *Clinical Sports Medicine,* pp. 161–168. McGraw-Hill, Sydney.

Bruno L. A., Genarelli T. A. & Torg J. S. (1987) Management guidelines for head injuries in athletics. *Clinics in Sports Medicine* 6, 17–29.

Cacayorin E. D., Petro G. R. & Hochhauser L. (1987) Headache in the athlete and radiographic evaluation. *Clinics in Sports Medicine* 6, 739–749.

Cannell H. (1986) Oral, dental and maxillo-facial injuries. In Helal B., King J. & Grange W. (eds) *Sports Injuries and Their Treatment,* pp. 71–99. Chapman & Hall, London.

Cantu R. C. (1986) Guidelines for return to contact sports after a cerebral concussion. *Physician and Sports Medicine* 14, 75–83.

Cantu R. C. (1988) Head and spine injuries in the young athlete. *Clinics in Sports Medicine* 7, 450–472.

Carson C. A. & Taylor H. R. (1994) The effects of sunlight on the eye and the role of prevention. *Modern Medicine* 37, 58–64.

Committee on Head Injury Nomenclature of the Congress of Neurological Surgeons (1966) Glossary of Head Injury including some definitions of injury to the cervical spine. *Clinical Neurosurgery* 12, 386.

Dicker G. (1991) A sports doctor's dilemma in concussion. *Sports Training, Medicine & Rehabilitation* 2, 203–209.

Easterbrook M. (1987) Eye protection in racket sports: An update. *Physician and Sports Medicine* 15, 189–192.

Easterbrook M. (1988) Eye protection in racket sports. *Clinics in Sports Medicine* 7, 253–267.

Ellis T. H., Streight D. & Mellion M. B. (1994) Bicycle safety equipment. *Clinics in Sports Medicine* 13, 75–98.

Fong L. P. (1994) Sports-related eye injuries. *Medical Journal of Australia* 160, 743–750.

Genarelli T. A. (1991) Head injury mechanisms. In Torg J. S. (ed.) *Athletic Injuries to the Head, Neck, and Face,* 2nd edn, pp. 232–240. Mosby Year Book, St Louis, MO.

Gisolfi C. V., Rohlf D. P., Navarude S. N., Hayes C. L. & Sayeed S. A. (1988) Effects of wearing a helmet on thermal balance while cycling in the heat. *Physician and Sports Medicine* 16, 139–146.

Greenberg M. S. & Springer P. S. (1991) Diagnosis and management of oral injuries. In Torg J. S. (ed.) *Athletic Injuries to the Head, Neck, and Face,* 2nd edn, pp. 635–649. Mosby Year Book, St Louis, MO.

Handler S. D. (1991) Diagnosis and management of maxillofacial injuries. In Torg J. S. (ed.) *Athletic Injuries to the Head, Neck, and Face,* 2nd edn, pp. 611–634. Mosby Year Book, St Louis, MO.

Hodgson V. R. (1991) Impact standards for protective equipment. In Torg J. S. (ed.) *Athletic Injuries to the Head, Neck, and Face,* 2nd edn, pp. 28–43. Mosby Year Book, St Louis, MO.

Jahre C., Pavlov H. & Deck M. D. F. (1991) Computed tomography and magnetic resonance imaging for evaluation of head trauma. In Torg J. S. (ed.) *Athletic Injuries to the Head, Neck, and Face,* 2nd edn, pp. 256–269. Mosby Year Book, St Louis, MO.

Jones N. P. & Tullo A. B. (1986) Severe eye injuries in cricket. *British Journal of Sports Medicine* **20**, 178–179.

Jordan B. (ed.) (1992) *Medical Aspects of Boxing.* CRC Press, Boca Raton, FL.

Levy I. S. (1986) Eye injuries. In Helal B., King J. & Grange W. (eds) *Sports Injuries and Their Treatment,* pp. 61–69. Chapman & Hall, London.

McCarthy P. (1988) Athletes' headaches: Not necessarily 'little' problems. *Physician and Sportsmedicine* **16**, 169–173.

McCrory P., Maddocks D. L. & Dicker G. D. (1994) Head and brain injury in sport. *Australian Sports Medicine Federation Position Paper,* Canberra.

Vinger P. F. (1986) How I manage corneal abrasions and lacerations. *Physician and Sportsmedicine* **14**, 170–179.

Vinger P. F. (1991) The eye and sports medicine. In Duane T. D. & Jaeger E. A. (eds) *Clinical Ophthalmology,* pp. 1–51. Harper & Row, Philadelphia, PA.

Vinger P. F. & Knuttgen H. G. (1988) Eye injuries and eye protection in sports (International Federation of Sports Medicine Position Statement). *Physician and Sports Medicine* **16**, 49–51.

White M. J., Johnson P. C. & Heckler F. R. (1989) Management of maxillofacial and neck soft-tissue injuries. *Clinics in Sports Medicine* **8**, 11–23.

CHAPTER 16

DENTAL PROBLEMS

J. P. Fricker and M. L. O'Neill

The purpose of this chapter is to inform the non-dentist of the common problems athletes have with their teeth and the tissue surrounding them. It deals mainly with traumatic injuries to the teeth and supporting tissues and dental pain in the regions of the maxilla and the mandible. The following material is intended to assist in a better understanding of the above problems so that informed decisions can be made with relation to definitive care by a dental practitioner.

ANATOMY OF THE TEETH AND FACE

The maxilla houses the upper teeth and is bounded superiorly by the inferior rim of the orbit and laterally by the anterior section of the zygomatic arch (Fig. 16.1). The other major region of the face is the mandible which is the only movable segment, and thus the only portion of the face that involves a joint, the temporomandibular joint (TMJ). The mandible consists of a horseshoe-shaped body that is the tooth-bearing section of the mandible, and two rami.

The inferior dental or mandibular nerve and associated blood vessels enter the mandible on the internal surface and pass along the intra-osseous canal. A majority of these nerves and vessels then exit through the mental foramen to supply the chin and lips.

The condylar process makes up the mandibular portion of the TMJ, while anterior to this are the

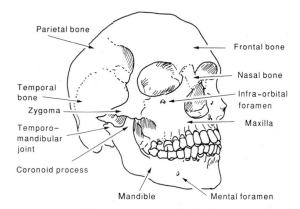

Fig. 16.1 The anatomy of the skull.

mandibular notch and coronoid process. The TMJ allows the opening and closing of the jaws and the articulation of the dental arches during mastication. The joint itself consists of the head of the condyle and the temporal fossa and eminence of the temporal bone. Interposed between these two surfaces is an articular cartilaginous disc and two synovially filled articular cavities. Several ligaments, with nearby muscle attachments enable safe movement of the joint during function.

Teeth are living, hard tissues, similar in composition to bone and are arranged in the dental arches of the maxillae and the mandible (Fig. 16.2). The clinical crown of the tooth is that part which is exposed in the oral cavity and the clinical root is the region in the supporting bone.

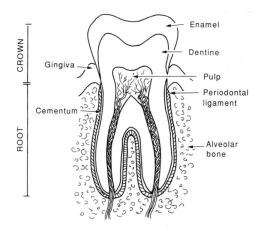

Fig. 16.2 The anatomy of the tooth.

The outer layer of the crown is enamel with cementum forming the external layer of the root. The internal structure of the tooth is dentine surrounding the pulp chamber, which contains the neurovascular bundle of the dental pulp.

OROFACIAL AND DENTAL TRAUMA

Orofacial and dental trauma are classified according to the tissue involved and the magnitude of the trauma (Andreasen 1981). The following injuries are common in collision sports, such as the various codes of football and hockey, or are sustained in accidents when the athlete falls or comes in contact with equipment or facilities while competing, such as in cricket or baseball.

Injuries to Tooth Structure

Tooth trauma can be categorized in relation to the various structural levels of the tooth itself and subclassifications are defined according to these anatomical subdivisions.

CROWN FRACTURES (FIG. 16.3)

This is the most common area of trauma to dental tissues (Martin *et al*. 1990). Injuries to the crown of the tooth can be further subclassified according to the amount of structural damage sustained during the trauma.

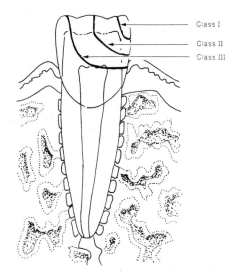

Fig. 16.3 Classes of crown fractures.

A Class I fracture involves the enamel layer of the tooth, the damage often being to the cutting edge or its corner. Usually no symptoms occur, although immediately after the injury there may be some tenderness on percussion (tapping) as a result of bruising of the periodontal ligament. No immediate treatment is required, but the chipped area should be seen by a dentist to aesthetically restore it.

A Class II fracture is more extensive and the underlying dentine is exposed at the site. This fracture usually presents with an obvious reaction to the exposure of the dentinal tubules containing the nerves, which communicate reactions from the junction of the enamel and dentine to the pulpal tissues. The immediate treatment involves plugging the dentinal tubules to avoid loss or damage to the nerves and these injuries require prompt treatment from a dentist.

A Class III fracture involves the exposure of the enamel, dentine and the pulpal tissues at the fracture site. The exposure of the pulpal tissues may be minimal or extensive; however, in either case immediate treatment is required by a dentist.

CROWN-ROOT FRACTURE

These injuries range from the simple to the complex,

depending on the amount of tooth lost and the position of the fracture line.

A simple fracture involves the enamel, dentine and cementum, but not the pulp. Generally, this type of crown-root fracture is seen on the mesial or distal edge of the tooth. Initial treatment is to approximate the crown of the tooth and the fractured piece, since the fractured section will be generally attached to the gingival tissues. A simple fracture necessitates the dentist plugging the exposed dentinal tubules and building up the tooth in acid-etch composite restoration.

A complicated fracture involves exposure of the dentine and the pulpal tissues, with the fracture line descending below the gingival attachment. Treatment is similar to the Class III crown fracture unless the fracture line descends well below the attached gingiva or if the fracture is full length through the mid-line of the tooth. In the latter situations it may be necessary to extract the tooth as there may be no chance of rebuilding it.

ROOT FRACTURES

Root fractures are less common and the treatment varies with the site of the fracture and its angle. Usually teeth that are traumatized by root fracture appear to be repositioned further back in the mouth than their neighbours. Clinically, the patient is very aware of this repositioning because of its interference with the bite. Unless the fracture is near the gingival cuff, clinical manipulation to a near-as-normal position and then splinting are all that needs to be done initially. Radiographs will easily substantiate the area and angle of any fracture that occurs. Follow-up radiography will demonstrate if stabilization has been achieved for the root fragment and pulp testing will clarify the integrity of the pulpal tissues. The site of the fracture and the angle of the fracture line will determine whether root canal therapy or extraction is indicated. Alternatively, it may be possible to orthodontically extrude the root fragment so that a crown buildup may be carried out as for a simple crown fracture (Wong & Fricker 1991).

Injuries to the Periodontal Ligament

The term luxation refers to the movement of a tooth within the periodontal ligament over and above normal physiological limits, as a result of trauma. The most common area to be involved in this type of injury is the upper anterior region of the mouth, specifically the upper incisor teeth. Luxation injuries may be classified as follows.

CONCUSSION

This refers to an injury to the teeth's supporting membrane, the periodontal ligament, without physical signs of mobility. The tooth is tender to percussion, but is otherwise unaffected. Radiographically, the periodontal ligament appears relatively normal and the usual treatment is to adjust the loading from the opposing teeth and carry out periodic vitality testing to ensure the integrity of the pulpal tissues.

SUBLUXATION

This is similar to concussion, except that there is marked mobility of the tooth in the socket. There may be some haemorrhage from beneath the gingival cuff, indicating damage to the periodontal ligament. Radiographically, the periodontal space appears normal, but the tooth may react abnormally to clinical percussive testing. Treatment is again palliative, with follow-up radiography and pulpal testing.

INTRUSIVE LUXATION

This occurs when the tooth is forcibly pushed further into the socket along the crown apex line and involves simultaneous comminution and possible fracture of the alveolar bone. Clinically, the intruded tooth appears shorter than those around it and the crown may in fact completely disappear within the soft tissue from the force of impact. Radiographically, there is a missing or greatly reduced periodontal space around the root of the tooth. As has been already mentioned, most luxations appear in the upper central incisors, with the lateral incisors being the next most commonly affected. If an upper central incisor is intruded sufficiently to cause the tooth to disappear into the soft tissues, there is a possibility that the apex of the tooth may appear physically within the nasal cavity mucosa or even pierce the nasal mucosa itself.

The treatment should attempt to reposition the tooth after the injury over a 3–4 week period, using orthodontics. This allows the bone to heal and to keep up with the re-eruption of the intruded tooth. Immediate repositioning leads to a much greater risk of subsequent root resorption and loss of marginal bone support for the tooth.

EXTRUSIVE LUXATION

This is also called partial avulsion as the tooth is partially displaced out of its socket. Clinically, a partial avulsion appears as an elongation of the tooth in the arch and usually has a palatal or lingual deviation. There is always haemorrhage about the gingival cuff and radiographically the periodontal space appears widened, with some obvious deviation of the axial position compared with neighbouring teeth. It is essential to physically reposition the tooth by splinting, using an acid-etch bond of the traumatized tooth to its neighbouring teeth. Orthodontic banding and the use of an arch wire are successful alternatives.

All the types of luxation injuries can irreparably damage the pulpal tissues, with necrosis of this tissue a common sequela to the injury. If the patient is young the apical foramen of the tooth is still wide and the chances of at least some of the pulpal tissues remaining vital and intact are greater than in the case of adult teeth, where the apical foramen is narrow and no development of the root of the tooth is possible. If deciduous teeth are luxated, the usual course of treatment is to leave them in place or to extract them.

Avulsion

The definition of avulsion is the complete displacement of a tooth from its bony socket with complete severance of the tooth's apical tissues from the bone.

The most commonly involved teeth are the maxillary central incisors while the mandibular teeth are rarely avulsed. It is also uncommon for more than one tooth to be injured in this way. Avulsion is rarely an isolated injury, as it is usually accompanied by other luxation injuries and soft tissue damage.

Influencing the healing process will be the presence of any bone fragments within the socket itself or any dirt or debris from the sports field. Bone fragments should be removed using forceps and the operator should never irrigate the socket vigorously to remove debris, as this has an adverse effect on the prognosis of a reimplanted tooth.

EMERGENCY TREATMENT OF AN AVULSED TOOTH

The following procedure should be carried out in the treatment of an avulsed tooth:

- Rinse the avulsed tooth in a saline solution or water without physically handling the root of the tooth (so as not to remove the periodontal ligament)
- Reposition the tooth in its socket in as-near-as-normal a position as is possible using firm pressure to displace any blood clot. The socket should not be irrigated
- The tooth should then be stabilized in position with a temporary splint using adhesive tape. Adjacent teeth should be thoroughly dried on their outer surfaces with gauze to aid adhesion of the adhesive tape
- Send the patient to a dentist as soon as possible. Where immediate replacement of the tooth cannot be done, it should be stored in milk and taken with the patient to the dentist. Alternatively, the tooth can be stored in the patient's mouth until a dentist can be located

When presented with a case of an avulsed tooth, the therapist must consider the following pertinent questions:

- How long has the tooth been avulsed? If it is for more than 2 h, or if the tooth has not been kept moist in saliva, saline solution or milk, there is little chance of successfully reimplanting it
- What is the condition of the tooth itself? If it is grossly traumatized or broken, reimplantation should not be attempted.

It should further be noted that a local anaesthetic is rarely indicated for reimplantation.

Injuries to the Alveolus

As mentioned earlier the alveolus (Fig. 16.2) is the

plate of compact bone whose main function is to support the teeth and maintain and retain them. Fractures of the alveolar bone can be divided into categories according to the position and involvement of the fracture.

COMMINUTION

This occurs when the tooth is forcibly pushed further into the socket and the periodontal ligament is compressed.

FRACTURE OF ALVEOLAR SOCKET WALL

Such an injury occurs to the labial or palatal wall of alveolar plate bone and almost always occurs with lateral luxation — often with extrusive luxation or complete avulsion of the tooth. The usual site of injury is the upper anterior region of the mouth. Clinically, testing for tooth mobility also demonstrates fracture of the alveolar plate, as the plate is usually attached to the tooth via the periodontal membrane. Treatment involves proper repositioning of the tooth in the socket and splinting. Follow-up radiography of the area will allay fears of mal-union of the alveolar plate or infection in the area. Healing usually takes place in a clean environment over a period of 3–4 weeks.

FRACTURE OF THE ALVEOLAR PROCESS

Such injuries are usually found in adults, where mobility testing of a loosened tooth or teeth will show 'block' movement of teeth and alveolar bone. The upper molars are most often involved.

Necrosis of the pulpal tissues of the tooth or teeth involved is almost certain and treatment is initially by reduction of the fracture, immobilization and then subsequent pulp testing for the integrity of the pulpal tissues. If the teeth involved in the fracture have chronic periodontal disease, the teeth may need to be extracted. This should be deferred, however, until the alveolar bone fragment is stabilized.

Very young children with any of the above-mentioned injuries should be treated slightly differently. Usually, reduction of the fracture is sufficient in most cases, with dietary advice to the parents to restrict the child to a soft or liquid diet. In severe cases, reduction under a general anaesthetic may be carried out by an oral surgeon, with stabilization achieved by an overlaying acrylic splint wired into position over the alveolar crests for approximately 3 weeks.

Facial Bone Fractures

Facial bone fractures may be direct, where the fracture occurs at the point of contact of the blow, or indirect, where the fracture occurs at some distance from the point of contact. Fractures may be single, fissural or comminuted, where the bone is fragmented into two or more pieces. A compound fracture occurs when the fractured bone communicates with a wound to the skin or mucous membrane. Where a tooth is involved in the fracture line, the fracture is almost certainly compound, communicating with the mouth via the periodontal membrane.

FRACTURES OF THE MANDIBLE

The most common sites of fracture of the mandible are the condylar neck, the angle of the mandible and in the pericanine area (Macalister 1985). Displacement of the fracture is common due to the effects of a muscle pull or the force of a traumatic blow. Verification of all fractures must be done by a series of radiographs.

Condylar fractures

The most common site of fracture is the neck of the condyle resulting from a blow to the point of the chin and such fractures may be unilateral or bilateral (Macalister 1985).

In unilateral condylar fractures the lateral pterygoid muscle pulls the condylar head forward while the other muscles of mastication tend to move the ramus of the mandible superiorly so as to cause an open bite on the opposite side to the fracture. Opening of the mouth causes the entire mandible to shift to the opposite side of the face.

In bilateral condylar fractures the two lateral pterygoid muscles move both condylar heads anteriorly; the other muscles of mastication pull both rami of the mandible superiorly so that when closing the two dental arches together only molar contact is possible and front teeth cannot meet.

The effect of the muscles of mastication on angle fractures is to produce depression of the anterior mandible, elevation of the ramus and medial displacement of the angle of the mandible behind the fracture. Displacement of angle fractures is resisted by the teeth in occlusion and the periosteum. The angle of the fracture line will determine whether displacement of the sections occurs when the muscles contract.

Pericanine fractures occur in the region of the canine teeth, which have the longest roots of all the teeth and are therefore prone to fracture. Unilateral fractures in this area can generally be prevented from displacement by occluding the teeth. Bilateral fractures can become displaced by a muscular pull, of the loose anterior section downwards and backwards, with a subsequent loss of control of the tongue. This may result in the tongue falling back towards the pharynx and blocking the airways, which must be cleared immediately.

Mid-line mandibular fractures

Symphyseal fractures can lead to the halves of the mandible becoming displaced inferolingually, or in rare cases, overlapping of the two sections in the mid-line area. These should be treated by a specialist maxillofacial surgeon immediately.

Fractures of the Maxilla

Fractures of the maxilla are usually called the fractures of the middle third of the face, the area being bounded by the occlusal plane of the maxillary teeth and a line drawn through the pupils of the eyes. The bones involved are primarily the paired maxillae, with the alveolar processes and teeth, the paired palatine bones, the paired zygomatic or cheek bones and the paired nasal bones.

Classification of fractures of the middle third of the face are universally separated into five categories.

ALVEOLAR PROCESS FRACTURES

These have already been discussed with luxations.

GUERIN'S OR LE FORT I FRACTURES

The palate and the alveolar process are separated from the maxillae by a fracture line just above the floor of the antra and the floor of the nose. Signs and symptoms include blood in the antra and a deranged occlusion. Treatment involves temporary stabilization and consultation with an oral and maxillofacial surgeon as soon as possible.

LOW PYRAMIDAL OR LE FORT II FRACTURES

The fracture line passes through the lateral and anterior walls of both the maxillary antra and continues through the infra-orbital ridges to join across the bridge of the nose. Often this is called the 'full floating maxilla'. Clinically, the patient presents with the following symptoms: gross oedema; bilateral infra-orbital paraesthesia (altered skin sensation); subconjunctival bleeding; diplopia (double vision); and a maxillary dental arch pushed back with an anterior open bite. If the maxillary arch is retroposed this can occlude the airways. Immediate treatment involves pulling the maxillary process forward to open the airways and the patient should be immediately transferred to an emergency clinic at a hospital.

HIGH PYRAMIDAL OR LE FORT III FRACTURES

The clinical signs are the same as the Le Fort II fracture, with the addition of cerebrospinal fluid leakage from the nose and general signs of head injury. As with Le Fort II fractures, maintenance of the airways is a priority, with arrangements for immediate transfer to hospital being made.

Zygomatic bone fractures

A blow to the side of the head may cause impaction of the zygomatic bone and zygomatic arch, with antral involvement. Signs and symptoms include an obvious step deformity in the infra-orbital ridge, subconjunctival bleeding, diplopia, infra-orbital paraesthesia, blood in the antra and interference with opening and closing the mouth due to the contact of the coronoid process of the mandible with the displaced zygomatic bone. These fractures account for about 30% of injuries to the facial skeleton (Macalister 1985). Immediate transfer to hospital is recommended, with no palliative treatment necessary. The patient should avoid blowing the nose or sneezing, as these will force air bubbles into the soft tissues in the area of the antral fracture. The surgical procedures for treatment of the above fractures are beyond the scope of this chapter, but the reader is referred to the recognized standard texts on the subject for further information (Archer 1975)

COMPLICATIONS OF JAW FRACTURES

The most obvious complication relates to the protection of airways, especially in Le Fort II and III cases. When teeth are in the fracture line it is best to delay extraction, as this will almost certainly lead to further displacement of the fracture. The teeth that are retained allow repositioning of the fragments to be achieved as closely as possible to the pre-trauma position.

Infection is another major complication which must be addressed. It is advisable in the case of any luxation, avulsion or jaw fracture to administer prophylactic antibiotics in order to avoid the onset of infection, which is the major cause of prolonging or preventing the normal healing processes.

Soft Tissue Injuries

The majority of the bony injuries that have been discussed present with some form of accompanying soft tissue injury. The intra-oral tissues (mucosa, gingiva and tongue) are most often involved, with the external and vermilion surfaces of the lip being the next most commonly involved.

Intra-orally there are generally four types of soft tissue injury, which are as follows:

- A wound resulting from a tear of the gingiva or mucosa, which generally results from a blow with a sharp instrument or tongue bite
- Bruising which may result from a blow by a blunt instrument, causing submucosal haematoma, but with no surface break
- The 'scrape' or 'graze' resulting in a raw, bleeding area
- Multiple and sometimes extensive lacerations noted in conjunction with luxation or avulsion of the teeth, or in conjunction with a compound fracture of the jaw

If severe, the first type of soft tissue injury may need suturing, while the latter may requires treatment which is secondary to the treatment of the luxation, avulsion or fracture.

The oral cavity has a well developed blood supply and thus bleeds profusely when traumatized. Wound healing, however, is rapid and it should be stressed that, unless the injury to the soft tissue is major, the more important problems that arise from the trauma should receive priority. The more severe tooth and bone injuries are those which can lead to aesthetic and functional difficulties later in life.

ORAL AND FACIAL PROTECTION IN SPORT

Mouthguards

A 4 year study of anterior dental trauma recently carried out in Australia (Martin *et al.* 1990) demonstrated that sports-related dental injuries accounted for 15% of cases which presented to the hospitals chosen for the survey. Crown fractures and luxations are the most common injuries, with the most susceptible individuals aged between 12 and 23 years (Figs 16.4 and 16.5).

In sports where collisions with opponents or their equipment occur, it is important to wear a mouthguard which should function in the following way (Fricker 1983; Hunter 1989; Johnsen & Jackson 1991):

- Cushion and distribute forces from a direct blow
- Protect soft tissues from laceration
- Protect opposing teeth from fracture as a result of an upward blow
- Protect the player against concussion
- Protect against a condylar fracture
- Protect against neck injuries
- Provide psychological support

A mouthguard should cover the occlusal surfaces of the upper teeth and extend almost to the junction between the attached and free mucosa on the buccal sulcus. This ensures that the lips and gingiva are protected, as well as providing maximum retention without impinging on muscle attachments or fraena.

The mouthguard should also extend behind the

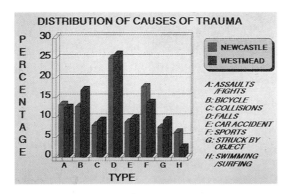

Fig. 16.4 A distribution of the causes of dental trauma (Martin *et al.* 1990).

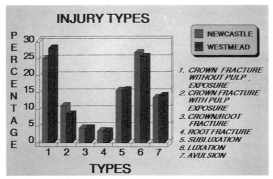

Fig. 16.5 The types of dental injuries occurring in sport (Martin *et al.* 1990).

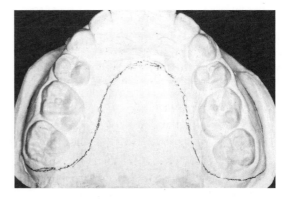

Fig. 16.6 The outline of the correct peripheral border on the palatal surface of a mouthguard.

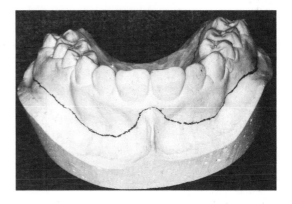

Fig. 16.7 The outline of the correct peripheral border on the outside surface of a mouthguard.

last tooth on each side and on to the palate. The palatal cover should be kept to a minimum, reaching a compromise between retention around tooth undercuts and interference with speech and breathing (Figs 16.6 and 16.7). If the palatal cover goes back too far, it will trigger the 'gag' reflex making it impossible to wear.

It is important that even occlusal (bite) prints are placed in the mouthguard when fitting it in the mouth. This may be done by heating the areas over the teeth, placing it in the mouth and gently closing the teeth to about 2 mm from the position of maximum tooth contact. This braces the muscles of the head and neck as the teeth uniformly contact the mouthguard. It also holds the condylar heads out of the glenoid (temporal) fossae reducing the risk of concussion. The tooth prints also restrict lateral sliding of the mandible in the event of a blow to the side of the jaw and reduce the risk of condylar fracture (Chapman 1989).

Types of Mouthguards (Guevara & Ranalli 1991)

STOCK

These mouthguards are made from rubber or plastic and 'one size fits all'. The mouthguard is retained in the mouth by supporting it with teeth clenched. It gives some protection against lacerations, but is of little use otherwise and is not recommended.

MOUTH-FORMED

They generally consist of a tough horseshoe-shaped shell of firm rubber or plastic and an inner resilient liner that is fitted to the teeth. The outer shell provides a smooth durable surface with the liner adapted by heating to fit over the tooth and soft tissues to provide retention. These mouthguards can provide some protection but are limited in comfort and retention.

CUSTOM-MADE

This type of mouthguard is individually manufactured on plaster casts made from the individual's teeth. Thermoplastic material is adapted to the cast to provide the best fit for comfort and retention. The mouthguard material may be built up where teeth are missing to provide better rigidity to the appliance.

Another type of custom-made mouthguard is the pressure laminated form. Mouthguard material is adapted in layers on casts of the teeth which are mounted on a dental articulator that simulates jaw movements. These can be used to provide the tooth prints in the biting surfaces similar to those in the mouth-formed type (Fig. 16.8).

The greatest advantage of the custom-made mouthguard is that the design is flexible and may be varied depending on the following:

- The anatomy of the athlete's mouth
- The nature of the sport

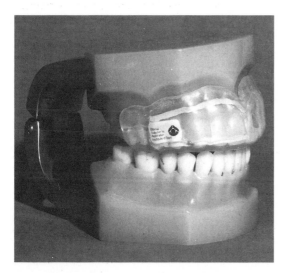

Fig. 16.8 A custom-made pressure laminated mouthguard.

Higher-risk sports such as hockey, boxing or football require thick firm support around the outside and between the occlusal surfaces of the teeth and the athlete receives this support from the laminated type.

BIMAXILLARY MOUTHGUARDS

These are made to cover both upper and lower teeth and make breathing and speech difficult as they lock the jaws into a predetermined position. Any advantages they give are usually outweighed by the disadvantages they cause the wearers.

Ill-fitting mouthguards can cause ulceration of the soft tissues and continued use may result in chronic fibromas, which usually resolve themselves once the cause is removed. In rare cases a fibroma will not resolve and will require surgical removal by a suitably qualified surgeon.

In all sports involving either direct or indirect contact a mouthguard should be worn. These include the following:

- Netball
- Basketball
- Hockey: field and ice
- Boxing
- Lacrosse: field or box
- Cricket
- Martial arts
- Squash
- Baseball: softball
- Water polo
- Football: rugby union, rugby league, soccer, Gaelic, Australian and American football
- Wrestling
- Individual sports: horse-jumping, motor cross, competitive skiing (water and snow), trampolining

Care of Mouthguards

Should be stored in a perforated plastic box. Before wearing, they should be rinsed with a mouthwash or antiseptic and washed again in warm water and soap after use. Mouthguards should not be allowed to overheat (e.g. left in the glove box of a car) as the material will suffer stress release and all retention will be lost.

The cost of a custom-made mouthguard is significantly higher than one 'off the shelf'; however, the advantages of the custom-made type justify the cost and these are strongly recommended.

Facial Protectors and Helmets

Those who need full face and helmet protection include goalkeepers of sports such as hockey, lacrosse, cricket (when facing up to fast bowling or when fielding in positions close to the bat) and baseball (catchers), as well as American footballers. These protectors are more fully discussed in Chapter 15.

DENTAL PAIN

Toothache

Toothache may be of tooth origin or from supporting soft tissues or bone. Other conditions which may present as toothache are maxillary sinusitis and temporomandibular dysfunction (Hutchison & Nally 1991).

Dental Caries

Dental caries is caused by acid resulting from the action of micro-organisms on carbohydrates. It is characterized by decalcification of the inorganic portion of the tooth and by a disintegration of its organic substances. Caries is the major cause of discomfort and is the primary cause of tooth loss prior to age 35.

The acids that initially decalcify the enamel have a pH of 5.2 or less and are formed in dental plaque, which is defined as an organic nitrogenous mass of micro-organisms firmly attached to the tooth structure. Dental plaque is present on all teeth and forms within 24 h of tooth brushing. Micro-organisms within dental plaque provide enzymes which act on the carbohydrates to produce lactic acid and if sufficient lactic acid remains in contact with the tooth structure, it will initiate the development of carious lesion.

Fluoride ions incorporated into the tooth enamel alter the structure of hydroxyapatite making it more resistant to lactic acid attack. Fluoridation of drinking water has been found to be the most effective method to reduce dental caries.

In addition to fluoridation, adequate oral hygiene and a controlled diet reduce the chances of dental caries. Further, a reduction in sucrose-containing foods, particularly the sticky types, will control the lactic acid production in dental plaque.

The caries process progressively destroys tooth structure leaving the pulp and dentine unprotected from external stimuli. Once the pulp is exposed micro-organisms may invade it and produce pulpitis (Fig. 16.2).

Although prevention is the preferred option, topical fluorides are helpful in remineralizing areas of lost enamel in the early stages of the dental caries. Once caries has extended into the dentine a restoration or filling of the deficient tooth structure is required. Restorative materials such as amalgam, quartz-filled resins, porcelain or gold are commonly used to restore normal masticatory function.

Pulpitic Pain

As caries spreads to the pulp chamber, micro-organisms can produce an acute pulpitis. Pulpitic pain is severe and the patient often cannot localize it to a particular tooth (Moule 1988). Such a severe throbbing pain is typically precipitated by extremes in temperature; however, in some cases the pain may be considerably relieved by cold fluid being held over the aching tooth. Pulpitic pain may persist for several days, and usually stops quite suddenly, implying necrosis of the pulp. It may then be replaced by the pain from acute inflammation due to a periapical abscess.

Acute pulpitis may also follow the filling of teeth, either immediately or after an interval of several years. Often this is the result of physical irritation such as excessive heat and trauma in cavity preparation and/or the use of pulpally irritating restorative techniques and materials. Placing poorly sealed restorations over residual bacteria can also result in a severe pulpitis. A careful history of recent fillings and their relationship to the pain is essential, but if the pain is diffuse and many teeth are heavily filled it is often difficult to establish which tooth is the cause of pain. Sharp pain on biting may be indicative of a cracked tooth.

Chronic Pulpitis

This may induce a dull pain and can be very difficult to diagnose. The causes basically are the same as in acute pulpitis and the diagnostic methods are similar.

Pain of Bone Origin

ACUTE PERIAPICAL ABSCESS

An acute periapical abscess may follow acute pulpitis but usually develops in connection with a tooth in which the pulp has asymptomatically necrosed following either caries, trauma or restorative treatment. When combined with the invasion of micro-organisms, the pain is very severe, while the acute inflammatory process is contained within the supporting bone (Gayford & Haskall 1979).

The tooth becomes mobile and is very sensitive to percussion. Soft tissue inflammation and oedema can result from an acute periapical abscess. Suppuration occurs early and if pus extends outside the bone it forms an abscess cavity which is likely to be in the attached gingiva and rarely outside the mouth, that is the so-called dento-alveolar abscess. There may be trismus ('lockjaw') if a posterior tooth is involved and X-rays will usually reveal an area of periapical radiolucency. The treatment of periapical infections consists of drainage and root canal therapy. Antibiotics are useful if immediate treatment by a dentist is not possible.

Periodontal Disease

The periodontium is comprised of the gingiva (gums), periodontal ligament and alveolar bone surrounding the teeth. Periodontal disease is characterized by the inflammation of gingiva and the loss of bony support of the teeth and is the major reason for tooth loss in people over age 35 years.

The most common causes of periodontal disease are dental plaque and calculus (tartar) resulting from poor oral hygiene. Bacterial toxins stimulate inflammation and immunological mechanisms are

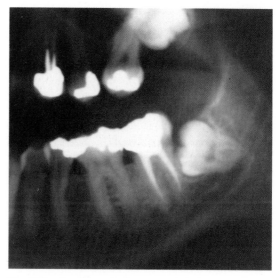

Fig. 16.9 A radiograph showing an impacted lower third molar.

also implicated. There is significant individual variability in host susceptibility to periodontal disease.

Diabetes mellitus also predisposes individuals to periodontal disease because hyperglycaemia suppresses local defence cell systems which control bacterial proliferation and inflammation.

Early periodontal disease may go unrecognized as it is often asymptomatic; however, it is readily confirmed by X-rays to assess bone loss and by clinical examination. As bone loss continues, there is increased tooth mobility as well as gingival erythema and pain associated with a gingival exudate. If the bone loss is allowed to continue, the tooth will eventually be lost.

Acute Periodontal Abscess

An acute periodontal abscess arises in the depths of a periodontal pocket and presents as an acute painful swelling, often on the palatal side of the upper molars or in the lower incisor region. Swelling is more localized and confined to the alveolus.

Pus can always be released by cleaning down the periodontal pocket to the abscess. The affected tooth is always loose and radiographs show irregular

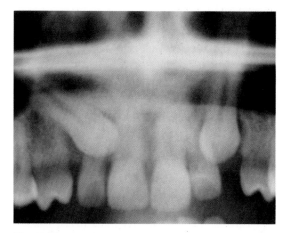

Fig. 16.10 A radiograph showing impacted maxillary left and right canines.

bone destruction due to periodontal disease (Gayford & Haskall 1979).

Treatment consists of drainage by vertical incision in the gum margin, followed by periodontal treatment aimed at the removal of toxins and cleaning of root surfaces. The teeth should be extracted only if the above treatment fails.

Acute Post-extraction Osteitis (Dry Socket)

A dry socket occurs only after tooth extraction. The pain usually starts 2 days after and peaks after a further 48 h. The pain can be severe, dull, gnawing, persistent or throbbing and is usually associated with a foul taste in the patient's mouth. A dry socket takes approximately 2 weeks to become symptom-free (Fazakerley & Field 1991).

Examination reveals an empty (hence 'dry') socket in which food debris has accumulated and the blood clot broken down. The surrounding mucosa is inflamed and very tender, but swelling is rare. Regional lymph nodes are swollen and sensitive to touch.

Radiographs usually reveal only a socket, but occasionally part of a tooth will be identified or a piece of foreign matter may be found in the socket. Treatment is required by a dentist and local dressings of the socket must be carried out. Antibiotics are of little value in such cases.

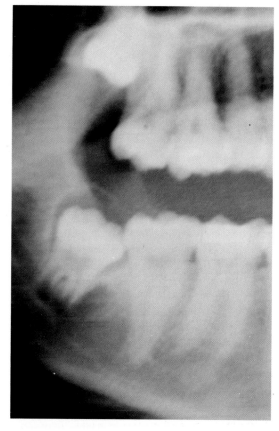

Fig. 16.11 A radiograph showing pericoronitis around a partially erupted lower third molar.

Impacted Teeth

An impacted tooth is an unerupted tooth, which is prevented from completely erupting due to the pressures from adjacent teeth or bone. The most commonly impacted tooth is the lower third molar or wisdom tooth. Pain from impacted teeth is diffuse and dull and may occur spontaneously or on biting and radiate to adjacent teeth. Wisdom tooth pain should not be confused with TMJ pain, which will be discussed later in this chapter.

As the offending tooth erupts the overlying gum recedes. However, often the lower third molar may retain some gingival cover resulting in a food trap and a focus for infection called pericoronitis. Less commonly the upper permanent canines (eye-teeth) may be impacted with similar symptoms of pain.

This latter condition occurs between the ages of 12 and 16 years and occasionally results in resorption of adjacent permanent teeth, which is normally accompanied by pain (Figs 16.9 and 16.10).

Unerupted third molars may weaken the mandible at the angle and contribute to jaw fractures in this area. Prophylactic removal of impacted third molars in a time of non-competitive sport is recommended for those playing contact or collision sports, such as boxing or football (Schwimmer et al. 1983).

Acute Pericoronitis

Acute pericoronitis results from inflammation around the crown of the tooth and is most frequently related to the erupting lower third molar (wisdom tooth). Acute pain, swelling over and beneath the angle of the mandible, severe trismus and tender submandibular or upper cervical lymph nodes are common symptoms. Oral examination reveals considerable inflammation with swelling and maceration of the gum in the lower third molar region. The wisdom tooth may not be visible but is at least palpable and pus can usually be expressed from around the overlying flap of gingival tissue (operculum).

The maxillary third molar can usually be seen to be biting on the inflamed lower gum and this tooth often initiates and aggravates acute pericoronitis (Fig. 16.11). Treatment consists of the removal of both the third molars.

Acute Maxillary Sinusitis

This disorder commonly follows a mild nasal infection but may also arise from periapical infection of the upper teeth.

Inflammation of the maxillary sinus is characterized by pain centred in the cheek which radiates to the region above the eye (Moule 1988). Swelling appears clinically as a unilateral nasal obstruction and mucopurulent nasal discharge. There is rarely any swelling of the face and the pain may appear to originate in the upper teeth which, in any case, are often extruded and sensitive to pressure. The surrounding gingiva may also be sensitive to pressure and the pain characteristically worsens towards the evening or if the subject bends forward or lies down. Jumping or running will also precipitate pain.

Treatment is by the use of antibiotics and the imidazole group of vasoconstrictors to promote mucosal shrinkage (Stevens 1991).

SOFT TISSUE DISEASE

Acute Ulcerative Gingivitis (Vincent's Gingivitis, Pyorrhoea, Trench Mouth)

Acute ulcerative gingivitis is a fusospirochaetal infection that usually affects the gingival margin but is occasionally more extensive. The gingival margins become inflamed and the tissues between the teeth are ulcerated and pocketed with areas of grey necrotic tissue. Symptoms are pain in the teeth and gums on eating, accompanied by bad breath and a metallic taste.

The most important factor in aetiology is poor oral hygiene. Other factors which contribute to the onset of the disease include those which reduce the host's immune defences, for example smoking, fatigue, stress or undue exertion (Gayford & Haskall 1979).

Treatment is by an improvement in oral hygiene and by the use of metronidazole (Flagyl). When the condition is not responsive to conservative therapy, a physician should be consulted to investigate the possibility of an underlying condition such as a blood dyscrasia (leukaemia, lymphoma, etc.).

Primary Herpetic Gingivostomatitis

Primary herpetic gingivostomatitis, mostly involving herpesvirus type I, is usually subclinical, but a small percentage of patients present with classic symptoms (Gayford & Haskall 1979).

Initially there is fever, malaise, headache and enlarged lymph nodes of the neck and jaw. This is followed within a few days by intense redness and swelling of the gums and by vesicles (small blisters) distributed throughout the mouth. The vesicles rupture soon after forming, leaving painful small ulcers surrounded by a red border. Treatment is palliative; symptomatic and supportive analgesics and topical anaesthetics may provide temporary relief. Tetracyclines used as a mouth rinse may also assist by controlling secondary infections.

Dentures

Ill-fitting dentures may cause discomfort by rocking on the mucosa and causing ulceration. Pain may radiate to adjacent areas and occasionally present as TMJ pain. Usually younger athletes will not be wearing dentures; however, veteran athletes often have them.

ANGULAR CHELITIS

This results from a fungal infection (*Candida albicans*) at the corners of the mouth arising from inadequate vertical support of the lower third of the face and lips. This is commonly related to severely worn down dentures. The corners of the mouth become cracked and the area is constantly moist due to poor lip seal, allowing the opportunistic *Candida* organism to infect the area, which may be quite painful.

Preferred treatment is to replace the denture, together with topical applications of antifungal agents to eliminate the *C. albicans*.

DENTURE SORE MOUTH

The mucosa under the upper denture may become irritated due to poor fit and allow infection by *C. albicans*. The denture-bearing area may be inflamed and swollen.

Treatment involves correcting the fit of the denture and the use of topical antifungal agents. Antifungal paste may be placed on the tissue-bearing surfaces of the denture, which should be worn during the day only. Dentures should never be worn during sleeping hours.

Temporomandibular Joint Dysfunction (Myofacial Pain Dysfunction Syndrome)

The TMJ are non-weight-bearing articulating joints between the mandibular condyles and the glenoid fossa of the temporal bone. The movement of the mandible is integrated by proprioceptive feedback from the muscles of mastication, the periodontal membranes of the teeth and the capsule of the joint. High fillings in the teeth or an occlusal interference between natural teeth may cause an 'avoiding' action by the mandible, leading to altered neuromuscular relationships with subsequent 'condylar displacement'. The syndrome can also occur in patients with a normal occlusion and it may be due simply to excessive and abnormal condylar movements.

With the loss of the molar teeth, the possibilities of the development of TMJ dysfunction are enhanced as condylar displacement may be due to the lack of posterior occlusal support.

There is no set pattern of bite problems consistently associated with TMJ dysfunction and many patients with large interferences in the bite or loss of molar support do not develop joint symptoms. In many cases 'stress' and or depression may play a part. Correct diagnosis and successful treatment of this syndrome is one of the most challenging aspects of modern dentistry.

CLINICAL FEATURES OF TMJ DYSFUNCTION

Sufferers are more frequently female and aged from 15 years to old age, but there is a sharp peak incidence in the early twenties. The major symptoms are as follows (Gayford & Haskall 1979):

- Pain
- Trismus (limitation of movement of the mandible due to muscle spasm) and episodes of TMJ locking
- 'Clicking' of the TMJ

One or more of these symptoms may be present for some time before the patient presents for treatment. The severity of symptoms often fluctuates and diagnosis of TMJ dysfunction should not be on the basis of one symptom alone.

Pain

The pain is a dull ache, which may be limited to the region of the joint but may radiate to the temple or down over the ascending ramus of the mandible and frequently behind the ear. Occasionally, the pain is felt purely as an earache.

It is characteristically increased by movement of

the jaw and particularly by chewing, which may lead to sharp pain radiating widely around the region of the TMJ.

Trismus

This varies considerably and in the most severe cases it may not be possible to open the mouth. The limitation of movement may be unilateral, leading to deviation of the jaw on opening towards the affected side. The trismus is often worse after sleep. 'Lockjaw' may occur when the mandible becomes immobile usually in the half to three-quarters open position. Such locking is transient and most patients are able to manipulate the joint so that normal movement is restored.

Click

This is a common symptom and may precede the development of pain and trismus by months or years. The click usually occurs with the incisors being separated by a few millimetres, as the condyle starts its movement in the lower joint compartment. It also occurs at the corresponding point in the closure of the jaw.

TREATMENT

Referral to a dentist is indicated to determine any occlusal discrepancies in masticatory function and to establish a definitive treatment plan (Moule 1988). Explanation and reassurance are the first and most important aspects of treatment. It is necessary to explain the muscular nature of the symptoms to the patient and consideration should be given to the patient's home circumstances, job, finances and other stresses.

ANALGESICS

Analgesics form a major part in dental therapy and the control of pain. Aspirin, paracetamol alone, or combined with codeine are now commonly prescribed.

CONCLUSIONS

Dental problems, either of a traumatic or infectious origin can limit the performance of an athlete both directly and indirectly.

Traumatic injuries to the teeth and facial bones can 'sideline' an athlete for several weeks and it is recommended that custom-made mouthguards be fitted and worn where appropriate to minimize these injuries.

Toothache and related pain should also be recognized by the athlete, coach and sports physician for their debilitating effects. Regular dental screening is important to prevent these problems arising and liaison with a 'sports dentist' is desirable for advice and/or treatment.

REFERENCES

Andreasen J. O. (1981) *Traumatic Injuries of the Teeth*, 2nd edn, Ch. 3–8. Munskaard, Copenhagen.

Archer W. H. (1975) *Oral Surgery: A Step by Step Atlas of Operative Techniques*. W. B. Saunders, Philadelphia, PA.

Chapman P. J. (1989) Mouthguards and the role of sporting team dentists. *Australian Dental Journal* 34, 36–43.

Fazakerley M. & Field E. A. (1991) Dry socket: A painful post-extraction complication (a review). *Dental Update* **January/February**, 31–34.

Fricker J. P. (1983) Mouthguards. *Australian Journal of Sports Medicine and Exercise Science* 15, 22–23.

Gayford J. J. & Haskall L. R. (1979) *Clinical Oral Medicine*, 2nd edn, pp. 176–225. John Wright & Sons, Bristol.

Guevara P. A. & Ranalli D. N. (1991) Techniques for mouthguard fabrication. *Dental Clinics of North America* 35, 667–682.

Hunter K. (1989) Modern mouthguards. *Dental Outlook* 15, 63–67.

Hutchison I. & Nally F. (1991) Management of orofacial pain. *The Practitioner* 235, 72–77.

Johnsen D. C. and Jackson E. W. (1991) Prevention of intraoral trauma in sports. *Dental Clinics of North America* 35, 657–660.

Macalister A. D. (1985) Dental and facial injuries in sport treatment and prevention. *Patient Management* **June**, 77–78.

Martin I. G., Daly C. G. & Liew V. P. L. (1990) After-hours treatment of anterior dental trauma in Newcastle and Western Sydney. A four year study. *Australian Dental Journal* 35, 27–31.

Moule A. (1988) Dental pain. *Dental Outlook* 14, 102–111.

Schwimmer A., Stern R. & Kritchman D. (1983) Impacted third molars: A contributing factor in mandibular fractures in contact sports. *American Journal of Sports Medicine* 11, 262–266.

Stevens M. (1991) The diagnosis and management of acute and chronic sinusitis. *Modern Medicine of Australia* April, 16–26.

Wong P. D. & Fricker J. P. (1991) Treatment of traumatic injuries to an anterior tooth. Case report. *Australian Dental Journal* 36, 44–46.

CHAPTER 17

INJURIES TO THE SPINE

K. F. Maguire

Spinal injuries can be a devastating consequence of sports participation and injuries presenting to hospital spinal injury units may come from occupational, recreational, motor vehicle or sporting accidents (Hochschuler 1990). Traumatic injuries to the spinal column are relatively common and may result from either a single incident trauma such as a fall, or be the result of repetitive stress.

The majority of injuries are relatively minor involving the soft tissue structures, resulting in either a sprain or a strain. More severe injuries usually result from motor vehicle accidents, falls or heavy contact sports such as the various codes of football. Major trauma may result in fractures or dislocations and, in a small number of cases, cause damage to the spinal cord or peripheral nerves. Sporting accidents account for nearly 5% of patients (Menzies Foundation 1987) being admitted to spinal cord injury units in Australia. The range of problems includes death, quadriplegia or paraplegia and chronic pain and disability as well as self-limiting strains.

This chapter discusses injuries of the cervical, thoracic and lumbar spine and major neurological sequelae are reviewed as well as techniques for evaluation and transportation of the athlete with spinal injury. Comments on congenital and developmental problems which may become manifest as a consequence of sports participation are also presented.

The complex issue of low back injury and pain is reviewed with particular attention to examination techniques, diagnostic evaluations including advances in imaging techniques, and a review of recent developments in pain relief strategies. The aim of this chapter is to describe the various aspects of biomechanics, anatomy and pathology that are important in the diagnosis and treatment of the most common spinal injuries.

FUNCTIONAL ANATOMY

The spine consists of a number of individual mobile segments, each with an intervertebral disc and two posterior zygapophyseal joints. The stability of these mobile segments depends on the anatomical arrangement of the facet joints and intervertebral discs, as well as the soft tissue structures which surround them. It should be remembered the atlanto-occipital and atlanto-axial joints do not have intervertebral discs.

The anatomy of the spine can be considered to be either static or dynamic. Static structures are those whose constitution cannot be changed, although they can move or change shape. These structures, which may undergo degenerative change, include the intervertebral disc, the ligaments and the tendons which provide support to the spine. The dynamic structures are those whose constitutional make-up can be altered by diet and/or exercise and both bone and muscle will respond to stress. Bone will increase its volume in response to activity, notably in the pars interarticularis, which will hypertrophy if repetitive extension movements are undertaken, particularly in the immature spine. This hypertrophy results in pars interarticularis sclerosis, but with further stress may eventually go on to become a stress fracture.

Reversible changes in the intervertebral discs can occur in sport activities. Ahrens (1994) has demonstrated a reduction in vertebral column height (VCH) from C7 to T2 after running 6 miles. The change in VCH varied from 0.2 to 2.0 cm. Changes in disc hydration have been implicated.

From a sportsperson's viewpoint, the main structures that can be altered are the muscular tissues that circumferentially surround all joints and provide a protective function to each mobile segment. Therefore muscle can be considered to be the major structure which athletes can alter when trying to improve their performance. The analogy can be made with instability in the limbs, where rehabilitation programmes are aimed at over-strengthening muscles that support a particular joint, in an endeavour to overcome any instability of that joint. This principle can be applied to the spine, be it the cervical or lumbar region. The thoracic spine has its own inherent stability, but the thoracolumbar area, which is primarily involved with rotatory movements, can often benefit greatly from a muscle strengthening programme aimed at improving rotatory muscle strength, with particular respect to the abdominals.

The primary function of musculotendinous units is to contract, so that closure of the joint occurs, but they also have a secondary role as stabilizers during other movements. The abdominal muscles are the prime flexors of the trunk, while the erector spinae act as stabilizers of the individual motion segments during this flexion movement. During extension the abdominals become the stabilizers, while the erector spinae become the prime movers in combination with the gluteals. That is, as the spine extends, the abdominals use the so-called 'laying out' principle controlling this movement.

In sports where repetitive movements occur it is important to minimize the extremes of movement in flexion, extension and rotation. In this situation the pelvis can become very important in order to prevent some of the rotary forces that may occur. The pelvis can be rotated through approximately 90° in the majority of people, and by using rotation in this region one can reduce the repetitive forces on the spine which may result in injury to the various soft tissue structures, or even prevent a resultant stress fracture.

In considering back pain and spinal injuries in children an extremely careful evaluation for organic causes is required. The situation of back pain in children (especially pre-adolescents) that persists more than 1–2 weeks has been associated with occult fractures, spondylolysis, spondylolisthesis, symptomatic kyphosis or scoliosis, infection, tumour, disc herniation, discitis, slipped vertebral apophysis and juvenile arthritis (Thompson 1993).

GENERAL BIOMECHANICS OF SPINAL INJURY

The forces which act on the spine are flexion, extension, rotation, axial compression, distraction or combinations of some of these.

Spinal Movement

Spinal flexion causes the anterior structures, including the anterior two-thirds of the intervertebral disc, nucleus pulposus and vertebral body to be compressed, whereas the middle column (posterior annulus and posterior longitudinal ligament) with the adjacent neural structures and the posterior column are exposed to tensile forces. The reverse occurs with extension. Further, as the spine flexes rotation may occur at the facet joint, but in full extension the facet joint locks and no rotation occurs unless there is underlying instability.

Sagittal Plane Forces

The structures that will fail under flexion (compressive) forces include the intervertebral disc and the vertebral body, while simultaneous tension on the posterior structures, particularly if rotation is combined, may cause rupture of the posterior elements. A significant force is required in a single incident type injury for these structures to fail,

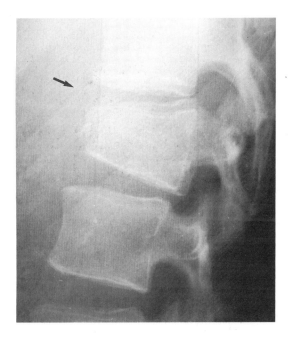

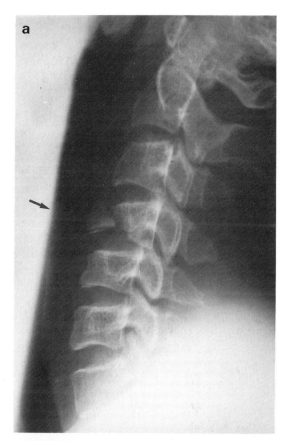

Fig. 17.1 A stable wedge compression fracture of L1.

unless there is pre-existing degenerative change, instability or osteoporosis. Tensile forces acting on soft tissues such as the posterior facet capsule, interspinous ligament and muscle can cause tearing of one or more of these structures, resulting in a strain or sprain, which is probably the most common injury sustained by a sportsperson. Although many of these minor soft tissue injuries will heal, if there is degeneration or instability in that segment, the symptoms are much more likely to be protracted.

Injuries to the bony structures of the spine can occur in the following situations (Holdsworth 1970).

- Pure flexion injuries may cause anterior wedging of the vertebral body, but are rarely associated with neurological damage and are usually stable (Fig. 17.1)
- Axial compression injuries result from falls and the force is more centrally directed and can cause compression of the vertebral body, resulting in a fracture with dispersion of the fragments, which in some cases may retropulse into the spinal canal causing neurological deficit (Fig. 17.2)

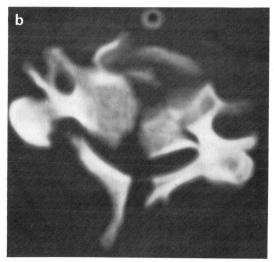

Fig. 17.2 (a) A lateral X-ray of an axial compression fracture of C4 after a fall with complete paralysis. (b) A CT scan of the above fracture showing more than a 50% loss of the intracanal diameter due to intracanal fragments.

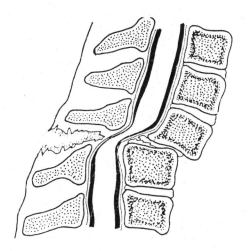

Fig. 17.3 A diagram of a flexion rotation injury usually obvious on X-ray and often associated with neural damage.

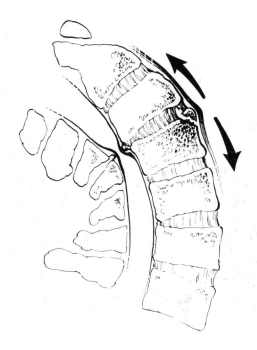

Fig. 17.5 A diagram of a hyperextension injury where there is usually a small piece of bone avulsed from the anterosuperior margin of the lower vertebrae. In osteoarthritic spines a compression of the spinal cord can cause neurological damage (central cord syndrome).

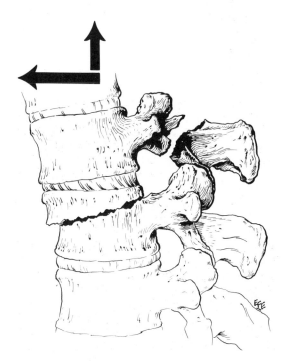

Fig. 17.4 Distraction injury usually related to lap seat-belts where sudden deceleration causes distraction of the upper torso in relation to the lower torso, which is fixed by the seat-belt.

- If flexion is combined with rotation then disruption of the posterior structures is more likely and dislocation may occur in association with the fracture causing an unstable injury, sometimes associated with neurological damage (Fig. 17.3; Lin *et al.* 1993)
- Distraction injuries occur in vehicular accidents with lap-type seat-belts. When the vehicle comes to a sudden stop, the lower torso is held by the lap-belt and the cranial half of the torso is thrown forward due to sudden deceleration, resulting in an unstable fracture–dislocation (Fig. 17.4)
- Extension injuries are generally stable and rarely associated with neurological signs or instability except in the upper cervical spine, or if there is pre-existing degenerative disease particularly in the cervical spine (Fig. 17.5)

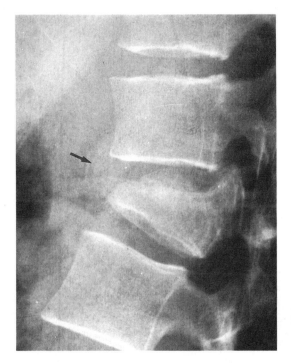

Fig. 17.6 A severe compression fracture which is mechanically and neurologically unstable.

Spinal Stability

Denis (1983) classified first, second and third degree spinal instability as follows:

- First degree instability is mechanical
- Second degree instability is neural
- Third degree instability is a combination of the two

Mechanical instability is seen in seat-belt injuries or compression injuries where there is a 50% compression of the anterior vertebral body. Neural instability occurs in burst compression injuries where there are two or more columns involved and they are associated with intracanal involvement (Figs 17.6 and 17.7). A combination of the two instabilities occurs with severe burst compression and flexion–rotation injuries.

Although most sporting injuries do not involve instability, it is important in the early assessment to have a knowledge of it so that appropriate treatment can be given at an early stage. When a suspected

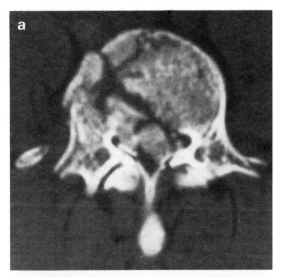

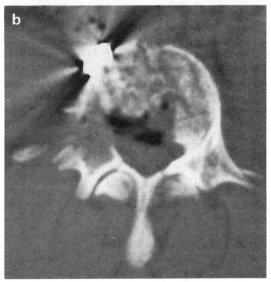

Fig. 17.7 (a) A CT scan of an L4 burst dispersion injury with almost complete loss of the intracanal diameter but incomplete paralysis. (b) Early surgical decompression via the anterior approach has restored the intracanal dimensions and some further neurological recovery has occurred.

instability does occur, appropriate early splinting and transportation to a specialized centre should take place without risking further neurological damage. Unstable injuries are unlikely to occur with direct blows, twisting, extension (except in

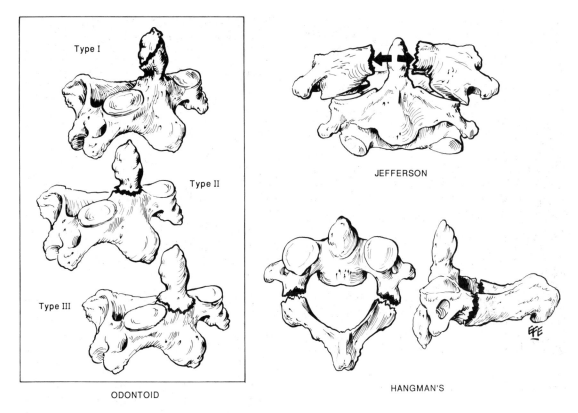

Fig. 17.8 Common fractures of the atlanto-axial articulation: odontoid, Jefferson and Hangman's fractures.

the upper cervical spine) or pure flexion. However, vehicular accidents, falls, flexion–rotation-type injuries (a collapsing scrum in rugby), or axial compression injuries such as a spear tackle in rugby can cause instability.

Extension Injuries

SINGLE INCIDENT

In single incident injuries, these are usually stable in the thoracic and lumbar spine. However, in the cervical spine, forced hyperextension may cause complete disruption of the anterior longitudinal ligament and resultant instability. Recent magnetic resonance imaging (MRI) studies of hyperextension–dislocation injuries of the cervical spine have shown many clinically pathological sequelae. These include disruption of the anterior longitudinal ligament and of the annulus of the intervertebral

disease, separation of the posterior longitudinal ligament from the subjacent vertebra and some cases of widening of the disc space, posterior bulging or herniation of the nucleus pulposus and disruption of the ligamentum flavum (Harris & Yeakley 1992). Hyperextension of the upper cervical spine may cause a fracture through the odontoid and the types of fractures which occur are as follows (Anderson & D'Alonzo 1974) (Fig. 17.8):

- In a Type I injury the fracture occurs in the mid part of the odontoid and is often a congenital anomaly called an os odontoideum, or it may be an avulsion of the tip of the odontoid where the apical ligament inserts
- Type II is where the fracture line runs through the base of the odontoid and can almost be considered a spondylolisthesis (disruption of the bone between two joints). In this situation

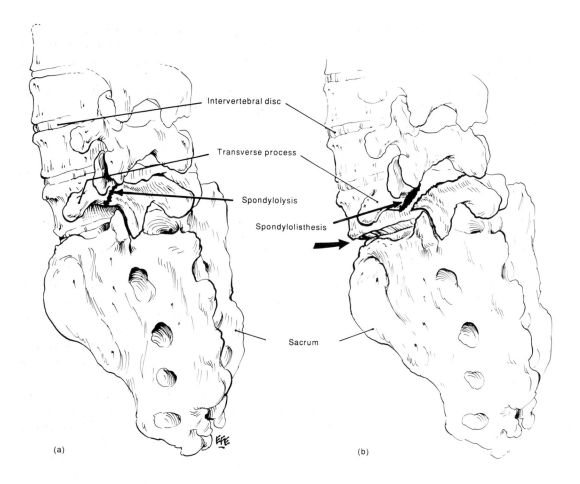

Intervertebral disc

Transverse process

Spondylolysis

Spondylolisthesis

Sacrum

(a)

(b)

abnormal movement does occur between the C1 and C2 mobile joints and is considered unstable

- In Type III, the fracture line runs within the body of C2 in a various pattern, and this is considered a relatively stable injury and will heal with minimal movement on flexion–extension

REPETITIVE INJURIES

Repetitive extension, particularly with rotation, may cause the development of a stress fracture through the pars interarticularis (Fig. 17.9). Although the mechanism of stress fractures has been debated from an anatomical aspect, when the spine is placed into full extension the inferior tip of the inferior facet will abut the pars interarticularis where it joins the adjacent superior facet of the

Fig. 17.9 (a) A fracture of the pars intra-articularis which is initially undisplaced (spondylolysis). (b) If the fracture is due to repetitive stress and it does not unite then a forward displacement of the vertebrae may occur resulting in a spondylolisthesis.

adjacent caudal segment. Those sports that have repetitive hyperextension movements such as fast bowling in cricket, gymnastics, javelin throwing and high jumping have a much higher risk of developing a stress fracture in the lumbar spine, particularly at the L5 or L4 level (Hardcastle 1991).

CERVICAL SPINE INJURIES

Congenital Anomalies

These are unusual in the cervical spine. Os odontoideum is a separation of the cranial part of the odontoid peg with associated atlanto-axial instability. Contact sports should not be played with this anomaly.

Atlanto-axial instability occurs in 10–40% of children with Down syndrome. Some sports have been deemed 'risky' for such individuals (Cremers *et al*. 1993). Recent studies show that there is no reason to stop children with Down syndrome from playing certain sports and no need to screen them by radiography before they take up such sports activities. Sports with perceived risk include: diving, wrestling, judo, gymnastics, high jump, trampoline, soccer, skiing, horse riding and rugby. Sports without perceived risk include: hockey, athletics, swimming (no diving), tennis, skating, jazz ballet, canoeing, curling, bicycling, folk dancing and walking.

Congenital fusion (block vertebrae) occurs but should not prevent a person playing sport. Conditions such as absent pedicle and spina bifida occulta are rare and can be associated with spondylolisthesis.

Biomechanics of Injury

Most injuries to the cervical spine are relatively minor sprains or strains. However, more severe injuries to the ligamentous, osseous or neural structures may occur. The usual mechanism is as follows:

- Sudden forced flexion of the neck as in a collapsed scrum may cause a wedge compression fracture
- Axial compression injuries result from falls, diving into shallow water, or hitting the vertex of the head directly into the ground (spear tackle etc.), or sliding head first into the boards, for example ice hockey (Reynen & Clancy 1994)
- High velocity motor or bike accidents can result in fracture dislocations
- Forced hyperextension injuries from falls, contact sports (head high tackles) and deceleration injuries usually cause damage to the upper cervical spine

Rule modification in contact sport (football codes) is aimed at preventing head high and spear tackles as well as stopping deliberate collapsing of the scrum. This has resulted in a significant reduction in the number of neck injuries in these sports. The most likely cause of injuries in football is axial loading in the neutral position but other forces including hyperextension, lateral flexion and rotation can also cause damage (Torg 1982).

Diving injuries constitute approximately 10% of those seen at large spinal cord injury treatment centres, often being next in frequency behind motor vehicle accidents and industrial or work-related accidents. Unfortunately, a high percentage of diving accidents result in neurological injury (up to 70%), and the actual incidence of diving injuries may be underestimated because they sometimes result in drowning.

Because the damage to the spinal cord usually occurs as an isolated event involving hyperflexion or axial compression of the neck, affected patients tend to have few other associated injuries. Pulmonary involvement is the major source of morbidity, owing to aspiration and near-drowning or to subsequent neurological compromise of ventilatory mechanisms.

Injuries to the cervical spine are uncommon but are catastrophic occurrences to those participating in athletic events. Classifications of athletic-induced cervical spine injuries can be a result of:

- Participation in non-supervised activities, such as diving, surfing, trampolining, skiing and other recreational activities
- Motor or equestrian accidents
- Contact sports

Injuries of the cervical spine in children and adolescents are rare; however, those under 11 years old have a higher incidence of upper cervical cord injury and increased mortality (McGrory *et al*. 1993).

The body contact injuries occur primarily to athletes competing in football codes such as rugby, American football, Australian rules football, wrestling and other martial arts and may constitute up to 4% of the total admissions to spinal injury units. The American experience with 'gridiron' football is important, in that the incidence of spinal injuries has been reduced because of improvements to equipment, rule changes, pre-season conditioning and the teaching of safer body contact techniques.

Syndromes of Spinal Cord Injury

Trauma to the spinal column may cause a variety of clinical syndromes depending on the type and severity of the impact and bony displacement, as well as secondary problems such as haemorrhage, ischaemia and oedema (McSwain et al. 1989). The consequences of cervical intervertebral disc injuries can cause cord damage (Kinoshita 1993).

Complete spinal cord injury results in a transverse myelopathy with total loss of function below the level of the lesion. This is caused by either anatomical disruption of the spinal cord or haemorrhagic or ischaemic injury at the site of injury. Complete injury patterns are rarely reversible; however, with long-term follow-up, improvement of one spinal level may be seen as a result of resolution of initial traumatic swelling of the spinal cord.

SPINAL SHOCK

The more severe injuries which involve the spinal cord result in the initial phase of a complete inhibition of reflexes known as spinal shock. The duration varies and seems to parallel the degree of development of the cerebrum, so that it may last several weeks in humans, but in lower species it is only transient, lasting a matter of minutes or hours (Bedbrook 1981).

The pulse rate is usually normal but there is a fall of blood pressure, with the systolic pressure below 100 mmHg due to the vasodilation that results from spinal shock. It is very important to realize that this is a normal consequence of injury to the spinal cord and not due to internal haemorrhage. In the initial phase motor, bladder, bowel, sexual and vasomotor reflexes are absent. The flexor response is the first to return and denotes the end of spinal shock.

There are several patterns of incomplete spinal cord injury, usually produced on a vascular basis. About 70% of these patients with incomplete lesions will make some degree of recovery and recent evidence suggests that with the use of megadoses of methylprednisolone (Bracken et al. 1990) and early decompressive surgery as well as stabilization, neural recovery may improve if there is an intracanal fragment causing compression on the spinal cord or corda equina (Willen et al. 1990).

Incomplete Spinal Cord Injuries

CENTRAL CORD SYNDROME

This results in an incomplete loss of motor function with disproportionate weakness of the upper extremities compared with the lower ones. It is considered to be the result of haemorrhagic and ischaemic injury to the corticospinal tracts because of their somatotropic arrangement and the long tracts for the lower limbs being more peripherally situated. Non-specific bladder and sexual dysfunction also occurs. Two types of injury pattern are recognized:

- Hyperextension (Fig. 17.5) in the spondylitic spine causing central haemorrhage and necrosis
- Flexion and axial compression with or without rotation in younger patients can result in central cord damage

The prognosis for the younger age group is much better for neural recovery. MRI assessment is indicated in both age groups to exclude extradural compression which may require surgical decompression.

ANTERIOR SPINAL CORD SYNDROME

Injury to the anterior two-thirds of the spinal cord in the area supplied by the anterior spinal artery can cause complete loss of all motor function below the level of the injury, in addition to loss of sensation conveyed by the spinothalamic tracts, that is, pain and temperature. There is usually an equal amount of deficit in the upper and lower extremities and anterior cord syndrome usually includes impairment of sphincteric and sexual function.

BROWN-SEQUARD SYNDROME

This is classically described as a hemisection of the spinal cord by a penetrating knife, with loss of ipsilateral motor function and contralateral spinothalamic (pain and temperature) modalities. This latter finding occurs because of a cross-over of the spinothalamic fibres one or two spinal levels above the entry site into the cord, whereas the corticospinal tracts have already crossed higher in the medullary pyramids and maintain their ipsilateral course to spinal levels of innervation of the anterior horn (motor) cells. The Brown-Sequard syndrome usually occurs not in a pure form, but in combination with other types of incomplete injury. Most common is a mixture of central cord and Brown-Sequard syndromes, in which the patient has some degree of unilateral motor weakness and contralateral sensory deficit, but with relatively greater weakness of the upper extremities.

POSTERIOR SPINAL CORD SYNDROME

In this rare clinical phenomenon there is a loss of dorsal column function with preservation of the corticospinal and spinothalamic tracts. It is believed to be due to selective ischaemia in the distribution of the posterior spinal artery.

NON-CLASSIFIED PATTERNS OF SPINAL CORD INJURY

There are many patients who have an incomplete injury not classifiable into any particular group. These injuries usually consist of a loss of all or nearly all their useful motor function below the level of the injury, with a sensory loss that does not fit any specific pattern. This sensory pattern does, however, portend a better recovery than does complete functional loss.

Terminology which is used is as follows. The level where normal sensation and motor function ends is stated, that is C5. If there is preservation of any movement or sensation below this it is called 'C5 incomplete'. Where all function is lost the word complete is used. That is, 'C5 incomplete motor and C7 complete', means there is weakness in C6 and C7 but no function in C8. Similar terminology is used for sensation. Atypical syndromes caudal to the injury site in patients following spinal cord injury have been subject to clinical, neurophysiological and MRI study by Tosi *et al.* (1993).

'BURNING HANDS' SYNDROME

This syndrome is characterized by a burning sensation and altered feeling of both hands and is seen in athletes who participate in contact sports (especially the various contact football codes and martial arts) with repeated cervical trauma. It is thought that the syndrome is a variant of central cord syndrome, in which there is a selective injury to the central fibres of the spinothalamic tract that subserve pain and temperature to the upper limbs. This injury does not result in permanent loss of either function or awareness of pain and is probably a result of oedema or vascular insufficiency. Credence to this theory is given with studies in which somatosensory evoked potentials and MRI following cervical injury have demonstrated a reversible injury to sensory pathway conduction in the spinal cord, implicating a confusion of sensory signals as the pathogenetic mechanism. The burning hands syndrome has been known to occur both with fractures and dislocations of the cervical spine and in patients with no demonstrable radiographic abnormality.

VASCULAR INJURIES CAUSING NEUROLOGICAL DAMAGE

There is a small group of patients at risk from neurological injury on the basis of vascular damage. The carotid and vertebral arteries are vulnerable from direct compression or as a result of traumatic fracture with subluxation. However, a patient with a vascular injury may radiographically show only chronic degenerative changes or a normal spine. The carotid arteries are rarely injured in athletic competition, but this injury must be kept in mind whenever signs or symptoms suggest cerebral hemispheric dysfunction as in hemiparesis, hemiplegia, hemianaesthesia, dysphagia and homonymous visual field defects. A delay in appearance of the neurological defect, even up to several days, is most characteristic.

Injury to the vertebral artery can occur with a fracture or fracture–dislocation at or above the C6 vertebra. Louw *et al.* (1990) found the vertebral artery occluded in five of seven patients with bilateral dislocation, and in four patients of five with unilateral dislocation. Two of their nine patients had neural deficits above the level of their injury and this was thought to be due to the vertebral artery occlusion.

Such an injury to the vertebral artery could be symptomatic immediately after the trauma, with a developing neurological deficit ranging from gradual and mild to sudden and severe. The clinical manifestation may be any of a variety of cerebellar and brain stem syndromes. The signs of vertebrobasilar insufficiency or infarction include:

- Dysarthria
- Vomiting
- Ataxia
- Vertigo
- Diplopia
- Long tract deficits

Complete brain stem infarction is rare but may occur. There is a lower incidence of altered level of consciousness and lateralizing signs compared with ischaemia of the anterior cerebral circulation. Computerized tomography (CT) scanning is less likely to show an abnormality in hind brain ischaemic injury than in anterior circulation ischaemia, but in either case, if a vascular injury is suspected urgent angiography must be performed to determine a diagnosis.

Cervicomedullary injury has been demonstrated in American football injuries and two possible mechanisms have been proposed. The first involves vertebrobasilar artery insufficiency from occlusion or underperfusion of either the major arteries (vertebral or basilar), or the smaller vessels and microcirculation, especially in the zones of poor collateral blood flow. With vertebrobasilar artery insufficiency, either temporary neurological deficits or complete lesions may be seen. The diminution or lack of circulation to the cervical and upper thoracic spinal cord can produce intramedullary circulation and haemorrhage.

A second cause of these serious injuries is an impact to the top of the skull (the vertex). As the relatively freely movable brain travels first towards the top of the skull, then rebounds in the opposite direction, the cerebral hemispheres may be displaced, so that there is a herniation of the uncus of the cerebral cortex through the tentorial notch. This may cause either acute arterial inflow or venous outflow obstruction leading to acute cerebral stroke or oedema and death. In addition, a shift of the brain stem and cerebellum through the foramen magnum may cause direct compression on the medullary centres for respiration and cardiovascular control. Also, high velocity vertex impact can cause a pressure discrepancy that produces petechial haemorrhages of the C1 and C2 region of the upper cord which is tethered by the dentate ligaments (Torg 1982).

Other causes including intracranial mass lesions need also to be considered if there is a deterioration in mental status following craniocervical injury.

FRACTURES OF THE UPPER CERVICAL SPINE

Three different types of fractures are common in this region (Fig. 17.8). The first are odontoid fractures which have previously been discussed. The second are Jefferson fractures, which are characterized by a compression extension injury involving disruption of the vertebral arch at C1, with dispersion of both lateral masses of the atlas with resultant joint incongruity between the atlanto-axial joints. These fractures are best seen on the open mouth view and are usually stable.

The hangman's fracture is a traumatic spondylolisthesis with a fracture through the vertebral arch at C2. This is an extension injury which is quite stable and will heal with immobilization, even in the presence of 1 or 2 mm of displacement. If there is more displacement or significant movement on the flexion–extension views halo immobilization is recommended.

These injuries will rarely be associated with neurological signs, and if damage to the spinal cord does occur it usually results in death due to asphyxia.

IMMEDIATE EVALUATION

When injury to the nervous system is suspected, the on-field assessment of the athlete begins with the preparation for cardiopulmonary resuscitation (Parks & Livoni 1986). An examination of the following should be made immediately:

- Airways — are they obstructed?
- Breathing — is it rhythmical and spontaneous?
- Circulation — is the heart beating?

OFF-FIELD TRANSPORT

Usually the circulation is not disturbed and the primary objective is to establish and maintain the airways. Conscious injured athletes who complain

slight force in the axial direction along the spine. Enough personnel should be used in order to move the injured athlete easily without the person at the head being distracted from the sole responsibility of maintaining proper cervical alignment (Dickson & Tonkin 1987; Fig. 17.10, Grundy & Swain 1993).

EXAMINATION

The evaluation of conscious patients begins with questioning about extremity numbness, painful sensation or paraesthesiae, weakness and neck pain. A limited examination can determine whether there is an obvious neurological deficit. If any neural symptoms are present on questioning or examination, or if the injured person is unconscious, the athlete should be carefully transported on a spinal board with the head and cervical spine in a neutral and immobilized position, retained either by hand or with sandbags and tape.

In injured athletes with an altered level of consciousness, the initial evaluation should check for the possibility of head trauma. Evaluation should include an examination of the level of consciousness and cranial nerve function, and Babinski response. The reader is referred to Chapter 15 for a more detailed discussion of the management of head injuries.

Once the patient has been removed from the playing field, time is available for a more detailed inquiry into nervous system function. The patient can be questioned in greater detail about the presence of neurological symptoms (motor and sensory). The cervical spine is examined in the following way:

- Check the overall appearance of the athlete as well as the presence of deformity, bruising, etc.
- Palpate the anterior and posterior structures for tenderness, swelling or ligamentous gaps between the spinous processes
- Move the cervical spine and shoulders (independently) through a passive then active range and note any restrictions
- Apply gentle compression and distraction to see if this aggravates pain
- Carry out a neurological examination, including the cranial nerves

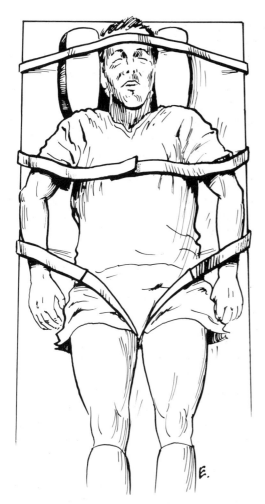

Fig. 17.10 If a fracture of the spine is suspected the patient should be totally immobilized.

of numbness, weakness, paralysis or neck pain and all unconscious people should be handled as if they have a cervical fracture, and thus an unstable spine. Moving and off-field transport should take place with sufficient personnel (usually four) so that the athlete's spinal column is supported and will not move in any plane. In particular, flexion and extension movements must be avoided since they are most likely to compromise the size of the cervical spinal canal. The most experienced person should be responsible for stabilizing the cervical spine and transferring the patient by cradling the shoulders and neck in the forearms while applying a

Any patient with a cervical injury should have a radiological evaluation with a cervical spine X-ray series which must include the T1 vertebrae. If this does not reveal an abnormality but the clinical setting suggests that the spinal column or cord is involved, further examination is indicated, including flexion–extension lateral X-rays to assess stability. Undisplaced fractures may not show on X-ray, so a CT scan of any painful areas should be performed as well. Do not hesitate to repeat the X-rays if the symptoms persist or do not respond to treatment.

CT scanning should be used to view the axial plane of the spine for fractures and to examine the relationship of bony injury to the spinal canal. With the use of water soluble contrast media and sagittal reconstruction formatting, the presence of spinal cord and canal compromise may be better appreciated on X-rays.

MRI is used in the diagnostic evaluation of the spinal-injured patients with incomplete neural lesions. With these lesions the MRI will give a much better assessment of any neural compression from a bony or disc fragment which may require surgical decompression in the early stage of management. In addition, it would appear that MRI can provide prognostic value of outcome in such cervical spinal cord injury (Sato et al. 1994).

Gadolinium enhancement of MRI can be used to detect intraneural lesions and is also particularly useful for diagnosing recurrent disc protrusion after previous surgery (Runge and Gelblum 1990). Although rare, acute traumatic rupture of the intervertebral disc or haematoma must also be considered.

At times there is uncertainty whether an injury represents involvement of the central nervous system or peripheral nerves. This can be seen in brachial plexus injuries sometimes found in wrestlers. Such an injury results from head and shoulder contact in which the head is laterally flexed with downward traction applied to the 'opposite' shoulder, causing traction on the upper trunk of the brachial plexus. For up to 15 min there may be a searing pain and ensuing temporary paralysis of the arm. Residual pain or neurological deficit corresponding with the upper trunk of the brachial plexus or cervical nerve root may persist for days or months.

In assessing athletes with these problems, the doctor must attempt to discern whether the complaints and any detectable abnormalities characterize involvement of the nerve root, brachial plexus or spinal cord. Nerve root symptoms include pain radiating into a specific dermatomal pattern, with the possibility of neurological deficits related to that dermatomal sensory pattern or to the muscle innervated. Plexus involvement is predicted by persistent pain in the entire upper extremity, in multiple sensory dermatomes, or by weakness of more than one muscle. One must discern the likelihood of a more serious spinal cord injury, which is more common if the symptoms are bilateral, or if they occur in the lower extremities, have long tract signs and symptoms, or include bladder or sexual dysfunction. Electromyographic (EMG) studies may help in distinguishing nerve root and plexus injury from spinal cord involvement.

TREATMENT

The treatment of spinal injuries which occur in contact sport begins with the withdrawal of the patient from further participation until the exact nature and risk of the injury is known. In the case of the severest injury, that is, spinal column and neurological injury, the athlete should be transferred to a definitive care hospital with adequate facilities for diagnosis and treatment of such problems.

Most cervical injuries are relatively minor and the symptoms will resolve quickly. Management of the more severe injuries, however, is described below. In most instances, after clinical status has been stabilized, those with severe spinal trauma appear best managed in a multidisciplinary acute spinal cord injury unit (Tator et al. 1994).

Following admission to the hospital the following steps are taken to deal with cervical spinal cord injuries:

- The insertion of a nasogastric tube because of the associated paralytic ileus and potential inhalation
- Intravenous infusion (i.v.i.) inserted; with cervical injuries fluids should be restricted to no more than 2 L·day^{-1}
- Thrombo-embolic stockings should be fitted on both legs

- Indwelling urinary catheter inserted
- Appropriate management of the cervical bony injury should be carried out
- Consideration of methylprednisolone given intravenously, with a bolus dose of 30 mg·kg^{-1} and then 5 mg·kg^{-1} for the next 23 h (Bracken *et al.* 1990)
- Oxygen should be given
- Patients with C4 neural lesions should have an immediate tracheotomy and be ventilated

Specifically, cervical traction with a halo should be applied to unstable injuries to reduce and maintain alignment in the anatomically neutral position. This must be accomplished with regular radiographic assessment and repeated neurological examination of the patient. Medical practitioners need to be cognisant of the respiratory and cardiovascular alterations that may occur after spinal cord injury and be prepared to treat them effectively as they arise. An intensive care setting is the best place to care for such injuries in the acute phase.

Once the patient has been initially evaluated and placed in cervical traction to reduce the fracture, a decision must be made whether surgical fusion, an external orthosis or traction will be used for spinal stabilization. The current trend in the majority of neck injury cases is to treat them conservatively. For approximately 90% of patients treated in this manner adequate bony healing will occur with 12 weeks of immobilization. In cases of traumatic subluxation without a fracture being demonstrated by CT scanning or X-ray tomography, adequate healing with halo-immobilization has been reported in 82% of patients (McSwain *et al.* 1989). Surgical treatment, however, is indicated in the following cases:

- Inadequate reduction of the fracture or dislocation which would cause an unacceptable deformity
- Incomplete neural lesions where there is greater than 30% reduction in intracanal diameter in the cervical and thoracic regions, or 50% reduction in the lumbar region
- Neurological deterioration following initial assessment
- With grossly unstable injuries, particularly in the presence of multiple injuries, it may be

preferable to internally fix and stabilize these injuries to allow easier nursing management

If surgical management is undertaken the best time is approximately 48 h post-injury, though in some emergency situations earlier fixation may be indicated. Decompression of the spinal canal to remove intracanal fragments must be through the anterior approach. If conservative treatment is instigated and after a period of 8–12 weeks spinal instability is present, then surgical stabilization will be necessary. If during the period of conservative treatment the initial reduction is lost or deformity progresses, then earlier surgery may be indicated to realign the spine and stabilize it in an adequate position.

RETURN TO NORMAL LIFE

Patients with fractures that are stable radiographically when determined by flexion–extension films and who do not have spinal cord injury should be allowed to return to their normal daily activities. Athletes with brachial plexus trauma or 'burning hands' may also be considered healed when their symptoms have resolved and they no longer have any neurological abnormalities.

Those athletes who do not have recovery of their neurological deficit can still be considered for a career involved with sporting pursuits. The long-term sequelae of chronic spinal cord injury will not be reviewed in this chapter; however, an excellent overview is provided by Ditunno and Formal (1994).

RETURN TO TRAINING AND COMPETITION

The question of whether to allow an athlete to return to training and competition after a documented or suspected spinal injury has always been contentious. Certainly, it is advisable that any athlete who suffers a neurological injury to the spinal cord should not be allowed to play contact sport again. Furthermore, athletes who have had fractures and dislocations of the spine requiring halo-brace or surgical stabilization probably do not have the strength to withstand further competition in contact sports.

However, there are some spinal fractures which are inherently stable and when they have occurred without neurological injury, need not preclude the

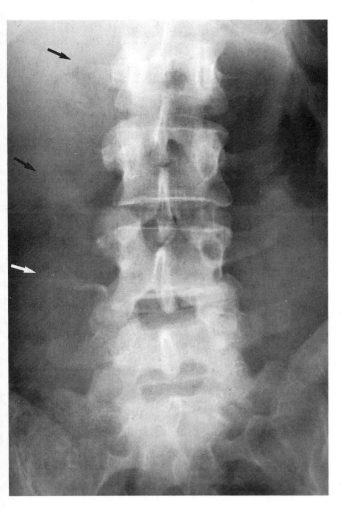

Fig. 17.11 An anteroposterior X-ray of the lumbar spine showing avulsion fractures of the lateral or transverse processes of L2, L3 and L4.

athlete from further participation in contact sports. Such fractures include isolated laminar, spinous process, wedge compression fractures of the vertebral body (Figs 17.1 and 17.11) or fractures in the upper cervical spine which heal without any neurological sequelae or instability (Fig. 17.8).

THE HIGH-RISK GROUP

There are a group of patients with a heterogeneous assortment of abnormalities which by themselves do not require treatment, but which may be associated with a higher risk of injury in contact sports than other individuals (Wilberger & Maroon 1990). Such patients include those with the following lesions:

- Congenital spinal canal stenosis
- Posterior ligamentous compromise
- Resolved transient neurological deficit (either surgically or medically)
- Congenital vertebral body fusion

Likewise, a patient with cervical spinal canal stenosis, that is a spinal canal less than 13 mm (C3–C7) in diameter, should no longer participate in contact sports because of the risk of spinal cord compression if the bony spinal column is injured.

THORACIC SPINE INJURIES

The thoracic spine is the most stable section of the vertebral column. The 12 thoracic vertebrae together with the ribs and sternum combine to form the bony thorax and the entire structure is such that it tends to limit the motion of the spine. Its general contour is one of dorsal convexity with the normal kyphosis ranging between 10 and 40°. The spine itself has good intrinsic stability with the vertebrae being very firmly bound together by the various ligaments. The articular processes are vertical and face each other in such a manner that the inferior processes of the vertebrae above lock behind the superior processes of the vertebrae below. This prevents any forward displacement unless there is a fracture of the arch. The nerve supply from the spine is direct, coming from the spinal roots, which are very well protected and seldom damaged. It should be noted, however, that there is increased mobility from T10 caudally and the thoracolumbar junction is where rotation occurs and this can be a common site for fracture dislocations.

Contusion

Contusion of the thoracic spine in sport is relatively common but not often severe. The subcutaneous spinous process may receive a blow that crushes the skin against the protruding bone beneath or may damage the underlying bone. The most common contusion of the spine is of the muscles lateral to the spinous processes. One should make an effort to determine whether there is some underlying pathological condition, as the contusion may cause a haematoma within the muscle. If this has occurred then the patient will require the usual treatment with cold therapies, local injection and pressure, followed by heating modalities.

The most common complication of a contusion of a muscle in this region is residual stiffness, which causes an aching pain and restriction of motion for several days after the injury. This can be treated with heating modalities, pain-free massage and gentle exercise. If the contusion is over the spinous process there may be some periosteal reaction, or reaction in the supraspinous ligament which will leave a painful, tender area which is very sharply localized. If very painful it could indicate a fracture and may be a crack in the spinous process which cannot be demonstrated by X-ray, but which may be visible on a radionuclide bone scan. The resultant painful area can usually be treated by the following:

- Physiotherapy
- Local injection of a long-acting anaesthetic with or without a corticosteroid preparation

If athletic participation is to be continued following contusion, a localized protective pad can be placed over the affected area.

Muscle Strain

The spine is particularly susceptible to muscular strain because of the multiplicity of muscles involved in holding the body erect and constant strain on these muscles may be uncomfortable. In the early stages it may be difficult to distinguish a strain from contusion, as the contusion may cause some haemorrhage within the muscle and pain on movement. The early history may be a valuable guide in diagnosis as the athlete may mention some unusual occurrence which took place during the game or event. Basically, a strain is caused by overstretching the muscle and is usually located at the musculotendinous junction or at the tendon bone interface.

On examination it may be difficult to identify the exact muscle involved. There may be muscle spasm and acute tenderness over the injured muscle and pain caused by passive stretching or active contraction. If, for example, the spinalis group is involved on the right side, one will often find tenderness just to the right of the spinous process. Pain is elicited by passive forward flexion, whereas active forward flexion, even against forceful resistance, is pain-free. Passive spinal extension will be painless since the involved muscle relaxes in this motion, whereas active extension against resistance (as for example with the patient lying prone and raising his or her chest from the table) may cause acute discomfort. Passive flexion to the right is pain-free while active flexion to the right against resistance will cause it. To the left side passive flexion is painful and limited active motion, even against resistance, is not. If the condition is fairly severe and well established there is tenderness and spasm in the whole group of spinal muscles as they endeavour to resist motion in order to reduce discomfort. In this instance the spastic muscles themselves may become painful, even though not originally involved, and diffuse pain in the back is the result. The athlete presents with a rigid spine that resists motion in any direction.

TREATMENT

Treatment is general as well as local and includes the following:

General treatment

- Muscle relaxants
- Anti-inflammatory agents

Local treatment

- Initial icing or ice massage
- Local physiotherapy
- Local injection to the painful area
- Isometric exercises and depending on the severity of the injury, institution of a graduated isotonic programme
- Local heat used 1–4 days after the initial injury to promote better blood supply

As soon as the muscle spasm has subsided, usually between 1 and 10 days, rehabilitative measures may be commenced but carried out strictly within the limits of pain. Far too often the athlete is urged to compete earlier than he or she should and the sports physician should resist this. It is difficult to protect the thoracic spine by any protective device or a thoracic corset, but adhesive strapping of the thoracic spine to limit motion, notably forward flexion and lateral flexion, can sometimes be of value to relieve pain in light training and during rehabilitation.

If pain persists after adequate treatment the diagnosis should be reconsidered. Further investigations may be indicated to exclude more significant pathology such as a disc protrusion, isthmic fracture, discogenic or facet pain lesion.

Chronic back strain represents a major problem and is frequently the result of an acute strain that has not been adequately treated, particularly if there is underlying degeneration. Every recurrence of the condition makes the final cure more difficult and it may only resolve after prolonged absence from sporting activity. The best overall treatment is intensive physical therapy and avoidance of a further injury to that area.

Sprain

Sprains and muscle strains are often present in the same region as a result of a similar injury mechanism. The same force that causes muscular strain may tear some of the many ligaments in the area of the spine. Many of them are deeply placed, such as those located around the articular processes and between the lateral processes, or those extending between the lamina and vertebrae. The only ligament that can be palpated easily in the thoracic spine is the supraspinous, which extends along the tips of the spinous processes. Injury to this ligament can be determined by localized palpable tenderness either along the course of the ligament itself or at its attachment to the bone. Extension of the spine should be pain-free but forward flexion will cause pain at the involved area if the supra- or interspinous, or interlaminal ligaments are involved.

The direction of motion that causes pain is the key to diagnosis of sport-related spinal ligament injuries. Given right side involvement with damage to the capsular ligament, one would expect the local tenderness and spasm to be on the right side in an effort to prevent stretching of this ligament. Forward flexion, either active or passive, is painful. Either active or passive extension may also be painful. Ipsilateral flexion should relieve the symptoms and indeed the athlete usually stands with a lean to the right side. Contralateral flexion will increase the pain unless it is prevented by the spastic muscle. X-rays are of little value in the diagnosis of sprain, but may be used in a serious injury in order to exclude bone injury. In a rupture of the supra- and infraspinous ligaments, forward flexion X-rays may reveal greater separation of the spinous processes than at segments above and below the injury. This is an unusual injury to the thoracic spine but does occur from time to time in sport.

Treatment for thoracic spine ligament injury is similar to that of ligamentous injuries elsewhere. Protection of the ligament against excessive stretch is required until healed and a short period of bed rest may be necessary. Most sprains or strains will heal within 10–14 days; however, if symptoms persist after this period the diagnosis should be reconsidered.

Dislocation

Dislocation of the thoracic spine is extremely rare in sport since it is inherently very stable. It may be associated with severe neurological complications involving the spinal cord and reduction of a dislocated segment, with or without neurological complications, is usually required. Dislocation leading to instability may require a surgical procedure to stabilize the unstable segment.

Fracture

Fracture of the thoracic spine is more common than dislocation, but is unusual even in heavy contact sports such as ice hockey or the football codes. The incidence is higher, however, in motor sports or equestrian activities, for example showjumping, polo, horse-racing, etc. Fractures may affect the vertebral body, the arch or the spinous or lateral processes.

COMPRESSION FRACTURE OF THE VERTEBRAL BODY

Fracture of the vertebral body is usually caused by sharp forward flexion or a fall. The athlete gives a history of sudden forward flexion of the spine, having the head forcibly pushed between the knees, or falling violently on to the buttocks. This flexes the very rigid thoracic spine, and because the posterior ligaments hold, the force is taken by the anterior portion of the body of the vertebra. The cancellous bone fractures or impacts to a variable degree and the anterosuperior corner of the vertebra may be broken off. More commonly there is compression of the vertebra so that the cancellous bone is impacted into itself (Fig. 17.1).

A compression fracture of the thoracic spine does not always prevent walking, so the athlete may actually be back on his or her feet in spite of severe back discomfort. On examination, forward flexion will usually be painful, although it may be difficult to determine the exact degree of the injury. This may be elicited by having the athlete lie in a supine position. The examiner then flexes the athlete's neck to force the chin against the chest, which will then usually cause localized pain in the fracture area. This test may also be positive if there is a ligament injury. Spinal motion in any direction usually causes some pain, even in an impacted fracture.

X-ray evaluation can demonstrate a compression fracture, but it can be missed if the deformity is mild on a lateral X-ray. In this case the vertebrae should be carefully measured anteriorly to determine whether any vertebra is narrower than the others. Of particular importance is the appearance of the bone itself and a fracture line may be visible. The bone may be compacted so that this particular vertebrae not only appears smaller but seems more dense than those around it.

TREATMENT

In the young athlete if the compression fracture causes more than 30° of kyphotic angulation or 10–15° of scoliosis or lateral deviation, then surgical reduction may be indicated depending on the site of the fracture. Provided there is no forward displacement and the kyphosis is less than 30° without intracanal involvement the compression fracture is probably stable.

X-ray follow-up is necessary to determine when union is complete and athletic competition should not be permitted for at least 4–6 months unless it is a relatively minor fracture. Rehabilitation should include a strengthening programme, which can usually be started within 1–2 weeks of the injury. There is some danger of late aseptic necrosis of the vertebra if vigorous weight-bearing exercise (such as running, weight-lifting) is permitted too soon.

POSTERIOR ELEMENT INJURIES

Fracture of the posterior structures of the dorsal spine is extremely infrequent since they are well protected by the ribs. Fracture of the laminae, inter-articular portion of the bone or of the articular processes themselves require examination by a CT scan for diagnosis. Adequate support by brace is usual for 6–8 weeks to prevent excessive formation of a painful callus or non-union of the fracture.

Fractures of the spinous process do occur and should be protected against forward flexion. If there is a separation of a fragment of the bone, a good deal of time will often be saved by its early removal as a primary measure, rather than waiting for non-union to occur and then removing the fragment at a later time if pain occurs. Separation is much more frequent in the upper dorsal spine, and may be the result of an avulsion of the tip of the spinous process by forward flexion of the neck and upper spine or by a direct blow. It is occasionally caused by a muscle 'jerk'.

SCHEUERMANN'S DISEASE (DORSOLUMBAR KYPHOSIS)

This condition in adolescence is essentially a disturbance of the growth of the vertebrae and usually occurs in males. It may be localized or more extensive and is evidenced by wedging of several dorsal vertebrae, with osteochondritis of the bodies which sometimes progresses to fragmentation. Occasionally, only a single vertebra may be involved and this may cause some confusion in the diagnosis in the early stages. However, it appears that malformation of the vertebrae appears definitely increased by active or passive forward flexion.

Dorsolumbar kyphosis, although often prominent, is frequently overlooked in the differential diagnosis of back pain in the active adolescent. The current major radiological criteria for the diagnosis of Scheuermann's disease have been delineated by Bradford (1981) and are as follows:

- Irregular vertebral end-plates
- Narrowing of the intervertebral disc space
- One or more vertebrae wedged at 5° or more
- An increase in normal kyphosis beyond 40°

There is an increased incidence of spondylolisthesis in the lumbar spine in association with Scheuermann's disease.

TREATMENT

Provided the kyphosis is less than 45°, treatment consists of a hyperextension exercise programme, education on posture and regular radiological assessment.

Hyperextension braces may correct the deformity over a period of time in the growing child and are recommended if the kyphotic angle is above 45°. These braces need to be worn all day but can be removed at night, and for extension exercises and swimming. Surgical correction of the deformity is indicated if the kyphosis is more than 60° and growth has been complete.

As the replacement phase of the osteochondrosis develops, demonstrated by improved density of the vertebrae, coalescence of the fragmented areas and a reduction in pain, the athlete may be allowed to gradually return to sport. In some cases he or she may need to wear the protective brace to minimize flexion until the bodies are completely reconstituted.

More difficult diagnostically is the localized manifestation of the same condition in which one, two or three of the vertebrae may be involved with quite major changes and yet be essentially pain-free, until an injury draws attention to the area, or the area becomes spontaneously painful. It may be, however, that the injury is entirely coincidental and should not be confused with an acute fracture. Bone scanning (technetium ^{99}m) may be required to assist in a diagnostic evaluation of the above problem.

It will be necessary to reduce the athlete's activity and by serial X-rays determine when the bone has repaired sufficiently to permit the stress of athletic competition to recommence.

LUMBAR SPINE INJURIES

Injuries to the lumbar spine are common in many sports. Such injuries range from strains and contusions to severe spinal fractures associated with paraplegia.

Anatomical Considerations

The lumbar spine is designed to provide greater mobility than the thoracic spine but has more inherent stability than the cervical spine. Lumbar lordosis results from the thoracic kyphosis and the lumbosacral angle, which varies between different individuals. The posterior arch is large, with heavy lateral or transverse processes extending well away from the mid-line to add additional leverage for muscle attachments. The laminae or arches of the vertebrae are heavy and the articular facets are in the sagittal plane. Hence the mobility in the spine is largely in flexion and in extension, in which the intervertebral joints serve more or less as an axis, with motion permitted by compression and distraction of the intervertebral disc and by separation and opposition of the spinous processes. There is little rotary motion in the lumbar spine.

The muscles attaching to the lumbar spine are large and are supported in their function to control lumbar spine movement by the abdominal musculature. The sacrospinalis group are interdigitated up into the dorsal spine and consist of large muscles arising from the pelvis to attach to the spinous processes and vertebral bodies and act as firm stabilizers of the lumbar spine. The abdominal muscles complete the stabilizing effect in the front. Anteriorly, these muscles extend from the pubis to the ribs and serve to provide active forward flexion and prevent overextension of the lumbar spine. The large mass of the paraspinal muscles also serves to protect the posterior portion of the abdominal cavity and prevent injury to the kidneys, spleen and liver.

In assessing an athlete with a lumbar spine injury, one must also consider the anatomical structures that may have been injured. Critical to this assessment is a careful clinical examination and the recording of information.

CONGENITAL ANOMALIES

Congenital deformities are much more commonly found in the lower spine than in the upper spine, specifically about the fourth and fifth lumbar and the first sacral segment vertebrae. These deformities can become a problem to the athlete since they require a decision on the advisability of the athlete continuing in sport and indeed on treatment of the acute condition. The great majority of these conditions do not affect the function of the spine enough to require restriction of activity.

Spina bifida occulta

Spina bifida occulta is relatively common and occurs in approximately 5–10% of the population (Fig. 17.12b). It is caused by the failure of the neural arch to fuse in one or more of the vertebrae. This is not a dangerous condition and withdrawal from activity is usually not necessary. Exceptionally wide spina bifida, involving several vertebrae, may be of sufficient concern to require the use of additional support, or the recommendation that some less strenuous activity be followed. A well placed sacral pad may give some reassurance to the individual. Nearly 30% of people with a spondylolisthesis have this anomaly.

Variations on sacral fusion (sacralization)

The sacrum is originally made up of five bones which during adolescence fuse into a solid mass; however, various anomalous conditions may arise as a part of this process. The lower lumbar vertebrae may participate to some extent in the sacral fusion and indeed may completely fuse, so that there is sacralization of the fifth lumbar vertebra, though this usually causes no problem. If the fusion is incomplete with one side fusing and the other not, then some imbalance may arise in the lower back and occasionally pain may be present. Occasionally it is necessary to complete the fusion surgically, after which unlimited activity is permitted.

Most cases of unilateral sacralization are symptom-free, and the same is true of lumbarization of the first sacral vertebra. If a portion of the sacrum fails to fuse, this is of no significance because the fibrous fusion is extremely firm and unlikely to be damaged by any type of athletic competition.

A sprain of the lumbar spinal ligament in which there is a congenital anomaly may be somewhat more resistant to treatment than an uncomplicated sprain and protection should be given, not for the congenital anomaly, but for the accompanying sprain.

Other anomalies

Other conditions such as hemivertebra, scoliosis, kyphosis and increased lordosis must be managed on an individual basis. In some instances such as lordosis, where a minor deformity is present, such a posture may even enhance athletic performance. See Chapter 1 for further details. The athlete must be judged symptomatically, as a deformity in itself may not necessarily be disabling if not accompanied by signs of secondary involvement, such as nerve root pressure and muscle contracture.

Contusions

The lumbar spine is frequently contused in sport. Such an injury is not usually very severe. The only subcutaneous bones in this region are the tips of the spinous processes which lie in a sulcus between the two erector spinae muscles and usually absorb shock from a blow to the back. Contusions of these muscles are treated in the same way as other similar muscle injuries. The patient's history is often that of a blow to the area with localized tenderness and moderate pain on movement. After several hours, muscle spasm supervenes, tightening up a group of muscles on the injured side, apparently in an attempt to prevent painful motion. At this time differentiation from strain may be very difficult. In simple contusions, active muscle contraction is not especially painful.

TREATMENT

If any treatment is necessary, application of ice followed by heat is indicated. If a massive haematoma appears to be present, an attempt can be made to aspirate it, although the exact location is often difficult to determine in these large muscles. Diagnostic ultrasound may be useful to delineate the haematoma and assist in guiding the aspirating needle. If the contusion seems to be severe, an X-ray of the underlying structures to determine the possibility of a fracture of the transverse or spinous process should be undertaken.

Muscle Strains and Ligamentous Strains

Ligamentous sprains and muscle strains can be considered the same in terms of treatment and prognosis. The only time it is possible to distinguish clinically between the two is if the supraspinous ligament is torn and mid-line pain is elevated. These injuries result from overstretching or overuse and may be difficult to distinguish from other causes of pain such as a facet joint strain.

The actual pathology of these injuries is uncertain as they are not explored surgically. Peripheral injuries that have been explored, that is hamstring and biceps injuries, show the muscular tear to occur at the musculotendinous junction or the osseotendinous interface. It would seem reasonable to hypothesize that the same occurs in the spine.

Muscle spasm appears to occur as a response to acute pain. Changes in muscle tension and position can be detected by the sensory ending such as muscle spindles, tendon organs and Ruffine endings. These sensory endings may be activated by certain positions and silenced in other positions. The activated ones can cause local muscle contraction or so-called spasm. Studies on myoelectric activity in patients with pain are conflicting and there is no evidence to suggest that electrical activity is increased in patients with low back pain and spasm. There are few reports on the pharmacological management of muscle spasm. Basmajian (1967) found that although muscle relaxants changed myoelectricity, there was no difference in the clinical results from patients treated with or without muscle relaxants. Despite the frequent diagnosis of muscle spasm in acute or chronic low back pain, little has

been established to confirm that this entity does occur through objective assessment.

TREATMENT

Strains and sprains are managed initially with local ice and analgesics. Heat can be used 1–4 days later once the acute initial muscle spasm has resolved. The period that the athlete should avoid sport will depend on the clinical symptoms, though isometric exercises can begin almost immediately as well as isotonic exercises in the painful range.

Sport should not be recommended until local tenderness has resolved and a full range of motion present. Protective corsets, wet suits or other devices may be used initially on returning to sport. These should be non-restrictive but provide local pressure as a protective measure.

Recurrent strains may require further investigation to assess the cause.

Additional forms of therapy for chronic muscle and myofascial pain include:

- Acupuncture or acupressure
- Transcutaneous nerve stimulation
- Massage techniques
- Local injection

The possibility of muscle pain being referred from the lumbar zygapophyseal joints can be evaluated by selective joint blocks.

REHABILITATION

Rehabilitation is extremely important, not only in complete recovery of a sprain or strain, but in avoiding its recurrence. Appropriate exercises which are continued for many months may well prevent the recurrence of the strain, which is, in effect, as a result of using the muscle beyond its capacity. Hence, the greater the strength of the muscle, the less likely it will be that the same injury will occur again.

Bone Injuries

FRACTURES

Fractures may occur in the body of the lumbar

vertebra, transverse process, spinous process or in some portion of the vertebrae.

FRACTURE OF THE BODY OF THE VERTEBRA

Fracture of the body of the vertebra is extremely rare as an athletic injury. X-ray examination reveals the injury and fractures causing minimal deformity do not need reduction. In the lower lumbar spine, compression fractures resulting from falls may show only a small degree of bony damage, but the CT scan can demonstrate significant retropulsion of fragments into the canal. Therefore it is recommended that all fractures are evaluated using CT scanning.

FRACTURE OF THE TRANSVERSE PROCESS OF THE VERTEBRA

Fracture of the transverse process is quite common in athletes (Fig. 17.11). It should be noted that the lumbar vertebrae have spike-like transverse processes, some of which are quite thin or have a narrow neck. These processes are ruptured by the following mechanisms:

- A direct blow as a complication of a contusion
- A violent exertion of the muscle attachment
- Or by a combination of the above two mechanisms

There is a difference of opinion as to the relative frequency of the two causes since the combination of a blow and exertion occur simultaneously. It is suggested that a direct blow may account for the fracture of a single lateral process, whereas fractures of multiple processes are of the avulsion type and may be associated with avulsion or damage to the adjacent nerve roots and trunks. In either event, the significance of the fracture is not the broken bone but the muscle injury. The distal fragment frequently separates quite widely and non-union is the result. This causes immediate pain in the lumbar region which may be quite severe or relatively minor. If participation continues, the pain increases, muscles become more spastic and the athlete's body is pulled towards the injured side. This is more noticeable after a period of rest and then resumption of activity. There is localized tenderness over the area of injury and stretching of the injured side by contralateral bending often causes acute pain. Ipsilateral bending against resistance is also painful, as is passive forward flexion and active backward flexion. Neurological signs may be present.

TREATMENT

Isolated fracture

Acute pain usually subsides within a few days and treatment is symptomatic. Exercises can begin as soon as the athlete is comfortable and return to sport is possible when pain resolves in a few weeks.

Avulsion fractures

The pain and initial disability is more severe, and a longer period of initial rest is indicated and some may require hospitalization. Isometric exercises can begin within a few days and mobilization usually on crutches is possible once the acute pain has resolved. A graduated strengthening and hydrotherapy programme can begin within a few weeks. Sport should not recommence for at least 5–6 weeks and only if asymptomatic. Specialist referral should be made if there is any associated neurological deficit.

FRACTURE OF THE SPINOUS PROCESS OF THE VERTEBRA

A fracture of the spinous process in the lumbar region usually has three different causes which are as follows:

- Hyperflexion that pulls off the tip of the process; for example a gymnastic forward or backward roll, or a fall
- Hyperextension that impinges one process against the other and breaks one or the other; for example a gymnastic back walk-over or a fall
- A direct blow that mechanically breaks off one of the projecting processes; for example in the martial arts or in wrestling

This condition may be diagnosed clinically by a sharp localized mid-line pain and confirmatory X-rays (including flexion and extension views) of the

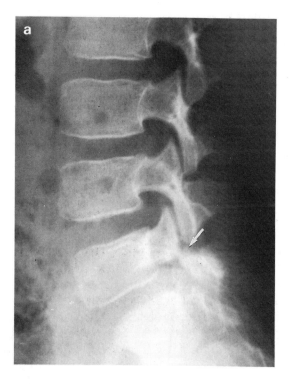

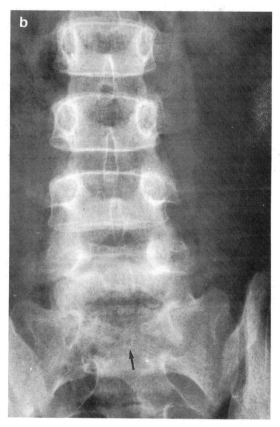

Fig. 17.12 (a) A lateral X-ray of a 7 year old girl with a spondylolisthesis. (b) An anteroposterior X-ray showing an associated spina bifida occulta in the same patient.

area are required. If there is actual separation of the fragment in the distal 2 cm of the process, a great deal of time and trouble will be saved by removing the fragment, since it is very slow to heal and the athlete is likely to have a recurrence of the pain on violent exertion. If the fracture is near the base of the process or in the arch, it heals much more rapidly and completely, provided the spine is immobilized in extension, preferably in a plaster cast or rigid bracing system for 3 weeks. Athletic competition is not recommended until complete healing has occurred.

Follow-up X-rays should be taken at weekly intervals for 3 weeks and again at 6 and 12 weeks, with the later X-rays including flexion–extension views.

VERTEBRAL ARCH FRACTURE

Any fracture involving the arch of the vertebra is potentially very serious because of the danger of neurological involvement. The fracture may be located at any of the following sites:

- Between the articular processes (pars interarticularis)
- Through the arch at the base of the process
- Within the articular process

Once such a fracture is recognized, the athlete must be immobilized to permit healing of the fracture, as painful function may result if the union is imperfect. This is a serious injury which should be treated as such and athletic competition is forbidden until healing is complete usually within 6 weeks. CT or technetium ^{99}m bone scan are the best for diagnosis and assessing union.

SPONDYLOLYSIS OR SPONDYLOLISTHESIS

Debate still continues as to whether defects of the

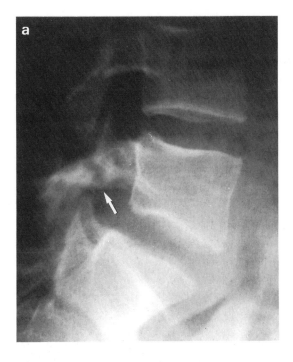

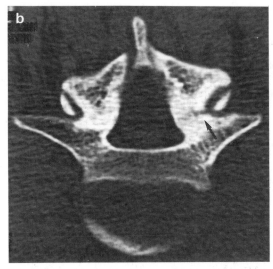

Fig. 17.13 (a) A lateral X-ray of a spondylolysis with very slight elongation of the pars interarticularis. (b) A CT scan showing a pars sclerosis and on the right side a stress fracture.

pars interarticularis are traumatic or developmental (Micheli 1983). Spondylolisthesis may be either:

- Dysplastic due to an underlying congenital anomaly
- Isthmic where there is a fracture through the pars interarticularis which is thought to be traumatic and may displace with age

These isthmic defects are rare before the age of 6 or 7 (Fig. 17.12a,b) and anatomical studies in newborn children have failed to demonstrate a spondylolisthesis at birth (Balis 1939). It appears that a proportion of such problems are related to a fusion failure of the arch of the vertebra. However, a proportion do occur as a result of trauma to the pars interarticularis with subsequent non-union and the development of a bony defect. The resultant pseudoarthrosis has a well developed ligamentous structure rather than mere scar tissue (Eisenstein *et al.* 1994). This ligament is well innervated and studies have shown immunoreactivity to calcitonin gene-related peptide, the C-peptide of neuropeptide Y and vasoactive intestinal peptide in the ligament and adjacent adipose tissue. This provides further

evidence of another source for pain in a mechanically disordered segment and thus why denervation procedures may have a part to play in treatment.

The prevalence of defects of the pars has been recorded as 5% in the normal population, rising to 11% in groups of gymnasts (Jackson *et al.* 1981). Rates higher than 30% have been noted in certain sports groups, including Australian Olympic soccer representatives of which 55% of the players had radiologically confirmed pars defects, but very few were symptomatic. Hardcastle (1991) have reported an incidence of 48% in young fast-bowlers playing cricket. Acute stress fractures of the pars interarticularis have been well documented in these athletes and the research has implicated repetitive overuse of the spine in a rotated and hyperextended position during bowling as a factor in stress fracture aetiology (Fig. 17.13a,b). Rates of stress fractures in young fast-bowlers appear to be increasing.

Spondylolisthesis is spondylolysis in which there is forward displacement of one vertebra on the one below. The laminal defect does cause instability of the spinal segment, but to a variable degree. Many athletes have spondylolysis and spondylolisthesis all their lives and are asymptomatic. However, if an athlete has lumbar pain and spondylolysis is discovered, one is justified in directing the athlete away from sports involving hyperextension (Micheli 1985) or considering surgical repair of the defect (Hardcastle *et al*. 1990) in chronic situations.

DIAGNOSIS

Acute lesions of the pars interarticularis are best diagnosed with bone scanning showing increased uptake of the radionuclide. To accurately localize the uptake within the posterior elements of the vertebra, SPECT (single photon emission CT) may be used to pin-point uptake in the pars interarticularis. CT scanning, using a reverse gantry angle to give more accurate bone cuts through the pars interarticularis, provides useful information about the fracture. MRI scanning is of limited value in the detection of acute fractures, but with newer technology the T1-weighted images may show early fractures associated with haemorrhage and oedema and thus are useful in early diagnosis without subjecting the athlete, especially female athletes, to radiation exposure (Yamane *et al*. 1993).

TREATMENT

Acute pars interarticularis fractures should be treated with relative rest, bracing to minimize hyperextension and thereafter a graduated exercise programme in the pain-free range. Occasionally, a plaster jacket or light-weight complete spinal brace (for example, a Boston Brace) may be indicated. Healing can be followed with reverse gantry CT scanning at 12 weeks; however, complete healing may take up to 6 months. Failure to show good healing or persistence of pain may suggest consideration for surgical intervention and repair of the pars interarticularis fracture can be undertaken.

Chronic lesions appear as follows:

- A negative bone scan
- CT scan shows sclerosis at the fracture ends
- Defect is more than 1–2 mm wide

These lesions are best treated symptomatically as they rarely unite. Injury or pain to these segments may be caused by the following:

- Discal shear stress and injury at the level of the defect
- Zygapophyseal joint strain and associated pain syndrome
- Other ligamentous strain or muscle sprain

THERAPEUTIC OPTIONS

Conservative measures include:

- Local physiotherapy to relieve acute symptoms
- Graduated muscle strengthening
- Non-restrictive spinal supports
- Assessment of the athlete's technique in repetitive movement sports, for example fast bowling, high jump, field games

Zygapophyseal joint injections

Injection of joints above and at the level of the defect with local anaesthetic and corticosteroid can lead to dramatic improvement, as there is a direct communication between the fracture and the adjacent facet joints (McCormick *et al*. 1989). Once pain is controlled the athlete can proceed to spinal exercise and gradual rehabilitation.

Recurrence of joint pain can be treated with dorsal primary rami denervation procedures including radiofrequency or cryoprobe denervation.

Disc procedures — blocks

These may be annular blocks where the needle is placed within the periphery of the annulus, or discography, where the needle is placed within the nucleus pulposus to outline the internal structure of the intervertebral disc, or detect any peripheral tears arising from the internal aspect of the annulus (Fig. 17.14a,b). A corticosteroid can be added to the dye and may in some cases cause relief of pain. New techniques using radiofrequency to denervate the periphery of the annulus are being used, but no definitive results are yet available (Stolker *et al*. 1994).

Surgical considerations

If an athlete has had an adequate trial of conservative treatment and is still unable to pursue their sport due to a spondylolysis then consideration should

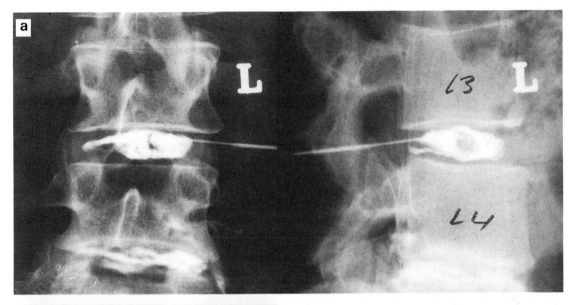

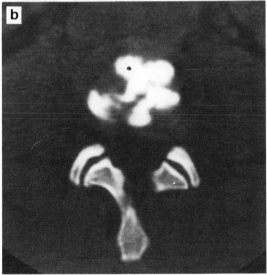

Fig. 17.14 (a) Spondylitic or stress fractures shown on a CT scan. Recurrent backache prevented this first class cricketer from fast bowling. (b) Surgical bone grafting of the defects resulted in the fractures uniting and the patient returned to first class cricket with an improved performance and no further back problems 3 years after his operation.

be given to surgical stabilization and bone grafting. It is suggested that the L4–5 isthmic spondylolisthesis more frequently justifies for surgical stabilization in comparison with the L5–S1 lesion (Grobler *et al.* 1993). In severe isthmic spondylolisthesis in adolescents *in situ* fusion is preferred rather than undertaking a reduction procedure followed by a fusion procedure (Schlenzka *et al.* 1993). Radiological investigations sometimes do not demonstrate the degree of instability that may be present. This can sometimes only be assessed at the time of surgery. Provided there is less than 1–2 mm of forward slip of one vertebra on another, then direct repair of the pars interarticularis defect should be considered. The procedure involves curetting the fracture site and removing the inferior tip of the adjacent inferior facet. The bone graft is placed within and around the fractures which are stabilized with screw fixation from the lamina through the fracture into the pedicle (Fig. 17.15a,b).

Four to 6 weeks after surgery a swimming, walking and bicycle riding programme is commenced. These fractures are assessed by reverse gantry CT scans 3 and 6 months after surgery. Once there is radiological evidence of complete union, full sporting activities can resume. If union has not occurred on the CT scan by 6 months it is recommended that these fractures be re-explored and further bone grafting performed if necessary.

In all cases of spondylolysis or spondylolisthesis, once pain control has been achieved, a comprehen-

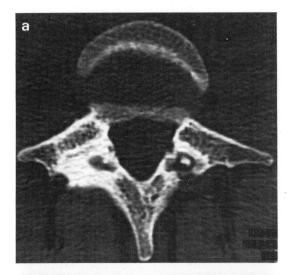

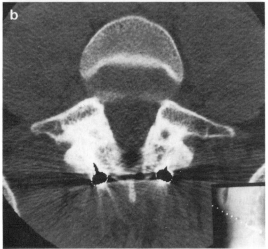

Fig. 17.15   (a) Anteroposterior and lateral X-rays of an L3–4 and L4–5 discogram. (b) The post-discogram CT scan (L3–4) gives a better definition of the internal annular tears located in the mid-line and laterally. This is not complete, however, as dye is contained within the annulus and has not extravasated into the epidural space.

sive exercise programme is required. Even in those in whom surgery is required a return to sporting activity is highly likely.

Discal Injuries

The diagnosis of disc pathology with or without attendant nerve root injury has become a major

area of study in recent years. The association of intervertebral disc disease with lumbar pain and referral of pain to the lower limbs has become well recognized in medicine. Data on disc disease and its relationship to athletic activity suggest that athletic participation is not associated with an unduly high incidence of discal injuries. In fact, exercise and sports participation has been strongly recommended for those with intervertebral disc disease.

Intervertebral disc lesions may result in pain from the following causes:

* Strain on the annulus fibrosus after internal disruption of the disc
* Tears of the anterolateral portion of the annulus fibrosus
* Tears in the posterior annulus fibrosus
* Pre-rupture of the nucleus pulposus

Protrusion of the nucleus pulposus through a posterior annular tear may be mid-line or postero-lateral and may cause compression of the neural structures in the following ways:

* Contained within the confines of the annulus
* Sequestrated where a fragment of the nucleus pulposus ruptures through the annulus
* Intradural location is rare but does occur

Disc protrusions usually occur at L4–5 or L5–S1 but can occur above these levels and protrusions at L2–3 and L3–4 are more likely to be associated with neurological signs.

However, it is to be noted that disc bulges and disc protrusions are extremely common in pain-free individuals whereas disc extrusions are not (Deyo 1994). Disc extrusions are almost always symptomatic in the acute phase.

In evaluating the pathophysiology of discal lesions, the three phases have been described as follows:

* Phase I — microtrauma/internal annular tears
* Phase II — development of anatomical lesions within zygapophyseal joints and discs/instability/hypermobility
* Phase III — organization/osteophytes/stenosis

Degeneration of the spine occurs even in very young people, and in a recent study carried out in

Western Australia, MRI assessment demonstrated that 70% of young fast bowlers playing cricket had evidence of degenerative disc disease (Hardcastle 1991). This very high incidence in young cricketers may be attributable to their sport, but despite this, some of them had no painful symptoms, which may be explained by the fact that they were still very young.

Often an advanced intervertebral disc degeneration is not painful in itself if mobility has been lost, which often occurs as people age. However, if instability is present, episodic pain may continue which may in some cases be quite severe, necessitating consideration of a spinal fusion.

The diagnosis of discal lesions includes a physical examination and further investigation and these are summarized in Tables 17.1 and 17.2.

MRI has become increasingly popular in the evaluation of patients with low back pain, because it is non-invasive and images the intervertebral discs, spine and spinal cord in multiple planes. It has been advocated as an important modality in identifying disc injury and degeneration.

Table 17.1 Low back pain physical examination distinguishing between zygapophyseal joint pain and discal pain patterns

	Zygapophyseal joints	Disc
Flexion	−	+
Deflexion*	−	++
Extension	+	−
Tenderness	+	+
Back pain with straight leg raise	±	+
Sympathetic signs	−	+
Neurological signs	−	±
Slump test†	−	+

*Deflexion: return to the neutral position after forward flexion.

†Slump test: This test is performed with the athlete sitting on the examination couch with the hands behind the back and neck in neutral position. The patient slumps forward with the pelvis fixed then flexes the neck. The athlete then extends one knee and subsequently dorsiflexes the foot. Neck flexion is then released. A positive test response is characterized by reproduction of the athlete's symptoms with knee extension and ankle dorsiflexion followed by alleviation of the positive signs by releasing the neuromeningeal tension (with extension).

Table 17.2 Imaging techniques to assess disc disease

- Plain radiology including functional views to assess for segmental instability. Computer analysis of functional X-rays may be considered since pain and mobility may be closely correlated with the early stages of degenerative disease
- CT scanning
- MRI which may detect internal disc abnormalities by changes in hydration of the disc, or the disc may also show protrusion
- Myelography + CT scan
- Discography to show internal disc abnormalities of the nucleus pulposus, followed by CT scanning which shows more clearly the internal disc disruption. It may also be used as a provocative test to simulate symptoms. Instillation of local anaesthetic and steroid to abate pain can be performed concurrently. Antibiotics should be injected at the same time to reduce the incidence of post-discogram discitis

However, a structural abnormality of the disc, such as that seen in internal disc disruption, may be missed on MRI (Brightbill et al. 1994). In injured athletes with unrelenting low back pain of apparent discogenic origin, lumbar discography should be strongly considered.

It can be very difficult particularly in the acute phase to distinguish between discogenic pain and zygapophyseal pain unless there are definite nerve compression or neurological signs. Zygapophyseal injections can be useful in diagnosis and should be performed before discograms because of the potential complications with discograms.

NEURAL COMPRESSION SIGNS

The femoral and sciatic nerve roots may be under tension as a result of a disc protrusion. The femoral stretch test is performed with the patient lying prone and by fully flexing the knee; one stretches the femoral nerve and a positive response is when pain is referred to the anterior aspect of the thigh. Usually, associated with this lesion is a wasting of the quadriceps muscle and an absent knee jerk reflex.

The sciatic nerve can be stretched classically with the patient lying supine and performing a straight leg test comparing one side with another. There are a number of tests to assess whether there is any nerve root tension on the sciatic nerve. Lasegue's manoeuvre is when the ankle is dorsiflexed just short of a maximal straight leg raise on the involved side, and is positive if pain down the leg is reproduced. The flip test is performed in the sitting position with each leg raised to 90° of hip flexion and the ankle fully dorsiflexed. If the patient leans backwards on the involved side only this is a sign of nerve compression. The slump test is described in Table 17.1.

Physical diagnostic manoeuvres for evaluating sciatic tension in patients with documented lumbar disc herniation have a high correlation with surgical pathology (Supik & Broom 1994). These diagnostic signs of sciatic stretch can be reliable guides that lead to more aggressive modes of evaluation. Correlation between specific sciatic stretch manoeuvres regarding location of disc herniation relative to the nerve root, does not appear good.

Further advances in delineating the site of functional nerve root compressions may be found with the epidural recording of nerve conduction studies (Sine *et al.* 1994).

TREATMENT

Initial conservative treatment options include the following:

- Bed rest for up to 3 days following acute pain, particularly if significant violence is involved
- Analgesics, non-steroidal anti-inflammatory medications, muscle relaxants
- Electrotherapeutic modalities
- Spinal mobilization techniques in cases of minor trauma associated with local joint stiffness
- Spinal brace or strapping may be considered

Once the acute inflammatory phase has been resolved, exercises and treatment options to improve mobility need to be considered, though a further clinical assessment should be performed and if nerve compressive signs are present a CT or MRI performed. Further treatment may involve spinal traction and manual therapy, with mobilization and manipulation (see Chapter 13). Manipulation and mobilization are better suited to minor injuries resulting in locked facet syndromes and stiff joints after periods of immobilization, rather than discal

injuries (Shekelle 1994). Two methods are currently available, one utilizing a manual therapist and the other doing a formal manipulation under general anaesthetic and full muscle relaxation.

Athletes with discal injury and associated abnormalities in other tissues (including zygapophyseal joints) appear to benefit from manual therapy. The influence of manual therapy manoeuvres on pure disc pathology is unknown; however, manipulative techniques have a potential to worsen internal disease derangements or disruptions. Pain from the intervertebral disc or zygapophyseal joint may give rise to trigger point pain over different muscles. Trigger point therapy may prove useful in athletes with discal injuries, perhaps by relieving pain in referred pain sites.

Spinal exercises must be carefully performed within the pain-free range as for ligamentous injury. Improvements in spinal muscle function are important for restoration of normal spine rehabilitation. A better understanding of paraspinal muscle dysfunction is now being achieved to provide further guidance for rehabilitation (Cooper 1993). Exercises in extension as described by Mackenzie (1989) are useful.

Hydrotherapy and swimming, as well as other aerobic conditioning exercise (Brennan *et al.* 1994), can play an important part in the rehabilitation of athletes with discal disease but careful supervision is required and correct swimming technique is essential. If an athlete is a poor swimmer, the use of flippers, buoyancy devices, goggles and a snorkel may be used to maintain a good horizontal position in the water until his or her swimming skills improve.

Other techniques need to be considered if the above regimens are not working; for example, lumbar epidural injection using the following:

- Local anaesthetic and corticosteroid
- Local anaesthetics and opiate
- Local anaesthetic alone
- Normal saline solution

Nerve root or dural sleeve injections are useful in athletes with radicular symptoms and with minimal evidence of disc prolapse on imaging techniques (Hasue 1993). Of particular note is the variable anatomy of foraminal nerve root lesions (Sato & Kikuchi 1993). Diagnosis of nerve root entrapment in the foraminal zone can be made only through both morphological and functional findings by nerve root infiltration. Deformation of the nerve roots in the foraminal zone may be shown by nerve root infiltration with contrast medium.

Disc block or denervation procedures (Sluijter 1990)

- Annular disc blocks using local anaesthetic blocks plus corticosteroid or radiofrequency annular lesioning
- Discal denervation by using a radiofrequency sympathetic block for pain emanating from the anterior part of the annulus fibrosus, or radiofrequency lesion of the communicating ramus for pain emanating from the anterolateral part of the annular fibrosus (Aprill 1990)

Reduction in nucleus pulposus mass

Instillation of chymopapain into the nucleus pulposus via the posterolateral approach, after confirmation of lack of communication with the epidural space on discography is useful. Proof of lack of communication minimizes the risks of transverse myelitis due to chymopapain leakage into the intradural space. Chymopapain is not indicated if disc sequestration has occurred or if spinal stenosis is present. In approximately 65% of cases relief of sciatic pain is achieved. It is a procedure, however, which can cause severe muscle spasm for several weeks after the injection, and as complications (anaphylaxis, transverse myelitis) have been recently recorded, it is now much less popular in managing these conditions, though it has a place in managing contained disc protrusions.

Percutaneous discectomy by mechanical suction and curettage of the nucleus pulposus has been found to be useful in discal lesions associated with nerve root (radicular) symptoms (Mochida & Arima 1993; Sakou et al. 1993). However, this procedure has the disadvantage of not removing the actual protrusion and its part in the management of these disc protrusions is uncertain, as no specific control trials are as yet available to assess its efficiency.

Microsurgical discectomy is now used to minimize any trauma that may result from the operative procedure itself. Microlumbar discectomy has been shown to be a safe and cost-effective procedure and can be performed as an outpatient procedure (Zahrawi 1994). In sportspeople it is recommended that the entire nucleus pulposus is removed, as it has no role in spinal stability once it has degenerated to the point where it ruptures, and it is much better to remove all the nuclear material to prevent recurrent protrusion. Repeat decompression of lumbar nerve roots has been indicated in the past due to further disc herniation, lateral spinal stenosis, central spinal stenosis and periradicular fibrosis (Jonsson & Stromqvist 1993). Sciatica due to nerve-root scarring seldom improves by repeat operation.

Spinal fusion of the spinal segment at which the laminectomy for disc protrusions have been performed is considered controversial and should be reserved for those cases not responding to previous surgical procedures, or those who have significant segmental hypermobility or instability.

Spinal fusion of the spinal segment at which the laminectomy for disc protrusions has been perments are found but in which no major spinal or nerve root compromise is noted. Disc excision and posterior lumbar interbody fusion has proved successful (Lee et al. 1993).

After undertaking the above procedures, including surgery, to reduce spinal pain, the athlete should return to the exercise programme discussed earlier.

Zygapophyseal Joints

Injuries to the zygapophyseal joints may cause pain in the following situations (Bogduk 1990):

- Capsular tears
- Haemarthrosis
- The small meniscus which attaches to the capsule may be torn or locked within the joint
- The fat pad at the inferior aspect of the facet joint may be contused or locked within the joint
- Chondromalacia of the hyaline cartilage covering the facet joint occurs in the dysfunction stage and small pieces may become dislodged and

either locked within the joint or the synovium, causing an inflammatory response
- Subchondral fracture
- The long-term sequelae of the above including osteoarthritis

In sports and dance, which may involve repetitive posterior element loading, atypical stress fractures of the lumbar facet joints may occur (Fehlandt & Micheli 1993).

The interaction between discal and zygapophyseal disorders as a cause for lumbar pain after spinal injury is complex, since the integrity of each structure is dependent on the other. However, in athletes as in other patients with chronic low back pain, the combination of discogenic pain and zygapophyseal joint pain appears uncommon (Schwarzer *et al.* 1994).

The zygapophyseal joints are innervated by the medial branches of the lumbar dorsal rami, with each joint receiving dual innervation from the nerve above and below the joint.

The zygapophyseal joints may be studied by direct injection techniques and arthrography can define the size and shape of the joint space, as well as the integrity of the articular capsule. Pain patterns provoked by joint injection may implicate or exclude a given joint from consideration as a significant pain generator. Lumbar zygapophyseal joints are most easily injected by a posterior or posterolateral approach.

Injuries to the zygapophyseal joints may be associated with the following:

- Pain radiating to the buttock, groin or down the leg to the ankle
- Local tenderness
- Any movement may aggravate pain and, if mechanical, it is usually two or three directions that cause pain (usually extension), but if inflammatory, movements in all planes will be reduced
- Occasional back pain with straight leg raising which may be restricted but neural compressive signs are absent
- Neurological signs may be present but are non-specific (non-myotomal and dermatomal) with sensory changes occasionally involving the whole leg

Treatment is with relative rest, anti-inflammatory medication and local physiotherapeutic electro-modalities and supported by a brace to limit extension and treatment of associated factors, such as muscle spasm and trigger point tenderness. Manual therapy techniques often prove useful to improve pain relief and increase the range of segmental motion with concomitant reduction of pain. Thereafter spinal exercises include flexion with a restriction of extension. Pelvic shift exercises to minimize lumbar lordosis can also reduce pain.

Poor response to such conservative therapies necessitate further evaluation, including bone scanning to assess for arch fractures or intra-articular zygapophyseal joint fractures and CT scanning to assess joint subluxations and concomitant disc lesions.

Treatment for persistent zygapophyseal joint pain may involve zygapophyseal joint injections of local anaesthetic and corticosteroid or radiofrequency blocks of the medial branch of the dorsal ramus (North *et al.* 1994). The dorsal primary rami innervate the zygapophyseal joints and temporary blocks with local anaesthetic can assist in assessment of the contribution of the zygapophyseal joints to the overall pain pattern. Longer-term blocks using radiofrequency denervate the medial branch of the dorsal ramus (Esses & Moro 1993).

SURGICAL PROCEDURES

Zygapophyseal arthroplasty may be contemplated in some cases. This is a rarely used procedure that may have some value in the patients with zygapophyseal joint dysfunction. Thereafter an intensive physical therapy exercise programme will be required before returning to sports participation. Spinal fusion can provide relief of pain in patients whose joints are resistant to conservative treatment, as these cases usually have associated segmental instability.

Spinal fusion may be anterior or posterior. Even with a two-level fusion one can resume full normal activity or sport once union has occurred. Internal fixation with a Hartskill rectangle or a spinal plate is recommended as an adjunct to spinal fusion. Newer types of fusion systems are being evaluated: systems such as the Graf system which is a flexible pedicle fixation system aimed to restrict segmented vertebral motion rather than eliminating it (Strauss *et al.* 1994). Additional procedures may need to be considered for the athlete who has developed chronic intractable back pain. Neurosurgical implantation of a spinal cord stimulator may be appropriate in such cases (Watkins & Koeza 1993).

Spine-related Syndromes

SACRO-ILIAC SYNDROME

This may present with pain over the sacro-iliac joint, which radiates down into the leg and the ankle (Fig. 17.16a,b). The exact mechanism of injury and the cause of pain is uncertain, but it may be associated with stiffness of the joint and radiographs are usually normal unless there is an underlying inflammatory disorder such as ankylosing spondylitis, or an infective process (White & Cooper 1994). CT scans give a better definition of the sacro-iliac joint than plain X-rays. Although the cause of sacro-iliac pain is uncertain, it does respond well to local injections and manipulation.

PIRIFORMIS SYNDROME

This results from a minor twisting injury to one leg, usually when the patient is in an awkward position, or lifting. Pain is felt in the buttock over the piriformis and can be referred down the leg because of the close proximity of the sciatic nerve. The pain is usually the result of tearing of muscle fibres. Clinical features include local tenderness medial to the greater trochanter and pain on muscle contraction by performing resisted adduction of the involved hip in the sitting position. Rectal examination demonstrates some tenderness medial to the spine of the ischium. This syndrome usually responds well to local injection of marcaine and a longer-term benefit may be found if a corticosteroid preparation is added to the local anaesthetic.

QUADRATUS LUMBORUM SYNDROME

This causes pain between the 12th rib and the iliac

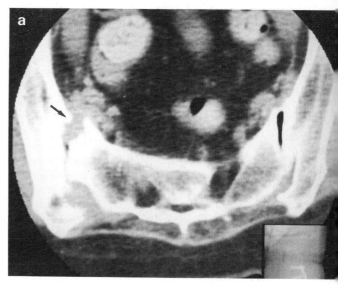

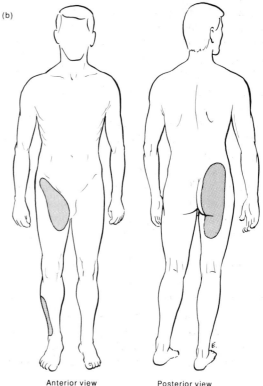

Anterior view   Posterior view

Fig. 17.16 (a) A CT scan of the sacro-iliac joint showing an erosive lesion anteriorly which would not be seen on plain X-rays due to infection. (b) A pain drawing of a patient with a sacro-iliac syndrome demonstrating the potential areas of referred pain.

crest lateral to the erector spinae. Often there is no history of trauma, though it is thought to be due to a rupture of the muscle fibres. The pain may be anywhere in the muscle and the pain may radiate into the groin or down into the thigh. Local tenderness is present and the pain is aggravated by stretching the muscle to the contralateral side. Local anaesthetic to the area will abolish pain and a corticosteroid added to the local anaesthetic may give long-lasting benefit.

OTHER CONDITIONS

There are other causes of low back pain, but these are not usually associated with trauma, and it is not the purpose of this chapter to describe them in detail. Referred pain from intra-abdominal or intra-pleural structures may cause pain and tenderness over the posterior spine, mimicking a zygapophyseal joint syndrome. Tumour or infection can occur and usually involve the vertebral body and the inter-vertebral disc. Tumours also occasionally involve the posterior elements, and if this is the case they are usually benign.

CONCLUSIONS

Traumatic sporting injuries to the spine can result in a wide variety of different pathologies, depending on the force involved, the position of the spine at the time the force is applied and the underlying anatomical and pathological constitution of the individual. The injuries involved may in many cases be trivial; however, more significant injuries do occur, and it is paramount to recognize them at an early stage. An accurate diagnosis must be made as soon as possible before treatment regimens are applied to the athlete. With recurring disability the cause should be investigated more fully, implementing a more multidisciplinary approach, including assessment of the athlete's technique, muscle strength and any underlying pathological problems he or she may have.

REFERENCES

Ahrens S. F. (1994) The effect of age on intervertebral disc compression during running. *Journal of Orthopedic and Sports Physical Therapy* **20**, 17–21.

Anderson L. D. & D'Alonzo R. T. (1974) Fractures of the odontoid process of the axis. *Journal of Bone and Joint Surgery* **56**, 1663–1674.

Aprill C. (1990) Provocation discography and modern imaging. *Proceedings of VIth World Congress on Pain, Official Satellite Meeting 'Spinal Pain', Precision Diagnosis and Treatment*. Perth, Western Australia.

Balis M. Jr. (1939) The aetiology of spondylolisthesis. *Journal of Bone and Joint Surgery* **21**, 879–884.

Basmajian J. U. S. (1967) *Muscles Alive: Their Functions Revealed by Electromyography*, pp. 52, 206–211. Williams & Wilkins, Baltimore, MD.

Bedbrook G. M. (1981) *The Care and Management of Spinal Cord Injuries*, pp. 20, 255–269. Springer-Verlag, New York.

Bogduk N. (1990) Neurology and pathology of spinal pain. *Proceedings of VIth World Congress on Pain, Official Satellite Meeting 'Spinal Pain', Precision Diagnosis and Treatment*. Perth, Western Australia.

Bracken M., Shepard M., Collins W. *et al.* (1990) A randomised controlled trial of methyl-prednisolone or naloxone in the treatment of acute spinal cord injury. *New England Journal of Medicine* **322**, 20, 1405–1412.

Bradford D. S. (1981) Vertebral osteochondrosis. *Clinical Orthopaedics* **158**, 83–90.

Brennan G. P., Shultz B. B., Hood R. S., Zahniser J. C., Johnson S. C. & Gerber A. H. (1994) The effects of aerobic exercise after lumbar microdiscectomy. *Spine* **19**, 735–739.

Brightbill T. C., Pile N., Eichelberger R. P. & Whitman M. (1994) Normal magnetic resonance imaging and abnormal discography in lumbar disc disruption. *Spine* **19**, 1075–1077.

Cooper R. G. (1993) Understanding paraspinal muscle dysfunction in low back pain: A way forward? *Annals of the Rheumatic Diseases* **52**, 413–415.

Cremers M. J. G., Bol E., de Roos F. & van Gijn J. (1993) Risk of sports activities in children with Down's syndrome and atlantoaxial instability. *Lancet* **342**, 511–514.

Denis F. (1983) The three column spine and its significance in the classification of acute thoracolumbar spinal injuries. *Spine* **8**, 817–831.

Deyo R. A. (1994) Editorial. *New England Journal of Medicine* **331**, 115–116.

Dickson H. & Tonkin J. (1987) *Spinal Injuries Handbook*. The Prince Henry Hospital, Ciba Geigy, Sydney.

Ditunno J. F. & Formal C. S. (1994) Chronic spinal cord injury. *New England Journal of Medicine* **330**, 550–556.

Eisenstein S. M., Ashton I. K. & Darby A. J. *et al.* (1994) Innervations of the spondylolysis 'ligament'. *Spine* **19**, 912–916.

Esses S. I. & Moro J. K. (1993) The value of facet joint blocks in patient selection for lumbar fusion. *Spine* **18**, 185–190.

Fehlandt A. F. & Micheli L. J. (1993) Lumbar facet stress fracture in a ballet dancer. *Spine* **18**, 2537–2539.

Grobler L. J., Novothay J. E., Wilder D. G., Frymoyer

J. W. & Pope M. H. (1993) L4–5 isthmic spondylolisthesis: Biomechanical analysis comparing stability of L4–5 and L5–5 spondylolytic defect. Proceedings of the International Society for the Study of Lumbar Spine. Orthopaedic Transactions. *Journal of Bone and Joint Surgery* 17, 281.

Grundy D. & Swain A. (1993) *ABC of Spinal Cord Injury,* 2nd edn. BMJ Publishing Group, University Press, Cambridge.

Hardcastle P. H. (1991) Lumbar pain in fast bowlers. *Australian Family Physician*, 20, 943–951.

Harris J. H. & Yeakley J. W. (1992) Hyperextension-dislocation of the cervical spine. Ligament injuries demonstrated by magnetic resonance imaging. *Journal of Bone and Joint Surgery* 74, 567–570.

Hasue M. (1993) Pain and the nerve root: An interdisciplinary approach. *Spine* 18, 2053–2058.

Hochschuler S. H. (1990) (ed.) *The Spine in Sports.* Mosby Year Book, Philadelphia, PA.

Holdsworth F. (1970) Fractures, dislocations and fracture dislocations of the spine. *Journal of Bone and Joint Surgery* 52, 1534.

Jackson D. W., Wiltse L. L., Dinegman R. A. & Hayes M. (1981) Stress reactions involving the pars interarticularis in young athletes. *American Journal of Sports Medicine* 9, 304.

Jonsson B. & Stromqvist B. (1993) Repeat decompression of lumbar nerve roots. *Journal of Bone and Joint Surgery* 75, 894–897.

Kinoshita H. (1993) Pathology of cervical intervertebral disc injuries. *Paraplegia* 31, 553–559.

Lee C. K., Vessa P. & Lee J. K. (1993) Internal disc derangements: The results of surgical treatment by disc excision and posterior lumbar interbody fusion. Proceedings of the International Society for the Study of the Lumbar Spine. Orthopaedic Transactions. *Journal of Bone and Joint Surgery* 17, 340.

Lin R. M., Panjabi M. M. & Oxland T. R. (1993) Functional radiographs of acute thoraco-lumbar burst fractures. Proceedings of the International Society for the Study of the Lumbar Spine. Orthopaedic Transactions. *Journal of Bone and Joint Surgery* 17, 320.

Louw I. A., Mafoyane N., Small B. & Noser C. (1990) Occlusion of the vertebral artery in cervical spine dislocations. *Journal of Bone and Joint Surgery* 72, 679–681.

MacKenzie R. (1989) *Treat Your Own Back.* Orthopedic Physical Therapy Products.

McCormick C., Taylor J. & Twomey L. (1989) Facet joint arthrography in lumbar spondylolysis. *Radiology* 171, 193–196.

McGrory B. J., Klassen R. A., Chao E. Y. S., Staeheli J. W. & Weaver A. L. (1993) Acute fractures and dislocations of the cervical spine in children and adolescents. *Journal of Bone and Joint Surgery* 75, 988–995.

McSwain N. E., Martinez J. A. & Timberlake G. A. (1989) *Cervical Spine Trauma: Evaluation and Acute Management.* Thieme Medical Publishers, New York.

Menzies Foundation Technical Report (1987) *Towards Prevention of Spinal Cord Injury,* 1, 17–20, Melbourne.

Micheli L. J. (1983) Overuse injuries in children's sports: the growth factor. *Orthopedic Clinics of North America* 14, 337.

Micheli L. J. (1985) Back injuries in gymnastics. *Clinical Sports Medicine* 4, 85–93.

Mochida J. & Arima T. (1993) Percutaneous nucleotomy in lumbar disc herniation. A prospective study. *Spine* 18, 2063–2068.

North R. B., Han M., Zahurak M. & Kidd D. H. (1994) Radiofrequency lumbar facet denervation: Analysis of prognostic factors. *Pain* 57, 77–83.

Parks R. E. & Livoni J. P. (1986) Detection of cervical spine injury in the multitrauma patient. In Blaisdell F. W. & Trunkey D. D. (eds) *Trauma Management, Cervicothoracic Trauma,* Vol. III, pp. 56–65. Thieme Medical Publishers New York.

Reynen P. D. & Clancy W. G. (1994) Spinal cord injuries rise dramatically in ice hockey. *American Journal of Sports Medicine* 22, 167–170.

Runge V. M. & Gelblum D. Y. (1990) The role of gadolinium diethylenetriamine-pentoacetic acid in the evaluation of the central nervous system. *Magnetic Resonance Quarterly* 6, 85–107.

Sakou T., Masuda A., Yone K. & Nakagawa M. (1993) Percutaneous discectomy in athletes. *Spine* 18, 2218–2221.

Sato K. & Kikuchi S. (1993) An anatomic study of foraminal nerve root lesions in the lumbar spine. *Spine* 18, 2246–2251.

Sato T., Kokubun S., Rijal K. P. *et al.* (1994) Prognosis of cervical cord injury in correlation with magnetic resonance imaging. *Paraplegia* 32, 81–85.

Schlenzka D., Roussa M., Seitsalo S., Ylokoski M., Hurri H. & Osterman K. (1993) Operative treatment of severe isthmic spondylolisthesis in adolescents: Reduction and fusion versus fusion *in situ*. Proceedings of the International Society for the Study of Lumbar Spine. Orthopaedic Transactions. *Journal of Bone and Joint Surgery* 17, 299.

Schwarzer A. C., Aprill C. N., Derby R., Fortin J., Kine G. & Bogduk N. (1994) The relative contributions of the disc and zygapophyseal joint in chronic low back pain. *Spine* 19, 801–806.

Shekelle P. G. (1994) Spine update. Spinal manipulation. *Spine* 19, 858–861.

Sine R. D., Merrill D. & Date E. (1994) Epidural recording of nerve conduction studies and surgical findings of radiculopathy. *Archives of Physical Medicine & Rehabilitation* 75, 17–24.

Sluijter M. (1990) Radiofrequency denervation of the discs. *Proceedings of VIth World Congress on Pain, Official Satellite Meeting 'Spinal Pain', Precision Diagnosis and Treatment.* Perth, Western Australia.

Stolker R. J., Vervest A. C. M. & Groen G. J. (1994) The

management of chronic spinal pain by blockades: A review. *Pain* **58**, 1–20.

Strauss P. J., Novotny J. E., Wilder D. G., Grobler L. J. & Pope M. H. (1994) Multidirectional stability of the Graf system. *Spine* **19**, 965–972.

Supik L. F. & Broom M. J. (1994) Sciatic tension signs and lumbar disc herniation. *Spine* **19**, 1066–1069.

Tator C. H., Duncan E. G., Edmunds V. E., Lapczak L. I. & Andrews D. F. (1994) Complications and costs of management of acute spinal cord injury. *Paraplegia* **31**, 700–714.

Thompson G. H. (1993) Back pain in children. *Journal of Bone and Joint Surgery* **75**, 928–938.

Torg J. S. (1982) *Athletic Injuries to the Head, Neck and Face*. Lea & Febiger, Philadelphia, PA.

Tosi L., Righetti C., Terrini G. & Zanette G. (1993) Atypical syndromes caudal to the injury site in patients following spinal cord injury. A clinical, neurophysiological and MRI study. *Paraplegia* **31**, 751–756.

Watkins E. S. & Koeze T. H. (1993) Spinal cord stimulation and pain relief. *British Medical Journal* **307**, 462.

White P. G. & Cooper A. M. (1994) Sacro-iliac joint sepsis. *Annals of the Rheumatic Diseases* **53**, 440–443.

Wilberger J. E. Jr & Maroon J. C. (1990) Cervical spine injuries in athletes. *Physician and Sportsmedicine* **18**, 56–70.

Willen J., Anderson J., Toonaka K. & Singler K. (1990) Burst fractures at the thoracolumbar junction. *Journal of Spinal Disorders* **3**, 1.

Yamane T., Yoshida T. & Mimatsu K. (1993) Early diagnosis of lumbar spondylosis by MRI. *Journal of Bone and Joint Surgery* **75**, 764–768.

Zahrawi F. (1994) Microlumbar discectomy: Is it safe as an outpatient procedure? *Spine* **19**, 1070–1074.

CHAPTER 18

INJURIES TO THE CHEST AND ABDOMEN

W. Johnson

Injuries to the chest and abdomen are more common than suspected. They fall into two major groups, those to the walls of the thorax and abdomen which are often painful, but relatively minor, and those to the vital organs within the thorax and the abdomen. The sports medicine specialist needs to be skilled at recognizing the signs and symptoms of the life-threatening injuries, as well as having an appreciation of the less dangerous ones in order to give the patient prompt and safe treatment.

GENERAL PRINCIPLES: MECHANISMS AND DIAGNOSIS

Thoracic Injury

Thoracic injury is caused by localized or diffuse compression of the rib cage or sternum, either from a collision with other athletes in high-speed sports, such as in football or hockey, or from a collision with walls or perimeter fences of the facilities in which they compete. A haemothorax, pneumo-thorax or haemopneumothorax may develop as a result of chest wall trauma with or without fractures. Anterior or parasternal insults may damage the myocardium, although in contact sports the injury is usually mild. Cardiac arrhythmias, including ventricular fibrillation, have been reported following direct blows over the precordium by a ball travelling at 'high speed', especially in sports like baseball and

cricket. These arrhythmias are more common when myocardial susceptibility is increased, such as in viraemia, or following myocarditis or chemotherapy. Myocardial injury and aortic rupture may occur in motor sports and ski racing, where high-speed deceleration is the major contributing factor.

ASSESSMENT OF THORACIC INJURY

- Pain is the principal factor in all thoracic injuries involving the diaphragm and shoulder tip pain is a feature
- Dyspnoea may be secondary to pain or may be due to decreased lung capacity from compression by air or blood

Rapid assessment (i.e. on the playing field) should determine airways patency, chest wall stability and air entry into the lungs. The cardiovascular status, position of the trachea and apex beat, together with air entry and respiratory rate may indicate the presence of a tension pneumothorax, which is a medical emergency.

Assessment of the cardiovascular status is important when myocardial injuries are suspected. A high jugular venous pressure in the presence of hypotension in a fit young athlete may indicate tamponade. Shock will intervene in any acute large blood loss injury, but in athletes indicates that severe decompensation has occurred, as a healthy cardiovascular system compensates well for mild to moderate blood loss.

The principal aim in the management of thoracic trauma is to re-establish normal ventilation and cardiovascular function. This ranges from analgesia in the case of fractured ribs, to the insertion of an endotracheal tube in persistent respiratory failure. Haemopericardium with cardiac tamponade will require a pericardial aspiration. Evacuation of blood and air from the pleural space is required in most cases of chest trauma with respiratory decompensation.

The history and mechanism of injury will help predict the severity and type of trauma. In injuries caused by high-speed collision, thoracic aortic rupture must be suspected even with a stable cardiovascular system. Treatment of thoracic injuries and the urgency of such treatment, will be determined by repeated physical examinations.

Abdominothoracic Injury

It is important to emphasize the anatomical relationships between these two areas. Injuries should be considered as thoracic, thoracoabdominal, abdominal and/or retroperitoneal. While 'chest' is taken as the area covered by the ribs, the abdomen projects up to the diaphragm at the surface level of the sixth intercostal space and important abdominal structures such as the spleen on the left and the liver on the right lie under the ribs (Fig. 18.1). Posteriorly, both kidneys are located close to the lower ribs, although part of their surface marking projects below the 12th rib into the relatively unprotected 'renal angle'. While the ribs offer protection for underlying structures, if fractured, they can cause trauma by lacerating liver, spleen, pleura or other viscus.

ASSESSMENT OF ABDOMINOTHORACIC INJURY

To reach a diagnosis, it is important to have a clear idea of the mechanism of the injury. At the point of impact was the athlete prepared, or was he or she off-balance, unable to take evasive action, and consequently liable to sustain a major injury? Severe injuries tend to occur in the latter situation, when the athlete is unprepared or unable to take evasive action or brace to absorb energy transfer, which occurs in an accident such as a collision.

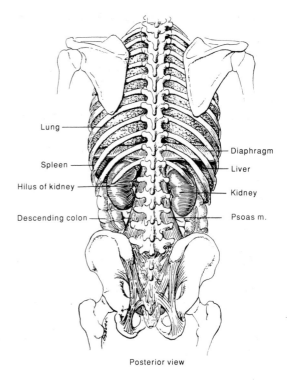

Posterior view

Fig. 18.1 The anatomy of the chest and abdomen (posterior view). Note that a significant portion of the abdomen is covered by the rib cage (from O'Donoghue 1976, with permission).

In addition, it is important to know the area of force transfer and what the athlete was doing in relation to it. A knee or elbow may transmit much more force per unit area than a hip or shoulder collision. The athlete impaled on a handle bar to the epigastrium may sustain deep retroperitoneal damage to the pancreas or the duodenum. A kidney may be avulsed by violent contact between the knee of an opponent and lumbar region of the patient, such as in high marking in Australian football or where a player drops with his/her knee into the kidney of another player in a rugby ruck.

- Pain is the most significant feature with abdominothoracic and abdominal injuries, while its changes with time are also important
- Peritonism with abdominal wall rigidity and lack of bowel sounds, indicates peritoneal irritation due to ruptured viscus or intraperitoneal blood

- Shock with acute blood loss denotes an emergency

The management of abdominothoracic and abdominal injuries rests with accurate early diagnosis and prompt definitive treatment. Preventing blood loss may require surgical intervention, while a perforated viscus definitely will. Hence, both must be treated in a specialty centre.

Haematuria may be the only indicator of renal trauma, but severe injuries may occur without its presence. Suspicion of renal trauma should be investigated radiologically.

CHEST INJURIES

Rib Fractures

Rib fractures are always painful, and relief of pain is the basis of their management. It is not advisable to strap or in any way restrict chest expansion, and analgesia must be adequate to allow full chest movement, thus preventing secondary atelectasis or infection.

Single fractures of multiple ribs may not interfere with ventilation if pain is adequately controlled. Multiple fractures of ribs occasionally produce a 'flail segment', which moves paradoxically (i.e. in when the chest expands) with respiration, sometimes significantly decreasing air entry on the injured side. The result is a gas/pressure mismatch as the non-aerated lung is perfused, causing hypoxia and/or possibly respiratory failure. In most cases pain will localize the site of the fracture(s) and this will allow detailed radiography of the area to confirm the diagnosis in the majority of cases. However, fractures of the costal cartilages or costochondral separations will not be visible on X-ray.

Once the diagnosis is made, the effect on ventilation should be assessed. In elderly athletes, or where there are multiple injuries and/or a flail segment, where gas exchange is reduced despite adequate analgesia, the question of respiratory support may arise. Most patients require analgesia alone. Pain usually settles after 2–3 days, but analgesia will be required for about a week. Intercostal nerve blocks with long-acting anaesthetic (1–2 mL Bupivacaine 0.5% per level) can provide excellent control; however, local anaesthetic at the fracture site is risky and is not advised. Fractured ribs need time to heal, and avoiding contact sports for 4–6 weeks or sometimes more is recommended. A player who returns 2 weeks early for example and reinjures his or her ribs will be out of sport for much longer than the one who waits until complete recovery has been attained (Dronen 1983).

Fractured Sternum

Sternal fractures occasionally occur from a direct anterior blow of considerable force. Local pain is the usual feature, and a palpable step may be felt if the swelling around the area allows it. Generally, sternal fractures cause little problem, because they do not interfere with ventilation and pain control is easily achieved. Their significance lies in the other potentially serious injuries that occur as a result of a heavy blow, which will affect the deeper structures such as the myocardium or the great vessels (Snow et al. 1982).

Pneumothorax

Pneumothorax is the presence of air in the pleural space. It may be 'spontaneous' (including after trauma), or, more commonly, secondary to rib trauma, with underlying damage to the lung parenchyma. The air which leaks from the lungs results in a progressive reduction in lung volume, as the lung then fails to fully expand during inspiration.

If a large leak develops in the lung, a 'trapdoor' mechanism may result in a rapid increase in pressure, which leads to mediastinal distortion and pressure on the atrial walls with decreased cardiac filling (and consequently decreased ventricular output). This change in cardiovascular dynamics is in addition to the profound effects on ventilation, and is called a tension pneumothorax (Fig. 18.2), an acute emergency requiring immediate release. The trachea, which is located on the mid-line in the sternal notch, will be forced away from the affected side. Release is accomplished by inserting a 12- or 14-gauge needle into the pleural space through the lower half of the fourth or fifth intercostal space around the mid-axillary line of the affected hemi-

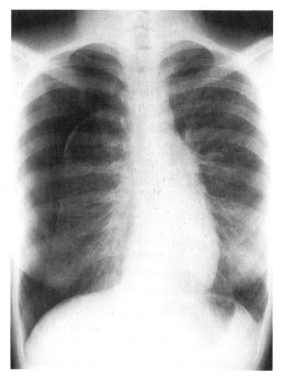

Fig. 18.2 A chest X-ray of a tension pneumothorax.

thorax, and a rush of air indicates that the problem has been converted to a simple pneumothorax.

In most cases, however, the pneumothorax is more subtle and increases slowly. This should be suspected in all cases of fractured ribs, and X-rays should be used to exclude the diagnosis where it is suspected. A single negative X-ray does not preclude later deterioration, so repeated X-rays in the case of deterioration and close monitoring in the early post-injury phase is mandatory. Clinical presentation varies from very few mild symptoms to respiratory failure and circulatory collapse.

TREATMENT

Treatment of pneumothorax involves insertion of an intercostal tube (via thoracostomy), which is then connected to underwater sealed drainage or low pressure suction. The tube is best inserted in the sixth intercostal space in the mid-axillary line, which appears quite high when marked on the surface; however, this site gives the most direct access to the pleural space and will drain air and fluid equally well. It also protects against the potential for damage to mediastinal structures when placed too far medially.

The technique of thoracostomy is performed under local anaesthetic which is infiltrated down to the level of the pleura using a 23-gauge needle, passing around the neurovascular bundle in the superior part of the intercostal space as it relates to the inferior rib edge. A skin incision is made and extended through the intercostal muscles and blunt forceps are then passed into the thoracic cavity. A finger should then be passed down the track into the pleural space. The intercostal tube is introduced only when the operator is confident that the space has been entered and is connected to underwater sealed drainage, and secured to the chest wall with sutures. While penetrating the chest wall with an intercostal tube and trocar without dissection seems simple and rapid, it frequently results in the catheter being inserted into the lung itself.

A tension pneumothorax requires initial release by the insertion of a needle, followed by intercostal catheterization in a more leisurely manner. Small pneumothoraces may be treated expectantly with frequent observations and regular X-rays. In some cases aspiration alone may be used, but requires careful monitoring and X-ray review. Pneumothoraces of all types should probably be catheterized before operation due to ventilation risks (Hughes 1965).

Haemothorax

Blood accumulates in the pleural space after trauma. Most commonly this is chest wall bleeding, but may also be visceral. When associated with a pneumothorax, a haemopneumothorax should be drained by the insertion of an intercostal tube as previously detailed. The best treatment of pure haemothorax is early and complete drainage, either by aspiration or tube drainage depending on the volume. Drainage tubes should always remain on low pressure suction, keeping blood out of the pleural space and the lung expanded to achieve haemostasis (even if ventilated). Ongoing losses in the drainage bottle can be measured and if substantial may warrant open thoracotomy.

Pulmonary Contusion

The importance of pulmonary contusion lies in the significant trauma required to produce it, and associated injuries should be sought. Its own clinical significance varies with the extent of the contusion. The patients are usually hospitalized because of associated injuries, and the area of contusion often seems to expand while under observation. The need for ventilatory support will depend on the size of the contusion, other thoracic injuries and their effect on the patient's respiratory function. There is no active treatment for pulmonary contusion, and time must be allowed for complete recovery.

Cardiac Trauma

Direct blows to the heart can cause various arrhythmias including ventricular fibrillation. For example, this can occur when a ball or other object strikes the precordium, and if not recognized quickly the player may die. Pre-existing viraemia or previous cardiac pathology, perhaps associated with chemotherapy, makes the myocardium more susceptible. Before instituting cardiopulmonary resuscitation, a repeat of the blow, this time with a fist, can reverse the fibrillation (Christensen & Sutton 1993).

Myocardial contusion and subsequent myocarditis may also occur and is usually associated with high-speed collisions where the heart slams against the sternum. A sternal fracture may occur, but is not a prerequisite and an electrocardiogram is mandatory when such trauma is suspected (Hood 1983).

Myocardial laceration may occur in association with rib fractures. This rare event results in cardiac tamponade, recognized by circulatory decompensation in the presence of raised jugular venous pressure and muffled heart sounds in a patient with a history of pericardial trauma. Decompression of the pericardium is urgent, and can be performed with a 14-gauge needle inserted through the left fourth intercostal space parasternally. This may be sufficient to reverse the situation; however, surgical decompression of the pericardium is required if tamponade persists or recurs, or if the laceration requires direct attention.

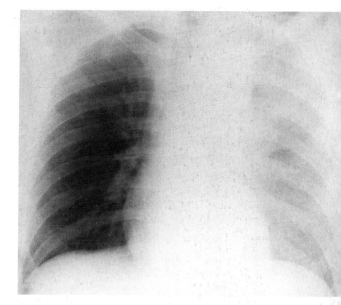

Fig. 18.3 A chest X-ray of a ruptured aorta. Note the wide mediastinum, blood over the left lung apex, loss of the aortic knuckle, depressed left main bronchus and tracheal displacement.

Rupture of the Thoracic Aorta

This is a deceleration injury where a shearing force causes rupture of the intima and media of the thoracic aorta at the junction of the arch and descending aorta in the region of the pulmonary ligament. The forces required are great and do not occur in most contact sports. However, they are seen in motor sport accidents and occasionally in downhill skiing (on colliding with a tree).

Clinical diagnosis is not simple, but should be suspected in all front-on high-speed deceleration injuries. The patient at first may appear clinically stable and have few signs of a serious injury; however, associated injuries such as fractures of the first and second ribs indicate that a major force transfer has occurred and may lead to further complications.

Loss or expansion of the aortic shadow on the left side of the mediastinum on chest X-ray or the so-called 'double shadow' which can be seen in relation to the aorta, as well as apical 'capping' (haemothorax) can provide radiological clues (Fig. 18.3), and should lead to arteriography or contrast scanning to confirm the diagnosis. Surgical repair is urgent and lifesaving (Mattox & O'Gorman 1988).

Rupture of the Diaphragm

Diaphragmatic rupture results from compression injuries of the chest or more commonly the abdomen, with a resulting diaphragmatic tear. High-energy forces are generally involved and associated injuries may be significant (Meyers & McCabe 1993). This, however, is not inevitable, as the rupture of the diaphragm significantly disperses the forces involved. The diagnosis may be difficult, especially on the right side where the liver may 'plug' the rupture. On the left side small ruptures are difficult to identify and it is often not until herniation of abdominal contents into the chest occurs that such a diagnosis is considered.

If the patient exhibits an irregular contour of the diaphragm in the chest X-ray, then a diaphragmatic rupture must be considered, especially if the injury involved considerable impact, such as, equipment falling on to an athlete. If herniation of the abdominal contents has occurred, the diagnosis is simple, if not, screening of the diaphragm, computerized tomography (CT) scans and serial X-rays should be done. Thoracoscopy and even laparotomy may be required to confirm or refute the diagnosis. If the injury is not diagnosed in the early stages, these patients may present many years later with complications (Aronoff et al. 1982).

The diaphragmatic rupture characteristically occurs at the junction of the central tendon and the diaphragmatic muscle and its repair by simple suture is effective in solving the problem.

ABDOMINAL INJURIES

Abdominal injuries are relatively uncommon in contact sports and this may at first seem surprising, but in most instances the athlete anticipates the contact and takes evasive action to minimize its effects or 'sets' his or her body to absorb the impact. In most instances, therefore, injuries to the abdominal region occur when the athlete is unable to react to the impending collision. There are two exceptions, which are as follows:

- The first is when there is a pre-existing condition making the organs more vulnerable, such as the spleen in infectious mononucleosis (glandular fever)
- The second is when a force is applied over a limited area, such as a knee sinking into the abdomen to rupture the liver or gall-bladder, or into the loin to avulse or contuse the kidney

Assessing abdominal injuries requires a clear picture of the circumstances leading to the injury in order to identify the passive injuries that are associated with significant damage. Pain is almost always associated with sporting abdominal injuries, and this assists in an accurate diagnosis. Further, it is also helpful to know when the last meal was ingested, as a full stomach is more susceptible to rupture. This also applies to urinary bladder injuries, and should be considered in pre-competition preparation by coaches.

Ruptured Spleen

Splenic rupture often occurs in association with left lower rib fractures or other thoracic trauma. With diseases such as infectious mononucleosis, direct anterior trauma may rupture the enlarged spleen, but the normal spleen is generally protected from anterior assault.

The potential for splenic rupture should always be considered in cases of left-sided thoracoabdominal trauma. Abdominal pain is always present, although it is often localized and can be surprisingly mild. Peritonism is not a prerequisite, and hypotension may be present, but not always in fit young athletes who may underestimate or down-play their complaint or discomfort.

Once a ruptured spleen is suspected, immediate investigations should be instituted to support or refute the diagnosis. The two most useful mediums are the CT scan of the upper abdomen (Fig. 18.4), or the technetium ^{99}m spleen scan. If the findings of the investigation are positive this does not mean automatic splenectomy, but if a conservative approach of splenic preservation is decided upon, then it will mean a period of hospitalization of up to 2–3 weeks and a further 6 weeks absence from

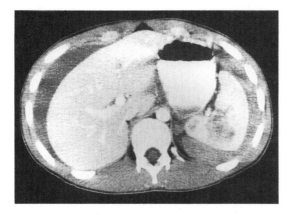

Fig. 18.4 A CT scan of a ruptured spleen.

contact sport. During this time resolution of the damage can be followed by serial scans (Kohn *et al.* 1994).

If a patient has left upper quadrant tenderness associated with hypotension, especially postural hypotension, then a diagnosis of a ruptured spleen is most likely. Profound shock must, of course, lead to an immediate laparotomy. If laparotomy is performed, the initial aim should be of splenic preservation if possible and this may require partial splenectomy or repair of capsular lacerations (Moore *et al.* 1984).

If the spleen is totally removed there is a slight but increased risk of post-splenectomy sepsis, which may be life threatening. As a consequence the patient should be given pneumococcal vaccine and should be told to seek immediate medical advice in all cases of systemic infection.

Ruptured Liver

Injury to the liver occurs usually in association with right lower rib fractures, although anterior contact may also cause damage. While rupture is uncommon, the formation of a haematoma may occur more frequently than anticipated.

Rupture is usually dramatic, often occurring in association with significant right lower chest injuries, abdominal pain and haemodynamic instability. Bruising, which is often described as a subcapsular haematoma, is not generally so dramatic. Such haematomas are always associated with deep liver

injury and the capsule can rupture at a later date, therefore requiring early diagnosis (Ochsner *et al.* 1993).

When a question of liver injury exists, a CT scan will usually resolve the dilemma (Fig. 18.5). If a rupture has occurred, early surgical intervention is then required. The presence of a subcapsular haematoma or intrahepatic haematoma should be followed by serial scanning. The athlete should be prevented from participation in all sports until resolution is confirmed (Pachter *et al.* 1990).

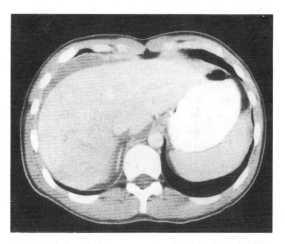

Fig. 18.5 A CT scan of a ruptured liver with a subcapsular haematoma.

Pancreatic Injury

Pancreatic injury is uncommon because of the organ's relatively protected position. The most common injury is that of transection occurring where the pancreas crosses the vertebrae, resulting from either a blunt injury by a narrow object such as a bicycle handlebar, or distraction injury over a fulcrum which sometimes occurs with non-harness seat-belts. In these situations pain is dramatic, and the circumstances of the injury make diagnosis relatively easy. Early laparotomy is necessary and a distal pancreatic resection required. The results of early surgery are usually excellent.

Injury to the head of the pancreas is often more difficult to diagnose and repair. The diagnosis is best made by CT scan or ultrasound and treatment is by surgical decompression, resection and/or diversion. Again, it often results from a blunt trauma with a narrow object and is restricted to sports which use such equipment as in gymnastics and equestrian sports. In other sports, such athletes as downhill skiers, racing car drivers and cyclists, who not only use equipment but also compete in dangerous surroundings are at risk if a collision occurs and run the definite risk of sustaining such injuries. In this context the injury is frequently associated with duodenal injury.

Gall-bladder Injuries

These injuries are rare, and include rupture and bruising with late bile leakage. They have been seen in various codes of football and are the result of a direct blunt trauma, and require laparotomy and cholecystectomy. The differential diagnosis is that of a duodenal injury.

Duodenal Injury (Asensio *et al.* 1993)

This injury occurs as a result of an anterior trauma with a significant force transmitted over a small area, in the unprepared athlete. Again, as in other localized injuries, a knee or fist in contact football or equipment in other fast moving agility sports or even a handlebar in cycling are the causes of such problems. The result is either haematoma or rupture of the duodenum.

A duodenal haematoma results in obstruction in many cases, and is slow to resolve with conservative management. It may require laparotomy for differentiation from a duodenal rupture. Such a rupture is either intraperitoneal, or more commonly extraperitoneal. Intraperitoneal (anterior) rupture is obvious in that the associated peritonitis leaves no doubt that a major intraperitoneal catastrophe has occurred and surgery is necessary. More sinister is the retroperitoneal (posterior) duodenal rupture, where pain is present and significant, but signs of intraperitoneal rupture are absent. It is, however, interesting that a posterior perforation may irritate the sympathetic supply of the testis, giving rise to right testicular pain as an associated referred symptom. If this injury is not diagnosed early, and there

is a delay before surgery, the mortality rate is high (Corley *et al.* 1975).

If a duodenal rupture is suspected, an early 'gastrograffin meal' should be administered, looking for extravasation of contrast into the peritoneal cavity or retroduodenal tissues. If there is still a question of the presence of duodenal rupture then a CT scan should precede laparotomy, providing this can be arranged urgently.

Small Intestine and Colon Injuries

It is very unusual to injure the bowel in contact sports, although perforation can sometimes occur. Knowledge of the mechanism and site of impact are important clues to the diagnosis. Direct blunt anterior trauma in high-speed sports is the most likely cause, such as in downhill snow sports, cycling and motor sports.

Colonic perforation is associated with much free gas in the peritoneal cavity, whereas small bowel injury is not. Indeed, in the latter there may be no gas present outside the bowel. In both injuries, the signs remain localized for some 4–6 h and bowel sounds may initially be present. With time these fade as peritoneal irritation increases. Peritoneal irritation is usually greatest with colonic perforation and may be surprisingly mild with small bowel perforation. Observation in cases of abdominal trauma where perforation may have occurred is necessary unless signs are dramatic. If pain does not subside and the likelihood of perforation is present, then a laparotomy is necessary.

Mesenteric haematoma is uncommon as an isolated sporting injury. It is rarely clinically significant, although it can present as a cause of delayed obstruction of the small intestine due to the development of an ischaemic segment. Presentation varies from 7 days to several months after injury, when secondary stricture may have occurred.

Rectal Injury

Rectal injury occurs either when an athlete is impaled on a pointed object or when fluid is forced into the rectum causing acute distension, such as in water-skiing accidents.

In the case of rectal impalement, the fact that the injury has occurred is obvious but its extent is difficult to estimate. All such patients require assessment for intraperitoneal rupture, then a careful examination under anaesthetic to assess the extent of the injury to the rectum, anal canal or anal sphincters. If the anal sphincters are damaged, immediate repair is essential. If rectal lacerations have occurred this can usually be managed with adequate antibiotic cover, initially in hospital. Intraperitoneal rupture will require laparotomy and faecal diversion (stoma).

High-speed water-skiing falls can lead to colonic perforation by water insufflation under pressure. This usually damages the rectosigmoid junction rather than the rectum. Signs of peritoneal rupture are obvious and dramatic, and early surgery is indicated. No attempt at initial repair of the rupture should be undertaken but faecal diversion via colostomy should be instituted.

URINARY TRACT INJURIES

Renal Injury

Injuries to the kidney result from posterior blows in the renal angle, which lies inferior to the 12th rib, lateral to the erector spinae, and superior to the posterior iliac crest. These are common in contact sports, including Australian football, rugby union, soccer and basketball where players are often jumping or pushing in packs with poor landing control. The force is significant and the result dramatic.

The kidney may be avulsed from its vascular pedicle, ruptured or contused. In avulsion there is usually no haematuria as the kidney remains intact, whereas in a rupture or with a contusion, haematuria is present, and its degree may indicate the extent of the renal trauma. All renal injuries must be investigated thoroughly with an intravenous pyelogram (IVP), which is the first investigation to be carried out (Fig. 18.6) and followed where necessary by an arteriogram or a CT scan if available (McAndrew & Corriere 1994).

Renal avulsion requires early surgery and usually a nephrectomy, because a warm ischaemic time of

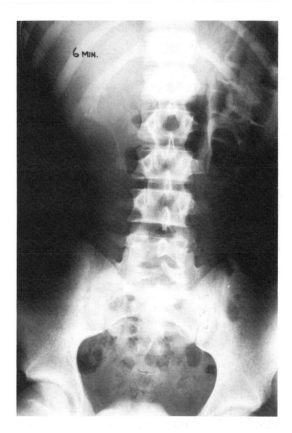

Fig. 18.6 An intravenous pyelogram (IVP) of a ruptured right kidney. Note the delayed appearance and filling of the upper renal pelvis only (indicating lower pole rupture).

12 h or more, generally precludes salvage. Rupture of the kidney in most cases is managed expectantly, and it is only when the perinephric tamponade is lost that early surgery is indicated because of hypovolaemia. In all other circumstances time should be allowed to fully define the problem with a view to partial or complete renal salvage. Early nephrectomy for a ruptured kidney is rarely indicated, but observation and complete investigation is essential so that an accurate picture of the damage can be obtained, and precise surgery undertaken if indicated (Cass 1982).

Problems can occur at a later time following renal injury, with resistant hypertension secondary to the renal hormonal balance upset. Athletes should be regularly followed up with blood pressure checks.

Bladder Injury

It is only the full bladder that is injured in contact sports. The result of compression of the full bladder is rupture which may be intraperitoneal or extra-peritoneal. Pain is dramatic and the diagnosis is suggested by the circumstances of the injury and the site of impact. Investigation is by performing a cystogram which fully distends the bladder, but two additional features should be observed. The first is the appearance of a nephrogram during the cystogram, suggesting that contrast has escaped into the peritoneal cavity, been reabsorbed and excreted by the kidney. The second is that at the completion of the cystogram the bladder should be completely emptied, and a further X-ray taken, looking for the 'shadow' of the bladder, which is due to extravasation into the pericystic tissues.

Intraperitoneal rupture requires laparotomy and repair. Extraperitoneal rupture can be managed by bladder drainage alone in the majority of cases. However, the site and size of the defect must be considered when making a decision on conservative management.

Urethral Injuries

Trauma to the male urethra usually occurs by the athlete falling astride some object, such as a cycle bar, or alternatively he may be kicked in the lower groin. This lesion should be suspected by the athlete's inability to void or by the appearance of blood at the urinary meatus. Full and early investigation of this injury is mandatory. If the athlete is able to pass urine, the urgency is reduced but in all other situations an early urethrogram should be performed. No attempt to pass a catheter should be made until a diagnosis is reached, to avoid the risk of creating a false urethral passage.

Testicular Injuries

Injuries to the testes are common and obvious. The most dramatic result of testicular injury is a haematoma, which is both large and painful. It is important to investigate the injury by ultrasound to determine whether the problem is a large haematoma of a normal testis or the first presentation of a testicular tumour.

ABDOMINAL WALL INJURIES

Hernia

Sudden increase in abdominal pressure occurs in all sporting activities but is perhaps more common in power lifting and weight training. Acute pain with and without swelling occurs in the common sites: epigastric, umbilical, inguinal or femoral. A persistent painful lump is most commonly associated with an acute epigastric or para-umbilical hernia. In these cases fat or omentum is obstructed in the hernial sac, with or without infarction. It is less common for an acute inguinal hernia to remain obstructed. In the case of an acute indirect inguinal hernia, it may be difficult to reproduce it clinically as the athlete presents only with acute pain localized to the deep inguinal ring.

Ruptures can occur elsewhere in the inguinal canal. Its medial aspect which is formed by the conjoint tendon can be associated with a rupture or tear which precipitates localized pain at the medial end of the inguinal canal above the pubic tubercle. This injury classically occurs in the complex resisted motion of kicking, as in Australian football. The pain, while initially localized can become more diffuse as the ilio-inguinal nerve becomes involved, giving referred pain down the medial aspect of the thigh and scrotum.

In the case of the acute injury involving the deep inguinal ring when no hernia is obvious, a conservative approach should be taken and this means complete rest for a period of up to 6 weeks. If the injury has not resolved itself by then, surgical exploration should be undertaken.

The situation regarding the conjoint tendon injury is more controversial. In the first instance a prolonged period of controlled rest for 6 weeks should be undertaken and a graduated retraining programme under supervision should follow. Failure of conservative treatment is an indication to explore the medial attachment of the conjoint tendon, repairing any tear and excising chronic inflammatory tissue. Again, prolonged postoperative rest and retraining is required. Conjoint tendon injuries are discussed in detail in Chapter 20.

When an irreducible hernia is present it should be repaired. In the case of epigastric, umbilical and femoral herniae good results can be anticipated. The femoral hernia is the most urgent, as the anatomy of the femoral canal has the potential for strangulation, particularly if the bowel is contained in the hernial sac. In many cases the patient presents 24 h later, by which time it is obvious whether or not the small bowel is involved.

Groin Pain

The term 'groin pain' is an extremely broad clinical description. Injuries to this area should be divided into those above the inguinal ligament, those below it and those involving the symphysis pubis (Fig. 18.7). Injuries below the inguinal ligament involve either the adductor muscles, iliopsoas (rare) or muscles around the femoral triangle. Those above the inguinal ligament will usually involve it in some way. This will either be in the form of a medial rupture of the conjoint tendon, a direct inguinal hernia or an acute indirect inguinal hernia. The differential diagnosis is to distinguish osteitis pubis from a muscular or ligamentous injury. In the former a bone scan is useful and X-rays of the symphysis using alternate leg weight-bearing views for instability are essential. However, instability may be coincidental and asymptomatic. Osteitis pubis is discussed in detail in Chapter 20. In injuries below the inguinal ligament it is important to place stress on the muscle involved to localize, accurately, the site of injury. Injuries to the adductor muscles are usually a result of flexion and internal rotation of the hip moving forcefully and suddenly, such as in sprinting or kicking a football. The site of the pain is well localized over the adductor muscles and the treatment of adductor muscle injuries is outlined in Chapter 20.

Postoperative rehabilitation is an essential part of the programme and should be rigidly controlled, as many athletes apply the illogical principle of 'no pain, no gain' to their rehabilitation. It is of no value repairing the injury only to have the athlete set out on a 9 km run to 'test things out' after 3 weeks.

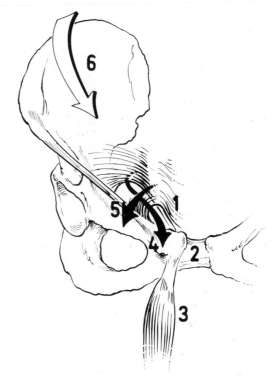

Fig. 18.7 The structures affected in groin pain. (1) Conjoint tendon tear. (2) Osteitis pubis. (3) Adductor longus strain/tear. (4) Indirect inguinal hernia. (5) Direct inguinal hernia. (6) Referred pain (back, kidney, etc.).

Rehabilitation for any abdominal wall repair must be supervised strictly. Swimming should be encouraged early and non-weight-bearing deep water running should follow. Without sensible supervision the athlete may overstrain himself and undo the good which has been done by the surgery.

Hip 'Pointer'

This injury is a haematoma trapped between the layers of the abdominal musculature at their insertion to the iliac crest (Fig. 18.8). The commonest cause is a direct blow, such as kick with a boot in contact sports. The pain may be excruciating, and may even require narcotic analgesia. Aspiration may relieve the pressure, but is technically difficult and risky. The outlook is good, but requires 2–3 weeks rehabilitation before the athlete is able to run and twist without discomfort.

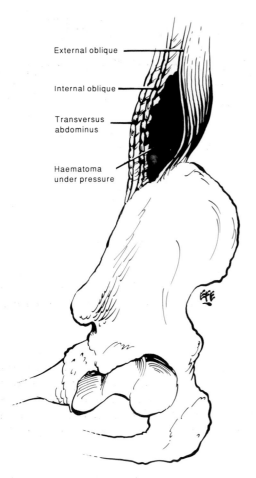

External oblique

Internal oblique

Transversus abdominus

Haematoma under pressure

Fig. 18.8 The anatomy of the hip 'pointer'.

CONCLUSIONS

It is important to recognize that many of the preceding injuries should be managed very carefully and with a high degree of suspicion. In the current professional sporting climate athletes may try to mask various signs and/or symptoms of injuries to enable them to participate as much as possible. Not only should this be discouraged, but appropriate specialist care must be sought when there is any doubt about the diagnosis or the prognosis.

REFERENCES

Aronoff R. J., Reynolds J. & Thal E. R. (1982) Evaluation of diaphragmatic injuries. *American Journal of Surgery* **144**, 671.

Asensio J. A., Feliciano D. V., Britt L. D. & Kerstein M. D. (1993) Management of duodenal injuries. *Current Problems in Surgery* **30**, 1021.

Cass A. S. (1982) Immediate radiologic and surgical management of renal injuries. *Journal of Trauma* **22**, 361.

Christensen M. A. & Sutton K. R. (1993) Myocardial contusion. New concepts in diagnosis and management. *American Journal of Critical Care* **2**, 28–34.

Corley R. D., Norcross W. J. & Shoemaker W. C. (1975) Traumatic injuries to the duodenum: A report of 98 patients. *Annals of Surgery* **181**, 92.

Dronen S. C. (1983) Disorders of the chest wall and diaphragm. *Emergency Medical Clinics: North America* **1**, 449.

Hood R. M. (1983) Trauma to the chest. In Sabiston D. C. & Spencer F. G. (eds) *Gibbon's Surgery of the Chest*, p. 299. W. B. Saunders, Philadelphia, PA.

Hughes R. K. (1965) Thoracic trauma. *Annals of Thoracic Surgery* **1**, 778.

Kohn J. S., Clark D. E., Isler R. J. & Pope C. F. (1994) Is computed tomographic grading of splenic injury useful in non-surgical management of blunt trauma. *Journal of Trauma* **36**, 386–389.

Mattox K. L. & O'Gorman R. B. (1988) Injury to the thoracic great vessels. In Mattox K. L., Moore E. E. & Feliciano D. V. (eds) *Trauma*, p. 385. Appleton and Lange, Norwalk, CT.

McAndrew J. D. & Corriere J. N. Jr. (1994) Radiographic evaluation of renal trauma: Evaluation of 1103 consecutive patients. *British Journal of Urology* **73**, 352–354.

Meyers B. F. & McCabe C. G. (1993) Traumatic diaphragmatic hernia. Occult marker of serious injury. *Annals of Surgery* **218**, 783–790.

Moore F. A., Moore E. E., Moore G. E. & Millikan J. S. (1984) Risk of splenic salvage following trauma. Analysis of 200 adults. *American Journal of Surgery* **148**, 800.

Ochsner M. G., Jaffin J. H., Golocovsky M. & Jones R. C. (1993) Major hepatic trauma. *Surgical Clinics of North America* **73**, 337–352.

O'Donoghue D. (1976) (ed.) *Treatment of Injuries to Athletes*, 3rd edn. W. B. Saunders, Philadelphia, PA.

Pachter H. L. & Spencer F. C., Hoffsetter F. R. *et al.* (1990) Experience with selective operative and non-operative treatment of splenic injury in 193 patients. *Annals of Surgery* **211**, 583–589.

Snow N. J., Richardson J. D. & Flint L. M. (1982) Myocardial contusion: Implications for patients with multiple traumatic injuries. *Surgery* **92**, 744.

CHAPTER 19

INJURIES TO THE SHOULDER GIRDLE AND UPPER LIMB

P. A. Fricker and G. Hoy

This chapter discusses the problems athletes face in their daily training and competition. It reviews soft tissue injuries in particular, but fractures, dislocations and subluxations are briefly discussed where the incidence of these injuries is high.

In sports where the shoulder girdle and upper limb are placed under extreme physical stress, it is important that the health professionals who assist the athlete ensure that this region of the body is strong and flexible. Shoulder joint hypermobility can be even more serious than hypomobility in sports with a moderate to high risk of dislocation (such as in wrestling and football).

Injuries to the shoulder girdle and upper limb have three major causes. They can result from external violence (a fractured clavicle), internal violence (an acute tear of the rotator cuff tendons or subluxation of the glenohumeral joint), or from overuse (as seen in the impingement syndrome producing a supraspinatus tendinitis).

The reader is referred to Chapter 13, which contains a detailed discussion of the rehabilitation of injury, as this complements the management of problems outlined below.

THE SHOULDER GIRDLE

The shoulder girdle comprises the scapula, clavicle and humerus. The glenohumeral joint allows extraordinary movement but relies heavily on muscular support, as well as on ligaments, for stability. By contrast, the clavicle relies on ligamentous support.

The Clavicle

Inherent in the actions of the arm is the need for a strut to stabilize the shoulder, and to prevent it from coming forward and across the chest. The clavicle performs this role and is attached to the sternum and first rib medially and to the acromion laterally.

FRACTURES OF THE CLAVICLE

Fractures are a common occurrence in contact sports such as the football codes and the martial arts, as well as in sports with a risk of falls from a height or at speed such as horse riding, motorcycling, cycling and snow skiing. The clavicle most often fractures across its middle third, resulting in a distal fragment which displaces inferiorly and anteriorly.

Clinical signs are obvious and an X-ray confirms the diagnosis. Treatment of an undisplaced fracture should utilize a sling to support the weight of the arm at the shoulder for 3 weeks. For the more serious fracture with displacement, a figure-of-eight bandage around the shoulders and axillae may be applied for 3–4 weeks.

Fractures of the outer third of the clavicle are less common and generally respond well to a supportive sling for 2–3 weeks, unless associated

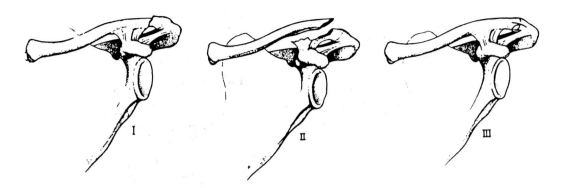

Fig. 19.1 Fractures of the distal clavicle. Type I, non-displaced, ligaments intact. Type II, displaced, separation of the coracoclavicular ligaments from the proximal fragment, unstable. Type III, fracture through the articular surface, may predispose to arthritis.

instability renders the strut incompetent (Fig. 19.1). Type 2 lesions require reduction and fixation and Type 3 injuries require fixation or excision of the joint.

CLAVICULAR LIGAMENT INJURIES

Sternoclavicular joint sprain

A force thrusting the shoulder forward as in a rugby tackle or a fall in judo produces this injury by driving the medial end of the clavicle medially and upwards. The clavicle may be anteriorly subluxed and treatment may be attempted by traction on the shoulder posteriorly with direct manipulation of the clavicle. Recovery over the next few weeks is aided by a sling for the shoulder (for the first 5–10 days in most cases), anti-inflammatory medication, ice and physiotherapy. If the costoclavicular ligament is torn, the medial end of the clavicle may remain subluxed. This is common but rarely requires surgical fixation. Although rare, posterior dislocations of the clavicle can occur at the sternoclavicular joint and can cause vascular and respiratory compromise (Hunter & Fricker 1992).

In all cases, X-ray tomography or computerized tomography (CT) of the sternoclavicular joint is vital to evaluate the degree of subluxation and to exclude a fracture. If a fracture occurs it may require fixation surgically (O'Donoghue 1976).

Acromioclavicular ligament sprain

The acromioclavicular joint has little mobility and relies on ligaments for stability (Fig. 19.2). A blow or force which moves the acromion down and/or away from the clavicle produces ligament injury. Similarly, a fall on to the outstretched arm may move the acromion up and produce ligament damage. This joint is commonly injured in football, cycling, judo and ice hockey.

A classification of acromioclavicular joint injuries has been proposed by Allman (1967) and revised by Rockwood and Green (1984). In a Type I injury, the joint is stable and X-rays are normal in the acute phase. There is pain and tenderness of the joint and localized soft tissue swelling may occur with some limitation of abduction of the shoulder joint because of pain. Type II injuries involve tearing of the acromioclavicular ligament and capsule, with the coracoclavicular ligament stretched but intact (Fig. 19.3). On X-ray, elevation of the clavicle is noted to be less than the width of the clavicle. It is important to remember that there may be only posterior displacement of the clavicle (because the coracoclavicular ligaments are intact) and an antero-posterior standing X-ray of both shoulders should be taken for comparison. Stress views are recommended and are carried out with weights attached to the patient's wrists. A Type III injury is the same as a Type II with the addition of a torn coracoclavicular ligament. An X-ray examination demonstrates an elevation of the clavicle above the superior surface of the acromion.

In Type II and III injuries a deformity of the joint is evident with associated soft tissue swelling, pain and tenderness. Shoulder movement is painful and limited.

Type IV injuries have posterior displacement through the trapezius and require stabilization.

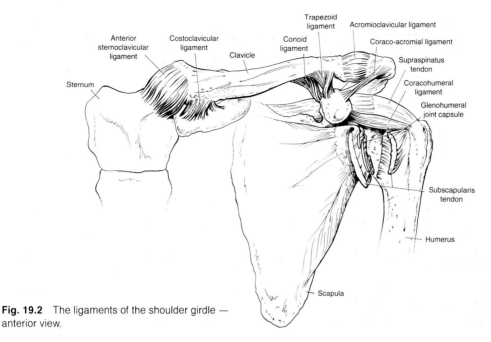

Fig. 19.2 The ligaments of the shoulder girdle — anterior view.

Type V (the 'ear-tickler') injuries have lost the deep fascial sling and also require surgical stabilization. Type VI injuries (subcoracoid dislocations) are rare.

Treatment of Type I injuries is usually carried out by the use of a supportive sling for 7–10 days, and by anti-inflammatory medication, electrotherapy modalities and early active exercises for the shoulder region.

Type II injuries generally respond to similar care. A sling may be worn for 10–14 days, and the shoulder rested from sport for 3–6 weeks. Treatment as outlined previously is followed with par-

ticular attention to the recovery of shoulder strength, flexibility and power prior to return to sport.

The treatment of Type III injuries is open to some debate. The conservative method of management is by the use of a sling for 6 weeks, complemented by anti-inflammatory medication and electrotherapy modalities, followed by a graded strengthening exercise programme and protection of the shoulder for 3–4 months. Some orthopaedic surgeons advise surgical reconstruction.

Surgery is otherwise reserved for those patients who have not had a satisfactory resolution of the

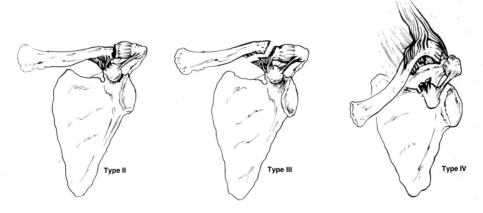

Fig. 19.3 The three most common types of A-C joint disruption seen in clinical practice (Rockwood classification).

signs and symptoms after a period of 6 months. There are many surgical techniques available and these are beyond the scope of this chapter; however, surgery aims to stabilize the distal end of the clavicle.

Osteolysis of the clavicle

This condition is one of uncertain aetiology and affects the lateral (distal) end of the clavicle only. Cahill (1982) reported osteolysis of the distal clavicle in 46 male athletes, none of whom had suffered acute injury to the affected acromioclavicular joint, and all but one were either competitive weight-lifters or indulged in weight training. The diagnosis of osteolysis is made on the findings of local pain and tenderness, together with radiographic evidence of osteoporosis, loss of subchondral bone detail and cystic changes at the lateral end of the clavicle. The mechanism of osteolysis in athletes appears to involve relatively minor repetitive trauma (such as bench pressing weights) to the acromioclavicular joint in the majority of cases, but can result from occasional trauma sustained in activities such as judo or football, which involve falls or blows to the shoulder. Cahill (1982) proposes that the lesion results from microfracture of the subchondral bone with subsequent attempts at repair, while other work has implied that synovial mechanisms are involved. A comprehensive discussion on this is provided by Lyons and Rockwood (1994).

Treatment consists of either rest from aggravating activities, or surgery to excise the distal end of the clavicle. The conservative option can be tried with the support of electrotherapy modalities and non-steroidal anti-inflammatory drugs for symptomatic relief, but recovery is invariably slow. Surgery is indicated where the patient can no longer tolerate the condition (and its impact on training) and the results of surgical excision of the distal clavicle appear to be good (Cahill 1982).

Other chronic acromioclavicular joint lesions

Repeated trauma to the acromioclavicular joint is commonly seen in contact sports and produces thickening and swelling of the ligaments about the joint, often with some degree of joint mobility. There may also be calcification or ossification of the soft tissues.

If the fibrocartilage within the acromioclavicular joint is damaged, the joint may be very irritable and any movement of the arm at the shoulder joint can be painful. Treatment therefore depends upon the amount of functional disability. If necessary, a local injection of corticosteroid and physiotherapy modalities may be administered and if symptoms persist, surgery may be justified to excise the fibrocartilage and contiguous bone. It should be noted that ossification of ligaments such as the coracoclavicular ligament is not infrequent and a decision to treat this surgically must depend on symptoms.

Complications of recurrent acromioclavicular joint injuries include osteoarthritis of the joint with typical radiological features and the need for appropriate management.

The Scapula

The scapula bears many muscle attachments and sits as a mobile bone over the posterior portion of the chest. It is often involved in both acute and overuse injury as a key functional unit in the shoulder girdle. Fractures of the scapula are uncommon and stress fractures are rare. Both types of fracture are generally treated with rest, but occasionally a displaced fracture of the 'neck' of the

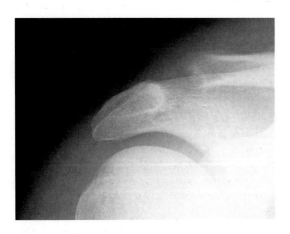

Fig. 19.4 Osteolysis of the distal clavicle. X-ray changes are of loss of subchondral bone and cystic changes (courtesy of I. Anderson).

scapula requires reduction, especially if the articular surface of the glenoid is disrupted.

ACUTE STRAIN OF SCAPULAR MUSCLES

Large powerful muscles with relatively small insertions are susceptible to acute strain and these are typically associated with throwing activities such as baseball pitching, javelin, discus and fast bowling in cricket. Muscles most frequently involved are those of the rotator cuff: the infraspinatus and the teres minor in particular.

Diagnosis is made on history and local signs and the treatment is orthodox, using the principles of rest, anti-inflammatory medication and physiotherapy for functional recovery and minimal scar tissue formation.

Occasionally, one of the major axillary muscles (pectoralis major or latissimus dorsi) can rupture at their insertions. Pectoralis major requires surgical repair, but latissimus dorsi ruptures heal without disability.

CHRONIC STRAIN OF THE SCAPULAR MUSCLES

Chronic strain of the muscles of the glenohumeral joint is considered later in this chapter; however, other scapular muscles may be injured through repetitive forceful movements. The teres minor and infraspinatus muscles are often injured in throwing activities, and the rhomboid muscles and levator scapulae may be injured by weight training. These settle quickly with appropriate anatomical and functional diagnosis and stretching and strengthening exercises, which address 'muscle balance' where appropriate and compensate for relative weakness. Anti-inflammatory measures can be used occasionally with corticosteroid injection being particularly useful.

BURSITIS

There are numerous bursae in the region of the scapula. Subacromial bursitis is discussed together with rotator cuff injuries later in this chapter; however, one should not forget that any bursa in this region may be involved where a muscle passes across a bone or other muscle.

One bursa which is often affected lies deep to the scapula at its inferomedial angle and overlies the muscles of the posterior chest wall. This may become inflamed through overuse, producing a local pain and tenderness elicited by compressing the scapula against the chest wall and by abducting the shoulder to 60° with 30° of flexion.

Bursitis generally responds well to anti-inflammatory medication, removal of any irritating factors and to physiotherapy modalities. Treatment by injection(s) of corticosteroid almost always produces relief.

Grating scapula is often the result of bursitis, but benign tumours must be excluded by X-ray or CT scan.

The Glenohumeral Joint

With respect to the practice of sports medicine, this section is discussed under the following headings:

- Joint subluxation and dislocation
- Superior labrum anteroposterior lesions
- Rotator cuff lesions
- The impingement syndrome and 'swimmer's shoulder'
- Tendinitis of the biceps

ANATOMY

The glenohumeral joint is essentially a ball and socket joint designed for extreme mobility at the expense of stability.

Patients with a relatively shallow glenoid fossa are generally believed to be at increased risk for instability and the glenoid labrum has a part in minimizing anteroposterior glenohumeral instability. The depth of the glenoid fossa is effectively doubled (from 2.5 to 5.0 mm) by the labrum, which is a fibrous structure intimately attached to the glenoid rim. It should be remembered that the biceps tendon attaches to the superior labrum and the inferior glenohumeral ligament attaches to the inferior labrum (Fig. 19.5). Also, the capsule of the shoulder joint attaches peripherally to the labrum.

The capsular ligaments are reinforced anteriorly by superior, medial and inferior glenohumeral ligaments, while the muscles of the rotator cuff —the supraspinatus, infraspinatus, teres minor and

Fig. 19.5 A schematic representation of the glenohumeral joint.

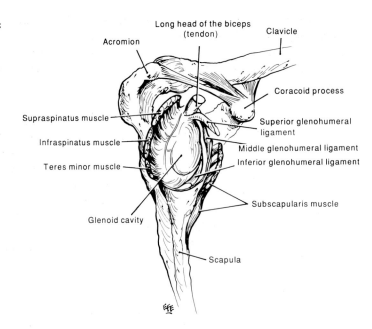

subscapularis — provide support to the joint superiorly, posteriorly and anteriorly via their common insertion about the head of the humerus (Fig. 19.5).

The rotator cuff also supports the head of the humerus against the glenoid cavity, while the deltoid and other muscles act above the shoulder. Without this support the humerus would sublux downwards with abduction of the arm.

GLENOHUMERAL DISLOCATION

Antero-inferior joint dislocation

This dislocation is the most common of these injuries (Fig. 19.6). It results from a force which pushes the arm into abduction and external rotation and is seen in contact sports such as football, wrestling and judo and in sports with a risk of falling such as skiing. The head of the humerus slips over the glenoid labrum and rests between the glenoid rim and the coracoid process. The arm then rests downwards and alongside, but not against, the chest wall, and the ruptured glenohumeral ligaments may in fact tuck in around the head of the humerus, preventing reduction. The risk of an associated fracture increases with age if the ligaments

are stronger than the bone, and a tear to the rotator cuff may also occur.

The diagnosis is made on the history of the injury and the typical appearance of a prominent

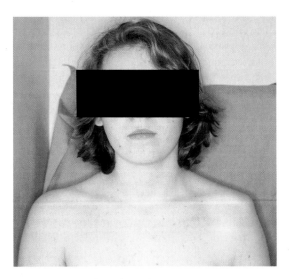

Fig. 19.6 The clinical appearance of the most common type of glenohumeral dislocation — anterior dislocation. (Williams 1980; with permission.)

acromion, a 'hollow' under the acromion and the 'dropped' arm being supported in slight external rotation. One must also assess the joint for neurological damage as a result of a brachial plexus lesion and exclude an associated fracture (as well as assess the dislocation) by means of an X-ray.

Treatment should be undertaken as soon as practicable and the following steps should be adhered to:

- Muscle relaxation (either with ice or by appropriate intravenous medication)
- Reduction of the dislocation by the Hippocratic method; by traction with the patient lying prone and the arm hanging down in a forward flexed position; or by the Kocher manoeuvre. Reduction must only be done by a suitably qualified person, such as an orthopaedic surgeon or specially trained medical practitioner. It is important to X-ray the joint after reduction and if there is any fracture an orthopaedic opinion must be sought
- Immobilization in a sling (to minimize abduction and external rotation) for 3 weeks
- Mobilization and rehabilitation thereafter as discussed below, should be undertaken as rapidly as can be tolerated by the patient

Arthroscopy in the management of initial dislocations is discussed later in this chapter.

Posterior dislocation

Posterior dislocation is infrequent and results from a severe blow to the front of the shoulder, an internal rotation and forced adduction injury as in wrestling, or a fall on the outstretched upper limb. No obvious deformity of the shoulder is seen as a rule; however, careful examination may show that the head of the humerus is in a posterior position and that the shoulder is very irritable and swollen. X-ray examination reveals overlapping of the head of the humerus and the glenoid in the antero-posterior view. However, special views such as the axillary view, are recommended for better diagnosis.

Treatment is by following the principles outlined for antero-inferior dislocation, except that the joint is restored by applying traction forward with simul-taneous forward pressure on the head of the humerus.

Fracture of the posterior glenoid is common with this injury and necessitates surgical management.

Inferior dislocation

Inferior dislocation results from a forced abduction of the arm which occurs in sports such as judo and wrestling. The head of the humerus slips down over the glenoid rim and then slides anteriorly to sit under the coracoid process. As a result it may be difficult to distinguish it from an antero-inferior dislocation. With a more severe injury the abducted arm may end in a position of full elevation — the arm held high above the shoulder. This injury is known as luxatio erecta and implies extensive rupture of the rotator cuff and capsule and the possibility of neurological damage.

Treatment of the more simple inferior dislocation is according to the principles of reduction outlined previously, with straight downward traction being used. Luxatio erecta demands surgical treatment to repair ligamentous and muscle structures and any possible fracture.

Rehabilitation

Rehabilitation of acute glenohumeral dislocations, after initial management as previously outlined, depends on strengthening the rotator cuff, deltoid and biceps musculature over a period of weeks and sometimes months, with comparisons being made against the opposite (non-injured) shoulder as a reference for strength and range of movement. Anterior dislocation, in particular, requires emphasis on adduction and internal rotation strength and power.

RECURRENT DISLOCATION OF THE GLENOHUMERAL JOINT

Recurrent anterior dislocation

This dislocation often recurs and may result either from recurrent trauma (often, after the initial injury, involving minimal force or during normal activity) or from defects of the glenohumeral joint. Such abnormalities include the Hill-Sachs lesion, which

Fig. 19.7 A Hill-Sachs lesion and the mechanism for recurrent anterior dislocation of the shoulder.

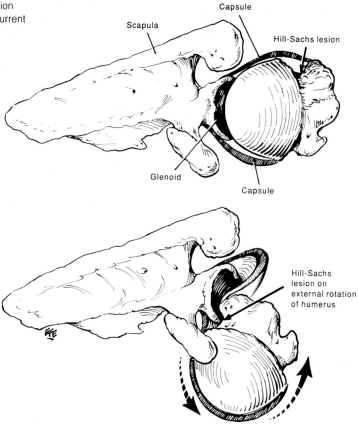

Capsule

Scapula

Hill-Sachs lesion

Glenoid

Capsule

Hill-Sachs lesion on external rotation of humerus

is a compression fracture in the head of the humerus posteriorly acquired by repeated dislocation or subluxation of the humeral head, allowing the humerus to slip or externally rotate off the glenoid cavity (Fig. 19.7); and the Bankart lesion which is an avulsion of the glenoid labrum and capsule. These lesions can be seen in Figs 14.6 and 14.7.

The apprehension test is useful in diagnosis. This test demonstrates an uncertainty by the patient when attempting to resist a force to the hand, while the patient's arm is held abducted at 90° and externally rotated.

Recurrent traumatic episodes produce a shoulder which may become loose and 'drop out' involuntarily. Repeated immobilization of the shoulder with each dislocation produces little benefit and surgery is usually the only real treatment. The principle of surgical correction is to strengthen the anterior capsule. At the time of the operation, laxity of the capsule, labral defects, loose bodies, etc. are also appropriately managed. Such associated lesions are common with this particular problem (Rolando *et al.* 1987).

Arthroscopy is a useful diagnostic tool for the unstable shoulder and arthroscopic reconstructions may have a role following traumatic first time dislocations in the young athlete. Its role in reconstruction of recurrently unstable shoulders is still controversial and as yet unproven.

Recurrent posterior dislocations

Recurrent posterior dislocations are less frequent and a similar approach to surgical management is taken to that of recurrent anterior dislocations, except that surgery uses the infraspinatus tendon to correct the posterior joint weakness.

Rolando *et al.* (1987) have highlighted the findings on CT arthrography of glenoid labral lesions, both anterior and posterior, together with capsular lesions in recurrent posterior dislocations.

A useful clinical test of posterior instability is as follows. The patient lies supine and relaxed and his/her arm is taken from abduction at 90° at the shoulder joint into flexion (across the body) and then back into abduction. Glenohumeral subluxation is felt by the examiner's hand behind the glenohumeral joint.

MULTIDIRECTIONAL INSTABILITY OF THE GLENOHUMERAL JOINT

The essential lesion producing instability of the shoulder in several directions at once appears to be laxity of the inferior capsule, particularly the inferior glenohumeral ligament, but including many structures within the shoulder joint.

Patients with multidirectional instability, where excessive laxity of ligaments becomes symptomatic, usually present with so-called '*atraumatic*' dislocations where minimal or no trauma was required for the first and all subsequent dislocations. Other forms of recurrent instability are with *repetitive microtrauma*, in which complete dislocations are uncommon, but patients still have apprehension in the at-risk position; and *traumatic* instability which is usually superimposed on ligamentous laxity in patients with multidirectional instability (Skyhar *et al.* 1990).

For patients without generalized laxity, a history of multiple injuries to the shoulder is usually obtained. Athletes with increased laxity often nominate repetitive activities such as swimming, throwing or lifting weights as the cause of their problem.

On examination there is usually evidence of the inferior laxity of the glenohumeral joint and there may be pain with or without a click with the arm held down in the dependent position. There may be a sulcus below the acromion and other directions of instability are revealed by specific movements. X-rays with weights attached to the wrist while the patient is standing should be taken and in some, CT arthrography may be further indicated.

Treatment for multidirectional instability is initially non-surgical. This comprises strengthening exercises (as mentioned for recurrent dislocation) and perhaps modification of activities to minimize the risk of repeated dislocations.

Surgery is indicated for those who do not achieve a satisfactory result from conservative treatment or for those who suffer this form of instability as a result of trauma (Skyhar *et al.* 1990). Often capsular plication is recommended and the particular technique varies with the direction(s) of the instability to provide comprehensive stability in all ranges of movement.

GLENOHUMERAL JOINT SUBLUXATION

Anterior subluxation

This subluxation occurs in the antero-inferior plane and is usually a result of the arm being forced backward and upward, or being caught in the overhand throwing position. This is commonly seen in the football codes, and in sports such as wrestling and judo. In the external rotation–abduction position, the humeral head is forced against the glenohumeral ligaments anteriorly, causing a tear of the anterior capsule and allowing the head of the humerus to ride over the rim of the glenoid. With the removal of the force, the head of the humerus then slips back into place.

The diagnosis is made on the history of the injury together with the presentation of a very painful, guarded joint which causes severe pain on movement. Often an athlete will state that 'the arm has slipped out of place and gone back in'. An X-ray is indicated to exclude fracture.

It is not uncommon to see an athlete such as a baseball pitcher or fielder in cricket present with a history of a subluxed glenohumeral joint (often resulting from a fall when attempting to catch a ball or steal a base, or brought on by a vigorous throw), with no preceding history of injury to the joint. In some instances laxity of joints is evident and may be a predisposing condition. In most cases, however, patients report a recurrent history of subluxation.

The treatment of a subluxation comprises rest in a weight-bearing sling for 1–2 weeks or for as long as the symptoms dictate. This is followed by progressive mobilization and rehabilitation of strength (particularly in adduction and internal rotation) and function over the ensuing weeks or months.

Some controversy exists as to whether prolonged immobilization of the shoulder after initial subluxation protects it against recurrent subluxation. Recent evidence appears to indicate that immobilization of the shoulder for 3–4 weeks or longer, does not provide such protection (Hovelius 1987). It is the author's practice not to immobilize the shoulder after subluxation as surgery in the form of a reconstruction is often required.

Inferior subluxation

Inferior subluxation of the shoulder is much less common. It is generally a result of an unusual injury or one where the support of the rotator cuff muscles is lost, either through paralysis or rupture (O'Donoghue 1976). A forced abduction injury such as in a rugby tackle or collapsing rugby scrum may lever the head of the humerus downwards and, depending on the force of the injury, it may cross the inferior glenoid rim. The patient holds the affected arm against the chest wall and palpation deep in the axilla reveals tenderness about the humeral head. X-ray examination is recommended to exclude fracture and treatment is carried out by placing the arm in a sling for approximately 3 weeks and allowing pain to determine a return to activity using rehabilitative exercises.

Posterior subluxation

This subluxation of the shoulder may result from a backward thrust of the arm while it is in a forward flexed position. On examination the posterior rotator cuff muscles are painful, tender and irritable.

Treatment, after an X-ray has excluded fracture, is by placing the arm in a sling for 2–3 weeks and then by gradual rehabilitation so that full strength, range of motion and function are achieved.

Recurrent glenohumeral subluxation

Recurrent anterior transient subluxation of the glenohumeral joint is widely manifest in players of contact sports who suffer repeated direct injury to the shoulder, or among pitchers or throwers whose arm 'goes dead' in the cocked position. It also occurs in tennis players who are unable to serve because of shoulder pain or in volleyball players who cannot spike the ball. The sudden loss of power in this latter group is typical and may follow an original injury to the joint when the shoulder was 'thrown' forward forcefully resulting in severe pain, or suffered an insult to the joint in a fall or by some other external force.

The apprehension test is useful in diagnosis. This test is described in the section on recurrent anterior dislocation of the shoulder.

On X-ray examination there may be a Hill-Sachs lesion and/or a Bankart lesion, also both previously described in this chapter. However, these are more commonly seen in dislocations.

Treatment consists of specific strengthening exercises of the shoulder, with emphasis on the internal and external rotators, over a period of 2 months. If the injured athlete still complains of episodes of 'dead arm' or other symptoms as described above, surgery may be necessary.

Surgery comprises repair of a Bankart lesion if present, with capsulorrhaphy, to tighten the joint capsule. Excellent results have been reported for this procedure (Rowe 1985).

Posterior instability occurs in throwing when the head of the humerus is placed against the posterior joint capsule and posterior tendons of the rotator cuff. This occurs at the phases of deceleration and follow-through in throwing. These posterior joint structures may be injured initially by throwing, weight-lifting or by trauma, as described in other sections of this chapter.

The diagnosis is made on a history of shoulder soreness and pain on throwing, together with palpable subluxation of the head of the humerus posteriorly while the patient is lying supine and relaxed, as previously described. An X-ray examination detects the presence of joint fractures which require specialist medical attention.

Treatment is by strengthening the supraspinatus, infraspinatus and teres minor muscles in particular, with involvement of the trapezius and deltoid muscle exercises as well. Bench pressing is contraindicated as it exacerbates posterior subluxation. Surgery is indicated for those who do not respond

Table 19.1 Classification of SLAP lesions (Snyder *et al.* 1990)

Type I	Fraying of the superior labrum. Firm glenolabral attachment
Type II	Superior labrum and biceps tendon stripped off glenoid. Instability of labral-biceps 'anchor'
Type III	Bucket-handle tear of labrum. Biceps insertion intact
Type IV	Bucket-handle tear of labrum extending into biceps tendon

to exercise therapy in 2–3 months, and consists of posterior capsule (and joint) reconstruction (Norwood 1985).

It should be noted at this point that chronic subluxation (or laxity) of the glenohumeral joint is a common predisposing factor to rotator cuff tendinitis, seen particularly in swimmers and throwers. This is discussed later in this chapter.

SLAP (SUPERIOR LABRUM ANTEROPOSTERIOR) LESIONS

In 1990, Snyder *et al.* described the SLAP lesion found in association with recurrent anterior instability. The lesion is 'an injury to the superior aspect of the labrum which begins posteriorly and extends anteriorly' and includes the biceps tendon at the glenoid. This lesion is most commonly caused by a fall on to the outstretched arm, in abduction and slight forward flexion at the shoulder.

SLAP lesions have been classified into four types (Table 19.1) and particular surgical correction is indicated for each type.

A strengthening programme may be tried in those patients who do not require (or are reluctant to undergo) surgery to the shoulder. A programme of exercises should be directed at developing strength and power of all the rotator cuff muscles in particular, throughout all ranges of movement.

INJURIES TO THE ROTATOR CUFF

The rotator cuff consists of the following muscles:

- Supraspinatus (superiorly)
- Subscapularis (anteriorly)
- Infraspinatus (posteriorly)
- Teres minor (posteriorly)

These muscles fuse with the capsule of the glenohumeral joint sharing a common insertion over the head of the humerus. As a result they contribute greatly to the stability of the shoulder joint.

The blood supply is provided by six arteries, but there are three areas of hypovascularity: the infraspinatus tendon, the subscapularis tendon and, notably, the supraspinatus tendon (Rothman & Parke 1965). This hypovascularity is a key factor in the aetiology of rotator cuff problems, as movement of the shoulder affects blood supply to the cuff. In particular, when the arm is adducted, there is avascularity of the tendon of the supraspinatus in the area of its insertion at the greater tuberosity (Hawkins & Kennedy 1980).

Neer (1972) demonstrated by cadaver studies impingement of the supraspinatus and biceps tendons, together with the greater tuberosity of the humerus against the coraco-acromial ligament, as the shoulder is flexed and internally rotated bringing the arm forward across the chest. This compression by impingement produces a 'wringing out' of blood supply from the tendons involved.

Pathophysiology and biomechanics

It is believed that ischaemia in the critical zones of hypovascularity mentioned may lead to cellular alterations and a cell-mediated inflammatory response, which results in the release of lysozymes and the consequent breakdown of connective tissue (Haleri 1980).

Rotator cuff injury in swimmers ('swimmer's shoulder')

Overuse is the principal cause of the tendinitis of the rotator cuff muscles in swimmers, commonly known as 'swimmer's shoulder'. Swimmers may train up to 16 km per day and, at the elite level, take very few rest days. Estimates of the number of strokes taken by each shoulder range in the order of 400 000–500 000 in 1 year of training.

With this enormous repetition, hypovascularity and ischaemia take their toll on the tendons and the factor of muscle imbalance becomes involved. As a result of normal stroke mechanics, swimmers generally increase their internal rotation strength and the head of the humerus becomes more internally rotated. This accentuates the process of impingement and 'wringing out' of the blood supply in the tendons.

By the very nature of their stroke mechanics, freestyle and butterfly swimmers produce more of these problems than breaststroke and backstroke swimmers and the pull-through phase of the stroke is very significant in producing injury.

The incidence of rotator cuff injuries has been reported by Kennedy *et al.* (1978) as affecting approximately 65–70% of competitive Canadian swimmers in 1 year; and at any one time about 15% of swimmers suffer shoulder pain.

Males are more often affected than females (70% of males, 65% of females) because males have lower buoyancy and increased muscle mass producing a more forceful pull-through (Ciullo & Stevens 1989).

'Swimmer's shoulder' refers to a rotator cuff injury particularly of the supraspinatus tendon, but may be associated with inflammation of the long head of biceps tendon and the subacromial bursa.

The impingement syndrome refers to a 'swimmer's shoulder' which has the following features:

- Shoulder pain associated with activity
- Focal tenderness of the supraspinatus tendon at the greater tuberosity
- A painful arc on abduction/elevation of the arm
- A positive impingement sign

A positive impingement sign is pain elicited by bringing the arm forward across the chest and then internally rotating it. The supraspinatus tendon and long head of biceps are squeezed against the coraco-acromial ligament and produce a local pain at the coraco-acromial ligament.

The impingement syndrome is a later development of swimmer's rotator cuff injury and depends on the restrictions on the rotator cuff structures

Table 19.2 Treatment of rotator cuff injury in swimmers

Grade	Management protocol
1	Maintain distance normally swum, limit painful strokes Warm-up, cool-down emphasized Stretching before and after exercise (Fig. 19.8) Ice applications Strengthening exercises for external rotators (Fig. 19.9) Technique correction (see Table 19.3)
2	Decrease distance and intensity of swims Avoid painful strokes, use kickboard (at chest) to maintain fitness in water Technique correction Ice, stretching, warm-up, cool-down Strengthening exercises for external rotators Anti-inflammatory medication and electro-therapy modalities
3	No swimming. Other activities (cycling, running in water, etc.) for fitness Ice, stretching, strengthening external rotators when tolerated Anti-inflammatory medication, electrotherapy modalities Corticosteroid injection in some cases If symptoms do not improve despite therapy, consider retirement from sport or surgical decompression (arthroscopy)

Note: The above grading is as outlined in Chapter 13.

Table 19.3 Prevention of rotator cuff injury in swimmers

Functional component	Stretching all muscles (using 'stretch slowly and hold' techniques) before and after exercise Should be no competition between swimmers to achieve greater ranges of movement
Strength	Strength training of external rotator muscles and scapular stabilizing muscles to achieve 'balance' with internal rotator muscles Use latex rubbers or weights
Technique	Encourage body roll on pull-through Early recovery from pull-through Hand leading elbow in recovery phase (Aim to minimize adduction and internal rotation at the shoulder.) Hold kick board close to the chest Avoid excessive use of hand paddles, allow gradual introduction and conditioning

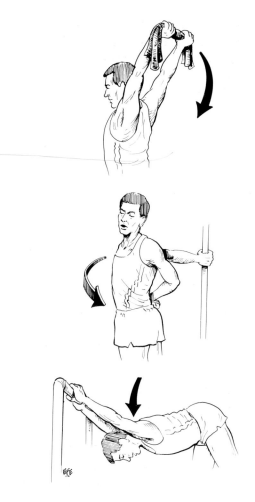

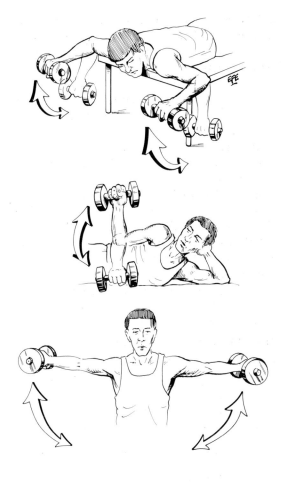

Fig. 19.8 Rotator cuff stretching exercises: hold each stretch for 10 s with 10 repetitions of each.

Fig. 19.9 Rotator cuff strengthening exercises — mainly for the external rotator muscles — use light weights with three sets of 10 repetitions per set.

imposed by the coraco-acromial arch. The coraco-acromial arch formed by the coracoid process, coraco-acromial ligament and acromion may impose upon the subacromial bursa, supraspinatus tendon and long head of the biceps. This exacerbates any inflammation brought on by overuse and the mechanical and physiological mechanisms discussed previously. In effect, the impingement syndrome is a vicious cycle.

MANAGEMENT OF ROTATOR CUFF TENDINITIS IN SWIMMERS

Grading of the injury is as described in Chapter 13

and underlies treatment of any inflamed shoulder. In particular, the modification of the swimmer's programme depends on the grade of injury. For example, a Grade 1 permits continued training while undergoing treatment, whereas a Grade 3 injury does not.

Tables 19.2 and 19.3 outline an accepted procedure of treatment and prevention of overuse injury to the rotator cuff in swimmers (Figs 19.8 and 19.9).

ROTATOR CUFF INJURIES IN NON-SWIMMERS

Rotator cuff injuries affect a wide range of athletes

413

including tennis players, gymnasts, baseball players, kayakers and canoeists, judokas, wrestlers and athletes who train with weights.

In most cases, overuse is the problem and is readily apparent when a history is taken. The procedures for diagnosis and management are the same as for 'swimmer's shoulder' as discussed in the previous section of this chapter.

The roles of flexibility, strength and power development, technique, anti-inflammatory measures and preventive strategies as discussed for swimmers, are all to be considered in the management of non-swimmers. Reference to Chapter 13 and to Table 19.2 in this chapter is recommended. Discussion with the particular athlete's coach is very useful in determining the strategy for recovery. The grading of the injury relates strongly to the modification necessary to the athlete's training programme and determines the pace of increases in duration and intensity of workouts and training sessions.

CALCIFIC TENDINITIS

Calcification of the supraspinatus tendon can be seen in the older athlete and may result from acute injury or from the repetitive microtrauma of overuse (Fig. 19.10). The shoulder may be very painful and abduction and rotation quite limited.

An X-ray confirms the diagnosis and management may be conservative, as calcification may disappear

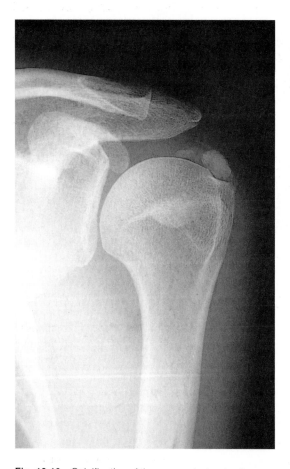

Fig. 19.10 Calcification of the supraspinatus tendon (courtesy of I. Anderson).

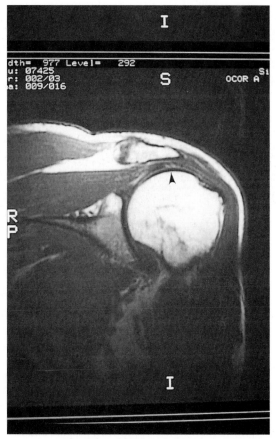

Fig. 19.11 MRI appearance of a tear (arrowed) of the supraspinatus tendon (courtesy of I. Anderson).

gradually or may require corticosteroid injections if the pain is particularly distressing (Norris 1990).

ACUTE TEARS OF THE ROTATOR CUFF

This injury is more common in the older age groups as a result of degenerative change. Acute tears of the rotator cuff are rare in athletes as isolated injuries and are almost always associated with a dislocation of the shoulder joint and with severe trauma.

The supraspinatus tendon is most often involved and the diagnosis is made on the history of the injury, local tenderness and pain on resisted abduction of the shoulder in particular. Persistent supraspinatus tendon pain in an older athlete should be suspected as a rotator cuff tear.

Tears of the cuff may be seen on an ultrasound scan, contrast arthrography, magnetic resonance imaging (MRI), CT or arthroscopically (Fig. 19.11). A surgical opinion should be sought as primary repair may be indicated. Full active rehabilitation of the shoulder is mandatory as dysfunction can be severe if untreated.

SUBACROMIAL BURSITIS

The subacromial bursa lies beneath the acromion and extends laterally under the deltoid muscle to cover the humeral head and rotator cuff. This bursa is distinct from the glenohumeral joint and provides for soft tissues to slide freely in the subacromial space (Fig. 19.12).

Bursitis in this area almost always accompanies overuse injuries of the rotator cuff, notably supraspinatus tendinitis, and contributes to the pain which designates the 'painful arc' and the 'impingement sign' described earlier. Bursitis is commonly seen in swimmers, tennis players, badminton players and gymnasts.

Treatment is carried out by the use of local ice applications, anti-inflammatory medication and electrotherapy modalities and may include local infiltration of corticosteroid into the subacromial space. Occasionally, surgery is performed to remove a thickened bursa (chronic bursitis), often associated with chronic tendinitis of the supraspinatus muscle and acromial osteophytes (bony spurs), which may require excision.

SUBCORACOID AND SUBSCAPULAR BURSITIS

These injuries are less frequent in athletes and usually result from overuse. Pain can be located anatomically by asking the patient to rotate the shoulder and treatment is as outlined for sub-

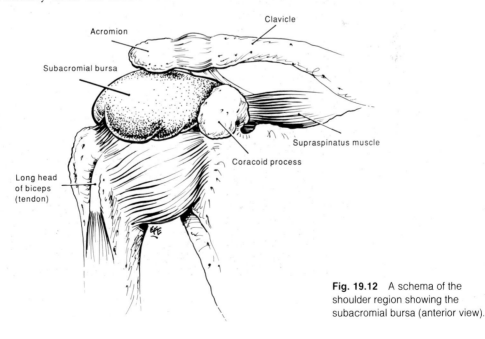

Fig. 19.12 A schema of the shoulder region showing the subacromial bursa (anterior view).

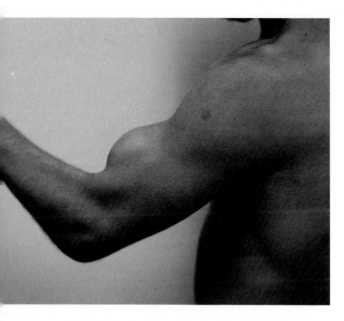

Fig. 19.13 A rupture of the long head of the biceps tendon. (Courtesy of A. S. Watson.)

acromial bursitis, except that local corticosteroid injections are directed at the appropriate bursa.

INJURIES TO THE LONG HEAD OF THE BICEPS TENDON

The biceps brachii muscle has two tendons: a short head, which attaches to the coracoid process and the long head which passes through the bicipital groove of the proximal end of the humerus. At this point it is bound by a thick fibrous band forming a 'roof' over the bicipital groove. It then traverses the head of the humerus to insert on to the superior lip of the glenoid rim. Movement of the shoulder joint with the elbow joint fixed, particularly in extension, results in the movement of the long head of the biceps brachii tendon through the confines of the bicipital groove. Overuse can produce a tendinitis or tenosynovitis (as the tendon has a sheath) and acute trauma can produce a sprain of the tendon at its glenoid attachment.

The diagnosis of a bicipital tendon injury is based on local pain and tenderness, accompanied by pain on rotation of the shoulder joint. Active contraction or passive stretching of the biceps is also painful. A useful test of the biceps tendon is to extend the elbow and the arm at the shoulder joint, or to resist supination of the forearm with the elbow flexed.

Treatment comprises applications of ice, anti-inflammatory medication and complete rest, or modified activities to partially rest the tendon. The prognosis for recovery of biceps tendinitis is usually good. Injections of corticosteroid over the tendon may settle pain but there is always the risk of tendon rupture to be considered.

Rupture of the long head of the biceps tendon

This occurs as a result of a forced extension of the shoulder and/or elbow with the biceps contracted, or from a forceful contraction of the biceps muscle. Examples of the latter include a biceps 'curl' while strength training, performing the 'cross', or 'crucifix', on the roman rings, or catching the bar while tumbling in mid-air during gymnastics training or competition. Rupture is common in the older athlete.

The diagnosis is usually obvious with a history of acute pain accompanied by a snapping sensation. This is immediately followed by the appearance of a distinct bulge in the upper arm where the biceps muscle 'belly' has collapsed (Fig. 19.13). Biceps muscle power is usually minimally affected in the long term because the short head of the biceps brachii compensates admirably. Specific treatment is therefore unnecessary, even for elite competitors.

Partial tears of the long head of the biceps tendon

These are occasionally seen and the history of the injury may be of acute or chronic tendon pain. An ultrasound scan may be useful in diagnosis and treatment is identical to that used for tendinitis, except that a corticosteroid injection may precipitate a tendon rupture.

Subluxation of the long head of the biceps brachii

This injury may occur acutely and then become recurrent. Diagnosis is made on the athlete's previous history and local tenderness may indicate an irritable tendon. The bicipital groove is often shallow on X-ray and an ultrasound scan may demonstrate the movement of the tendon (usually medially) on rotation of the arm. Surgical correction is indicated if the symptoms interfere with the athlete's training and performance.

SOFT TISSUE INJURIES TO THE UPPER ARM BELOW THE JOINT

Contusions to biceps and triceps brachii muscles are not uncommon, particularly in contact sports, but are generally uncomplicated.

Simple contusions respond well to ice applications and anti-inflammatory medication as well as electrotherapy modalities, with recovery over a week or two being the norm. Care must be taken with any injury to exclude significant haemorrhage, nerve damage and fracture. X-rays are therefore indicated to assess possible damage to bone.

Significant trauma to the arm can also produce myositis ossificans. This is readily visible on an X-ray after 4 weeks and usually necessitates no specific treatment except avoidance of further trauma.

Muscle strains in this region generally respond well to the usual anti-inflammatory and rehabilitation measures described for the treatment of soft tissues in Chapter 13.

Triceps tendinitis

Pain, tenderness and crepitus, all localized to the area of the triceps tendon proximal to the olecranon, are not infrequently seen among gymnasts and those who weight-train using forced elbow extension. Although a nuisance, the condition usually responds to modification of exercise, applications of ice, non-steroidal anti-inflammatory agents and physiotherapy modalities. Corticosteroid injection *over* the area of concern can be tried in more resistant cases, and usually produces relief within a few days. This condition should be carefully distinguished from olecranon bursitis (discussed below).

Rupture of the pectoralis major muscle

This muscle rupture can be induced by strength training (notably by bench pressing) and is seen in weightlifters and those athletes who use weights, such as wrestlers, throwers, rowers and players of contact sports. The rupture usually affects the muscle at its insertion on the humerus and is

diagnosed on the history and findings of local tenderness, swelling and bruising. An inability to contract the pectoralis major muscle on adduction and/or internal rotation of the arm against a resistance occurs when there is a complete rupture.

A partial tear is treated with the usual measures of rest, anti-inflammatory medication, electrotherapy modalities and a gradual programme of strengthening exercises over 6–8 weeks. In high performance athletes, however, a partial tear may require surgery. Complete rupture is an indication for surgery and an opinion from a specialist should be sought as early as possible.

THE ELBOW JOINT

Anatomy (See Fig. 19.14)

The elbow is composed of the articulations of the humerus and ulna, the radius and humerus and the radius and the ulna, and the integrity of the latter two joints in particular depends on their ligamentous support. The elbow joint is capable of flexion, extension, pronation and supination.

LIGAMENT INJURIES OF THE ELBOW

Medial ligament injury

Sprains of the medial ligament occur as a result of valgus stress and are the most common injuries to this region. They may present as an acute injury (caused by a fall) or as an overuse injury. 'Javelin thrower's elbow' refers to the repetitive stress imposed upon the medial ligaments by those who employ the 'round-arm' method (Williams & Sperryn 1976) and a similar injury can be seen in baseball pitchers and in gymnasts (Fig. 19.15).

Acute medial ligament rupture occurs with complete elbow dislocations and with some (but not all) serious radial head fractures. If unrecognized, medial ligament insufficiency has a poor prognosis for strength and sporting capability.

Local pain and tenderness of the medial ligament and pain on valgus stress of the elbow usually provide an accurate diagnosis. Treatment is by correcting a faulty technique and employing anti-inflammatory medication, electrotherapy and occasionally corticosteroid injection on to the ligament.

Valgus stress in the immature elbow produces widening of the medial epicondylar epiphyseal plate, and eventually stress fractures as part of the 'Little League elbow' spectrum of injuries. Displaced epicondylar fractures require surgical correction to maintain medial strength.

Valgus extension overload

Specific to baseball pitchers with excessive valgus stress and hyperextension forces in the throwing arm, this is a chronic condition with traction

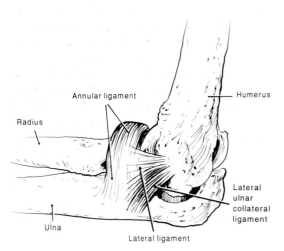

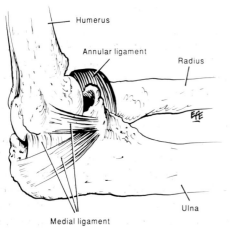

Fig. 19.14 The ligaments of the elbow joint.

osteophytes on the posterior and medial borders of the olecranon. Failure of conservative treatment leads to surgical excision of the osteophytes, but patients rarely get back to pre-injury level sport.

Posterolateral instability

An occasional complication of the 'perched' elbow dislocation (an incomplete dislocation with intact medial ligament), or of chronic stress, is insufficiency of the lateral ligament. This produces instability with supination of the forearm relative to the arm, with posterior radial head subluxation initially, and eventual elbow subluxation. Diagnosis clinically is by performing a 'pivot-shift' and the treatment is by surgical reconstruction of the ligament complex. Pure varus stress is less serious and responds usually to anti-inflammatory measures.

The 'pulled elbow' may be seen in sports such as judo and appears to be more common in the young athlete. It results from sudden traction on the forearm and is in fact a prolapse of the annular ligament into the radiocapitellar joint with, in effect, a radio-ulnar joint subluxation, which requires reduction of the head of the radius by rotation and axial compression of the radius (Williams 1980). Soft tissue inflammation is managed according to the principles described above.

OSTEOCHONDRITIS DISSECANS OF THE ELBOW JOINT

Osteochondritis dissecans (OCD) is a lesion of bone and articular cartilage commonly affecting the anterolateral surface of the capitellum.

OCD should be distinguished from *osteochondrosis*, or Panner's disease, which can be thought of as a benign lesion of bone that occurs in a young age group. It shows a characteristic fragmentation of the whole capitellum ossific nucleus, but does not form a loose body and goes on to reconstitute with conservative care (Jobe & Nuber 1986). However, OCD may be an extension of this process in the active athlete, with loose bodies, overgrowth of the radial head and early degenerative change. OCD is believed to be of either vascular or traumatic aetiology, or a combination of both.

This condition is prevalent among young baseball pitchers ('Little League elbow') and the trauma of

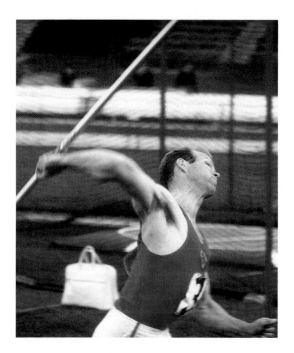

Fig. 19.15 The 'round arm' throw can produce a medial collateral ligament sprain of the elbow. (Williams 1980; with permission.)

throwing is thought to produce shear and compression across the radiocapitellar joint (Jackson *et al.* 1989). The valgus force which is applied to the elbow in throwing contributes to these forces and thus produces fragmentation of the capitellum, perhaps via disruption of the blood supply.

Three stages of OCD have been described, with particular reference to the radiocapitellar joint. Group 1 represents the original description of Panner's disease and affects children up to the age of 13 years and the prognosis for a favourable outcome is good. Group 2 involves adolescents aged 13 years to adulthood, who typically have a history of competitive, repeated activity and pain with elbow exercise. It is among this group that gymnasts are becoming more prevalent (Dixon & Fricker 1993). Both male and female gymnasts use their upper limbs as weight-bearing structures. Females, with wider carrying angles, tend to load their lateral elbow joints in extension and with manoeuvres such as handstands, round-offs and vaults they subject their radiocapitellar joints to

extremes of compression and shear. They may require rest, or surgery to the elbow to drill or bone graft a lesion to minimize progress of the disease. Group 3 comprises adults with chronic symptoms. There are loose bodies, joint incongruity, deterioration of the articular cartilage and often involvement of the entire elbow joint. Treatment may require arthroscopic removal of loose bodies, possible bone grafting and pinning of a partially detached fragment. Prognosis is generally poor.

OCD also commonly affects the olecranon/trochlear joint and is probably a result of repetitive forced extension of the elbow, with impingement of the olecranon against the olecranon fossa of the humerus. This is common among gymnasts and throwers in particular and is more often seen in adults. Bony changes include spur formation at the joint margins posteriorly and loose bodies within the joint (Fig. 14.5). There is often a history of catching or locking and pain associated with elbow exercise. Synovitis is common but swelling is not usually marked. Removal of loose bodies is indicated for relief of associated symptoms, but the prognosis for the elbow is generally poor.

X-rays are useful in providing an initial assessment, and CT scans and an MRI should only be considered if additional information is required, such as localization of chondral defects and loose bodies. Bone scanning is useful in assessing blood supply to a chondral lesion.

OLECRANON BURSITIS

Acute trauma to the point of the elbow produces inflammation, often with bleeding, of the olecranon bursa which lies superficial to the proximal end of the ulna at the olecranon (over the 'point' of the elbow). A marked, painful, tender, local swelling is evident and aspiration reveals a typically blood-stained synovial effusion.

Treatment with ice applications, anti-inflammatory medications, aspiration of the bursa (if enlarged), a compression bandage and electrotherapy modalities usually bring rapid relief. Occasionally, local infiltration of corticosteroid is needed and superficial padding, which reduces shear about the bursa, is also very useful.

Infection about the point of the elbow may

accompany bursitis and must be treated prior to any injection of the bursa. The bursa may also require drainage in this situation and a culture of the fluid is recommended prior to antibiotic therapy.

Chronic bursitis results from repeated injury and presents as a thickened, 'boggy', often tender swelling. There may be palpable loose intrabursal fibrous bodies which are quite irritating should the elbow be placed on a hard surface and leaned on. Surgery may be necessary if anti-inflammatory measures as described above are unsuccessful.

DISLOCATION OF THE ELBOW JOINT

Hyperextension of the elbow joint, caused by for example a fall from apparatus in gymnastics or a forced landing on a wrestling mat, can lever the ulna off the humerus. The humerus then rests distally to the coronoid and the capitellum rests on the neck of the radius. If there is a lateral component to the dislocation, the coronoid process of the ulna may come to rest behind the capitellum, displacing the head of the radius laterally. The elbow is held flexed at 120° and there is obvious posterior protrusion of the ulna with rapid swelling.

A dislocated elbow is an emergency and one must assess vascular supply to the forearm and hand by taking a radial pulse. Nerve damage often involves the median nerve and sensation to the palmar thumb, index and middle fingers must be checked. If reduction is to be attempted immediately after injury, the technique is one of gentle manipulation (exclude fracture prior to manipulation). Lateral displacement is reduced first by fixing the humerus and moving the forearm. Then traction into gradual extension of the elbow joint is employed.

If there is any doubt about the limb with respect to bone or nerve or vascular supply, specialist help must be sought immediately whether attempts at reduction have been made or not.

If reduction has been successful, repeated monitoring of nerve function and radial pulse are essential. Follow-up X-rays are important to exclude the possibility of bony fragments in the joint, incomplete reduction or delayed complications. The arm should be placed in a loose sling for 4 weeks and then actively rehabilitated to prevent the development of flexion deformity.

Associated fractures include those of the medial epicondyle, olecranon, the coronoid and the radial head. Coronoid fractures are an excellent marker of instability of the elbow, and are *not* an avulsion of the brachialis insertion, which is anterior to the coronoid tip. Larger coronoid fractures may lead to persistent or recurrent elbow instability, and should always be referred for specialist opinion. Medial epicondyle fragments may lodge within the joint preventing full reduction. These necessarily require specialist attention, as open reduction is often required and the complications described above must be guarded against. The less common supracondylar fracture and associated Volkmann's ischaemic contracture is worthy of note in this context.

HETEROTOPIC BONE FORMATION

Heterotopic ('new') bone formation can occur after injuries to the elbow joint and not only following severe injuries. Factors said to increase the likelihood are coexistent head injuries, previous history of heterotopic bone and forced passive range of motion exercises in the early postoperative period. High-risk individuals should be treated prophylactically with either single dose radiotherapy or a 6 week course of indomethacin (75 mg·day^{-1}) commencing immediately after injury. By the time bone is visible on X-rays, the bone is too well formed. Treatment is by avoiding physiotherapy and waiting up to 12 months for the new bone to mature (corticate) and if necessary excising it under cover of the above prophylactic measures.

POST-TRAUMATIC CONTRACTURES

Fixed flexion deformities of the elbow are extremely common after injury. Many are compatible with good sporting function, but some require attention. Anterior capsular contractures may respond to weight-assisted stretching programmes, but often require the addition of bracing. Turnbuckle splints, which act in a similar way to serial casting, usually correct the less mature contractures. Arthroscopic release is now a feasible option, but requires an elbow without degenerative changes. Open surgical releases are possible, but not compatible with many competitive sports.

EPICONDYLITIS OF THE ELBOW ('TENNIS ELBOW' AND 'GOLFER'S ELBOW')

There has been a great deal of discussion on the subject of epicondylitis. 'Tennis elbow' refers to epicondylitis of the lateral epicondyle and 'golfer's elbow' refers to medial epicondylitis.

Lateral epicondylitis

'Tennis elbow' affects the origin of the wrist extensor muscles, particularly the extensor carpi radialis brevis and is believed to be the result of a combination of factors. Repetitive 'micro-trauma' to the tendinous fibres of the extensor origin — particularly on backhand shots in tennis — is cited as the principal mechanism of injury. Secondary muscle spasm, poor vascular supply and inadequate techniques of recovery and prevention of further injury compound the problem.

A painful, tender lateral epicondyle and tenderness extending along the extensor muscle bellies is typical of this injury. A test whereby the epicondylar pain is reproduced can be performed by forcing the wrist and hand into flexion while the forearm is pronated and the elbow flexed. Resisted dorsiflexion of the wrist may also reproduce the pain.

There is usually very little swelling or bruising and histological changes are those of old and new scar formation, with areas of haemorrhage and fatty infiltration (Williams & Sperryn 1976).

Treatment consists of a series of simple exercises and preventive measures which are as follows:

- Ice applications to the painful epicondyle and muscle for 5 min are followed by wrist exercises. These exercises are performed with a light hand-held weight (0.5–1.0 kg). The forearm, wrist and hand are held in a pronated position off the end of a bench or table and the weight is then lifted slowly by wrist extension and lowered quickly to full wrist flexion, repeatedly for up to 10 min. Ice is again applied at the completion of the wrist exercises
- Grip size of a tennis racquet (if involved) is important. The correct grip size is the distance from the proximal transverse palmar crease to the tip of the ring finger
- An appropriate brace or splint for the forearm, applied distally to the elbow, is believed to dampen some of the shock that contributes to epicondylitis
- Adequate warm-up, muscle stretching and cool-down are always advisable
- A physiological heat retainer (thermal sleeve) may also be very useful and should be worn as often as possible

Corticosteroid injections (and/or surgery) should be reserved for those who fail to respond to the exercise programme outlined above after it has been carried out for 8 weeks or more. Physiotherapy modalities and acupuncture may assist recovery but the response is not usually dramatic. However, a change in racquet type (wood, metal, etc.) and grip size is sometimes useful and alteration of technique, such as adopting a two-handed backhand, may help.

An interesting feature of 'tennis elbow' is its association with C5/C6 segment pathology. Experience has shown that some patients often report relief of symptoms from lateral epicondylitis after appropriate manual therapy to the neck.

Medial epicondylitis

'Golfer's elbow' is a similar problem to that of 'tennis elbow'. The localized pain, tenderness and development through repeated injury is the same, although the medial epicondyle and associated wrist flexor muscle origin is involved. It is thought that hitting the ground with the golf club is one cause of the problem, while repetitive traumatic forehand shots at tennis may be to blame in others.

The treatment is the same as for 'tennis elbow', except that the wrist flexors are exercised with the hand, wrist and the forearm supinated.

THE FOREARM AND WRIST

Compartment Pressure Syndromes of the Forearm

Although not as frequently seen in the upper limb as in the lower limb, compartment pressure syndromes do appear among athletes who take part in vigorous exercise such as kayaking, canoeing and strength training (Ryan *et al.* 1987). The compartments most affected are the flexor muscles of the wrist and often both forearms are involved.

The condition is probably a result of exercise-induced ischaemia accompanied by swelling of the muscle(s) involved in the activity. Muscle compartment tenderness and tension, accompanied by local pain, are present and the diagnosis is confirmed by elevated compartment pressures. Fascial release provides relief when conservative measures of treatment such as ice, rest, anti-inflammatory medication and physiotherapy modalities fail.

Further reference to the treatment of compartment pressure syndromes is found in Chapter 20.

De Quervain's Disease

Stenosing tenosynovitis affecting the abductor pollicis longus and extensor pollicis brevis may be precipitated by repetitive hand and wrist motions such as in 10-pin bowling or racquet sports. There is local tenderness and swelling and pain on resisted abduction and extension of the thumb. There may also be palpable crepitus of the inflamed tendons. The superficial radial nerve passes directly over this sheath, and may be involved in the inflammatory process, giving symptoms of paraesthesia over the dorsum of the first web space. If this condition is treated early, rest, splinting and anti-inflammatory medication may provide relief. Corticosteroid in-

jection(s) into the sheath of the tendons can also be effective but, in chronic or refractory cases, surgical decompression of the tendons may be the only means of effecting a cure.

Intersection Syndrome

Rowers and weight-lifters may be affected by radial wrist extensor tendinitis where the abductor pollicis longus and the extensor pollicis brevis cross these structures (Fig. 19.16). Local pain, tenderness and crepitus make the diagnosis and treatment similar to that which has been described earlier, except that surgical decompression of the long extensor tendons of the forearm is undertaken to provide quick relief in the majority of cases (Williams & Sperryn 1976).

Carpal and Intercarpal Injuries

There are eight carpal bones, which act in a complex linked pattern, a triangular fibrocartilage (TFCC) and a ligamentous complex linking the distal radio-ulnar joint with the wrist joint. The lunate bone,

Fig. 19.16 Tenosynovitis in a rower: note the swelling on the dorsum of the forearm (Williams 1980; with permission.)

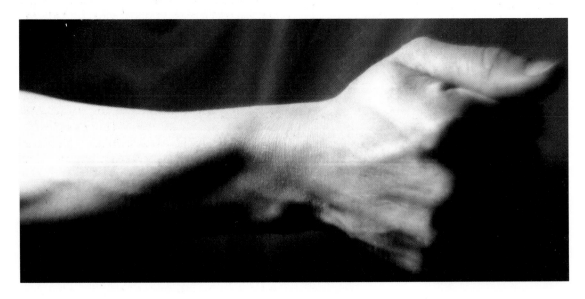

by its size and position, is prone to injury through mid-carpal force and the scaphoid in particular is noted for its tendency to fracture by falls on the outstretched arm, producing compression through the wrist. Stresses from falls pass through one of several recognized pathways, producing fractures with or without instability patterns. The carpal alignment on X-rays taken with wrist movements and gripping show many of these patterns.

Because the ligaments on the palmar surface of the wrist are much stronger than those on the dorsal side, dorsal, rather than ventral, subluxation of the carpal bones results more frequently from injury.

The carpal tunnel is an important structure and consists of the trapezium, trapezoid, capitate and hamate bones, which form an arch over the carpal ligament. This tunnel contains the median nerve and the tendons of the finger flexors (see carpal tunnel syndrome in this chapter).

Triangular Fibrocartilage Complex (TFCC) Injury

The triangular cartilage is the extension of the radiocarpal fibrocartilage which lies between the ulna and the carpus. Trauma to the wrist, which includes forced dorsiflexion, rotation, adduction or abduction, ruptures this structure and may produce local bleeding and calcification. Tears of the TFCC are classified according to whether they are degenerative, which are often central in the disc and related to chronic abutment of the distal ulna on the carpus, or shearing tears on the dorsal or volar margins, which are often associated with instability of the distal radio-ulnar joint itself. Local tenderness and wrist irritability on movement are easily detected and a CT arthrogram of the wrist may make the diagnosis clear. Treatment may be difficult with resistance to conservative (non-surgical) measures being quite commonplace. Surgical excision of the triangular cartilage may be necessary in protracted cases. Arthroscopy of the wrist joint now offers a less traumatic approach to treatment of these lesions, with diagnosis, partial excision and peripheral repairs all possible through or with the arthroscope.

Subluxation and Dislocation of Carpal Bones

Dislocation of the radiocarpal joint is uncommon, as is dislocation of the complete carpus. X-ray examination of an obvious deformity should provide a ready diagnosis and orthopaedic management should be instituted promptly.

The most commonly subluxed and dislocated bone in the wrist is the lunate. Forced dorsiflexion of the wrist produces this injury, for example, as in a fall on to the hand in contact sports such as rugby, basketball and volleyball. Examination of the painful wrist reveals tenderness of the dorsal wrist distal to the radius. Locking of the wrist may occur if the lunate is dislocated.

Compression of the median nerve may also occur and produce paraesthesiae and pain in the thumb and fingers supplied by this nerve. X-ray examination confirms the diagnosis of lunate dislocation and positive treatment depends on the reduction of the dislocated bone by manipulation under anaesthesia if seen early or by surgical means if presented later than 1 week after onset. Traditional treatment then consists of a period of rest in a splint, followed by rehabilitation as previously indicated. Recent advances in understanding the anatomy and biomechanics of the wrist have led to earlier surgical reconstruction with correction of subtle instabilities.

There are various other forms of dislocation and subluxation of the wrist and these include the carpal instabilities which involve the scaphoid bone and those which involve the lunotriquetral or midcarpal joints. Astute clinical observation of the wrist with a suspicious history, careful functional views on radiological examination using the opposite wrist for comparison (Fig. 14.2), or arthrography, usually provides a diagnosis. Management by an orthopaedic surgeon is recommended in these cases.

For a full discussion on instabilities of the wrist, the reader is referred to Culver (1986).

Fracture of the Scaphoid Bone

A fall on the outstretched hand is a common occurrence in most agility sports. Such a fall frequently produces a fracture across the waist of a scaphoid bone. There is pain and tenderness of the anatomical snuff-box of the thumb and X-rays may be negative for the first 2 weeks. Therefore it is sound practice to immobilize the wrist in a scaphoid plaster cast (splinting the first carpometacarpal joint) for this period and then repeat the X-ray. A technetium bone scan is useful in this early phase, but once the diagnosis is made the wrist must be placed in a scaphoid plaster cast for 6–8 weeks. On removal of the cast the scaphoid bone should be X-rayed again, as non-union of the fracture is common and may be associated with avascular necrosis of the proximal third of the scaphoid. This results from the fracture interfering with blood supply to the bone. Non-union is managed surgically in the majority of cases.

Kienbock's Disease (Avascular Necrosis of the Lunate)

This unusual condition occurs at any age and results in early stages in wrist inflammation, often confused with injury or overuse problems. The cause is unknown, but many cases have a relatively short ulna and a popular theory is that the stress of lunate translation across the 'edge' of the radius creates a stress fracture with subsequent loss of blood supply. Bone scanning shows a 'cold spot' and tomograms occasionally show a transverse fracture across the bone. MRI scanning is now the investigation of choice to confirm the diagnosis and stage of the disease. If the collapse of the bone is mild and early, operations to equalize the length of the forearm bones may relieve pain. The long-term prognosis is generally poor, with many patients needing later wrist fusion.

Fracture of the Hook of Hamate Bone

The hook of hamate is usually fractured while playing golf, tennis, racquetball, squash or baseball, or occasionally by a fall on to the hand during equestrian or cycling activities. The mechanism for injury with a club, racquet or bat may be by overuse or by direct trauma to the wrist associated with mishitting the ball or accidentally striking an object such as a tree, or the ground.

The hook is usually fractured near its base and mimics a wrist sprain. There may be little pain until activity with a racquet or club is undertaken. There is usually local tenderness at the fracture site but wrist motion is usually not painful. A plain X-ray must be taken with an oblique view of the wrist with the forearm supinated and the wrist dorsiflexed to show the lateral profile of the hook (Fig. 14.4). A CT scan may also be necessary, especially if plain X-rays are negative and/or a bone scan is positive.

The fracture may be treated in a plaster cast for 6 weeks but immediate surgical excision of a fractured hook provides excellent results and a return can be made to competition 6 weeks postoperatively (Zemel & Stark 1986).

Colles' Fracture of the Forearm

A fall on to the outstretched arm commonly produces a fracture of the distal radius and ulna with dorsal angulation of the distal fragments and occasionally impaction. This is known as a 'Colles fracture' and affects all age groups. Diagnosis is made on clinical signs and on an X-ray examination. Treatment is by closed reduction and immobilization in a cast, which covers the distal half of the forearm, the wrist and the hand, leaving the metacarpophalangeal (MCP) joints free. The cast is removed after 4–6 weeks and the prognosis is usually excellent.

HAND, THUMB AND FINGER INJURIES

The hand, thumb and fingers are notoriously prone to injury in sport. This should be no great surprise to anyone as the hand is used to throw, hit, catch, hold and support the body in an enormous range of activities from gymnastics to equestrian activities.

Dorsal Wrist Pain

Dorsal wrist pain is commonly seen in athletes such as gymnasts, who experience pain on wrist dorsiflexion while vaulting, tumbling or working on the pommel horse. The pain is also seen in divers (on entry into the water with wrists dorsiflexed) and in skaters who fall repeatedly on to the ice. Examination usually reveals a wrist that is painful to dorsiflex and is otherwise apparently normal. X-rays and a bone scan are usually quite normal, although there may occasionally be bony spurs on the lunate and distal end of the radius.

The problem may be one of impaction of joint margins of the wrist in an overuse setting. Treatment consists of limiting dorsiflexion by the use of a piece of foam taped to the dorsum of the wrist, limiting painful activity, anti-inflammatory medication and physiotherapy modalities, regular ice applications, increasing the range of motion of the wrist and strengthening wrist flexors and extensors. Technique correction should be encouraged where appropriate.

Other causes of wrist pain associated with overuse include stress fractures, which should be diagnosed on findings of local tenderness and a positive technetium bone scan and treated accordingly (see Chapter 20 for a detailed discussion on the management of stress fractures), and epiphyseal injury. Epiphyseal injury may be acute (as in Salter-Harris lesions, Fig. 22.8) or of gradual onset. Chronic injury to the epiphyses may be associated with disturbed bone growth and an ulnar drift of the wrist. In all cases of epiphyseal pain, referral to an orthopaedic surgeon should be considered and appropriate rest until tenderness disappears, supported by anti-inflammatory medication and selected electrotherapy modalities, should be instituted. It should be remembered that X-rays may be unhelpful in assessing epiphyseal injury and bone scanning shows increased uptake at normal epiphyseal growth plates. If X-ray changes are evident they usually consist of widening of the distal radial growth plates with irregular margins and perhaps marginal sclerosis with cystic changes and fragmentation within the growth plate (Carter et al. 1988). Comparison of epiphyses in the injured and non-injured limbs is always useful.

One cause of the dorsal wrist pain often forgotten is a ganglion. This is a herniation of the capsule of one of the many articulations about the wrist, sometimes with a long 'neck' to the site of the lump, or of a tendon sheath. Diagnosis by ultrasound is useful, especially in 'occult ganglion' cases where the lump is not palpable. Treatment options include aspiration, corticosteroid injection, and splintage to rest the implicated joint. In the past, surgery has had a poor reputation due to a high recurrence rate and poor rehabilitation, but current surgical techniques make this a curable condition.

Joint Injuries: Fractures, Subluxations and Dislocations

THUMB CARPOMETACARPAL (CMC) JOINT

The thumb CMC joint is the most mobile of the thumb joints, and is responsible for opposition and mobility of the thumb in many directions. Thus, the joint is a 'saddle' articulation and relies on ligamentous support for stability.

The base of the thumb may be injured by holding it within the closed fist and then punching the fist against a resistance. The dorsal or strong volar ligaments may be sprained, or worse, ruptured, resulting in a subluxation or dislocation at the base of the thumb.

Similarly, forced hyperextension of this joint may result in a sprain of the anterior fibres of the capsule, or subluxation/dislocation if more severe.

Fractures of the base of the first metacarpal involving the CMC joint are common ('Bennett's fracture'), and displace due to the pull of the strong tendon attachments to the shaft fragment. Treatment of fractures without displacement in a cast with thumb abduction for 4–6 weeks is possible, but any displacement requires surgical correction and pinning (open or closed).

Treatment for ligament injuries without persistent subluxation is by casting for 2–4 weeks and splintage to protect the joint. Ongoing instability of the joint may require tendon reconstruction.

OTHER CMC JOINTS

Dorsal dislocation or fracture/subluxation of the metacarpals on the carpals occurs usually in boxing or motorcycle injuries. Commonly, the ring and little fingers are involved, but any number of the four joints may dislocate. X-rays need to be accurate, and CT scanning is occasionally needed for confirmation. Treatment is by reduction with or without pinning.

THUMB METACARPOPHALANGEAL JOINT

In contrast to the CMC joint of the thumb, the MCP joint requires stability rather than range of motion. Thus injuries which rupture the stabilizing structures put this joint at risk. The ulnar collateral ligament (UCL) is covered by a stiff aponeurosis and if ruptured can be prevented from healing by tissue interposition. This can result from chronic stress, or acute injury ('skier's thumb') when the MCP joint is subjected to forced abduction during a fall on to the ground while holding a ski stock.

Sprains are treated with the usual means of reducing swelling and adhesive strapping may help to protect the joint until healing has occurred over the ensuing weeks after injury.

If X-ray examination reveals subluxation or dislocation, the joint should be reduced with traction and gentle manipulation and then immobilized in a splint for approximately 3 weeks. The thumb should be splinted in a thumb spica so that it is protected from further episodes of subluxation or dislocation. If the dislocation persists (with Grade 3 ligament tears), surgery is indicated to repair the joint, as pinch grip function is significantly impaired.

Avulsions of the distal attachment are not uncommon and require surgical reduction.

OTHER METACARPOPHALANGEAL JOINTS

Any forceful blow to a digit may sprain or rupture ligaments about the MCP joints. Hyperextension injuries are often involved and, if severe enough, may result in subluxation or dislocation.

The injury may be followed by spontaneous reduction or may require manipulation. This should be done by a qualified medical practitioner and must make use of traction, perhaps under anaesthetic, with appropriate manipulation. The joint should be protected by a splint, in a flexed position, for approximately 2 weeks and an X-ray examination must be done to exclude a fracture, particularly of the metacarpal neck, if a forced flexion injury has been involved. Rehabilitation should commence as soon as possible.

PROXIMAL INTERPHALANGEAL (PIP) JOINTS

Hyperextension or lateral forces to these joints may injure the anterior joint capsule or collateral ligaments, respectively.

Diagnosis depends on the history and evidence of local pain and tenderness. If subluxation or dislocation is suspected, the joint should be reduced by traction and appropriate manipulation.

The sprained, or now reduced, joint is then fixed in partial flexion for 7–10 days and thereafter actively rehabilitated. An X-ray examination is imperative to exclude fracture and if subluxation or dislocation is recurrent, surgical repair of the capsule should be considered.

Volar plate injury

This injury typically occurs as an acute traumatic episode in sport and results from forced hyperextension of the PIP joint. It may result from a kick to the hand or from clutching at an opponent's clothing or from catching a ball at cricket or baseball. Avulsion of a bony flake may occur from the middle phalanx, and the middle phalanx may be dislocated dorsally. Local pain, tenderness and inability to flex the joint is typical and X-ray demonstrates the presence of a dislocation and/or a fracture.

Dislocation should be managed by gentle manipulation with no traction, followed by immobilization in slight flexion in a splint for 3 weeks. Non-dislocated joints usually require similar splinting or surgical correction.

DISTAL INTERPHALANGEAL (DIP) JOINTS

Mallet finger

This results from a tear of the extensor expansion from its attachment to the base of the terminal phalanx and it may also be associated with a fracture. The finger is characteristically flexed at the DIP joint and cannot be extended at this joint.

Splinting the affected joint in extension usually gives good results and a protective splint should be worn for 6–8 weeks to ensure full recovery. It is important, however, that the splint is not removed during this period. If the splint has to be removed temporarily then the finger should be taped to hold the joint in extension.

Flexor profundus tendon avulsion

Avulsion of the profundus flexor tendon together with its bony attachment at the base of the distal phalanx is not an uncommon injury in sport. It may result from a direct blow such as a kick or from misfielding a ball at cricket. DIP joint flexion is lost and there is obvious swelling and pain. Early and direct repair is the best treatment and therefore X-ray and immediate surgical referral is advised.

TENDON RUPTURE

Ruptures of various tendons can occur as a result of a force which is applied to the flexed fingers, although these injuries are not common.

Diagnosis is made on the inability to flex the finger(s) and the presence of deep pain at the site of the lesion. Surgery is often indicated and a surgical opinion is recommended prior to instituting any treatment.

Rupture of the extensor expansion of the fingers over the PIP joint may result in a 'boutonnière', or 'buttonhole', deformity and this may also require surgery to correct the angular deformity of the joint.

TRIGGER FINGER/THUMB

Triggering of the PIP joints of the fingers or the interphalangeal joint of the thumb is usually due to entrapment of the flexor tendons through a thickened A1 pulley (volar to the MCP joint in the palm, and adjacent to the distal palmar crease). The cause is either a tendon nodule with secondary sheath changes or a sheath nodule with secondary tendon changes. Treatment in adults is often successful by injection of the sheath with a corticosteroid and local anaesthetic, but persistent symptoms respond well to a small surgical release in the palm.

LACERATIONS AND INFECTIONS OF THE HAND

Injury to the hand can produce laceration by various means — a footballer's cleated boot, an ice skater's skate, a hockey stick and even an opponent's teeth, can all contribute to such injuries. Any laceration should be treated seriously and all wounds should be attended to promptly, with care taken to exclude associated tendon or nerve damage requiring special attention.

Infection of the hand can have serious consequences for many athletes if left untreated and appropriate wound care and antibiotic therapy are of prime importance. The human bite is notorious for producing infections which are difficult to treat and a broad-spectrum antibiotic should be used with subsequent frequent review of the wound and the hand in general. If there is any suspicion of suppuration within the hand, drainage must be carried out and appropriate follow-up and rehabilitation measures must be taken.

Subungual haematoma

The 'blood blister', which forms under the nail is common and treatment is simple. A piece of wire such as an unfolded paper clip is heated over a naked flame until red hot. The hot wire is then quickly and firmly applied to the nail over the haematoma until the nail is burnt through and the blood released through the hole just created. The feeling of relief is instant and provided the finger is kept clean and dry there are usually no further problems.

Occasionally infection occurs, which necessitates antibiotic therapy and, infrequently, removal of the nail.

NEUROLOGICAL INJURY AFFECTING THE UPPER LIMB

Among the many causes of upper limb pain are entrapment and trauma to a peripheral nerve.

Brachial Plexus Lesions

The upper limb is often the source of symptoms from lesions of the brachial plexus by virtue of the fact that the lower plexus lesions produce referred pain to the shoulder and beyond. One of the most common conditions in this category is that of the *thoracic outlet syndrome*. This describes a combination of neurological and vascular features which result from compression of C8 and T1 nerve roots, in particular, together with compression of the subclavian vessels. Cervical ribs are the most commonly noted bony abnormality associated with this syndrome, and fibrous bands arising from the transverse process of C7 or from a short cervical rib are also often to blame. Abnormal fibromuscular bands associated with scalene muscles can also entrap the brachial plexus as can excessive callus formation following clavicular fracture (Baker & Liu 1993).

Clinically, the syndrome presents with paraesthesiae or sensory loss affecting the C8 and/or T1 dermatome on the affected side, together with venous engorgement of the upper limb (reflecting vascular obstruction). Symptoms may be exacerbated by throwing activities.

Diagnosis is made on the particular neurological and vascular signs described and an X-ray often shows an offending cervical rib. MRI may show a fibrous band when present and vascular studies can demonstrate the presence of obstruction.

Conservative treatment comprising avoidance of precipitating activities can be tried, but where mechanical obstruction or compression exists, surgery may be necessary for the benefit of the active or competitive athlete. Surgical intervention usually involves excision of a cervical rib and/or fibrous band, scalenotomy or release of fibrous bands. Recovery is generally good.

Suprascapular Nerve Entrapment

The suprascapular nerve, which is derived from the C5 and C6 nerve roots, supplies sensation to the posterior portion of the shoulder and acromio-clavicular joint. Its motor innervation is to the supraspinatus and infraspinatus muscles. The nerve passes through the suprascapular notch and enters the supraspinous fossa, a branch then passes around the base of the spine of the scapula to innervate the infraspinatus muscle.

Acute trauma, usually with traction, may damage the nerve, producing vague posterolateral shoulder pain and progressive wasting and weakness of the supraspinatus and infraspinatus muscles. Repetitive stretching of the branch to the infraspinatus muscle has been described in volleyball players, producing an isolated, painless wasting of the infraspinatus muscle (Ferretti et al. 1987). Recent attention has focused on the association of ganglia in the spino-glenoid notch and supraglenoid fossa with nerve dysfunction. These may be secondary to labral lesions of the shoulder, analogous to the meniscal cyst of the knee. Nerve conduction studies and electromyography usually confirm the diagnosis.

Management depends on rest and corticosteroid injections over the nerve at the suprascapular notch may be attempted by a specialist. Surgical division of the transverse ligament overlying the suprascapular notch may also be necessary.

Ulnar Nerve Entrapment at the Elbow

An entrapment neuropathy of the ulnar nerve in the cubital tunnel is common, especially after prolonged flexion of the elbow (Corrigan & Maitland 1983). The nerve is trapped by the arcuate ligament which runs from the medial epicondyle to the olecranon. Several factors have been cited to produce the neuropathy and these include trauma, repeated pressure on the elbow, valgus deformity of the elbow and subluxation of the nerve with elbow movements (Corrigan & Maitland 1983). A recent classification of the anatomical variants aids in identifying patients at risk of ongoing problems (O'Driscoll et al. 1992).

The diagnosis is made on the pattern of sensory change which affects the little finger and ulnar half of the ring finger. Weakness affects the hypothenar muscles and the intrinsic muscles of the hand. In advanced cases, hyperextension of the MCP joints may be seen, with extension of the ring and little fingers. Pressure on the nerve may produce pain in the distribution of the nerve, which it may palpably sublux over the elbow.

Nerve conduction studies demonstrate the site of entrapment and distinguish the problem from spinal causes. Management ranges from avoidance of aggravating factors to surgical decompression if symptoms and disability persist.

Median Nerve Entrapment at the Elbow

The median nerve occasionally becomes trapped under the ligament of Struthers, at the medial epicondyle or between the two heads of pronator teres. Sensation to the three and a half radial digits is affected (as in the carpal tunnel discussed later), but the motor symptoms are those of weakness of forearm pronation, wrist flexion, thumb opposition and flexion of index and middle fingers. Surgical decompression is necessary in order for normal function to return.

Radial Nerve Entrapment at the Elbow

The radial nerve may be trapped by the supinator muscle to produce superficial branch symptoms which are largely sensory, or deep branch symptoms which are mainly motor.

Sensory symptoms affect the radial aspect of wrist and thumb while the deep branch, the posterior interosseous nerve, may become affected by elbow or forearm trauma to produce a weakness of the wrist and finger extension, together with wrist and thumb pain. The condition may mimic lateral epicondylitis ('tennis elbow'). Surgery may provide a cure if the appropriate management of soft tissue swelling does not produce relief.

The Carpal Tunnel Syndrome

This is common, as numerous reasons exist for compression of the median nerve. Repeated wrist flexion and extension, trauma to the wrist with or without carpal bone subluxation or dislocation, fluid retention associated with pregnancy and the premenstrual phase are all commonly involved. Endocrine and rheumatological conditions such as hypothyroidism, acromegaly, tenosynovitis and rheumatoid arthritis must also be considered.

Diagnosis is made on the sensory loss affecting the radial three and one half digits, a positive Tinel's sign, wasting of the thenar muscles and weakness of thumb opposition and/or abduction.

Nerve conduction studies may confirm the diagnosis and management includes rest (sometimes in a splint), from aggravating factors, judicious use of corticosteroid injections and mobilization of the wrist. Surgical decompression may be necessary if all else fails and the condition becomes chronic, or if muscle wasting and weakness are evident at the time of diagnosis.

Ulnar Nerve Entrapment at the Wrist

The ulnar nerve traverses the tunnel of Guyon which lies between the pisiform bone and the hook of hamate. Trauma, tendinitis, ganglion formation and compression by prolonged or repeated dorsiflexion of the wrist may all produce entrapment of the ulnar nerve.

Cycling has produced its share of such ulnar nerve entrapments as a result of the hands resting dorsiflexed at the wrist on the handlebars during long road races (Fig. 19.17). Sensory changes affect the little finger and the ulnar half of the ring finger while weakness affects the hypothenar muscles, the interosseous muscles and adductor pollicis brevis. Nerve conduction studies are useful in confirming the diagnosis and the management is as outlined for the carpal tunnel syndrome. Prevention of the problem in cyclists is by regular shifting of hand position and posture, and by wearing padded gloves.

Vascular Injury Affecting the Upper Limb

There are numerous vascular and neurovascular syndromes which affect the upper limb, including

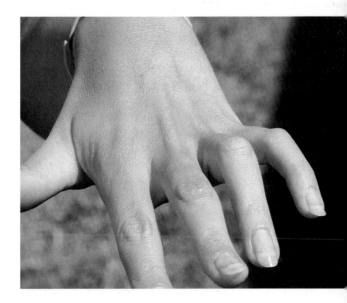

Fig. 19.17 Ulnar nerve entrapment in a cyclist. (courtesy of Dr A. S. Watson.)

the thoracic outlet syndrome described above. Other vascular injuries include occlusion of the axillary artery, seen in throwing athletes, the quadrilateral space syndrome (involving compression of the axillary nerve or its main branches and the posterior humeral circumflex artery adjacent to the scapula) also seen in throwing athletes, and the syndrome of effort thrombosis of the axillary/subclavian vein. Both the conditions affecting the axillary artery and the posterior circumflex humeral artery require surgical decompression in most cases. Effort thrombosis of the axillary/subclavian vein is described below.

Effort Thrombosis of the Axillary or Subclavian Vein (Paget-Schroetter Syndrome)

The axillary vein begins at the inferior edge of teres major, where it continues on from the basilic vein, to become the subclavian vein at the first rib. Compression of this vein occurs in the costoclavicular space, in most cases, and occurs with neck hyperextension and hyperabduction of the arm, or with a 'military brace' position with shoulders held back. The vein can be caught between the clavicle and first rib, the first rib and the costocoracoid ligament or the subclavian muscles and first rib. Athletes who develop compression and thrombosis of this vein usually do so as a result of repetitive activity rather than from acute or direct trauma, and come from sports such as basketball, baseball, weightlifting and gymnastics.

The diagnosis is made on finding a swollen upper limb which is cool, mottled, perhaps bluish in colour and covered by dilated superficial veins about the arm and shoulders. The patient complains of subacute development of an aching or painful limb with perhaps paraesthesia or numbness and a history of exercise-induced fatigue of the limb. Arterial pulses are usually normal.

Venography confirms the diagnosis and treatment depends upon anticoagulation to minimize progress of the thrombosis and time to allow resolution of the clot. Streptokinase has been effective in acute situations to dissolve the thrombus but this practice is not common. Surgery involving thrombectomy

and simultaneous decompression of the vein (by excision of the first rib) has also been proven effective (Baker & Liu 1993). Athletes are able to return to sport after complete recovery.

CONCLUSIONS

The approach to the diagnosis and management of disorders of the shoulder girdle and upper limb must include a thorough understanding of the unique structure and function of the glenohumeral joint in particular, as it is this region which often causes concern to the medical practitioner or therapist who treats injured athletes. A careful check of previous injury, attention to the site of any pain and investigation of the particular movement(s) which produce(s) the pain, may provide a diagnosis before any further investigation is carried out.

Also worthy of note are those neurological problems which affect the upper limb and the reader is encouraged to become familiar with the anatomy of these structures.

Rehabilitation is always of vital importance and simple regular exercise programmes, incorporating stretching and strengthening drills, are often all that are required to provide good functional recovery from injury.

REFERENCES

Allman F. L. (1967) Fractures and ligamentous injuries of the clavicle and its articulations. *Journal of Bone and Joint Surgery* 49, 774–784.

Baker C. L. Jr & Liu S. L. (1993) Neurovascular injuries to the shoulder. *Journal of Orthopaedic Sports Physical Therapy* 18, 360–364.

Cahill B. R. (1982) Osteolysis of the distal part of the clavicle in male athletes. *Journal of Bone and Joint Surgery* 64, 1053–1058.

Carter S. R., Aldridge M. J., Fitzgerald R. & Davies A. M. (1988) Stress changes of the wrist in adolescent gymnasts. *British Journal of Radiology* 61, 109–112.

Ciullo J. V. & Stevens G. S. (1989) The prevention and treatment of injuries to the shoulder in swimming. *Sports Medicine* 17, 182–204.

Corrigan B. & Maitland G. D. (1983) *Practical Orthopaedic Medicine*, p. 78. Butterworths, London.

Culver J. E. (1986) Instabilities of the wrist. *Clinics in Sports Medicine* 5, 725–739.

Dixon M. & Fricker P. A. (1993) Injuries to elite gymnasts over 10 years. *Medicine and Science in Sports and Exercise* 25, 1322–1329.

Ferretti A., Cerullo G. & Russo G. (1987) Suprascapular neuropathy in volleyball players. *Journal of Bone and Joint Surgery* 69, 260–263.

Haleri G. B. (1980) Ruptures of the rotator cuff. *Canadian Medical Association Journal* 123, 620–627.

Hawkins R. J. & Kennedy J. C. (1980) Impingement syndrome in athletes. *American Journal of Sports Medicine* 8, 151–157.

Hovelius L. (1987) Anterior dislocation of the shoulder in teenagers and young adults: Five year prognosis. *Journal of Bone and Joint Surgery* 69, 393–399.

Hunter D. & Fricker P. A. (1992) Case Report: Sternoclavicular dislocation. *Excel* 8, 111–117.

Jackson D. W., Silvino N. & Reiman P. (1989) Osteochondritis in the female gymnast's elbow. *Arthroscopy* 5, 129–136.

Jobe F. W. & Nuber G. (1986) Throwing injuries of the elbow. *Clinics in Sports Medicine* 5, 621–636.

Kennedy J. C., Hawkins R. & Krissoff W. B. (1978) Orthopedic manifestations of swimming. *American Journal of Sports Medicine* 6, 306–322.

Lyons F. R. & Rockwood C. A. Jr. (1994) Osteolysis of the clavicle. In De Lee J. C. & Drez D. D. Jr (eds) *Orthopaedic Sports Medicine*, pp. 541–542. W. B. Saunders Company, Philadelphia, PA.

Neer C. S. (1972) Anterior acromioplasty for chronic impingement syndrome in the shoulder. *Journal of Bone and Joint Surgery* 54, 41–50.

Norris T. R. (1990) Calcific tendinitis. In Nicholas J. A. & Hershman E. B. (eds) *The Upper Extremity in Sports Medicine*, pp. 59–61. C. V. Mosby, St Louis, MO.

Norwood L. A. (1985) Posterior shoulder instability. In Zarins B., Andrews J. R. & Carson W. G. (eds) *Injuries to the Throwing Arm*, pp. 153–157. W. B. Saunders, Philadelphia, PA.

O'Donoghue D. H. (1976) *Treatment of Injuries to Athletes*, 3rd edn, pp. 146 and 213. W. B. Saunders, Philadelphia, PA.

O'Driscoll S. W., Bell D. F. & Morrey B. F. (1992) Posterolateral rotary instability of the elbow. *Journal of Bone and Joint Surgery* 73A, 440–450.

Rockwood C. A. Jr. & Green D. P. (1984) (eds) *Fractures in Adults*, 2nd edn, pp. 719–721. J. B. Lippincott, Philadelphia, PA.

Rolando D. S., Feldman F. & Bigliani L. (1987) CT arthrographic patterns in recurrent glenohumeral instability. *American Journal of Radiology* 149, 749–753.

Rothman R. H. & Parke W. W. (1965) The vascular anatomy of the rotator cuff. *Clinics in Orthopedics* 41, 176–186.

Rowe C. R. (1985) Anterior subluxation of the throwing shoulder. In Zarins B., Andrews J. R. & Carson W. G. (eds) *Injuries to the Throwing Arm*, pp. 144–152. W. B. Saunders, Philadelphia, PA.

Ryan C., Fricker P. A. & Hannaford P. G. H. (1987) Muscle compartment pressure syndrome of the upper limb and shoulder: Two case studies. *Australian Journal of Science and Medicine in Sport* 19, 24–25.

Skyhar M. J., Warren R. F. & Altchek D. W. (1990) Instability of the shoulder. In Nicholas J. A. & Hershman E. B. (eds) *The Upper Extremity in Sports Medicine*, pp. 181–209. C. V. Mosby, St Louis, MO.

Snyder S., Karzel R., Del Pizzo W., Ferkel R. & Friedman R. (1990) S.L.A.P. lesions of the shoulder (lesions of the superior labrum both anterior and posterior). *Orthopedic Transactions* 14, 257–258.

Williams J. G. P. (1980) *Atlas of Injury in Sport*, p. 58. Wolfe Publications, London.

Williams J. G. P. & Sperryn P. N. (1976) *Sports Medicine*, 2nd edn, pp. 405, 407 and 411. Edward Arnold, London.

Zemel N. P. & Stark H. H. (1986) Fractures and dislocations of the carpal bones. *Clinics in Sports Medicine* 5, 709–724.

CHAPTER 20

INJURIES TO THE PELVIS AND LOWER LIMB

K. J. Crichton, P. A. Fricker, C. Purdam and A. S. Watson

Injuries from sport are frequently presented to medical practitioners and physiotherapists, and the pelvis and lower limb are the commonest sites of overuse sporting injury. Ankle ligament sprains and trauma to the knee are familiar problems in casualty departments and often present diagnostic challenges and problems in management. This chapter discusses the more common injuries to the pelvis and lower limb in sport and, while it is largely clinical, it also relates discussion to the principles of biomechanics and podiatry in particular, as well as to the principles of treatment and rehabilitation presented earlier in this book.

INJURIES ABOUT THE PELVIS

Osteitis Pubis

The pubic symphysis unites the two pubic bones. The articular surfaces are ridged and covered by a thin layer of hyaline cartilage, the joint containing a disc of fibrocartilage which is thicker in females. The joint is structured for limited motion (normal vertical movement is up to 2 mm) and consequently is injured when excessive movement is imposed upon it.

Athletes suffering osteitis pubis (inflammation of the symphysis pubis) are usually males. They present with a subacute or gradual history of pain which may be rather diffuse, extending from the pubic symphysis up into the rectus abdominis muscle, down along the adductor muscles to above the knee and often into the scrotum. Activity, particularly running and kicking, aggravates the problem and prolonged rest alleviates the symptoms. The problem is common to sports such as soccer,

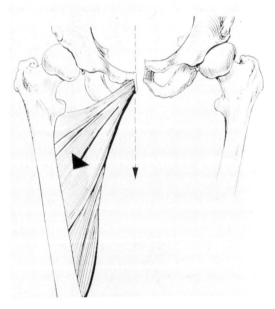

Fig. 20.1 Osteitis pubis is thought to result at least in part from the pull of the adductor muscles in activities such as kicking. (Courtesy of Allan McGavin Sports Medicine Centre, UBC, Vancouver.)

432

Australian football, ice hockey and endurance running (Fig. 20.1; Fricker *et al.* 1991).

In females the problem may be seen postpartum and precipitated by kicking and running activities. Examination may reveal tenderness of the symphysis pubis and often associated loss of full rotation of one or both hip joints. This lack of rotation is believed to be a causative factor, as it forces the symphysis pubis to 'open' when hip rotation is blocked during activities such as kicking and pivoting to change direction while running (Williams 1978). In some patients, limitation of hip rotation appears after osteitis pubis has developed and the mechanism for this is unclear. There may also be an associated dysfunction of sacro-iliac joints and lumbosacral spine and a leg length discrepancy. All of these may contribute to abnormalities of pelvic and lower limb mechanics and thus compound the problem.

Investigation of osteitis pubis is by X-ray and technetium [99]m bone scan. Increased isotope uptake along one or both of the joint surfaces occurs early and is diagnostic (Fig. 20.2). X-rays taken while the patient stands on alternate legs (the 'flamingo' view) may show subluxation of the pubic joint (pubic symphysis instability). Joint changes such as marginal erosions, sclerosis and joint widening may also be seen.

Management depends on settling inflammation of the symphysis, restoring full range of movement to the hip joints and on muscle strengthening to provide abductor and adductor support to the pelvis and hips. Rest from painful activities is advised and recovery may take 6–18 months. Activities such as cycling and swimming should be encouraged during recovery, followed by a gradual reintroduction of running and kicking over a period of weeks to months.

Anti-inflammatory medication and modalities can be useful, although the response is not usually dramatic and some sufferers find relief by wearing a 'physiological heat retainer' (e.g. 'Thermoskin' shorts). Injections of corticosteroids appear to contribute little to recovery.

The role of surgery for instability of the symphysis is much debated and an orthopaedic opinion must be sought in this respect.

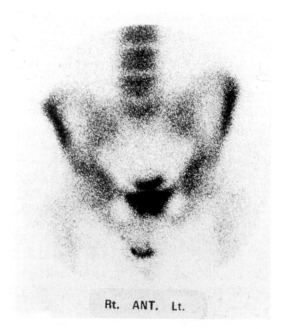

Fig. 20.2 A technetium [99]m bone scan showing increased isotope uptake at the pubic symphysis in osteitis pubis. Note the outline of the bladder above the symphysis. (Courtesy of Allan McGavin Sports Medicine Centre, UBC, Vancouver.)

The differential diagnosis of osteitis pubis includes adductor muscle origin strain, conjoined tendon lesion, pelvic infection, stress fracture of the pubic ramus and osteomyelitis.

Conjoined Tendon Lesions

The conjoined (or conjoint) tendon is formed by the common insertion of the rectus abdominis muscle, the internal oblique muscle and the transversalis fascia at the pubic tubercle, extending along the superior surface of the superior pubic ramus as a reflection of tissue to form the posterior wall of the medial end of the inguinal canal.

Activity in sport which involves kicking, jumping and twisting of the trunk, together with activities which contribute to raised intra-abdominal pressure (such as lifting weights for strength training), appear to produce a tear or defect in the posterior wall of the inguinal canal. This has been referred to as 'crypt-hernia', 'incipient inguinal hernia' and 'conjoined tendon tear' in recent years.

Patients present with pubic pain which may radiate up into the rectus abdominis or laterally along the inguinal ligament, accompanied by exquisite tenderness at the site of injury. The pain is often reproduced by coughing or sneezing. History is usually of a gradual onset but there may be an acute presentation associated with stressful abdominal muscle activity such as lifting weights.

Investigations are generally unrewarding but X-ray and radioisotope scanning of bone may serve to exclude conditions such as osteitis pubis or stress fracture of a pubic ramus. Intraperitoneal radiography (a technically difficult procedure with significant risk of complications) has demonstrated laxity of the posterior wall of the inguinal canal (crypt hernia) in many patients with symptoms of conjoined tendon lesions (Smedberg et al. 1985).

Management is difficult as most anti-inflammatory medications (including corticosteroid injection) and electrotherapy modalities appear to contribute little to a long, slow recovery, which is easily upset by any activity. Surgical repair of a defect in the posterior wall of the inguinal canal provides good results with a high percentage of success in terms of resumption of sport, particularly when supported by rehabilitation which provides for adequate healing and normal muscle strength (Malecha & Lovell 1990; Karlsson et al. 1994).

Adductor Muscle and Tendon Lesions

Adductor muscle strains are usually the result of an acute forced abduction at the hip (as in a rugby tackle or when trapping a ball in soccer), a sudden increase in intensity of sprinting or a sudden change in direction. Treatment is directed at reducing inflammation and muscle spasm with medication and electrotherapy. Local massage is useful for relieving muscle spasm and gentle stretching should be encouraged, although it is important that athletes do not overstretch as this may lead to tenoperiosteal problems. Acute muscle strains generally settle within 4–8 days with judicious care, but chronic adductor strain may require local corticosteroid injection and subsequent rehabilitation.

Adductor tenoperiostitis is generally secondary to adductor muscle strain, although in many cases on presentation the causative strain is asymptomatic and the tenoperiostitis is the principal presenting problem. In many cases the athlete does not present until quite late which makes management more difficult. It is important to recognize that stretching may aggravate the condition in its acute phase and is often the causative factor for chronic lesion. Management should be directed at reducing contributing factors, such as associated muscle spasm, and treating the tenoperiosteal lesion itself. Modalities that may be useful include pulsed magnetic field therapy and laser therapy. Acupuncture may also be of some value.

Exercises commence with hourly or second hourly isometric 'holds' in adduction (two sets of five repetitions) for the first 2–3 days until the 'holds' become pain-free. At this stage cycling or swimming with a pull-buoy between the knees is the only safe activity. Once the isometric exercises are pain-free, the athlete may then commence gentle stretching and isotonic exercise as well as resume normal training.

Follow-up treatment and management is directed at achieving full range of hip and pelvic motion as well as full stretch and strength in the adductor muscle groups. With tenoperiostitis it is important to recognize that modalities such as ultrasound and interferential therapy may aggravate the condition. In chronic cases corticosteroid injection or adductor tenotomy may be undertaken, although these are usually unnecessary with appropriate early conservative care.

Piriformis Muscle Syndrome

Buttock pain in cyclists and runners may be caused by spasm of the piriformis muscle. This muscle is an external rotator, an extensor and an abductor of the hip, and originates from the posterior aspect of the sacro-iliac joint, inserting on the superior and posterior aspects of the greater trochanter.

The pain is of gradual onset and may radiate to the hip and down the posterior thigh as a result of sciatic nerve compression by the piriformis muscle. Pain is exacerbated by activity, often appearing

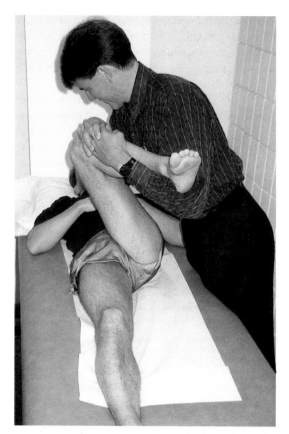

Fig. 20.3 The piriformis muscle spasm may be detected by placing the hip into adduction, flexion and internal rotation and then applying a force along the line of the femur. A painful response provides the diagnosis.

after cessation of exercise. Deep local tenderness and spasm of the muscle are diagnostic and stretching the piriformis reproduces the pain. This is done by positioning the hip in adduction, flexion and internal rotation and then applying stretch to the muscle (Fig. 20.3). Magnetic resonance imaging (MRI) may be of benefit in defining the sciatic nerve in the pelvis and observing constriction and at the same time assessing the lumbar spine.

Treatment is by decreasing painful activity, undertaking daily stretching and deep massage, physiotherapy modalities and anti-inflammatory medication. Recovery usually ensues over a period of weeks. It is important when dealing with chronic piriformis lesions to address any causative factors, the most common being lumbosacral disc or sacro-

iliac problems, or poor pelvic stabilization in the stance phase of gait.

Trochanteric Bursitis

There is a large bursa overlying the greater trochanter of the femur, which may be subjected to repetitive injury from the muscles, tensor fascia lata and gluteus maximus, particularly in running sports, or from direct trauma in contact sports such as the various football codes and wrestling.

Several biomechanical factors may predispose to the overuse injury. These include a tight iliotibial tract (which includes the tensor fascia lata), genu valgum and foot pronation, and most commonly poor horizontal stabilization of the pelvis in the stance phase of gait by the gluteus medius and minimus and tensor fascia lata, all of which accentuate the problem of tension across the greater trochanter and associated bursa.

A catching or snapping pain at the hip while walking or running is often noted and there is localized tenderness over the trochanter.

The differential diagnosis of trochanteric bursitis includes haematoma, stress fracture of the neck of the femur, arthritis of the hip and referred pain from the spine or sacro-iliac joint.

Management of the problem entails correction of any predisposing biomechanical factors with appropriate strengthening (in relation to pelvic strength) and possibly orthotics, stretching of the abductor muscles of the hip, rest from painful activities and management of inflammation with frequent ice applications, appropriate medication and electrotherapy modalities. Occasionally, an injection of corticosteroid into the bursa is necessary for persistent bursitis.

THIGH INJURIES

Hamstring Muscle Strains (Biceps Femoris, Semitendinosus and Semimembranosus Muscle Injuries)

ACUTE STRAIN

Acute hamstring strains are often the result of an increase in intensity of sprinting, hurdling or kicking. Wood (1986) demonstrated that eccentric hamstring strength is the major limiting factor to increasing sprinting speed. It is therefore no surprise that hamstring strains are among the most common injuries in sport.

Contributing factors to hamstring muscle tears include cold, fatigue, the presence of pre-existing injury, weakness, delayed muscle soreness, or neurological and biomechanical factors.

The history of onset is generally quite spectacular, although occasionally minor tears are difficult to differentiate from localized muscle cramp. It should be remembered that muscle cramp typically occurs in the inner range of hamstring contraction, whereas muscle tears generally occur in the outer range or at footstrike in the co-contraction phase with the quadriceps muscle group. Clinical assessment of local tenderness and muscle dysfunction determines the severity of the strain. A muscle defect (particularly in Grade 3 strains) may be palpable.

Initial treatment consists of ice, compression and elevation, anti-inflammatory medication and a short period of rest. Excellent results may be gained by early mobilization using continuous passive motion and ice (Stanton 1988). The athlete is placed on a continuous passive motion machine from day 1 or 2 of injury for periods of up to 3 h at a time, with applications of ice for 10 min every 40 min. Full range is often gained by the second day. Useful electrotherapy modalities at this stage may include pulsed magnetic field, laser and microstimulation currents.

Once full range is gained the athlete may commence early functional activity and gentle isotonic activities with weights. These can be complemented by concentric and eccentric exercises. A thermal (heat-retaining) sleeve worn as much as possible is a useful support to this phase of rehabilitation.

In elite athletes dramatic results may be achieved with a running programme for functional strengthening of the hamstring muscle group (Reid 1992). This consists of high volume running with a gradual increase in intensity over a number of days to maximal sprinting. Where possible dynamometer testing should be used to compare strength of hamstring groups. Full strength throughout the

extended range required by the sporting activity is the key to preventing recurrence.

Localized massage and/or acupuncture may be useful within these regimens to reduce muscle spasm and pain.

Time to full recovery is dependent on factors including the site of the injury and its vascularity, the severity of the initial injury and the initial condition of the patient. A Grade 2 tear of the middle third of the hamstring belly may repair in 8–10 days in an elite athlete, whereas a Grade 3 tear in the upper third of the hamstrings in a non-elite athlete may take 12 weeks or more.

CHRONIC STRAIN

Chronic muscle strains imply an ongoing inflammation, with incomplete tissue healing and organization. In many cases the organization of inflammatory oedema has resulted in the loss of homogeneous elasticity within the affected muscle group and produced areas of induration and tenderness. It is not uncommon to see impaired lumbosacral or sacro-iliac function associated with these lesions.

Treatment of inflammation is by electrotherapy modalities and medication. Reduction of muscle spasm and the induration associated with chronic inflammation is achieved by mechanical means such as deep connective tissue massage and stretching. Graded strengthening is also important, progressing from strength and power sets to specific eccentric work.

Recurrent hamstring strains may also require investigation of biomechanical factors which may be contributing to an increase in stress of the hamstring group. These include lumbar or sacro-iliac joint problems, pelvic or calf muscle weakness, or a faulty sprinting or hurdling technique.

Rectus Femoris Muscle Tears

A tear of the rectus femoris is usually the result of either sprinting or kicking in ball sports. The management is very similar to that of hamstring muscle tears, although it should be emphasized that the lack of synergists with rectus femoris action limits rapid recovery. In general, rectus femoris tears take 3–6 weeks to recover sufficiently to allow sprinting and may take another 2 weeks before the athlete can safely kick a ball.

While in adults rectus femoris tears usually occur mid-belly in the muscle, in adolescents avulsion of this muscle may occur at its origin on the anterior inferior iliac spine (Fig. 14.9).

Quadriceps Muscle Contusion (Haematoma)

Management of this injury may be divided into intramuscular and intermuscular haematoma. These may be diagnosed by ultrasound scan or MRI.

INTRAMUSCULAR HAEMATOMA

In this case trauma to the quadriceps muscle results in bleeding within a muscle belly. Restriction by the muscle belly itself and associated muscle spasm limit the amount of bleeding that occurs. The haematoma may be palpated as a tender, localized induration within a discrete muscle belly.

Intramuscular haematomas may be a frequent source of frustration to both the athlete and the therapist, because the rise in intramuscular pressure is difficult to manage conservatively. Early mobilization or ultrasound and interferential therapy may be fraught with the dangers of recurrent bleeding.

Once the danger period for re-bleed has passed (approximately 4–10 days), mobilization and electrotherapy may be introduced, with the patient slowly resuming activity as discomfort allows. Swimming and hydrotherapy are particularly useful in rehabilitation. Full weight-bearing is permitted as symptoms allow and an exercise programme is commenced and graduated up to full activity. Hopping and skipping are useful in the later stages of rehabilitation to regain muscular endurance.

INTERMUSCULAR HAEMATOMA

In contrast to the above, intermuscular bleeding affects an area between individual muscles. As a result there is little in the way of muscle spasm or pressure to restrict or minimize the bleeding that occurs. Such a lesion is susceptible to re-bleeding with injudicious use of heat, electrotherapy modalities or over-zealous massage. The presentation is typified by a poorly localized, painful swelling, which often gravitates to the knee and may produce subcutaneous bruising and an irritative synovitis of the knee joint.

Treatment in the initial stages comprises rest, ice, compression and elevation and mobilization may take place on the second day after injury, using a combination of ice and gentle stretching. Ultrasound and interferential therapy may be of some benefit in reducing the clot and associated muscle spasm. Athletes are generally able to jog without discomfort by days 3 or 4 after injury and resume training once full range of movement has been achieved. Athletes with intermuscular haematoma rarely miss playing the following week.

MYOSITIS OSSIFICANS

Ossification within a muscle may develop as a sequel to acute or chronic trauma with bleeding. The most common presentation is in the quadriceps femoris following contusion. Myositis ossificans may also be seen in the adductor muscle group or, less commonly, the abductor group of the thigh. The heterotopic new bone may be contiguous with normal bone, or free within the muscle.

The exact cause for myositis ossificans has not yet been established. The presentation of myositis ossificans is that of increasing irritability of the affected muscle group. The patient complains of increasing morning stiffness, aching within the muscle, and often there is a palpable increase in the muscle temperature. In the acute phase there is a progressive loss of range of movement of that muscle group. Any active attempt at regaining this loss of range of movement often results in an exacerbation of the condition and therefore all active events should be ceased. Calcification is evident on plain X-ray (Fig. 20.4) and a computerized tomography (CT) scan can help to differentiate the problem from malignancy.

Treatment initially requires rest of the injured muscle to allow reduction of inflammation and reabsorption of the by-products of injury. Almost without exception electrotherapy modalities are contra-indicated and return to activity is allowed

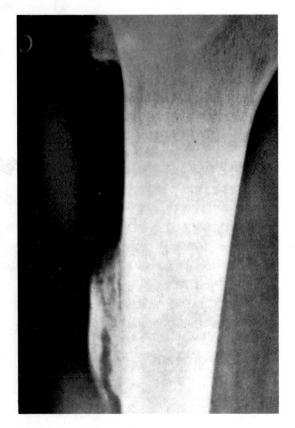

Fig. 20.4 An X-ray shows ectopic bone formation typical of myositis ossificans in the thigh. (Courtesy of Allan McGavin Sports Medicine Centre, UBC, Vancouver.)

when pain and tenderness have settled. Surgical excision is rarely necessary and is only performed after a bone scan indicates maturation of the calcified area.

OVERUSE KNEE INJURIES

Iliotibial Band Friction Syndrome

The iliotibial band (ITB) is described as a ligament or condensation of fascia. However, functionally it is a tendon within the fascia lata which arises from the iliac crest and inserts into Gerdy's tubercle on the anterolateral aspect of the tibia, just below the knee joint. Part of the gluteus maximus posteriorly and the tensor fascia lata muscle anteriorly form a V-shaped insertion into the ITB, serving to control

and tension the band and, as mentioned above, make it function as a tendon. With the knee flexed to 30° the ITB lies on or behind the lateral femoral condyle and with extension of the knee the ITB moves anterior to this bony prominence.

The ITB friction syndrome is common and results from inflammation of the distal posterior fibres of the ITB and the bursa which lies deep to the ITB and over the lateral femoral condyle. The syndrome is often associated with a single long hard run, a rapid increase in training distances, running on banked or cambered surfaces such as a beach or shoulder of the road, or excessive downhill running.

ITB friction syndrome also occurs in cyclists. Again it is the posterior fibres of the ITB (which contour more closely to the lateral femoral condyle) which seem to be susceptible to friction irritation. With each pedalling stroke the ITB is pulled anteriorly on the down stroke and posteriorly on the up stroke. The pain is often rhythmical in time with pedalling and may significantly reduce the power in the pedalling stroke. The factors which should be looked for in cyclists include active increased pronation, cleats which are excessively internally rotated, a saddle position either too high or too far aft, or training problems. The most common training problems are excessive hill work, an inadequate early-season training base or lack of stretching (Homes et al. 1994).

Stinging pain is usually noted over the distal 3 cm of the ITB and is notably worse running downhill. Reproduction of pain on compression over the lateral femoral condyle with the ITB stretched is confirmatory (Fig. 20.5). Crepitus may also be felt with the test. Tightness of the ITB, malalignment and leg length discrepancy may be contributory and there may also be excessive foot pronation and downward contralateral tilt of the pelvis during stance on the affected leg during running (which stretches the ITB).

Conservative management is usually successful, particularly if symptoms are of recent onset. Avoidance of painful activities, reduction in training distance, non-steroidal anti-inflammatory medication, daily stretching of the ITB and orthotic devices to control excessive foot pronation are all useful. Strengthening of the ipsilateral hip abductors is indicated for those who display pelvic drop or sway with running, as described above. Checking for optimum seat height and cleat orientation is essential in cyclists with ITB irritation.

If first-line treatment measures fail, a local infiltration of corticosteroid at the site of friction may be useful, and, for recalcitrant cases, surgery may be performed to divide the ITB 3 cm above the lateral femoral epicondyle, or to release the posterior

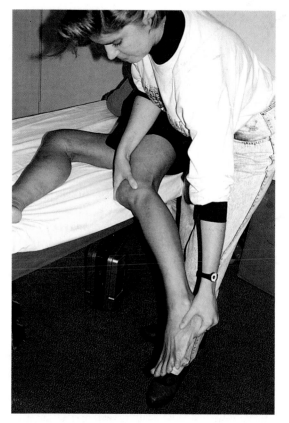

Fig. 20.5 A test for iliotibial band friction syndrome. The patient lies on the unaffected side with the back of his pelvis very close to the edge of the bed. He stabilizes his pelvis, preventing it from tilting in the frontal plane and the examiner then adducts the thigh over the edge of the bed in line with the trunk to stretch the iliotibial band. The knee is then flexed and extended around 15° knee flexion with the thumb over the lateral epicondyle of the femur. The test is positive if pain is felt by the patient or crepitus is felt by the examiner as the inflamed iliotibial band passes between the thumb and lateral epicondyle with movement of the knee.

2 cm of the ITB producing a 'V'-shaped defect in the band over the epicondyle. This procedure may be performed in an operating theatre using local anaesthetic and, if performed through a small incision, inflamed bursal tissue over the lateral epicondyle of the femur may be removed at the same time (Firer 1992).

ITB friction syndrome must be differentiated from popliteus tendinitis and lateral meniscal lesions of the knee.

Popliteus Tendinitis

The popliteus muscle winds around the posterolateral aspect of the knee and stabilizes the knee in flexion by resisting forward displacement of the femur on the tibia.

Tendinitis of this structure is less common than ITB friction syndrome but arises under similar circumstances. Local tenderness is found just posterior to the superior attachment of the fibular (lateral) collateral ligament, and pain may be reproduced by resisted knee flexion with the tibia held in external rotation.

Treatment comprises modification of painful activity, applications of ice, stretching of the knee flexors and the use of anti-inflammatory medication and electrotherapy modalities. Reduction of aggravating factors, notably inner range knee flexion activities, is also beneficial. Corticosteroid injection may be useful in chronic cases.

Patellofemoral Joint Pain Syndrome

Table 20.1 provides a differential diagnosis of anterior knee pain and of these conditions the patellofemoral joint (PFJ) pain syndrome is most often seen in athletes.

This syndrome, which affects females more often than males, presents in adolescence and into the fourth and fifth decades. The sufferer usually complains of diffuse pain 'under the kneecap', which may be aggravated by climbing or descending hills or stairs. The pain is more often of the medial PFJ than of the lateral one and may be associated with pain on sitting for long periods. Relief is sought by walking or extending the knee. Often the PFJ pain

Fig. 20.6 A schema of patellofemoral joint pain. VMO = vastus medialis obliquus muscle.

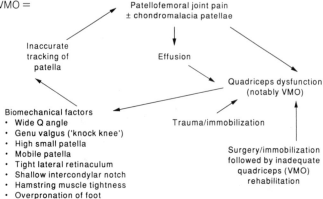

is associated with episodes of the knee buckling, occasionally with quadriceps muscle weakness and with crepitus.

Sufferers of this condition participate in a wide range of sports including running, tennis, squash, the football codes, skiing, skating and basketball.

Examination of the patient reveals notable irritability of the PFJ. Crepitus may accompany patellofemoral movement and there may be a small effusion of the joint. Quadriceps muscle weakness and wasting may be evident, notably of the vastus medialis muscle.

A range of biomechanical factors may be associated with PFJ pain syndrome and these include a wide Q angle (above 16° in males or above 18° in females), a high small mobile patella, genu valgus, a

Table 20.1 Differential diagnosis of anterior knee pain

Patellofemoral joint pain syndrome (including chondromalacia patellae)
Patellar subluxation
Synovial plica
Osteochondral lesions of patella or femur
Infrapatellar fat pad lesion
Patellar tendinitis
Sinding-Larsen-Johanssen disease
Osgood-Schlatter's disease
Anterior horn lesion of meniscus
Trauma to patella (including fracture)
Stress fracture patella
Bipartite patella
Prepatellar bursitis
Pain referred from the hip

shallow intercondylar notch and a pronated gait, which increases internal rotation of the tibia. All these factors are capable of adversely affecting patellar tracking. Radiographic examination may show tilting of the patella laterally and/or a shallow intercondylar notch on a 'skyline' view, as well as excluding osteochondritis dissecans of the PFJ, symptomatic bipartite patella or other patellar pathology.

These factors emphasize the proposed mechanisms of the PFJ pain syndrome. It is believed that pain may arise from the subchondral bone of the PFJ or tight retinacular structures. Either excessive or inadequate pressure to the articular cartilage may affect nutrition of this tissue and result in pain and degenerative change.

The tendency to lateral shift of the patella is compensated in the normal situation by the vastus medialis muscle. Under various conditions normal tracking of the patella is disturbed because of vastus medialis dysfunction and the PFJ pain syndrome results. With chronic maltracking of the patella, true chondromalacia of the patella occurs. Figure 20.6 provides a schema for the PFJ pain syndrome and Fig. 20.7 details patellofemoral mechanics.

The management of PFJ pain syndrome incorporates pain-free activity and quadriceps muscle rehabilitation, with emphasis on vastus medialis re-education and correction of biomechanical factors. One very successful rehabilitation programme uses tape to hold the patella so that it tracks correctly with quadriceps muscle contraction (McConnell

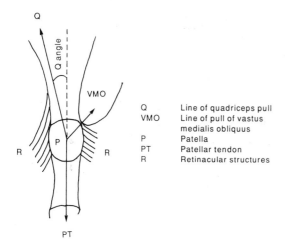

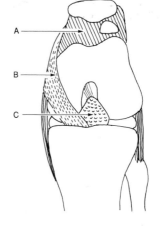

Fig. 20.7 A vector diagram of the patellofemoral joint. (Adapted from Williams 1980.)

Fig. 20.8 A diagram of the synovial plicae of the knee joint. (A) Suprapatellar plica. (B) Medial patellar plica (C) Infrapatellar fat pad.

1986). An important factor in quadriceps rehabilitation is the success of eccentric muscle drills, where the patient daily performs 'drop squats' to half knee flexion and then adds light hand-held weights, progressively heavier, for a period of 6–8 weeks. Biofeedback may assist muscle training in resistant cases.

Surgery is indicated when conservative measures fail. Arthroscopy may diagnose chondromalacia patellae (or otherwise) and provides the opportunity for chondral shaving, if appropriate, and/or lateral retinacular release of the PFJ. Very occasionally patellar tendon realignment is performed to correct a wide Q angle.

Patellofemoral Synovial Plica

Folds, bands or septa of the synovial lining of the knee joint may project into and partially divide the joint cavity. These plicae are remnants of the septa of the embryonic joint and although often present, are not usually tight, thick or large enough to cause problems. Plicae may become symptomatic if subjected to acute trauma or overuse.

The medial patellar plica runs from the medial suprapatellar pouch to the intrapatellar fat pad and

may impinge on the medial femoral condyle and PFJ in flexion (Fig. 20.8). If fibrotic and tight (due to repeated injury) it may cause joint surface abrasion.

Aching is felt anteriorly in the knee joint on sitting when the knee is flexed and this may be more intense during the first few walking steps in the morning. There may be a tender band felt under the medial retinaculum with catching or snapping with knee flexion. Occasionally, a mild effusion is present. The pain may be reproduced by resisted knee extension and is often made worse by the examiner gliding the patella medially.

A suprapatellar plica may completely divide the suprapatellar pouch from the joint cavity but is commonly deficient laterally (Fig. 20.8). This fold or partial septum may cause poorly localized anterior knee pain when stretched on knee flexion and, if large, the fold can be demonstrated by arthrography.

Treatment consists of rest from painful activities, ice applications, anti-inflammatory medication and, occasionally, lignocaine and corticosteroid injection if the tender medial plica is palpable. If pain and effusion persist despite appropriate treatment, arthroscopic excision of the symptomatic plica is recommended.

Infrapatellar Fat Pad Syndrome

The infrapatellar fat pad may be injured by direct trauma to the anterior aspect of the knee in collision sports or by impingement between the tibial and femoral condyles on forced knee extension. It may also result from arthroscopic knee surgery. Subsequent inflammation may cause anterior knee pain and occasionally an effusion. Pain may be reproduced by hyperextension of the knee with pressure over the fat pad.

Repeated injury or multiple surgical insults may cause progressive fibrosis with involvement of the deep infrapatellar bursa.

Relative rest, brief limitation of knee extension, anti-inflammatory medication and electrotherapy modalities are usually effective unless significant fibrosis has occurred. In rare cases of persistent problems, arthroscopic examination and partial fat pad resection may relieve the symptoms.

Patellar Tendinitis ('Jumper's Knee')

The patellar tendon is also known, perhaps more correctly, as the infrapatellar tendon or the patellar ligament. It is the continuation of the quadriceps femoris tendon to the tibia and is a flat band which is extremely strong. It attaches proximally to the lower margin of the patella and is continuous with fibres of the quadriceps femoris tendon (the patella is a sesamoid bone within this tendon). It inserts distally on to the tibial tuberosity.

Most often a result of overuse, patellar tendinitis is seen in basketballers, volleyballers, triple jumpers, long jumpers, high jumpers, the kicking athletes and, notably, in weight-lifters and those athletes who perform 'squats' with weights, such as rowers and throwers. It is related to the repetitive extensor action of the knee with the generation of large eccentric forces. Biomechanical analysis of jumping and landing has shown the greatest tensile forces in the patellar tendon in basketball activities are in landing. Patients present with a history of gradual onset of local pain and tenderness of the tendon at or below the mid-line of the patella at its lower pole (Torstensen *et al.* 1994). The pain is often associated with an increase in training load and may sometimes be exacerbated acutely. Occasionally, the tendon is injured by a fall on to a hard surface.

Examination reveals local tenderness and sometimes swelling or crepitus of the tendon, but otherwise the knee is unremarkable. There is often associated quadriceps muscle tightness, and occasionally bursitis of the superficial or deep infrapatellar bursa.

An ultrasound or MRI scan may show a defect within the proximal posterior part of the tendon.

Histologically, patellar tendinitis may involve a tenoperiostitis at the inferior pole of the patella, with advanced cases demonstrating a breakdown of the 'blue line' between mineralized and non-mineralized fibrocartilage. In others, evidence of degeneration of the tendon substance is seen with granulation of the tendon deep in its sheath. This degenerative change appears to coincide with the 'cystic' change seen on an ultrasound scan.

Acute tears are seen as disruption of the tendon with typical associated inflammatory changes.

Management relies on grading the injury (see Chapter 13) and applying active rest, ice and anti-inflammatory modalities and medications as appropriate. A thermal (heat retaining) sleeve may be useful. The synergists of the quadriceps muscles, the hip extensors and plantar flexors of the ankle should be exercised to reduce the load on the patellar tendon during rehabilitation. Remodelling of the connective tissue in the tendon can be enhanced by the use of eccentric exercises. This involves a 'drop squat' knee programme, with progression of the load on the knee induced by increases in the speed of drop of the body and by increases in the weight carried in the hands of the patient, for example, up to 5 kg in each hand (Curwin & Stanish 1984). With progress, the patient may jump (or 'drop') from a height of up to 40 cm, provided two-legged landing is used. Rehabilitation of a Grade 1 injury may take 6–8 weeks, and of a Grade 3 injury, 12–18 months.

Attention to biomechanical factors such as footwear, court or track surface, PFJ problems and taping of the patellar tendon is recommended.

Surgery to the tendon is indicated where conservative therapy has failed or where a significant degeneration of the tendon is demonstrated on ultrasound scan associated with symptoms. Rehabilitation using the techniques described is then prescribed for up to 6 months following surgery.

Pes Anserinus Bursitis

The pes anserinus ('goose foot') bursa lies deep to the common insertion of the tendons of the semitendinosus, gracilis and sartorius.

Repetitive injury to the bursa, through running in particular, produces a localized burning pain and tenderness, which may settle with rest and then be exacerbated by the next bout of exercise. Tight hamstrings, inadequate stretching, previous hamstring injury, and unaccustomed exercise such as hamstring strength training, may all predispose to pes anserinus bursitis.

Treatment comprises rest from painful activities, daily hamstring stretches and ice applications, anti-inflammatory medication, physiotherapy modalities and, occasionally, local infiltration of corticosteroid in persistent cases. Orthotics may be necessary for correction of contributory biomechanical faults such as overpronation of the foot or valgus knee alignment.

ACUTE KNEE INJURIES

The following discussion of acute knee injuries refers to the different ligamentous, meniscal, chondral and osteochondral lesions which are common in sport and, for the sake of clinical applications, patellofemoral dislocation and subluxation are also discussed. It is hoped that grouping these injuries together in this way will facilitate a better understanding of the acutely injured knee.

Anterior Cruciate Ligament Tear

Anterior cruciate ligament (ACL) rupture is one of the most disabling knee injuries for a sportsperson involved in 'pivoting and turning' activities such as basketball, football, netball and hockey (Fig. 20.9). A completely torn ACL in a young athlete who desires a return to competitive contact sports often requires surgical reconstruction and/or repair. Many ACL ruptures are missed during the initial diagnosis

and the feeling by many practitioners that the anterior drawer is important in diagnosis, clouds the early detection of this significant knee injury.

The ACL is intracapsular, covered by synovium and positioned within the intercondylar notch attaching proximally on the posterolateral femur with an oval-shaped 2 cm attachment and fans out in three bands to attach distally on the tibial spine (Fig. 20.10). The three bands of the ligament, that is anteromedial, intermediate and posterolateral, are taut in different degrees of knee flexion.

The ACL serves two main functions. The most important is to cause the 'screwing home' of the tibia on the femur by external rotation of the tibia on the femur as the knee extends. In the side-step, excessive internal rotation of the tibia occurs and the ACL is tightened. It is in this position that the

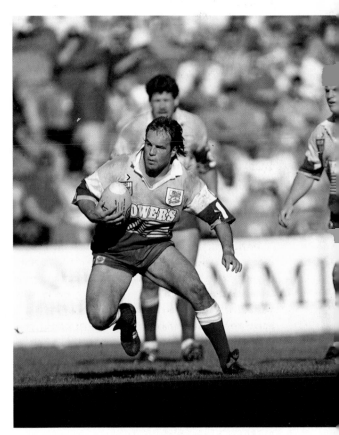

Fig. 20.9 Mechanism of injury of the anterior cruciate ligament. Deceleration associated with internal rotation of the tibia are two key factors involved.

Fig. 20.10 The anatomy of the anterior cruciate ligament.

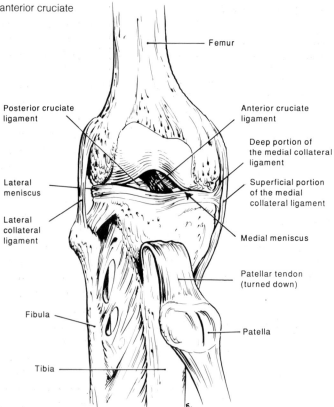

Femur

Posterior cruciate ligament

Anterior cruciate ligament

Deep portion of the medial collateral ligament

Superficial portion of the medial collateral ligament

Lateral meniscus

Lateral collateral ligament

Medial meniscus

Patellar tendon (turned down)

Fibula

Patella

Tibia

ACL is most commonly torn. Any forces acting against the 'screw home' mechanism compound the tear of the ACL. The second important function of the ACL is to resist anterior displacement of the tibia on the femur.

Less common mechanisms of injury include an external tibial rotation force, which causes a third degree tear of the tibial collateral ligament followed by a rupture of the ACL; a direct anterior drawer, particularly if assisted by a quadriceps contraction, such as a skier falling backwards; a varus force applied to the inside of the knee resulting in disruption of the lateral capsular structures, the fibular collateral ligament and the ACL; and a hyperextension force which causes disruption of the ACL first and then the posterior cruciate ligament (PCL).

The majority of people who present with an ACL tear state that they turned, pivoted or landed from a jump with a subsequent giving way. Many note an audible crack or pop at the time, followed by an immediate swelling (haemarthrosis) of the knee. Very occasionally a complete ACL tear will swell overnight or not at all. This history represents a ruptured ACL until proven otherwise.

The typical examination findings of an isolated acute rupture of the ACL are as follows:

- A painful knee
- A moderate to gross effusion of blood (haemarthrosis)
- Loss of extension of the knee, due to the bundle of the ACL within the intercondylar notch. This produces a 'soft end feel'
- Tenderness, which may be diffuse but most obvious over the posterolateral joint line due to lateral capsular tearing or lateral meniscus damage. Tenderness along the medial joint line may indicate an associated medial meniscus tear
- A negative anterior drawer
- Lachman's test positive, with a 'soft' or 'no'

Table 20.2 Clinical tests of knee injury

Lachman's test

The patient lies supine and relaxed with the knee supported and flexed to 30°. The examiner places one hand behind the upper tibia and the other over the front of the lower femur. The tibia is then brought anteriorly in a gliding fashion to test the integrity of the ACL. A positive test denotes ACL injury and allows excessive tibial excursion anteriorly and with no definite 'end-point'. To perform this test the examiner's left knee should support the patient's right thigh and vice versa. The examiner's 'femoral' hand can then fix the thigh on their knee while performing the Lachman's test on the tibia with the other ('tibial') hand.

Pivot shift test

The patient lies relaxed and supine. The patient's knee is then brought from full extension into full flexion repeatedly while held in valgus with internal rotation of the tibia. As the knee moves into flexion from full extension there is a 'clunk' and notable shift of the tibia posteriorly accompanied by external rotation.

McMurray's test (modified)

The patient lies relaxed and supine and the knee is brought from full flexion into extension while the tibia is circumducted with valgus stress to assess the lateral meniscus and varus stress to assess the medial meniscus. The test is positive if a painful click is elicited.

end-point (Table 20.2). Often a little increase in movement can be detected at this early stage

- 'Jerk' or 'pivot shift' test is positive in experienced hands with the patient relaxed (Table 20.2)

Many other tests exist to detect anterolateral instability, but all require a high level of expertise. It should be noted that 60–80% of acute haemarthroses are due to ACL lesions. X-ray examination of the knee is usually normal, although avulsion of the tibial spine in the younger patient, a Segond fracture (pathognomonic of a ruptured ACL), or depressed lateral tibial plateau may be present.

CONSERVATIVE MANAGEMENT OF ANTERIOR CRUCIATE LIGAMENT RUPTURE

This involves settling of joint effusion with anti-inflammatory medication and electrotherapy modalities, restoration of painless range of motion of the knee over 4–6 weeks with mobilizing tech-

niques applied to speed recovery, restoration of full muscle power (with emphasis on the closed kinetic chain in rehabilitation of muscle strength about the knee) and proprioceptive training, which includes running 'figures of eight', trampoline drills and side-stepping exercises.

Depending on the athlete's aspirations, one may then elect to gradually introduce the 'at-risk' sports, being aware of any minor episode of knee joint giving way and seeing this as a signal to decrease that activity and seek advice, or alter the way of playing the sport. For example, one may recommend not turning on the affected leg or advise altering the position of play, such as moving a right winger with a right-ruptured ACL to the left wing to allow pivoting mainly on the left leg, or suggest changing to a different activity, such as running, swimming or cycling.

Derotation braces are controversial, as it has been suggested that absolute laxity of an ACL-deficient knee is unchanged by the wearing of a derotation brace. By contrast others have found braces such as the Lenox Hill, the Don Joy and the Generation II to be useful in sports with relatively low-velocity twisting of the knee, such as tennis, squash and skiing, as well as in high-velocity sports such as ice hockey, field hockey and football. Practitioners should be aware that there are many inadequate knee braces on the market and care must be taken to prescribe an appropriate appliance.

If a conservative programme has been successful in allowing a patient to maintain sporting activity, a maintenance programme of exercises is required to ensure the best function.

In summary, patients opting for conservative management may:

- Maintain an adequate sporting activity and be happy with knee function
- Avoid surgical management even though they are unhappy with their level of activity
- Continue on to surgical reconstruction after failure of the knee in sporting or everyday activities
- Continue sport with frequent episodes of instability. This should be strongly discouraged by all treating practitioners, as recurrent insults

to the knee may damage the menisci and result in degenerative change of the articular cartilage (osteoarthritis)

SURGICAL MANAGEMENT OF ANTERIOR CRUCIATE LIGAMENT RUPTURE

ACL repair and/or reconstruction is preferred by many patients. The age of the patient, his or her sporting aspirations, anatomical make-up (particularly with relation to ligament laxity) and the stability of the other knee are all factors to be considered. Family history of ligament injuries and the personality of the patient are also important.

Procedures available to the surgeon include one or a combination of:

- Primary repair
- Intra-articular graft
- Extra-articular stabilization
- Allograft
- Synthetic ligament

These may be performed arthroscopically or via open joint surgery (arthrotomy).

Arthroscopic patellar tendon graft or hamstring (semitendinosus and gracilis) grafts sited arthroscopically are the most popular with those experienced in ACL surgery for both acute ruptures and chronic instability (Jackson & Jennings 1988).

After repair a prolonged rehabilitation period including all the points discussed under conservative management is undertaken.

CHRONICALLY UNSTABLE ANTERIOR CRUCIATE LIGAMENT DEFICIENT KNEE

Patients with a chronically unstable ACL-deficient knee complain of instability (i.e. knee giving way), pain, swelling or locking. Diagnostic signs are usually more obvious than in the acute rupture of the ACL and may include a positive anterior drawer test, a lack of 'end-point' to the Lachman test, a positive 'jerk' or 'pivot' test and perhaps signs of degenerative joint disease such as crepitus and compartmental pain on movement. There may also be signs of meniscal damage, and effusion may or may not be present.

Conservative management encompasses all the measures previously discussed for acute rupture of the ACL.

Arthroscopy may be required for partial meniscectomy or chondroplasty prior to full rehabilitation. An unstable knee may prevent successful meniscal repair.

The indication for ACL reconstructive surgery is instability on turning in sport or with day-to-day activities. At the time of writing there is the tendency toward performing the procedure arthroscopically using only patellar tendon grafting (Jackson & Jennings 1988). Rehabilitation is similar to the programme for acute repair or reconstruction.

Posterior Cruciate Ligament Tear

The PCL like the ACL is intra-articular but extrasynovial. It is twice as strong as the ACL, works reciprocally with the ACL, and is tightest in the mid ranges of motion. Because of its fan-shaped insertion, some parts of it are tight during each degree of knee motion. It becomes tighter with internal rotation of the tibia and it resists an anterior slide of the femur when the athlete is weight-

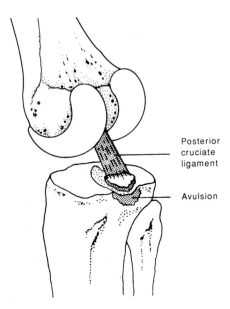

Fig. 20.11 Mechanism of injury of the posterior cruciate ligament. Hyperextension of the knee joint may produce an associated avulsion fracture of the tibial attachment of the posterior cruciate ligament.

bearing. The PCL also resists hyperextension and contributes to medial stability of the knee.

The two most common mechanisms of injury to the PCL are a direct blow to the anterior tibia in a flexed knee (Fig. 20.11), and during hyperextension of the knee.

The first mechanism is by far the most common. The athlete with this injury often presents later with secondary symptoms such as patellofemoral pain syndrome due to an increased patellofemoral stress, with the femur sliding forward on the tibia, or a feeling of 'giving way' when attempting to slow down from a run or when running downhill. Avulsion of the ligament at its tibial attachment is not uncommon.

Examination findings typically include a lack of haemarthrosis, as the ligament is extrasynovial and any blood tends to escape through an associated posterior capsular tear. This may cause calf pain and mimic a deep venous thrombosis. A delayed effusion is common.

There may be recurvatum of the knee ('bowing' of the leg backwards) particularly when the cause of injury is hyperextension, a posterior sag of the tibia (which may not be obvious initially) and a posterior drawer of the tibia. Again, this may not be obvious in the acute presentation as the posterior capsule may be intact and mask the drawer. With later stretching of this posterior capsule an obvious posterior drawer appears.

All such patients should have an X-ray to detect the rare cases of bony avulsion of the tibial insertion of the PCL and these cases may do well with primary surgical repair.

Many patients with a ruptured PCL present late with the symptoms of PCL insufficiency. These symptoms include persistent patellofemoral pain, medial joint line pain and tenderness related to shear stress in the medial compartment or an instability in attempting to decelerate.

An isolated PCL rupture may be treated conservatively achieving full range of movement of the knee by intensive quadriceps strengthening and improved hamstring flexibility. A graduated return to sport and a possible restriction of 'at-risk' sports such as distance running and 'stop–start' sports such as squash and netball should be considered.

Posterior cruciate surgical repair is usually reserved for cases where multiple ligament disruption has occurred, particularly if a third degree tear of the medial collateral ligament (MCL) exists, where there is an avulsion of the tibial spine, or if symptoms are unremitting after appropriate conservative care. PCL procedures, although becoming more popular, remain of variable success. Even so, with recent findings indicating that significant degenerative joint disease occurs with PCL insufficiency, these reconstructive procedures may become more common.

Medial Collateral Ligament Tears

The medial support structures of the knee consist of the deeper medial capsular ligament, with its attachment to the medial meniscus, and the more superficial, MCL.

The rugby player tackled from the side, two soccer players kicking the ball simultaneously and the downhill skier catching an inside edge of the ski are all likely to suffer a tear of the MCL. The two fundamental mechanisms of injury of the MCL are direct valgus force applied to the knee and external tibial rotation force. Most injuries to the MCL are due to a combination of these two forces.

It should be remembered that opening the medial side of the knee joint will also compress the lateral side; thus the lateral meniscus must always be checked as associated tears are not uncommon. Medial meniscal injury is rare and more likely to be meniscotibial ligament injury.

Tears of the MCL, like most other ligament injuries, can be divided into three degrees of severity and are as follows:

- First degree tear of the MCL (minimal numbers of fibres of the ligament torn and no laxity present). This is the most common downhill skiing injury but also occurs in the 'propping' sports like rugby, soccer and squash. The patient presents with a history of having twisted the knee, with medial pain exacerbated by further twisting. Swelling is usually not a problem, but if present, it is localized to the medial side of the joint at the site of the tear. Pseudolocking may occur due to hamstring spasm initiated by the pain from medial structures which tighten as the knee comes to full extension. Examination findings include a lack of effusion, pseudolocking of the knee, tenderness most commonly over the proximal MCL (at the medial femoral epicondyle above the joint line) and pain, but no laxity to the valgus stress test at 30° of knee flexion

- Second degree tear of the MCL. This injury may be produced by similar but larger valgus or external rotation forces with greater disruption of the ligament. Examination findings include a similar tenderness to the above but more localized swelling, a joint effusion due to capsular tearing and perhaps a small haemarthrosis. The valgus stress test at 30° of knee flexion shows laxity with an obvious end-point, and pain

- Third degree tear of the MCL. Under greater forces a complete tear of the medial structures occurs. Examination findings include marked tenderness, which is often more diffuse than is found with lesser degree tears, and a gross effusion, or no effusion due to its escape through large capsular tears. This may result in diffuse medial soft tissue swelling and obvious bruising.

Valgus stress at 30° of knee flexion lacks an end-point and is sometimes surprisingly painless because of the complete division of the ligament.

With these large forces it should be realized that a ruptured ACL is often present. Disruption of the PCL and the lateral ligament, along with fractures particularly of the lateral tibial plateau, may also occur. As such, a dislocation of the knee may have occurred with the risk of serious vascular damage.

MANAGEMENT OF MEDIAL COLLATERAL LIGAMENT TEARS

The management of the first degree tear of the MCL requires an initial healing time of 3–6 weeks, achievement of full range of motion with formal physiotherapy for full strength and proprioception, and maintenance of straight line activity. The patient should be encouraged not to twist on the knee, which is maintained by the patient using crutches at times when the knee is stressed. Within 2 weeks most patients are able to recommence some straight line exercise such as cycling or jogging on a smooth, flat surface.

Over the first 6 weeks as symptoms subside the patient is allowed gradual increases in activity and return to sport. This is facilitated by undertaking change of direction and 'cutting' drills, followed by specific sport skills at increasing levels of difficulty. Athletes required to kick 'side-on' (as in passing the ball at soccer) need careful evaluation before return to competition.

Management of a second degree tear is along similar lines to the above, although healing time may be longer. Second degree tears with significant laxity may benefit from the application of a limited range of motion brace for 4–6 weeks.

Management of third degree tears is contentious. Skill gained from experience in the management of this injury is required so as to assess those who can be managed conservatively and those to be managed surgically. Most third degree tears of MCL with an intact ACL progress well with conservative care. Some third degree tears, those with gross laxity or an avulsion fragment of bone, those with marked posteromedial structure disruption (indicated by marked tenderness in this area) or associated condyle fracture, may benefit from surgical repair. All require a limited range of motion brace from 4 to 6 weeks and then rehabilitation is as previously discussed for first and second degree tears.

Return to training for sport is recommended when there is:

- Full range of movement
- Full strength and proprioceptive function
- Minimal ligament tenderness
- Minimal symptomatology
- Pain-free stress to the end-point of knee joint movement
- Confident, pain-free running and changing direction

With the return to sport attention must be paid to maintenance of exercises for strength and proprioception, and accepted ligament healing time must always be heeded. This may be 12 months for full recovery.

PELLEGRINI-STIEDA DISEASE

A disruption of the femoral origin of the MCL may lead to heterotopic (abnormal) ossification in the proximal fibres (Fig. 20.12). The patient complains of marked pain and persistent tenderness medially with pain on twisting the knee, plus a restriction of both flexion and extension. Radiological changes become evident at 3–6 weeks, with obvious calcification at the proximal attachment of the medial ligament. Active mobilization of the joint is encouraged in this situation to prevent possible loss of range of motion. If gross calcification occurs this may require excision.

Lateral Collateral Ligament Tears

The lateral collateral ligament (LCL) provides resistance to varus stress on the knee and is usually more lax than the medial ligament.

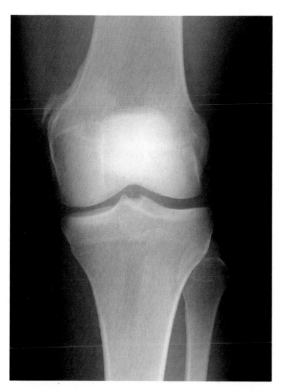

Fig. 20.12 Pellegrini-Stieda disease. This X-ray shows the typical calcification of the upper fibres of the medial collateral ligament of the knee following injury.

Tearing of the LCL is rare and is usually caused by direct varus force. First and second degree tears are managed along similar lines to first and second degree tears of the MCL. Third degree tears of the LCL typically involve disruption of associated structures and may result in external rotational knee recurvatum and posterolateral rotatory instability. The symptomatic knee with these instabilities often presents a difficult management problem.

It is important to note that with a rupture of the ACL, the posterolateral capsule is occasionally torn and thus specific tenderness is located at the posterolateral joint line. One must therefore be suspicious of an ACL rupture in the absence of a good history of LCL injury *per se*.

Internal Derangement

INJURIES TO THE MENISCI

Anatomically, the menisci are intracapsular structures which are attached to the tibia at the anterior and posterior horns of the intercondylar eminence and by the coronary ligaments to the tibial condyles. The middle third of the medial meniscus is closely attached to the joint capsule (deep layer of medial ligament) and is therefore less mobile than the lateral meniscus. The medial meniscus is 'C-shaped' and the lateral meniscus is more like an 'O'.

The most important function of the meniscus is as a load-bearing structure or shock-absorber. The integrity of the anterior and posterior horn attachments is important to help generate the 'hoop stresses' in the meniscus under load to provide this function. The complete removal of the meniscus (total meniscectomy) can result in an increased incidence of degenerative change due to loss of this load-bearing function, hence the modern tendency towards partial meniscectomy only or meniscal repair by suture. The menisci also reduce the disparity between femoral and tibial surfaces by acting as a wedge and thus help stabilize the joint. They also assist in articular cartilage nutrition and cushion hyperextension and hyperflexion by filling the triangular space between the periphery of the femoral and tibial condyles and the capsule, synovium and ligaments.

Meniscal nutrition is derived peripherally from a vascular plexus and centrally from synovial fluid. The middle third of the meniscus has a mixed nutritional supply. The vascular plexus extends deeper into the meniscus in young people and this is important when considering meniscus repair.

Medial meniscus tears

These usually occur in the posterior third of the medial meniscus, and in young people are of a longitudinal or vertical type often associated with major ligament injury, such as to the ACL. An incidence as high as 80% has been reported (Scott *et al.* 1986). With age, the meniscus becomes more brittle and tears more easily, especially with prolonged knee flexion such as in squatting, and flap tears and degenerative horizontal cleavage tears occur most commonly in this respect.

Lateral meniscus tears

The lateral meniscus is most often torn in its middle third in the form of radial, parrot-beak or flap tears and these can occur at any age. Horizontal cleavage and much less often, longitudinal vertical tears, also occur with ligament injury.

A tear of a meniscus occurs when the knee is forcibly flexed and twisted while weight-bearing. This can occur in football (tackling), netball, basketball and volleyball (landing from a jump) and skiing. As stated above, menisci can also be injured by prolonged squatting and rotating (which stresses the posterior horns in particular) or by overuse such as running long distances.

The single most important symptom of meniscal injury is pain localized to one side of the joint, which is made worse by activity. Patients with flap tears complain of catching or clicking, whereas patients with 'bucket-handle' tears complain of true locking and a sudden unlocking with a 'clunk', which relieves their pain. Meniscal tears may also cause swelling, buckling due to pain and wasting of the quadriceps.

The most important sign on physical examination is localized joint line tenderness on palpation and frequently there is also a small effusion. A bucket-handle tear may present as a 'locked knee' lacking full extension and flexion. McMurray's test (see Table 20.2) and Apley's compression test may also be positive. A pseudocyst may be observed on the lateral joint line at 45° of flexion due to a parrot-beak tear of the lateral meniscus (Cross & Watson 1981).

Posterior horn tears produce pain on full squatting, and asking the patient to squat and 'duck walk' often makes the diagnosis clear. There is rarely enough effusion to justify aspiration of knee joint fluid but if aspiration is performed the fluid is yellow 'reactive' fluid. In a major injury with significant swelling, there is also blood in the joint as this arises from a ligament tear. Plain X-rays do not demonstrate menisci and an arthrogram is reasonably accurate for both medial and lateral meniscus tears; however, CT arthrography may be a more accurate form of diagnosis. MRI is highly accurate for diagnosing meniscal tears but is expensive and not widely available. These tests are confirmatory and usually unnecessary with adequate history and experienced examination.

Figure 20.13 provides a classification and description of meniscal tears.

MANAGEMENT OF MENISCAL INJURY

When a patient presents with a recent onset of symptoms suggestive of a meniscal tear, conservative treatment may be appropriate. This consists of restriction of activity, and physiotherapy with electrotherapy modalities and a quadriceps exercise programme. After 4–6 weeks, if symptoms persist, orthopaedic referral and possibly arthroscopic surgery is appropriate.

With recent onset of true locking or a significant injury also involving ligaments, immediate orthopaedic referral is advised.

If there is a significant history of chronic or recurrent symptoms suggestive of meniscal pathology, arthroscopic surgery is indicated and usually involves resection of only the torn part of the meniscus. When performed arthroscopically this results in rapid recovery and early return to work or sport, with a decreased incidence of later degenerative change when compared with open knee surgery.

Meniscal repair has proved most successful in treating longitudinal acute tears in the vascular

Fig. 20.13 Types of meniscal injury.

1 *The medial meniscus*
   (Left) C-shaped
   The lateral meniscus
   (Right) O-shaped
2 *Flap tear*
   Common tear, usually medial occurring in late
   teens to old age
3a *Longitudinal vertical* (Partial thickness)
3b *Longitudinal vertical* (Full thickness)
   Are common with ACL injuries. May extend to
   a bucket handle tear and are frequently
   repairable by suture
4 *Bucket handle tear (BHT)*
   Can cause locking. Multiple BHT usually occur
   with chronic ACL instability
5 *Radial tear*
   A common tear on the lateral side and may be
   small or extend to the meniscosynovial junction.
   Can be associated with meniscal degeneration
   or meniscal cysts
6 *Horizontal cleavage*
   May be medial (usually in the older degenerative
   meniscal tear) or lateral (associated with ACL
   disruption)
7 *Complex tear*
   Long-standing tear with multiple pathology
8 *Meniscal cyst*
   Usually lateral and associated with a radial or flap
   tear
9,10 *Discoid meniscus*
   A vulnerable meniscus usually lateral. Is
   susceptible to tearing at a young age.
11 *Pseudocyst*
   Is unique to the lateral meniscus with a parrot beak
   tear causing the meniscus to bulge at 45° of
   flexion (Pseudocyst). (Cross & Watson 1979)

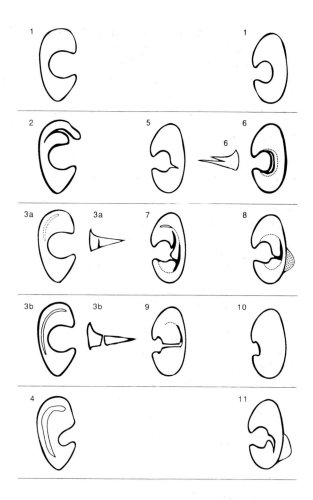

periphery of the meniscus in young individuals with stable knees, although other types of meniscal tears (radial, flap and complex tears) have been repaired. The long-term success of these types of repairs is less predictable. It is now commonplace for surgeons when performing anterior cruciate reconstructions to leave untouched small tears, particularly partial thickness, with the expectation that these will heal uneventfully.

CYSTS OF THE LATERAL MENISCUS

Cysts of the lateral meniscus can be removed as an open procedure via a small lateral skin incision, or removed arthroscopically by pushing a powered shaver through the body of the meniscus from within the joint and shaving out the contents of the cyst.

OSTEOCHONDRAL FRACTURE

Osteochondral fracture may mimic a meniscal tear. Examination findings may be very similar, although joint line tenderness tends to be more diffuse. The differentiation of these two diagnoses may be impossible without arthroscopic examination.

Osteochondritis dissecans

Osteochondritis dissecans may mimic a meniscal tear or PFJ pain. This condition develops usually between adolescence and the completion of growth and presents in three clinical phases. The first is that of a mildly irritable knee and is the reaction to early products of degeneration of the affected area of articular cartilage. The knee swells and aches after exertion and may be uncomfortable at night.

X-rays usually, but not always, reveal the lesion at this stage. The gradual separation of the fragment introduces the second clinical phase. When one edge is free the fragment may lift slightly and may thus cause catching, swelling and an increase in pain. By this time the X-rays are diagnostic. Once the fragment separates completely the picture is that of a 'joint mouse' with locking or mechanical catching. This condition is common and makes early X-ray examination of the painful swollen knee important, particularly in the younger patient. X-ray examination should include an intercondylar or tunnel view of the knee.

Management of this disorder can be assisted by bone scanning techniques to determine vascularity of the lesion and also by CT scanning to delineate more clearly the stages of development and separation outlined previously. If there is good blood supply evident on the bone scan, then conservative (non-surgical) management is indicated, whereas if separation of a fragment is seen on CT examination, surgery is indicated.

Conservative management depends on strict avoidance of painful activity with substitution of activities such as cycling and swimming to reduce load on the joint and to allow repair over a period of months. Serial X-rays are important in supervising this period. Graded return to activity with emphasis on strength and power development, proprioceptive function and regaining of sport-related skills is then instituted.

Arthroscopic internal fixation of a pedunculated or partially separated fragment may be indicated when first recognized and an orthopaedic opinion must be sought early. In later stages, arthroscopy may be necessary to remove loose bodies and attend to any cartilage defects.

The best results of treatment occur in the younger athlete, with juvenile osteochondritis. Although conservative therapy is usually effective, surgery may be indicated and should be performed before epiphyseal closure occurs to minimize the risk of degenerative change, which is seen more often in the skeletally mature adult.

Other causes of loose bodies include osteochondral fracture from a patellofemoral dislocation, a free meniscal tag, a fractured osteophyte and synovial chondromatosis.

Patellofemoral Instability

Patellofemoral instability is the most likely condition to mimic ACL rupture, resulting in recurrent instability, particularly in the young athlete. Patellofemoral instability may be gross where dislocation occurs, or subtle, with subluxation causing recurring episodes of instability with few ensuing clinical signs.

PATELLOFEMORAL DISLOCATION

Patellofemoral dislocation is a major knee injury with frequent continuing problems in the form of chronic patellofemoral pain syndrome, recurrent dislocation and loose body formation. Appropriate early management lessens these chronic problems.

The patella usually dislocates when the athlete twists, causing internal femoral rotation on the fixed tibia. Knee extension and/or valgus stress to the knee may exacerbate the force. Examples of this mechanism are a hook shot in cricket or suddenly turning on the knee in soccer. The patient states that he or she twisted and experienced a 'giving way' feeling with a subsequent deformity of the knee and severe pain with immediate swelling. The deformity is caused by the patella sitting laterally to the lateral femoral condyle. The dislocation may spontaneously reduce or require reduction.

Patellofemoral instability is often associated with hypermobility of joints or with a degree of 'malicious malalignment', as a result of femoral neck anteversion, genu valgus, hyperpronation of the feet, small flattened patella (patellar dysplasia), high patella (patella alta), a loose medial retinaculum and tight lateral retinaculum, shallow femoral groove (femoral trochlear dysplasia), poorly developed (dysplastic) vastus medialis and a wide Q angle ($>16°$ in males or $18°$ in females).

The assessment of each of these is important with regard to the likelihood of continuing problems and the best combinations of treatment methods. If the injured knee cannot be examined easily due to pain or swelling, one should examine the un-injured knee, looking for structural abnormalities which are most often bilateral.

Examination findings of patellofemoral dislocation include the following:

- A gross effusion (haemarthrosis) of the PFJ
- A tender medial retinaculum or medial border of the patella
- A lateral sitting patella
- An inability to contract the quadriceps
- An inability to flex the knee
- A positive apprehension test (Fig. 20.14)

Associated medial ligament tears are common with these injuries and it should be noted that the Lachman test has a solid end-point and the jerk/pivot shift test is negative, thus excluding ACL rupture.

Reduction of the dislocated patella should be achieved with as little force as possible and assisted by flexing the hip to relax the quadriceps and then by gradual extension of the knee. Relaxation or anaesthesia may be required. An X-ray, including anteroposterior, lateral and 20° skyline patellar views, is important to assess the possibility of a loose body which may require arthroscopic removal.

Initial management also involves aspiration of any haemarthrosis as it is inadvisable to leave a large amount of blood in the knee joint. Blood is chondrolytic and articular cartilage requires movement for nourishment. In the knee with a small effusion, protected movement may be achieved with the aid of a patellofemoral brace restricting the initial movement to 20°–60°. Once comfort is improved and swelling has decreased, further rehabilitation takes the form of gradual range of motion work and an intensive quadriceps strengthening programme concentrating specifically on the vastus medialis muscle and a gradual return to sport.

Sports should be restricted until full quadriceps rehabilitation has occurred and the knee is symptom-free with full range of motion and no effusion.

With return to sport a patellofemoral stabilizing brace is often required. Bracing may be provided in the form of a neoprene sleeve or a 'stocking' brace,

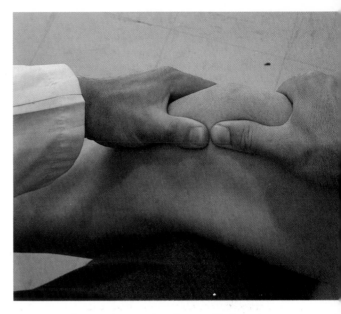

Fig. 20.14 The patellar apprehension test. The knee is flexed to 30° and moving the patella laterally elicits discomfort and a feeling by the patient that the patella will sublux or dislocate (as with episodes of the knee 'giving way').

with the selection being dictated by the sport involved. Braces do not offer any great resistance to the patella dislocating but may offer proprioceptive feedback, thus lessening subsequent dislocation after appropriate rehabilitation. If further dislocations occur with the use of a brace, or if dislocation becomes a problem with everyday activities, surgical reconstruction is appropriate.

Surgical management may comprise any combination of a lateral retinacular release (either arthroscopic or open), advancement of the vastus medialis, medial realignment of the tibial tubercle, altering patella height and plication of lax medial patellofemoral stabilizers (which may be performed arthroscopically or open).

PATELLOFEMORAL SUBLUXATION

Patellofemoral subluxation may be insidious and difficult to diagnose. It should always be suspected with a history of instability or a history of acute pain with turning on the leg. Diagnosis is achieved by eliciting a positive apprehension test (Fig. 20.14).

Management is as for rehabilitation of patello-femoral dislocation. Appropriate conservative management has a high level of success for subluxation of the patella; however, surgical management may be required if there are significant structural abnormalities.

OVERUSE INJURIES OF THE LOWER LIMB

Stress Fractures: General

Stress fractures are fatigue failure of bone as a consequence of overuse injury. McBryde (1976) defines stress fracture as a 'partial or complete fracture of bone due to its inability to withstand non-violent stress that is applied in a rhythmic, repeated subthreshold manner'.

Most stress fractures in athletes occur 3–5 weeks after a change in type or intensity of physical activity or training (Goldbert & Pecora 1994). This provides a signal for bone resorption and, if not enough rest is allowed to assist remodelling, a stress fracture may develop through the weakened bone. Similarly, muscle fatigue or dysfunction during the period of change in intensity may cause altered mechanics, permit greater applied stresses to the bone and failure of the protective function of the muscles.

Stress fractures occur at any site where the repetitive muscle action of sporting activity applies excessive stress to the skeleton. Thus, non-weight-bearing bones can be injured and present as first rib stress fractures in weight-lifters, or rib stress fractures in rowers for example. This highlights the fact that bones may be injured by means other than repetitive impact or shock absorption.

Some athletes exhibit individual biomechanical characteristics which predispose them to stress fractures. Greater bone bending moments, capable of causing stress fractures, have been noted in groups of athletes who have sustained stress fractures compared with matched groups who have not (Grimston & Zernicke 1993).

Most stress fractures occur in the lower limb and affect the tibia, tarsal bones, metatarsal bones, femur, fibula and sesamoid bones, in decreasing order of frequency (Matheson et al. 1987). Other sites of stress fracture include the lower lumbar spine, the ribs, humerus, radius and ulna.

Women athletes or dancers who have low body-weight and are amenorrhoeic appear to have a higher than normal risk of stress fracture (Kadel et al. 1992). This is discussed in more detail in Chapter 23.

The pain of a stress fracture initially presents acutely or subacutely and may be associated with a particular event or activity. Pain may then present after exercise only and disappears or eases after a short rest. If treatment is not undertaken the condition progresses so that pain is more marked after exercise and requires longer rest periods to settle. With further aggravation of the injury by continued repetitive activity the pain becomes worse during and after exercise and is only partially relieved by any amount of rest. The pain is often mechanical, occurring as the bone is stressed during the activity.

The pain may be localized to the area of injury or, if in a deeper structure such as the femur, may be more diffuse. There is focal tenderness and often some associated soft tissue swelling. If healing has commenced there may be callus palpable at the fracture site. Often there is an obvious limp and there may be muscle atrophy or weakness associated with the fracture. Adjacent joints are normal to examination.

Simple X-rays are rarely positive until 2 or 3 weeks after the onset of symptoms and at that time demonstrate the lesion in less than half the cases. On X-ray one may see a radiolucent line, periosteal or endosteal callus formation and soft tissue swelling.

Bone scanning, however, with technetium ^{99}m-labelled phosphate salts approaches 99% accuracy and can be positive as early as 2 or 3 days after the onset of symptoms.

CT scans may be useful in situations of doubt to exclude other pathology or to evaluate difficult sites of injury such as the tarsal navicular, the pars interarticularis or the neck of the femur.

The programme of management includes rest

from painful activities and substitution of non-impact or low stress (to bone) exercise such as swimming, cycling and fast wading in a swimming pool, to maintain cardiovascular and muscle fitness as much as possible. Ice and anti-inflammatory medication may be useful and electrotherapy modalities such as magnetic field therapy may assist bone healing. If biomechanical faults of the lower limb are considered to be contributing to the problem, then orthotic inserts may be necessary.

Once the symptoms have settled, gradual reintroduction of the activity should be undertaken over a 6–12 week period.

One must always be careful to consider other causes of bone pain such as infection, tumour, epiphyseal injury and referred pain and undertake appropriate investigations promptly to establish the diagnosis.

Stress Fractures of the Femur

Approximately 7% of all stress fractures occur in the femur (Matheson *et al.* 1987) and of these, about half occur in the femoral neck.

The mechanism of those occurring in the shaft involves increased bone tensile stress on the medial femoral cortex caused by bending of the bone with impact or muscular action by the adductors.

Stress fractures of the femoral neck may be divided into two main types: failure in compression (normally occurring on the inferior cortex) or tensile fractures (occurring on the superior cortex). Tensile fractures tend to be transverse, more rapidly propagated and more prone to complete fracture and displacement. This can result in aseptic necrosis of the femoral head. Compression stress fractures often occur as a result of heavy individuals subjecting themselves to high running mileage and these fractures tend to be oblique and more slowly propagated (Fig. 20.15).

Femoral shaft stress fractures produce a vague ache on the anterior or medial aspect of the thigh, made worse by running. Stress fractures of the femoral neck present with diffuse pain on the medial aspect of the thigh which may extend to the knee and sometimes to the groin, and are similarly aggravated by activity.

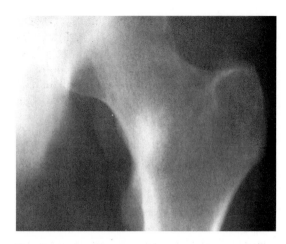

Fig. 20.15 A radiograph of the superior portion of the femur demonstrating a compressive oblique stress fracture of the femoral neck extending from the inferior cortex. This occurred in a 95 kg runner increasing his training distance suddenly from 30 to 70 km per week in preparation for running a marathon.

Fractures of both the femoral shaft and neck cause pain on internal rotation of the hip joint and those of the shaft characteristically show reproduction of the pain when the leg is supported at mid-thigh over the edge of the examination couch (the 'hanging leg' sign). If any doubt exists, pressure may be gently applied by pushing downward on both ends of the femur and reproducing the pain (Masters *et al.* 1986). Deep palpation of the femoral shaft may also elicit tenderness over the fracture site. A positive 'hop test' (hopping on the affected leg reproducing deep hip pain) is also found in a stress fracture of the femoral neck (Matheson *et al.* 1987).

Stress fractures of the inferior cortex of the femoral neck are treated by non-weight-bearing on crutches for a period of 3–4 weeks, progressing to partial weight-bearing (walking with stick) and then full weight-bearing according to symptoms. At the stage of partial weight-bearing the patient may be allowed to swim or 'run' in deep water while wearing a flotation vest. At the stage of walking with a stick the patient may be allowed stationary cycling within the limits of pain. Running may commence once the patient is able to walk 3 km without pain or limp, and then running is gradually increased with a session every 2–3 days.

It should be noted that if there is an area of increased uptake in the neck of the femur after a bone scan has been taken, a CT scan is indicated. If a complete fracture is evident the patient must be treated accordingly with immobilization and possible internal fixation of the fractured neck of the femur. The risk of displacement of the head of the femur is very real in this situation if it goes untreated.

Rehabilitation following a stress fracture of the femoral neck should involve a specific graded strengthening programme for the abductor musculature and individuals who are overweight should be counselled to lose weight before returning to a moderate to long-distance running programme.

Stress Fractures of the Tibia and Fibula

Over half the stress fractures seen in athletes occur in the leg and the majority of them are found in the tibia.

Tibial and fibular stress fractures occur most commonly in runners and dancers of all ages. The

pain is usually well localized and severe enough for sufferers to voluntarily cease activity before complete progression of the fracture. However, in anterior mid-shaft stress fractures of the tibia on the tension side of the bone, a complete fracture with displacement may occur during violent physical activity with very little warning.

Management is as outlined in the initial discussion on stress fractures and recovery usually takes place over 4–6 weeks. An 'Air-Cast' ankle brace can be very useful in the initial phase of weight-bearing until the patient can walk without a limp. Pulsed magnetic field therapy may also facilitate healing. Flexibility and strengthening of calf and anterior tibial muscles are important components of rehabilitation.

Stress Fractures of the Foot

Over a third of all stress fractures seen in runners occur in the feet. Most of these affect the second and third metatarsals, calcaneus and navicular (Fig. 20.16).

METATARSAL STRESS FRACTURES

The second metatarsal is subjected to the highest bone stress in the foot and is thus the most prone to stress fracture. This is because the base of the second metatarsal extends proximally into the distal tarsal row and is held stable and rigid (Fig. 20.16). If the first metatarsal ray is short (Morton's foot), the longer second metatarsal is subject to more stress and is therefore predisposed to stress fracture (Fig. 20.17).

The second metatarsal is also subject to more stress than usual if the forefoot is hypermobile, due to excessive and prolonged pronation, in which case the first and fifth metatarsals may move dorsally to avoid weight-bearing stress.

For these reasons, orthotic support and strengthening of extrinsic and intrinsic foot muscles are an important part of management and complement the treatment measures outlined previously.

A rare oblique stress fracture may occur at the base of the second metatarsal in ballet dancers and jumpers. This requires aggressive treatment, as it may develop delayed or non-union.

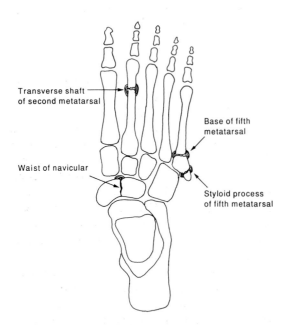

Fig. 20.16 Common sites of stress fractures in the foot.

Transverse shaft of second metatarsal

Base of fifth metatarsal

Waist of navicular

Styloid process of fifth metatarsal

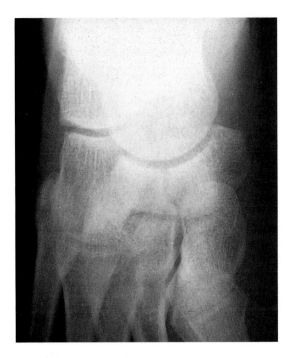

Fig. 20.17 A healing stress fracture of the shaft of the second metatarsal bone on an anteroposterior X-ray of the foot.

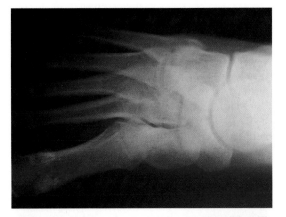

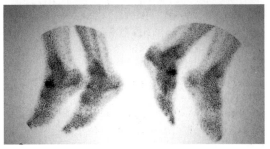

Fig. 20.18 (a) A plain X-ray demonstrating a stress fracture of the 'waist' of the navicular bone. (b) Stress fracture of the navicular bone as seen on a technetium-99m bone scan (delayed view).

Stress fracture of the proximal shaft of the fifth metatarsal just distal to the styloid process (Jones' fracture) also requires more radical treatment. This fracture does not unite readily and should be treated by immobilization in a non-weight-bearing plaster boot for 4–6 weeks. Delayed union may require longer application of a short leg cast. Medullary curettage and bone grafting, or internal fixation is essential in non-union.

NAVICULAR STRESS FRACTURES

Navicular stress fractures are notorious for their difficulty in diagnosis and management. Plain X-ray often misses an established fracture of this bone and a CT scan is essential if a bone scan is positive (Khan *et al.* 1992).

In nearly all cases the fracture is sagittal (Fig. 20.18a,b) and arises from the dorsal cortex of the navicular. The symptoms are often vague, with a dull ache over the dorsum and medial arch of the foot and local tenderness at the mid-point of the proximal border is typical.

Navicular stress fractures should be treated in a non-weight-bearing short leg cast for 8 weeks. If displacement, delayed union or non-union has occurred, bone grafting and/or internal fixation may be necessary, followed by 6–8 weeks in a non-weight-bearing cast. Upon removal of the cast, strapping of the foot, orthotics and a full rehabilitation programme, as outlined previously, is undertaken.

Inadequately treated, or missed, navicular stress fractures may proceed to complete fracture of the bone and result in avascular necrosis of the lateral fragment. This requires surgical management and a lengthy recovery.

COMPARTMENT PRESSURE SYNDROMES AND MEDIAL TIBIAL STRESS SYNDROME ('SHIN SPLINTS')

Soft tissue pain about the shin in endurance athletes is common (Clement *et al.* 1981). An understanding of such problems has led to the separation of true compartment pressure syndromes from the medial tibial stress syndrome.

Most compartment syndromes involve the lower leg, but it must be remembered that the posterior thigh, upper limbs and the shoulder muscles may also be affected (Ryan *et al.* 1987), and some reference will be made to upper limb conditions in this discussion.

A compartment pressure syndrome may be defined as a condition in which the blood flow and function of soft tissues within a closed space are compromised by increased pressure within that space.

Acute and chronic forms of compartment pressure syndrome exist. The acute form is most often related to trauma with or without muscle damage, and is not the form usually seen in sports medicine practice, while the chronic form of compartment pressure syndrome usually presents as exercise-related lower leg soreness.

The typical history of chronic recurrent compartment pressure syndrome is of a well localized tightness, with discomfort or pain of exercising muscles. This may occur during or after exercise and may last minutes to hours after activity. In a few cases, muscle pain and tightness is constant and made worse by any activity. There is typically no bruising or change of skin colour and peripheral pulses are normal. Some athletes relate a history of swelling of the particular muscle group involved, but this is usually not marked. By contrast flexor compartments of the forearms, however, may appear swollen after exercise and muscle tenderness is typical.

In some patients, the presenting complaint may be more of paraesthesiae affecting the anterior ankle and dorsum of the foot (by nerve compression) and occasionally a feeling of weakness with muscle tightness. The condition may be self-remitting over weeks to months or may gradually worsen until rest intervenes. With resumption of activity symptoms may return.

The commonest precipitating factors include a sudden increase in intensity and duration of muscle

Fig. 20.19 The muscle compartments of the lower leg.

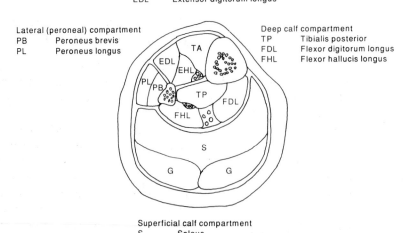

Anterior tibial compartment
TA   Tibialis anterior
EHL   Extensor hallucis longus
EDL   Extensor digitorum longus

Lateral (peroneal) compartment
PB   Peroneus brevis
PL   Peroneus longus

Deep calf compartment
TP   Tibialis posterior
FDL   Flexor digitorum longus
FHL   Flexor hallucis longus

Superficial calf compartment
S   Soleus
G   Gastrocnemius
    (medial and lateral)

activity or, in runners and court sports players, more time being spent on harder surfaces. Biomechanical factors play a role in the aetiology of compartment pressure syndrome and the use of new equipment (including shoes or boots) must be considered.

During exercise, an increase in transcapillary filtration of intravascular fluid occurs, which is not compensated for by increased drainage. As a consequence the volume of skeletal muscle may increase by as much as 20% during exercise (Levick & Fricker 1993). Symptoms and signs vary depending on the response of the particular compartment to this physiological process.

It is pertinent to consider the different anatomical compartments here (Fig. 20.19).

Anterior Compartment Pressure Syndrome

The anterior tibial compartment contains the tibialis anterior, extensor digitorum longus and extensor hallucis longus muscles, together with the anterior tibial artery and vein and deep peroneal nerve. The muscles are confined within a tight fascial envelope, including the interosseous membrane posteriorly. Exercise induces local compartment pain, tenderness and some dysfunction of the muscles, all of which tend to be resistant to attempts at 'running through the pain'. There may also be numbness of the first web space of the foot.

Lateral Compartment Pressure Syndrome

Similarly the lateral compartment of the lower leg, containing the peroneus longus and brevis muscles, may present with exercise-induced pain, tenderness and some dysfunction because of a tight fascial envelope.

Both anterior tibial and peroneal compartment syndromes are a result of abnormally elevated intracompartmental pressures.

Deep Calf Compartment Pressure Syndrome

The deep calf muscle compartment, containing the

tibialis posterior, flexor hallucis longus and flexor digitorum longus muscles, can also produce symptoms of exercise-induced pain and tenderness, and as such, is a true compartment syndrome with elevated compartment pressures which persist after exercise.

Tibialis Posterior Compartment Pressure Syndrome

In addition the tibialis posterior muscle may develop its own compartment pressure syndrome because of a separate fascial envelope. This must be distinguished from the medial tibial stress syndrome (periostitis) on the basis of bone scan findings and pressure studies.

Superficial Calf Compartment Pressure Syndrome

The fifth muscle compartment of the lower leg contains the gastrocnemius and soleus muscles: the superficial calf compartment. This may produce a compartment pressure syndrome as previously described with local pain, tenderness and dysfunction of the calf. Pressure studies also show abnormal readings in this compartment.

Compartment pressure syndrome may affect more than one compartment and symptoms are often bilateral and symmetrical.

Diagnosis and Management of Compartment Pressure Syndrome

The diagnosis of compartment pressure syndrome revolves around the measurement of intracompartmental pressures and several methods have been devised.

Styf and Korner (1987) recommend a range of resting pressure from 0 to 10 mmHg, returning to normal within 10 min of rest after exercise, as the reference for diagnosis. Pressures above this range are diagnostic of compartment pressure syndrome. However, one should be aware that compartment pressures can be normal in the presence of diagnostic symptoms and signs, and treatment including fasciotomy or fasciectomy should never be withheld on the basis of normal pressure studies alone.

Treatment of compartment pressure syndrome varies. Conservative measures include active rest, that is, easing up on workloads involved, followed by a gradual increase in workload over a period of weeks to months to allow for 'conditioning' and adaptation of the injured muscles, tendons and fascial attachments. Massage and anti-inflammatory medication, regular applications of ice, muscle stretching and strengthening exercises, orthotic devices, heat-retaining 'thermal protectors', physiotherapy modalities, massage and anti-inflammatory medication all have a role in management.

However, it is becoming increasingly clear that fasciotomy is the definitive treatment for compartment pressure syndrome in its usual, chronic form. Various studies (Detmer et al. 1985) report high percentages of success where athletes have returned to sport within weeks of surgery which has split the fascial sheath of the offending muscle compartment with minimal disturbance of other anatomical structures. Relapses are few and may be attributed to insufficient fasciotomy (or fasciectomy) or scarring and/or healing of the fasciotomized fascia in most instances. Occasionally, ischaemic changes to muscle have occurred prior to surgery, limiting full recovery.

Medial Tibial Stress Syndrome ('Shin Splints')

By contrast, the medial tibial stress syndrome involves the deep calf muscle compartment containing the tibialis posterior, together with the (separate) compartment containing the flexor hallucis longus and the flexor digitorum longus (and posterior tibial artery and veins, tibial nerve and peroneal artery and veins). These muscle compartments can expand with exercise and produce traction of the fascia around the compartments at the fascial attachment along the medial tibial border. This results in a typical pain and tenderness along the medial tibial edge; described as the medial tibial (stress) syndrome or, rather more generally, medial tibial 'shin splints'. Often there is accompanying tenderness of the posterior tibial tendon. A bone scan using technetium ^{99}m isotope may reveal evidence of a periostitis at the fascial attachment described, which must be distinguished from a stress fracture.

In the context of pressure studies, the medial tibial stress syndrome stands out as being generally a 'normal pressure' problem. The periosteal reaction evident on bone scan indicates stress at the fascial attachment and the concept of raised compartment pressure during exercise (and not prolonged thereafter) may fit this clinical picture. Another explanation of normal pressure studies may be that the symptomatic compartment in the calf may not be the one measured through technical error in placement of the pressure monitor catheter (Hannaford 1988).

Treatment of the medial stress syndrome is similar to that for the compartment pressure syndrome which affects the deep calf, and relies on modifying painful activities, maintaining calf strength and flexibility and employing the various anti-inflammatory measures available through medication and physiotherapy. Attention to biomechanical factors of the foot and ankle is also advised as appropriate correction of overpronation for example may affect rapid relief. Surgery to release the fascia at its attachment along the medial tibial border is indicated where measures as outlined previously are unsuccessful.

ACUTE INJURY TO THE LEG

Calf Muscle Strains (Gastrocnemius, Soleus)

The calf muscle is made up of the gastrocnemius muscle superficially and the soleus muscle below it. The plantaris, a small rudimentary muscle with a long tendon passes obliquely (laterally to medially) between the gastrocnemius and soleus muscles. All these muscles insert into, and form, the Achilles tendon.

Because the gastrocnemius muscle crosses two joints (the knee and the ankle), it is prone to injury, particularly when 'caught' between active contraction and stretch during running, jumping and landing.

Most calf strains occur at mid-belly, at the musculotendinous junction or at the origin (usually the medial head) of the gastrocnemius muscle. The soleus is rarely injured. Injury is usually acute and often dramatic. A lunge at tennis or squash, or a sudden sprint or change in direction at soccer, football or basketball, results in acute local pain, tenderness and swelling followed by bruising over the next few days. Calf muscle strain may also occur as an acute event in muscles that are fatigued or stiff from overuse, such as in marathon runners who have increased training distances and not allowed adequate time for recovery.

Muscle strains, at Grades 1, 2 or 3 level of severity, are treated in the same way as other soft tissue injuries, with rest from painful activities, daily applications of ice, anti-inflammatory medication, electrotherapy modalities and stretching and strengthening of the injured muscle as recovery takes place over 10 days to 6 weeks.

Eccentric muscle exercises such as 'drops' — standing backwards on a step and lowering the body to below the level of the step quickly, and then raising up slowly — are most important, and a heel raise can also be very effective in the first few weeks of recovery.

Return to full activity or competition should not be undertaken until the calf has regained full length, is pain-free when hopping and has full strength and power.

Achilles Tendon Injuries

A classification of Achilles tendon injuries is shown in Table 20.3.

The Achilles tendon is the common tendon of the gastrocnemius and soleus muscle of the superficial compartment of the calf. The tendon twists as it descends, rotating laterally, from 12 to 15 cm above the insertion where the soleus begins to contribute fibres to the tendon. This twisting produces a concentration of stress in the tendon from 2 to 5 cm above its insertion where rotation is most pronounced; in effect there is a 'sawing' action of one part of the tendon on the other. This area also has the least blood supply to the tendon.

At the insertion there are two bursae: a subcutaneous retro-Achilles bursa; and a retrocalcaneal bursa between the os calcis and the Achilles tendon.

Table 20.3 Classification of Achilles tendon lesions

Type of injury	Subtype of injury
Rupture	Complete
	Partial
	Laceration
Focal degeneration	
Tendinitis	Calcific
	Chondritic
Peritendinitis	Acute
	Chronic
Mixed lesions	
Origin/insertion lesions	Musculotendinous junction
	Insertion
Associated structures	Bursitis
Other mechanisms	Rheumatic
	Metabolic
	Infection

Adapted from Williams (1986).

The epitenon and paratenon are referred to collectively as the peritendon. This is not a synovial sheath and as such cannot produce a 'tenosynovitis'.

The Achilles tendon is subject to various forces, all of which may compound stress through the 'twisting' tendon at its point of decreased blood supply. The history of injury distinguishes the acute partial tear from chronic degeneration of the tendon. Nodular thickening of the tendon which moves with plantar flexion and dorsiflexion of the ankle suggests a tendon lesion such as a tear or focal degeneration. A nodule which does not move with ankle movement suggests a peritendinitis instead.

Factors in the aetiology of injury include inappropriate footwear (lack of rearfoot support or excessive lateral heel flare), terrain (cambered surfaces), excessive training loads, or particular strength training or conditioning programmes being employed which involve the Achilles tendon, and biomechanical factors of the foot and leg. A simple biomechanical assessment of the heel and forefoot is useful as overpronation, rearfoot varus or valgus, pes cavus and supination, and tight gastrocnemius and soleus muscles, may benefit from orthotic correction and appropriate stretching and strengthening exercises.

Assessment of the tendon and its associated structures is assisted by an ultrasound scan to delineate tendon morphology, in particular the presence of swelling, degenerative 'cysts', calcification, tears and associated bursitis. There may be the need to exclude rheumatological conditions such as the seronegative arthropathies (Reiter's disease, ankylosing spondylitis, etc.) or gout and serum uric acid estimation, and the presence of HLA-B27 histocompatibility antigen may be useful.

Recovery from chronic Achilles tendinitis takes time. A Grade 1 tendinitis implies a 6 week programme of rehabilitation, with Grades 2 and 3 requiring significantly longer.

Treatment involves active rest, daily ice applications, anti-inflammatory medication and electrotherapy modalities, the use of a heel raise (1–1.5 cm) to 'rest' the affected tendon, orthotics as necessary and a gentle stretching programme for the gastrocnemius and soleus muscles and the tendon.

The use of corticosteroids is controversial and should be limited to single doses at or around the tendon (never into the tendon) to settle inflammation. This minimizes the well-documented risk of tendon rupture secondary to the softening effect of corticosteriod, which may last for 14 days (Kennedy & Baxter-Willis 1976).

Eccentric stretching and loading of the tendon is a very useful means of rehabilitation once inflammation is controlled. This technique involves the patient lowering or dropping his or her bodyweight over the edge of a support — such as, by standing backwards on the edge of a step and 'dipping' slowly and then returning to a neutral stance repeatedly. Pain determines the rate of progress in the number of repetitions and speed of drop. It has been suggested that such eccentric work promotes collagen laydown along the lines of stress in the tendon, contributing to enhanced elasticity and tendon function (Curwin & Stanish 1984).

Treatment of associated bursitis includes the previously mentioned therapies, but corticosteroid injection with ultrasound or short-wave diathermy may be especially useful. Very occasionally surgery for chronic bursitis and/or the associated Haglund's deformity of the superior aspect of the calcaneus is indicated.

TENDON RUPTURE

The typical presentation of acute tendon rupture is by a male aged approximately 40 years or more with a history of acute pain in the calf (as if whipped or shot) while playing squash or tennis.

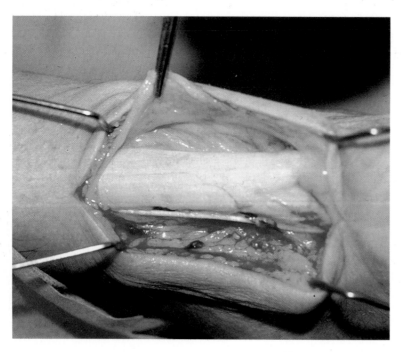

Fig. 20.20 The appearance of a partial tear of the Achilles tendon during surgery. (Courtesy of Allan McGavin Sports Medicine Centre, UBC, Vancouver.)

Kannus and Josza (1991) found all tendons have pre-existing pathology before spontaneous rupture, despite the fact that two-thirds of the patient population are asymptomatic prior to the event. Examination of the patient lying prone and relaxed reveals a notable lack of plantar flexion of the foot on the affected side when the calf muscle is squeezed firmly and briskly (Thomson's test). Ultrasonography can be very useful in the assessment of an injured tendon, and can distinguish partial from complete tears.

The management of a complete tear consists of immediate referral to a surgeon or, if this is not possible, application of a plaster cast below the knee with the foot plantar flexed to 30° for a period of 4 weeks, followed by reapplications of casts to bring the foot back to 90° of dorsiflexion over the following 1 or 2 months. Intensive rehabilitation should then follow to regain muscle and tendon length, strength and function. Surgical repair is the preferred option for the younger elite athlete; however, older, 'recreational' sportspeople achieve good function from conservative management.

SURGERY TO THE TENDON

Surgery is indicated for partial Achilles tendon rupture which is either acute or chronic (Fig. 20.20), adhesive peritendinitis where a thickened peritendon compromises the tendon which is usually inflamed and, depending on the individual surgeon's preference, complete tendon rupture. Rehabilitation then follows for 3–8 weeks for peritendinous problems, or up to 6–8 months for intratendinous lesions (Inglis *et al.* 1976).

ANKLE INJURIES

The ankle joint consists of the ankle mortise and the trochlea or dome of the talus and is essentially a hinge joint. As the ankle joint moves into plantar flexion the narrower posterior part of the trochlea is less stable in the mortise, and this predisposes the ankle to injury.

Three groups of ligaments provide stability to the ankle joint (Fig. 20.21a–c) and are as follows:

- The lateral ligament complex
- The medial (deltoid ligament)
- The syndesmosis

Ankle Sprains

Inversion sprains of the ankle are among the most common acute sporting injuries, comprising 20–25% of all time-loss injuries in every running or jumping sport. Sports which involve landing after difficult manoeuvres or contact in the air, such as

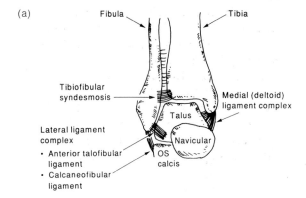

(a)

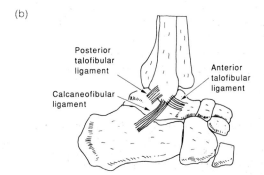

(b)

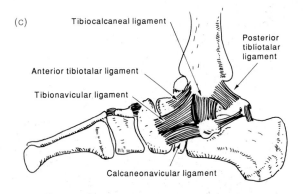

(c)

Fig. 20.21 (a) The three main ligaments of the ankle (anterior view). (b) The lateral ligament complex of the ankle (lateral view). (c) The medial (deltoid) ligament of the ankle (medial view).

soccer, Australian football, basketball, netball and volleyball, show a particularly high incidence. Other sports such as rugby and squash where rapid changes of direction are a feature of the game, and sports played on uneven surfaces, such as orienteering or field games played on poorly prepared surfaces, also contribute to such injuries.

The mechanism of injury is usually by inversion and plantar flexion of the foot when landing off balance or clipping another player's foot. This most commonly injures the anterior talofibular ligament; however, further force may also tear the calcaneofibular ligament and on occasions the posterior talofibular ligament. The musculotendinous units acting as dynamic joint stabilizers may also be injured, particularly the peroneal muscles and tendons.

Individuals with varus malalignments of the lower limbs (e.g. tibial varum), calf muscle tightness and those who have sustained previous incompletely rehabilitated ankle sprains (in particular, those left with subtalar joint restriction) are predisposed to this injury.

Less commonly, the strong deltoid ligament is injured in an eversion–abduction injury. The force required to produce such an injury is great and a fracture is more likely to occur.

Significant ligament rupture allows tilting of the talus in the ankle mortise on inversion stress. If this tilt is 7° greater than the uninjured ankle it is considered diagnostic of ligamentous instability and is evident on a 'stress' X-ray. A useful clinical assessment of ligament laxity is the anterior drawer test (Figs 20.22 and 20.23).

Plain X-rays should always be taken to exclude a fracture or epiphyseal injury in the younger athlete and management of ankle sprains incorporates the RICE (rest, ice, compress, elevate) protocol (see Chapter 13) until inflammation subsides and then varies according to the severity of the injury.

GRADE 1 (MILD) SPRAINS

These usually affect the anterior talofibular ligament, and occasionally the calcaneofibular ligament by inversion and there is minimal instability in this situation. The anterior drawer test to the ankle is normal and 'stress' X-rays show no talar tilt.

Treatment is carried out by encouraging early active movement often in conjunction with cryokinetics (see Chapter 13) as well as stationary cycling and then walking supported by protective taping or a semi-rigid brace, anti-inflammatory medication, electrotherapy modalities and strengthening exercises for the ankle everters. Daily proprioceptive exercises such as one-legged standing and balancing with eyes closed and exercises on a balancing board ('wobble board') or rebounder should also be done. Ligamentous recovery should take place over approximately 6 weeks; however, return to sport is usually possible between 1 and 2 weeks. Rehabilitation involves a functional progression of running, jumping, hopping, swerving and cutting. The achievement

Fig. 20.22 Performing of the anterior drawer test for the ankle.

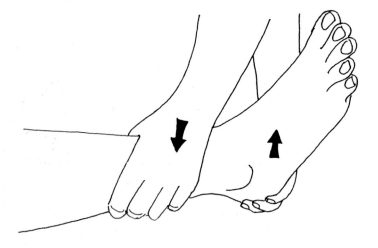

Fig. 20.23 An alternative method of performing the anterior drawer test for ankle instability. The foot is fixed firmly on the examination couch and the examiner then gently takes hold of the lower tibia, carefully avoiding the tender areas and gently pushes the lower tibia posteriorly on the fixed foot.

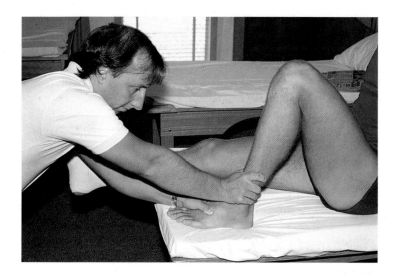

of full talocrural dorsiflexion and subtalar motion combined with the ability to hop pain-free and balance while throwing and catching should demonstrate a satisfactory outcome of treatment and permit a return to sport.

GRADE 2 (MODERATE) SPRAINS

These usually comprise complete tears of the anterior talofibular ligament with some damage to the calcaneofibular ligament. There may be some laxity of the joint capsule to anterior drawer and if X-rays are taken for talar tilt, these show little if any abnormal talar motion. Initial treatment may require 5 days of non-weight-bearing with the ankle taped or in a brace or cast, followed by rehabilitation as outlined for Grade 1 sprains, as pain permits.

GRADE 3 SPRAINS (SEVERE)

These are uncommon. They are dramatic and there is obvious laxity on an anterior drawer test, evident talar tilt on 'stress' X-rays and often an associated fracture and peroneal muscle and tendon injury. Management entails non-weight-bearing initially followed by limited weight-bearing in a brace for up to 6 weeks depending on pain and associated swelling, followed by aggressive rehabilitation as outlined previously.

Surgical reconstruction of an ankle may be performed with excellent results if conservative therapy

has failed. Late instability problems may also involve the subtalar joint and treatment should be directed appropriately.

Sprains of the medial (deltoid) ligament are treated along the same principles as for the lateral ligament injuries.

Small avulsion or chip fractures can be treated in the same manner as ankle sprains, but larger fractures must receive appropriate orthopaedic management.

Careful examination must be made of the X-rays, and if symptoms persist, further X-rays or bone scans may be necessary to exclude other injuries such as a fracture of the base of the fifth metatarsal (avulsed by peroneus brevis), a fracture

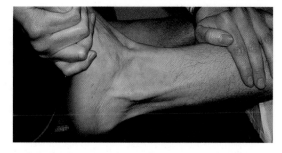

Fig. 20.24 Subluxation of the peroneal tendons over the lateral epicondyle. The subluxation is reproduced by attempting to evert further the foot against resistance from an already everted position

of the anterior process of the calcaneus (avulsed by the bifurcate ligament), or a talar dome fracture (see below).

Prophylaxis for ankle sprains has in the past been a subject of some considerable discussion. Although expertly applied athletic tape is effective in reducing the incidence and severity of ankle sprains, it appears that, particularly after the initial stages of an athletic competition or training session, the modern, non-stretch ankle braces are also effective in this regard (Shapiro et al. 1994). High top boots, if properly laced, also appeared to offer some increased protection over more low-cut designs.

Syndesmosis Ankle Sprains

Injuries to the ankle (tibiofibular) syndesmosis may appear benign initially but often cause considerable disability and require a long recovery period (Taylor & Bassett 1993). The normal mechanism of injury involves internal or external rotation of the weight-bearing foot on the ankle. Weight-bearing is immediately and significantly impaired. There is often minimal swelling, but tenderness over the anterior inferior tibiofibular ligament (often extending proximally up the interosseous membrane (Fig. 20.21a), and ankle range of motion is characteristically limited in dorsiflexion because of pain. Pain may also be reproduced by squeezing the fibula and tibia together at the mid-shaft. Delayed X-ray findings may include heterotopic ossification in the interosseous membrane as early as 4 weeks post-injury.

Grade 1 and 2 injuries are treated with an aggressive functional rehabilitation programme using the RICE principles and taping or an 'Air-Cast' to help stabilize the syndesmosis. Partial weight-bearing only may be necessary in Grade 2 injuries. Grade 3 injuries (diastasis) require referral to an orthopaedic surgeon for anatomical reduction of the talus in the ankle mortise. Typically, a weight-bearing X-ray view shows widening of the ankle mortise. Treatment in this instance may involve cast immobilization but often requires internal fixation with one or two screws.

Recovery times are often at least twice that of a lateral ankle sprain and in particularly high demand athletes, even with a Grade 2 injury, persistent pain and inability to push off on the toes because of pain, may require internal fixation.

This injury may proceed to a bony fusion between the distal tibia and fibula (synostosis). This significantly limits dorsiflexion and may be particularly disabling in certain sports. Often resection of the synostosis is required.

Peroneal Tendon Injuries

The peroneal tendons are important dynamic stabilizers of the ankle and are intimately related to the lateral ligament complex. The peroneal muscles are weak plantar flexors and strong everters of the foot.

Rarely, forced dorsiflexion of the ankle causes rupture of one or both of the tendons. More often, subluxation or dislocation of the peroneal tendons occurs and involves partial or complete rupture of the superior peroneal retinaculum and 'derailing' of the tendons from their pulley posterior to the lateral malleolus. Often the groove for the tendons in the posterior lateral malleolus is shallow or absent. The mechanism of injury is normally that of passive dorsiflexion, with slight eversion or inversion combined with violent reflex contraction of the peroneal muscles. Sprinting on uneven ground may produce such a mechanism without an inversion sprain of the ankle. Peroneal tendon injury may occur in football, basketball, ballet or in skiing and, if untreated, considerable disability (not simply limited to sporting activity) can result.

On examination there is often marked swelling and tenderness over the posterior part of the lateral malleolus. Subluxation may be reproduced by resisted extreme plantar flexion with eversion or resisted dorsiflexion with eversion (Fig. 20.24).

Occasionally, particularly in the case of subluxation, ankle strapping with adhesive, non-stretch tape and a pad over the lateral malleolus is successful. If soft tissue swelling is not too pronounced, a well-moulded, short non-weight-bearing cast may be very effective. If subluxation or dislocation is chronic or recurrent, surgical reconstruction is highly successful. This is followed by the application of a non-weight-bearing cast for 4 weeks and then by a graded rehabilitation programme similar to that for ankle sprains.

Rupture of a peroneal tendon requires surgical correction and a postoperative rehabilitation programme.

Disabling tendinitis of the peroneal tendons occurs in dancers, basketball players and volleyball players. It is related to the pulley action of the lateral malleolus on the tendons and may be the result of foot malalignment.

Treatment of peroneal tendinitis depends upon reduction or cessation of painful activity and temporary use of a lateral heel wedge. In severe cases the use of crutches and oral anti-inflammatory agents in addition to local cold therapy and physiotherapy modalities may be necessary. Injection with corticosteroid into the tendon sheath should be reserved for extremely recalcitrant cases. A graded programme of return to activity is mandatory with avoidance of rapid change of direction or sprinting

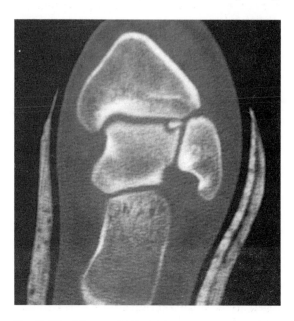

Fig. 20.25 CT scan of a Type IIA talar dome injury to the lateral edge of the talar dome (with subchondral cyst formation characteristic of a Type IIA lesion). This often causes significant ankle pain and aching post-activity following resolution of other symptoms of an ankle sprain. It usually requires arthroscopic treatment involving curettage of the cystic material and chondroplasty of any associated chondral flap tear (Shea & Manoli 1993).

for at least 6 weeks. Tenolysis of the peroneal tendons is reserved for chronic tenosynovitis that fails to respond to conservative management.

Talar Dome Fracture

Talar dome fractures are more common than previously realized and occur in approximately 6% of cases of persisting pain and disability following ankle sprain. They may present acutely or, more commonly, as a chronic sequela to ankle sprain. Compression or shearing force on the dome of the talus may damage the subchondral bone causing varying grades of bone injury, from symptomatic bone oedema to late separation and displacement of an osteochondral fragment. Anderson *et al.* (1989) proposed a staging system of talar dome fracture, from Stage I to Stage IV. Stage I implies subchondral trabecular compression. Stage II denotes incomplete separation of an osteochondral fragment and Stage IIA signifies resorption of necrotic trabeculae and the formation of a cyst. Stage III heralds the appearance of an unattached, undisplaced fragment of bone and cartilage. Stage IV is the end-point whereby a displaced fragment is evident.

Talar dome fracture may cause chronic pain, weakness, catching and a feeling of ankle instability. Early X-rays may be apparently negative and greater diagnostic accuracy can be achieved with a repeat X-ray at 6 weeks. Bone scans are positive with intense isotope uptake on either the medial or lateral edge of the talar dome and the bony injury can be confirmed and graded using a CT scan or MRI (Fig. 20.25). Osteochondritis dissecans with minimal or no definite trauma may result in a similar lesion in the adolescent or pre-adolescent athlete. In cases of separation of an osteochondral fragment, surgical removal of the loose body with arthroscopy or arthrotomy may be necessary with curettage of the defect.

Ankle Impingement Syndromes

ANTERIOR IMPINGEMENT

Repetitive traction or injury to the ankle joint capsule is believed to produce exostoses, which develop on the anterior margin of the tibia at the

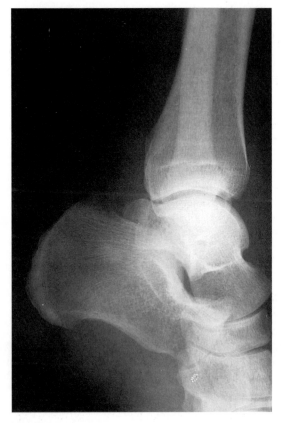 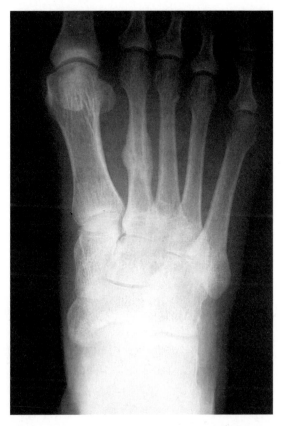

Fig. 20.26 (a) Lateral view on X-ray of an ankle and foot showing an os trigonum (posterior to the ankle joint). Plantar flexion of the ankle catches the ossicle between the os calcis and tibia and produces pain. (b) Posterior impingement of the ankle. This lateral X-ray is taken in forced plantar flexion. In this case posterior impingement is caused by a large posterior talar spur.

ankle and on the opposing area of the neck of the talus. These are commonly seen in soccer players, American and Australian footballers (from kicking and sliding on the ground with feet plantar flexed and under the body) and in basketballers and ballet dancers (from jumping and landing).

The anterior ankle is tender and sometimes stiff and painful after activity. Forced dorsiflexion at the ankle reproduces the pain but full range of movement is usually present.

X-rays, which should include a lateral view in forced dorsiflexion, demonstrate the impingement and exostoses, and may also detect exostoses which have become detached to form loose bodies within the joint.

Treatment such as talocrural mobilization and local massage and electrotherapy modalities is often successful with modified activity, anti-inflammatory medication and perhaps corticosteroid injection, but surgery may be indicated and includes excision of exostoses and removal of any loose bodies.

POSTERIOR IMPINGEMENT

Similar exostoses can be found in the posterior aspect of the ankle joint. These may be congenital, however, and usually take the form of a talar spur (trigonal process) or a separate un-united ossification centre of the talus, an os trigonum (Fricker & Williams 1979). Both of these may coexist in the ankle. Ballet, kicking footballs, kicking during swimming and fast bowling in cricket may all produce an impingement, where the talar process or os

468

trigonum behaves like a nut in a nutcracker (Fig. 20.26a,b). Posterior ankle joint pain is experienced on forced plantar flexion of the ankle, and there may be deep local tenderness at the posterior talus. Bone scanning may show increased isotope uptake at the site of a fracture of a talar spur.

Treatment includes avoidance of plantar flexion and inflammatory measures. Surgery is indicated in difficult cases to excise the os trigonum or talar spur. Recovery is usually prompt and complete.

FOOT INJURIES

Entrapment Neuropathies in the Foot

TARSAL TUNNEL SYNDROME

The tarsal tunnel runs posteriorly and inferiorly to the medial malleolus and contains the posterior tibial nerve and tendons of flexor digitorum longus, flexor hallucis longus and tibialis posterior muscles.

Entrapment of the posterior tibial nerve and its medial plantar, lateral plantar and medial calcaneal branches in the tunnel produces the tarsal tunnel syndrome. The pain produced is burning in nature and affects the medial ankle and plantar aspect of the foot and toes. It may be accompanied by paraesthesia or numbness and may be present at night. It is typically aggravated by prolonged standing or walking. The problem may present acutely after a fall on to the foot or may be related to overuse injury of the tendons nearby. The syndrome is also more common in those with over-pronated feet.

Tapping over the nerve often reproduces the pain (Tinel's sign) and compression may refer pain up the leg or into the foot. Nerve conduction studies may confirm the diagnosis and other causes of peripheral neuropathy such as diabetes mellitus, rheumatoid disease, hypothyroidism, neoplasm, a local ganglion or flexor tenosynovitis must also be considered.

Orthotic control of biomechanical faults may be very successful supported by anti-inflammatory measures and strengthening of the muscles of the foot. Surgical decompression is indicated if conservative measures fail.

MORTON'S NEURALGIA (NEUROMA)

Fibrous enlargement of a plantar interdigital nerve with entrapment between metatarsal heads (usually the third and fourth) produces this problem. The neuroma is thought to result from repetitive trauma and is compounded by 'dropped' metatarsal heads, tight shoes and playing sports on hard surfaces.

The pain affects the web between the affected toes and there may be an associated loss of sensation. Compressing the heads of the adjacent metatarsals produces a sharp pain and often there is local tenderness over the affected nerve.

Metatarsal pads to restore or stabilize the metatarsal (transverse) arch of the foot, together with correction of any other biomechanical abnormalities is often all that is required. Sometimes local injection about the neuroma with corticosteroid is indicated and surgical excision in persistent cases is curative.

Stress fractures of the metatarsal bones must also be considered in the differential diagnosis.

OTHER NEUROPATHIES

Other neuropathies include the dorsal cutaneous branch of the deep peroneal nerve on the dorsum of the foot and the sural nerve behind the lateral malleolus or over the styloid process of the fifth metatarsal (Pecina et al. 1993).

Sinus Tarsi Syndrome

The sinus tarsi is the lateral concavity between the talus and calcaneus and is at the lateral end of the tarsal canal which runs between the two halves of the subtalar joint. The syndrome is characterized by generalized pain in the anterolateral or posteromedial rear foot, occasionally associated with swelling just anterior to the lateral malleolus. It usually presents as an overuse syndrome following a change in the nature or intensity of running activity, or secondary to an ankle joint sprain.

Examination reveals increased local tenderness, and forced pronation often increases the pain. Careful palpation of the lateral ligaments differentiates this syndrome from chronic lateral ankle ligament pain.

Treatment of the syndrome is by control of overpronation with appropriate shoes and orthotics, mobilization of the subtalar joint within pain and, occasionally, local corticosteroid infiltration may be necessary. The use of a walking cast followed by a carefully supervised rehabilitation programme has been successful in very difficult cases.

Bursitis About the Heel

The subcutaneous posterior calcaneal bursa and the retrocalcaneal bursa, which lies between the Achilles tendon and the os calcis, may be inflamed by ill-fitting shoes and by overuse, notably in running. The retrocalcaneal bursa may be associated with a 'pump bump' (bony bossing) on the posterior aspect of the os calcis (Haglund's syndrome) and this may contribute to injury.

Treatment is as for bursitis with rest from painful activities, protective low-friction taping (e.g. 'leuco-silk'), anti-inflammatory medication and electro-therapy modalities, ice applications and perhaps injection of corticosteroid. Footwear must be care-fully selected to provide cushioned support without friction to the heel. Excessive padding of the heel may increase friction and aggravate the bursitis. Surgery is reserved for chronic bursitis which does not respond to any other therapy, and may also incorporate excision of a 'pump bump'.

Inflammation of the Achilles tendon at its in-sertion may be due to conditions such as Reiter's disease and these should be considered in the differential diagnosis.

Heel Fat Pad Syndrome (Bruised Heel)

This condition is characterized by pain under the heel and is caused by degeneration or acute dis-ruption of the fat pad under the os calcis. This complex fibrofatty structure is responsible for protecting the pain-sensitive periosteum of the under-surface of the os calcis from excessive pressure on heel strike. The normal ordered structure of fatty compartments with strong collagenous and elastic fibrous septa makes an efficient shock absorber. This problem is particularly common in veteran running athletes where age and repeated trauma cause thinning and disruption of the septa.

Treatment involves decreasing weight-bearing activity, weight reduction and the use of a semi-rigid moulded heel cup or rigid adhesive strapping to prevent dispersion of the fat pad. Shoes with a snug, firm heel counter are also useful in treatment of this condition. Heel pads, particularly those which are flat or convex are unhelpful in this condition and corticosteroid injections should not be used as they may hasten the degenerative process.

Plantar Fasciitis

Plantar fasciitis is a common condition which affects athletes of any age. Running on hard surfaces may be implicated, together with activity such as tennis, netball and jumping sports. The plantar fascia is repeatedly stressed by the transferring of weight forward on to the toes with metatarsophalangeal joint extension. Extension of these joints creates a 'windlass effect' with winding up of the anterior aspect of the plantar fascia, lifting the longitudinal arch of the foot (Kwong et al. 1988).

The plantar fascia is an important support of the medial longitudinal arch and excessive pronation can cause chronic irritation of this structure, usually at its posterior attachment to the calcaneus.

Periosteal reaction at the proximal attachment may produce a heel spur. It is important to consider the presence of a heel spur on X-ray as a sign of inflammation rather than the cause of the pain or target for treatment. Most heel spurs are asympto-matic and their presence or otherwise has no bearing on management.

Pain is normally felt under the medial aspect of the heel. Characteristically, this occurs with the first few steps taken on arising in the morning. Walking on the toes or climbing stairs may make the pain worse and there is tenderness over the medial tuberosity of the calcaneus. Occasionally, with long-standing symptoms the tenderness may extend along the entire course of the fascia.

Treatment should be directed towards relief of the pain and inflammation and control of adverse mechanical factors to prevent recurrence. Low dye taping often provides relief and is a very effective method of unloading the region. Footwear modifi-cation, orthotic control of excessive and/or pro-longed pronation, if indicated, stretching tight calf muscles and activity modification should be commenced early. Ice applications and deep massage may assist recovery and a 4–8 mm heel raise.

Rarely surgical management is indicated. It involves posterior release of the plantar fascia and removal of the bone spur if present.

It must be remembered that plantar fasciitis is a manifestation of seronegative arthritis in some patients and this should be carefully assessed.

Calcaneonavicular Ligament (Spring Ligament) Sprain

Acute twisting injuries to the foot as seen among soccer players, gymnasts and jumpers, may produce sprains of the various interosseous ligaments of the foot. The calcaneonavicular ligament in particular may be injured producing pain and tenderness along the medial arch of the foot, similar to plantar fasciitis.

Treatment is as for any ligament sprain with ice applications, anti-inflammatory medication and electrotherapy and perhaps supportive strapping or an orthotic device until the problem settles.

Tarsometatarsal (TMT) Joint Injuries

Injuries to the TMT joint occur in sports such as basketball, sailboarding, cricket, soccer or gymnastics. The mechanism often involves a quick turn with an abduction force being applied to the forefoot by the cleats or studs in the sports shoe. Sometimes this joint can be injured by a heavy landing on the flat foot, but often there is some abduction force on the forefoot as well. The nature and severity of the injury are frequently not recognized on initial treatment. Diagnosis is both clinical and radiological. There is swelling and tenderness over the TMT joint. Gentle passive pronation and simultaneous abduction of the forefoot with the hindfoot held still by the examiner often reproduces pain (Curtis *et al.* 1993).

Plain radiographs of the foot should be taken in the lateral view, a standardized 30° internal oblique projection and a weight-bearing anteroposterior view. In a third degree sprain there is evidence of diastasis at the TMT joint or between the bases of the first and second metatarsals and their adjacent cuneiforms. Particular attention is paid to small avulsion fractures from the lateral edge of the medial cuneiform. Unless recognized and treated appropriately and early, this injury may cause considerable and prolonged disability. In stable injuries treatment involves non-weight-bearing immobilization in a short leg cast (first and second degree sprains). The cast is removed when the symptoms become significantly improved following the institution of weight-bearing in the cast. Aggressive physiotherapy is commenced after removal of the cast. A third degree sprain of the TMT joint requires open reduction and internal fixation using a single screw inserted obliquely through the medial wall of the medial cuneiform into the base of the second metatarsal. The foot is protected for 2–4 weeks in a supporting cast. There is a period of non-weight-bearing for 10–12 weeks, removal of the screw between 12 and 16 weeks and then a gradual return to physical activity under physiotherapy supervision. Orthoses may serve to support the foot and speed up return to sporting activity. In severe cases with persisting symptoms, despite surgical intervention, a secondary arthrodesis of the TMT joint may be necessary to alleviate symptoms.

Cuboid Syndrome

The cuboid bone acts as a pulley for the peroneus longus tendon, which is the most important stabilizer of the transverse arch of the foot. This tendon changes direction sharply under the cuboid bone as it winds medially across the sole, bridging the transverse arch of the foot and inserting into the base of the first metatarsal and the adjacent medial cuneiform. 'Subluxation' of the cuboid (Newell & Woodle 1981) or irritation of the ligaments which stabilize it, particularly at the calcaneocuboid and cubometatarsal joints, by acute or repetitive injury, causes lateral mid-foot pain. Tenderness is reproduced by pressure over the dorsal and plantar aspects of the cuboid bone just proximal to the styloid process of the fifth metatarsal.

Manipulation or mobilization by flexing the cubometatarsal joint may relieve the pain and orthotic support and re-education of foot posture to control excessive pronation may be useful.

Reflex Sympathetic Dystrophy of the Foot

Reflex sympathetic dystrophy is a recognized complication of often minor strains, sprains, lacerations and surgery to the foot. The foot is painful, swollen, hypersensitive to touch, hot or cold, and often moist. If untreated the joints become stiff, muscles shorten and the skin becomes atrophic. X-ray examination reveals osteoporosis and soft tissue swelling. This condition, as the name implies, is due to sympathetic nervous system dysfunction and perhaps psychological factors may play a role. Weight-bearing is restricted or impossible. Thermography has been used in assessing treatment and progress, but technetium ^{99}m bone scan is perhaps more reliable in documenting the state of bony metabolism.

Treatment should be aggressive to prevent permanent loss of function. This includes a compression wrap proximally from toes to knee, gently resisted plantar flexion and dorsiflexion exercises, intermittent elevation of the foot, mild hot or cold applications which can be tolerated, stretching exercises of the foot and ankle and passive foot and ankle mobilization. In some cases chemical sympathectomy is necessary by epidural injection of long-acting local anaesthetic agents at L1–L2 levels. Intensive treatment as an in-patient may reduce recovery time from an average of 22 months to 8 weeks (Gregg & Das 1982).

Painful Conditions of the Forefoot

ANTERIOR METATARSALGIA

This is not an anatomical diagnosis but a syndrome of pain and tenderness of the plantar aspect of the metatarsal heads. This condition is usually caused by uneven weight distribution under the metatarsal heads and is common in feet which pronate excessively or which otherwise have excessive mobility of the first metatarsal ray. There is often a heavy callus under the second and third metatarsal heads which are 'dropped' (plantar subluxation of the heads) and tenderness may be reproduced by compressing the metatarsal head between the thumb and index finger.

Calluses should be soaked and pared down with an abrasive board or stone. If appropriate, weight reduction should be undertaken and metatarsal pads should be incorporated in a custom-made orthotic device, particularly for correction of excessive pronation. A graded, supervised, exercise programme for the intrinsic and extrinsic foot muscles should be combined with triceps surae stretches if these muscles are tight and attention should be directed to appropriately fitted shoes for all activities, preferably with low heels.

FREIBERG'S OSTEOCHONDRITIS

This condition is an ischaemic necrosis of the epiphysis of the second and rarely the third metatarsal head. It occurs in adolescence, rarely before the age of 12 years, but may not present until secondary degenerative changes occur in the metatarsophalangeal joint in early adulthood (Fig. 22.13). There may be pain and tenderness associated with swelling in the metatarsophalangeal joint. Treatment is symptomatic and orthotic support may be useful.

SESAMOIDITIS

The term sesamoiditis has, with usage, come to include a number of different clinical entities affecting the sesamoid bones in the tendons of the flexor hallucis brevis. These small ovoid bones slide under, and articulate with, the first metatarsal head. They increase the mechanical advantage of flexor hallucis brevis and take some bodyweight. In physical activity performed on the toes, or with impact loading with weight-bearing, the sesamoids are subjected to great tensile stress from maximum dorsiflexion of the great toe. For these reasons this problem is seen in dancers, ice skaters, gymnasts and basketball players.

The medial and lateral sesamoid bones are subject to contusion, crush fracture, proximal pole avulsion fracture, stress fracture, sprain of a bipartite sesamoid, osteonecrosis and osteoarthritis. The history, X-ray examination and a bone scan can all be helpful in the differential diagnosis. A positive scan differentiates between a stress fracture and a sprained bipartite sesamoid (at least one sesamoid is bipartite in over 30% of cases). Examination reveals tenderness over either or both sesamoids, best felt with the great toe fully dorsiflexed.

Most cases of sesamoid pain are effectively managed with custom-made orthotics. Shoes with elevated heels are avoided. Gymnasts and ballet or modern dancers present problems in this regard as they are unable to use an orthotic during performance, but may benefit from appropriately placed adhesive padding. Some require rest from their activity for 4–6 weeks with a gradual return to activity and an exercise programme for the other toe flexors.

Surgical excision of a sesamoid bone is rarely necessary and is most often required in cases of osteonecrosis. Only the involved sesamoid should be removed.

HALLUX RIGIDUS

This is characterized by diminished range of motion and degenerative arthritis of the first metatarsophalangeal joint. The normal range of movement in the first metatarsophalangeal joint is 30° of plantar flexion, to 80° of dorsiflexion. Normal walking requires 65°–75° of dorsiflexion and more range is required during running, particularly if it is done on uneven surfaces or on hills.

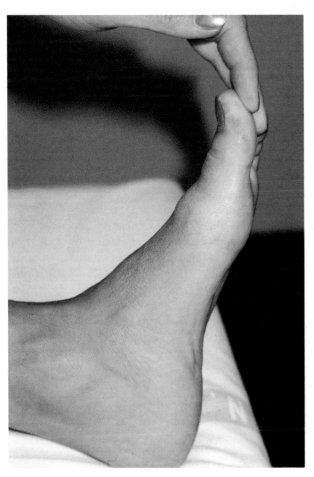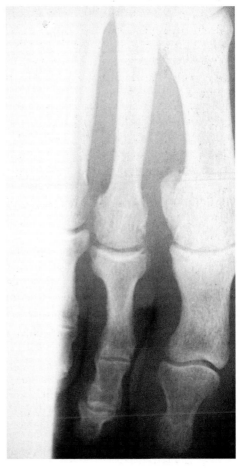

Fig. 20.27 (a) Hallux rigidus Full range of extension in the first MTP joint Note that when further extension is not possible this causes hyperextension of the interphalangeal joint of the big toe (b) Radiograph of the first MTP joint in the same patient as in (a) Note the loss of joint space and 'squaring off' of the joint margins

Hallux rigidus is caused by immobilization of the joint, destruction of the joint due to trauma, osteochondritis, infection or inflammation, or it may be hereditary. The first metatarsal is often longer than usual in the idiopathic cases. If this is associated with proximal migration of the sesamoids, the end of the first metatarsal is exposed more directly to weight-bearing forces which may hasten degenerative change.

The foot is characteristically widened with marked dorsal prominence of the first metatarsophalangeal joint (Fig. 20.27a). Pain becomes evident with severe restriction of joint motion and is usually worse with activity or prolonged standing. Activities which require a strong push-off, such as the football codes, tennis or basketball, exacerbate the pain, but there is usually no pain at rest. There may be skin irritation or bursa formation over the bony prominence. Shoe wear is often characteristic with wear down the lateral side of the sole, due to excessive supination during the gait cycle.

Radiological examination reveals narrowing of the joint space with widening of the articular surfaces on both sides of the joint (Fig. 20.27b). Dorsal osteophytic lipping is common. Weight-bearing lateral views of the foot may show a relative dorsiflexion of the metatarsal compared with the normal side. The great toe may also be slightly plantar flexed with a compensatory hyperextension of the interphalangeal joint.

Anti-inflammatory medication combined with passive joint mobilization may give some relief, as can shoes with a higher and wider toe box. Stiff-soled shoes, often with a small rocker in the outer sole underneath the metatarsal break (line of dorsiflexion of the foot on toe-off), may relieve pain. If symptomatic and degenerative change is severe, intra-articular injection of corticosteroid may be used. This condition is progressive and surgical treatment (cheilectomy) is often required to maintain function and reduce symptoms. This increases the range of motion and retains the stability of the metatarsophalangeal joint.

TOE SPRAINS

These are common, particularly in contact or collision sports. The first metatarsophalangeal joint is vulnerable to injury particularly if the toe section of a boot is too flexible. MCL sprains and sprains of the dorsal capsule may require strapping with adhesive non-stretch sports tape for some time to relieve pain and allow a return to sport.

'BLACK TOENAIL'

This sometimes occurs in distance runners. If the toe box of the shoe is inadequate or there is tenting of the forepart of the shoe over the toenail, friction and pressure are applied to the nail. A subungual haematoma then forms and the nail may become loose. The nail should be trimmed and bandaged with tape, but not forcefully avulsed as this may encourage infection. Attention should be paid to the athlete's shoes which probably do not fit well.

CONCLUSIONS

In this chapter information which provides a practical approach to the management of the more common problems affecting the pelvic girdle and lower limb in those persons who train intensively is presented.

An understanding of the biomechanics of the lower limb is invaluable as an aid to the prevention and management of injuries to this part of the body, especially where recommendations on appropriate orthotics and footwear are concerned. The reader is referred to the information on Podiatry in Chapter 28 of this book which provides more detail.

The role of stretching, strengthening and proprioceptive drills in the rehabilitation of injury is also emphasized, as well as modified activity, or 'active rest', both of which are integral parts of a complete programme of recovery for the injured athlete.

REFERENCES

Anderson I. F., Crichton K. J., Grattan-Smith T., Cooper R. A. & Brazier D. (1989) Osteochondral fractures of the dome of the talus. *Journal of Bone and Joint Surgery* 71A(8), 1143–1152.

Clement D. B., Taunton J. E., Smart G. W. & McNicol K. L. (1981) A survey of overuse running injuries. *Physician and Sports Medicine* 9, 47–58.

Cross M. J. & Watson A. S. (1981) Cysts and pseudocysts of the menisce of the knee joint. *Australian and New Zealand Journal of Surgery* **51**, 59–65.

Curtis M. J., Myerson M. & Szura B. (1993) Tarsometatarsal joint injuries in the athlete. *American Journal of Sports Medicine* **21**, 497–502.

Curwin S. & Stanish W. (1984) *Tendinitis: Its Etiology and Treatment*. Collamore Press, Lexington, MA.

Detmer D. E., Thorpe K., Sufit R. L. & Girdley F. M. (1985) Chronic compartment syndrome: Diagnosis, management and outcomes. *American Journal of Sports Medicine* **13**, 162–170.

Firer P. (1992) Results of surgical management for the iliotibial band friction syndrome. *Clinical Journal of Sport Medicine* **2**, 247–250.

Fricker P. A. & Williams J. G. P. (1979) Surgical management of os trigonum and talar spur in sportsmen. *British Journal of Sports Medicine* **13**, 55–57.

Fricker P. A., Taunton J. E. & Ammann W. (1991) Osteitis pubis in athletes: Infection, inflammation or injury? *Sports Medicine* **12**, 266–279.

Goldbert B. & Pecora C. (1994) Stress fractures — A risk of increased training in freshmen. *Physician and Sports Medicine* **22**, 68–78.

Gregg J. R. & Das M. (1982) Foot and ankle problems in the pre-adolescent and adolescent athlete. *Clinics in Sports Medicine* **1**, 131–147.

Grimston S. K. & Zernicke R. F. (1993) Exercise-related stress responses in bone. *Journal of Applied Biomechanics* **9**, 2– 14.

Hannaford P. G. H. (1988) Shin splints revisited: Medial tibial stress syndrome: The role of tibialis posterior. *Excel* **4**(4), 16–19.

Holmes J. C., Pruitt A. L. & Whalen N. J. (1994) Lower extremity overuse in bicycling. *Clinics in Sports Medicine* **13**, 187–203.

Inglis A. E., Scott W. N., Sculco T. P. & Patterson A. H. (1976) Ruptures of the tendo-Achilles — An objective assessment of surgical and non-surgical treatment. *Journal of Bone and Joint Surgery* **58A**, 990–992.

Jackson D. W. & Jennings L. D. (1988) Arthroscopically assisted reconstruction of the anterior cruciate ligament using patellar tendon bone autograft. *Clinics in Sports Medicine* **7**, 785– 801.

Kadel N. J., Teitz C. C. & Kronmal R. A. (1992) Stress fractures in ballet dancers. *American Journal of Sports Medicine* **20**, 445–449.

Kannus P. & Josza L. (1991) Spontaneous rupture of a tendon. *Journal of Bone and Joint Surgery* **73A**(1), 1507–1525.

Karlsson J., Sward L., Kalebo P. & Thomee R. (1994) Chronic groin injuries in athletes. Recommendations for treatment and rehabilitation. *Sports Medicine* **17**, 141–148.

Kennedy J. C. & Baxter-Willis R. (1976) The effects of local steroid injections on tendons: A biochemical and microscopic correlative study. *American Journal of Sports Medicine* **4**, 11–18.

Khan K. M., Fuller P. J., Brukner P. D., Kearney C. & Burry H. C. (1992) Outcome of conservative and surgical management of navicular stress fracture in athletes — Eighty-six cases proven with computerized tomography. *American Journal of Sports Medicine* **20**, 657–666.

Kwong P. K., Hay D. & Voner R. (1988) Plantar fasciitis: Mechanics and pathomechanics of treatment. *Clinics in Sports Medicine* **7**, 119–126.

Levick C. & Fricker P. (1993) Posteromedial tibial pain: The controversy surrounding diagnosis and management. *Technical Notes, No. 3.* National Sports Research Centre, Canberra (Australian Sports Commission).

Malecha P. & Lovell G. (1990) Inguinal surgery in athletes with chronic groin pain — the sportsman's hernia. *Australian and New Zealand Journal of Surgery* **62**, 123–125.

Masters S., Fricker P. & Purdam C. (1986) Stress fractures of the femoral shaft. Four case studies. *British Journal of Sports Medicine* **20**, 14–16.

Matheson G. O., Clement D. B., McKenzie D. C., Taunton J. E., Lloyd-Smith D. R. & Macintyre J. G. (1987) Stress fractures in athletes. *American Journal of Sports Medicine* **15**, 46–58.

McBryde A. M. (1976) Stress fractures in athletes. *American Journal of Sports Medicine* **5**, 212–217.

McConnell J. (1986) The management of chondromalacia patellae: A long term solution. *Australian Journal of Physiotherapy* **32**, 215–223.

Newell S. G. & Woodle A. (1981) Cuboid syndrome. *Physician and Sportsmedicine* **9**, 71–76.

Pecina M., Bojanic I. & Markiewitz A. D. (1993) Nerve entrapment syndromes in athletes. *Clinical Journal of Sport Medicine* **3**, 36–43.

Reid G. (1992) Hamstring tears. Lecture notes for post-graduate students. Curtin University School of Physiotherapy, Perth.

Ryan C., Fricker P. A. & Hannaford P. G. H. (1987) Muscle compartment pressure syndrome of the upper limb and shoulder: Two case studies. *Australian Journal of Science and Medicine in Sport* **19**(3), 24–25.

Scott G. A., Jolly B. L. & Henning C. E. (1986) Combined posterior incision and arthroscopic intra-articular repair of the meniscus. *Journal of Bone and Joint Surgery* **68A**, 847–61.

Shapiro M. S., Kabo J. M., Mitchell P. W., Loren G. & Tsenter M. (1994) Ankle sprain prophylaxis: An analysis of the stabilizing effects of braces and tape. *American Journal of Sports Medicine* **22**, 78–82.

Shea M. P. & Manoli A. (1993) Recognizing talar dome lesions. *Physician and Sports Medicine* **21**, 109–121.

Smedberg S. G. G., Broome A. E. A., Gullmo A. & Roos H. (1985) Herniography in athletes with groin pain. *American Journal of Surgery* **149**, 378–382.

Stanton P. (1988) CPM for muscle injuries. In Torode M. (ed.) *The Athlete Maximising Participation and Minimising Risk*, pp. 95–102. Cumberland College of Health Sciences Sydney.

Styf J. R. & Korner L. M. (1987) Diagnosis of chronic anterior compartment syndrome in the lower leg. *Orthopaedica Scandinavica* 58, 139–144.

Taylor D. C. & Bassett F. H. (1993) Syndesmosis ankle sprains. Diagnosing the injury and aiding recovery. *Physician and Sports Medicine* 21, 39–46.

Torstensen E. T., Bray R. C. & Wiley P. J. (1994) Patellar tendonitis: A review of current concepts and treatment. *Clinical Journal of Sport Medicine* 4, 77–82.

Williams J. G. P. (1978) Limitation of hip joint movement as a factor in traumatic osteitis pubis. *British Journal of Sports Medicine* 12, 129–133.

Williams J. G. P. (1980) *A Colour Atlas of Injury in Sport*, p. 101. Wolfe Medical, London.

Williams J. G. P. (1986) Achilles tendon lesions in sport. *Sports Medicine* 3, 114–135.

Wood G. (1986) Optimal performance criteria and limiting factors in sprint running. *New Studies in Athletics* 1 (2), 55–63.

SECTION 5

SPECIAL CONSIDERATIONS IN SPORTS MEDICINE

CHAPTER 21

THE TEAM PHYSICIAN

B. G. Sando

A team doctor requires good all-round knowledge and experience in sports medicine and general medical conditions. Team members present with as many general medical complaints, including dermatological, respiratory and gastrointestinal upsets, as they do with injuries from their sports. It is therefore important for the team doctor to maintain as much up-to-date knowledge of current trends in the diagnosis and treatment of everyday illness as it is in the sports injuries area.

PREVENTIVE ASPECTS

The opportunity exists for the team physician to have a large number of preventive measures implemented with the athletes for whom they care. Advice on hygiene and life-style can be given and pre- or early season assessments performed on team members to establish any potential or current problems. Remedial action may be taken, or specific training programmes devised to correct or avert any weaknesses or potential problems.

By attending training sessions and competitions in which a team participates, the practitioner has a better understanding of the following:

- The physical and psychological demands the sport places on the competitor
- The skills required of a competitor in that sport or event and the demands of the various team positions
- The protective equipment which is appropriate and permitted by the rules of the game

From the above knowledge the team physician is able to apply the various facets of training with relation to skill, strength, speed and endurance into his/her medical care of the individual.

ATHLETE EDUCATION AND ASSESSMENT

Early in the season, preferably during pre-season training, it is useful to address a team emphasizing the importance of such sports medicine matters as the following:

- The early reporting of any injuries and the importance of following treatment directions, particularly early first aid treatment
- The early reporting of illness and care in limiting the spread of any infection, so that sharing of drinking utensils, towels, etc. should be strictly avoided
- The need to complete treatment courses and adhere to the prescribed therapies which have been recommended
- The importance of fluid replacement in strenuous competition or training situations, particularly in endurance events in hot and humid conditions
- The need to observe sensible well balanced diets and specific diets in situations where they are specially prescribed
- The observance of good hygiene, including cleanliness and the wearing of correct well fitting apparel

- Care in the taking of over-the-counter preparations or medications prescribed by non-sports doctors which may infringe doping regulations
- The avoidance of advice or treatment from untrained, non-professional persons

Pre-season Assessment

The early season assessment should include taking a current and past medical examination and injury history. Inquiries should be made as to inoculations and appropriate boosters which have been previously administered, particularly in relation to tetanus and poliomyelitis. It is important to establish if any medication is being taken either regularly or occasionally, and if there is any history of allergy, and drug use including tobacco, alcohol and other agents. This is followed by a medical examination involving all systems, including a thorough musculoskeletal examination (Kulund 1988). Further investigations or assessments may be conducted as is deemed appropriate, for example muscle imbalance assessment, aerobic fitness, lung function, etc. Permission to obtain information from the practitioners and therapists who have previously treated the athlete for injury or illness must be sought and such information obtained when appropriate. A full blood count and serum ferritin are valuable baseline indices to establish at this time.

Consulting Area

While space may be limited, the layout of medical and treatment rooms should be as functional as possible. Equipment and furnishings must be kept clean and accessible and lighting be made as effective as possible. The range of equipment, dressings and strapping, various medications, etc. which will be required should be established and arranged in an 'essential', 'advisable', 'useful' priority list and obtained as the budget and space permit.

Record Keeping

Clinical case records must be kept for all competitors who are examined and treated. Such documentation is essential not only for medico-legal purposes but to provide an accurate medical and injury history for each competitor, and includes allergies, inoculations and treatments (Leach 1988). This information can assist in the collection of statistical data to determine injury patterns and their frequency, which may lead to training methods being modified, rules being examined and the sports medicine requirements for a particular sport being better understood.

MEDICAL EQUIPMENT

The equipment in the medical room and match day bag for 'away' competition will vary depending on the preference of an individual practitioner and the sport involved.

Diagnostic equipment for a body contact team sport is likely to include a torch (with spare batteries), stethoscope, auriscope, ophthalmoscope, sphygmomanometer, thermometer, tendon reflex hammer, visual acuity card, urine testing strips and eye fluoristrips.

Treatment items may include a range of dressings such as gauze squares, non-adherent dressings, skin closures, eye-pads, bandages, slings and splints. Antiseptic solutions, sterile saline solutions for eye-washes and wound irrigation, syringes, needles and suturing instruments and material are essential. Scissors and forceps are always required and a small tracheotomy set may be prudent for some sports.

A few drugs are often required and, in particular, analgesics, local anaesthetics, aerosol bronchodilators, anti-emetics and antidiarrhoeals are most frequently used. Care must be taken to include only those substances which will not give rise to doping infringements. One exception may be to have an opiate analgesic available in case of a very severe injury when its use may be essential for pain relief.

ROLE OF THE TEAM DOCTOR

The team doctor has the ultimate responsibility of establishing the diagnosis of the medical or injury problems of his team. It is the doctor's duty to determine, supervise and co-ordinate the type of management the athlete will be given and make the final decision on the fitness of the athlete to return to full training and competition.

A good working relationship should be developed between other medical staff associated with the team such as specialist doctors, physiotherapists, masseurs, podiatrists and trainers, and other sports science personnel such as the fitness adviser, sports psychologist and dietitian. Further, the team doctor must be able to relate to managers and selectors, particularly when providing advice as to the fitness of an athlete to compete. A good communication and relationship should also be developed with the coach.

Contact with a team member's usual medical adviser will be required from time to time. Team members in their home situation often have a long-standing relationship with a family medical doctor and care should be taken not to usurp this in relation to general medical conditions. In fact close co-operation is advisable in a number of instances, for example with the diabetic or asthmatic athlete.

RELATIONSHIPS

The Athletes

It is important to gain the confidence of all those persons associated with a team, but more particularly with the individual athletes themselves. This is obtained by offering an easy but confident approach and always demonstrating professional competence and a sincere regard for the athletes' health and welfare. As a team is made up of a group of individuals, the manner in which some team members are addressed and advised may differ from the way in which explanations are given to others. This of course occurs in all forms of medical practice.

The Coach

Many coaches are aware that a change in the performance of an athlete may be the consequence of an illness or injury and so may seek the assistance of the sports medicine physician for a quick assessment.

An understanding must be developed with the coach whereby it is left to the medical officer to decide whether an athlete is fit or not to participate in training or competition and, if there are limitations, what level and type of training is safe for the athlete.

There may be occasions when an athlete, although not fully recovered to the pre-injury level, is fit enough to resume training and competition without further aggravation of the injury. Under such circumstances the team doctor can advise the coach of the fitness level of the player and it then becomes the selector's decision as to whether or not such a competitor is best included in the team, to the exclusion of a fully fit, but less skilled, team-mate.

Selectors

The relationship with selectors is one where the fitness level or otherwise of the athlete to compete is supplied via the coach to the panel. The final decision is normally the responsibility of the selectors.

Other Team Members

Guarded comments should be made in relation to the severity and type of injury a team member may have when inquiries are received from concerned team-mates. The team practitioner's credibility is maintained by a conservative and non-alarmist response.

Management

The team manager is often charged with providing details to other persons and groups including the press, regarding injured team members. Professional confidentiality must not be breached in that the player should always be aware of the information being given and should agree with it. Details should be presented in simple terms and prognoses provided with care.

Other Team Personnel

It is courteous and prudent to meet the opposing team medical officer and offer appropriate assistance if any is required; or to obtain local knowledge in relation to special medical facilities when competing away from home, for example the accessibility of a telephone, ambulance, transport arrangements, back-up hospital and specialist support in case it should be required.

ETHICS

The International Olympic Committee medical commission has made a recent statement on ethics pertaining to sports medical care and this appears in Appendix A following this chapter. It is a useful document which fulfils almost all the situations which could confront a team physician.

TRAVELLING WITH TEAMS

In order to service the travelling athlete the sports medicine services should be well planned. Factors which must be addressed are:

- A knowledge of the region or country to be visited
- Medical support and facilities *en route*
- Pre-departure assessment of and advice to members of the touring party
- Necessary equipment and supplies
- Malpractice insurance and licence to practice (if necessary)

Area Being Visited

Ideally, the medical practitioner, particularly if accompanying a large team which is to spend a period of weeks in a distant location, visits the area to determine its facilities some time before the tour. Should this not be possible, this information can be obtained either from others who have visited it in the past or by communication with individuals in the area.

Information is required with regard to the following:

- Climate — temperatures, humidity, anticipated rainfall, etc.
- Altitude
- Air pollution

- Specific health risks — water, food, parasites, infections common to the area, etc.
- Local medical services

CLIMATIC CONDITIONS

Variations in temperature and humidity between the home base of a touring group and the area being visited will to some extent influence the time of arrival at the competition location. The climatic conditions are also of importance in deciding clothing, fluid intake, the need for sun-screening agents and clothes. The weight and thickness of tracksuits, the need for windcheaters or T-shirts and singlets and the type of uniform and casual clothes will all be governed by the climatic conditions of the areas being visited.

In hot or cold climates the type of artificial cooling or heating available at the accommodation sites and the protection from the weather at competition and training venues should be determined. Arrangements should be made to augment them if necessary.

Where there are significant climatic differences between the home training and the competition locations, for example maximum daily temperatures of more than 10°C variation or humidity of 20%, a week's acclimatization is advisable and hence arrival should be timed in order that the team can become steadily acclimatized. Some athletes, who are to compete in climatic conditions which are very different from those they normally experience, may find it helpful to have access to such a facility as a climate chamber for their pre-departure traning.

ALTITUDE

Where competition is to occur at high altitude, pre-departure altitude training or a longer period of acclimatization is recommended. This is required to condition the body to lower oxygen pressures and assist the physiological adjustments in relation to adaptation. See Chapter 6 for detailed information on altitude acclimatization.

AIR POLLUTION

The tendency to be affected by air pollution found in many industrial cities should be assessed (Fig. 21.1). Bronchoconstriction, rhinorrhoea and con-

Fig. 21.1 Air pollution is found in many industrial cities and should be taken into account when planning training and competition.

junctivitis are some of the complications which can result from smog and various forms of air pollution. Such pollution is most common in industrial centres or those with dense motorized road traffic, particularly in areas pocketed to some extent by surrounding hills. The most polluted cities are often those where the prevailing winds and breezes come in from the only open area in a near circle of hills surrounding the city and entrap the polluted air, preventing its dispersal.

Carbon monoxide, sulfur dioxide, ozone and hydrogen sulfide are some of the chemical pollutants which may create irritation to mucosal surfaces to produce an outpouring of secretions, oedema of such surfaces and bronchospasm (Shephard 1988). All such features can impair respiratory efficiency and performance.

Training and competition is best conducted at times of minor pollution and there is a need to take desensitizing or attenuating nasal sprays and bronchodilators for those who may require them. This can include athletes who have never had any previous symptoms and become affected by pollutants which they have never before encountered in such concentrations.

Allergens from different flora may be another source of allergic reaction producing irritation of respiratory and ophthalmic mucosa.

HEALTH HAZARDS

Drinking water

The quality of water from the local supply for drinking purposes must be thoroughly checked. Drinking water can frequently cause temporary gastrointestinal upsets because it may contain material to which the local population have become immune. Such parasites as *Giardia lamblia* and pathogenic *Escherichia coli* may be endemic in the area and cause major problems for athletes, and serious infections such as typhoid or cholera can cause death.

Where water is unfit for drinking, bottled or

purified water will be required. While there are some purifying tablets and filters available, boiling water is still the safest method of killing pathogenic bacteria. The addition of 0.25 mL of 2% tincture of iodine to a litre of clear water or 0.1 mL of 5% household bleach (hypochlorite) and allowing it to stand for an hour after gentle shaking, kills the majority of organisms (Looke 1990).

When purchasing bottled water in an overseas country the reliability of the brand should be established and one must ensure that the seal on the bottle has not been broken, because in some countries containers are refilled with local water and offered as the original product.

Ice should not be consumed as it is frequently made from non-purified water and care should be taken when drinking from bottles and containers which have been immersed in ice, as melted water from it may contaminate the outer surface of the container and trickle into the mouth or drinking utensil when the drink container is inverted. In order to prevent this, the container's outer surface should be dried before inversion or pouring.

Only water suitable for drinking should be used for toothbrushing, mouthwashing or gargling, as very small amounts may house large numbers of bacteria or parasites. Even fruit and salads which may have been washed with contaminated water must also be avoided. It is a wise precaution to only eat fruit and vegetables which one can personally peel.

Parasitic infections can be a problem in some countries and an awareness of infestations in various regions will assist in the prevention of diseases caused by them. Uncooked foods for example, like raw fish and shellfish, are among those which are best avoided.

Food

Food of similar type and quality to that which the athletes are used to consuming is usually available. In some cases Western food may be more difficult to obtain and local food may be of a quality which is not particularly pleasing. While compromises are sometimes required, it is usually possible to obtain satisfactory meals, perhaps with some negotiation and special advance requests.

It can be useful to take some special food items from home when travelling to retain contact with some familiar and enjoyed tastes. Teams sometimes travel with breakfast cereals from their home country, various spreads, etc.

Food problems of a different kind are sometimes encountered when the variety and availability of food is so attractive that athletes eat more than usual. Cautionary advice must be given to team members in such instances and the dietary balance maintained by careful supervision of the foods consumed (see Chapter 5 for further details).

Traveller's diarrhoea

Diarrhoea which occurs while travelling is common and is often due to the ingestion of the *E. coli* bacteria. It is usually of a different strain from the one to which the traveller is immune and will severely handicap the athlete's training and competition performance (Murtagh 1987). Regions of the world where such diarrhoea is more commonly experienced are Asia, Central and Latin America, the Middle East, Africa and the Mediterranean. Such pathogens are usually present in tap water and ice cubes and may be ingested in food such as seafood, unpasteurized milk, raw vegetables, some fresh fruit and salads. The local population who have been exposed to these pathogens over a long period of time have usually acquired an immunity to their effects.

When diarrhoea occurs it is usually a self-limiting condition and the procedure followed is that for any diarrhoea infection. That is, clear fluids for 24–48 h and avoidance of solid food and especially dairy products. Appropriate treatment such as anti-motility agents loperamide (Imodium) or diphenoxylate (Lomotil) may be administered but the most important treatment is the maintenance of adequate fluid and salt intake using soft drinks, fruit juices and dry biscuits which may be salted. A suitable oral rehydrating solution can be made by adding a level teaspoon of salt and eight teaspoons of sugar to 1 L of treated water.

Some medical personnel advocate the use of low-dose prophylactic antibiotics but their use must be balanced against the risks of producing allergic reactions in some individuals, an increase in the number of resistant organisms and possible photo-sensitivity effects from certain antibiotics which may be used for this purpose. Antibiotics which have been used for this purpose include trimethoprim and sulfamethoxazole, doxycycline, norfloxacin and ciprofloxacin. The first two have sensitivity or photosensitivity risks and the expense of the last named makes norfloxacin 400 mg once a day probably the best choice for athletes to take in areas where there is a high risk of developing traveller's diarrhoea (Scott 1990). Prophylactic therapy should commence a day before departure, be continued for 2 days after return and not exceed 3 weeks in duration. Doxycycline becomes an attractive option when journeying to malarial areas for a short period when it can present as a dual prophylaxis for both traveller's diarrhoea and malaria with the risk of photosensitivity having to be considered.

Should diarrhoea develop and be accompanied by a fever of 38°C or more then antimicrobial therapy using any one of the previous mentioned antibiotics can be used 12 hourly for 3 days — 160 mg trimethoprim and 800 mg sulfamethoxazole, or trimethoprim 200 mg alone, doxycycline 100 mg,

Table 21.1 Causative organisms of traveller's diarrhoea

Bacterial
  Escherichia coli, especially enterotoxigenic *E. coli*
  Salmonella species
  Shigella species
  Campylobacter jejuni
  Vibrio parahaemolyticus
  Vibrio cholerae
  Yersinia enterocoliticia
Viral
  Norwalk
  Rotavirus
Parasites
  Giardia lamblia
  Cryptosporidium
  Entamoeba histolytica
  Malaria
  Worms
'Food poisoning'
  Staphylococcus aureus toxin
  Bacillus cereus
  Clostridium perfringens

norfloxacin 400 mg and ciprofloxacin 300 mg (Looke 1990).

Persisting severe, or bloody diarrhoea, requires hydration, electrolytes and investigation to determine its nature, so that appropriate treatment can be implemented immediately. Possible organisms causing diarrhoea are listed in Table 21.1.

To summarize traveller's diarrhoea, which has a range of pseudonyms which include 'Bali Belly', 'Delhi Belly', 'Turkey Trots', 'Montezuma's Revenge', 'Inca Quick-step' can be largely avoided by following the saying 'Boil it, cook it, peel it or forget it'.

Athletes should be advised to avoid:

- Tap water, that is any drink not from a sealed bottle
- Unpasteurized milk products or dairy products including ice-cream
- Using unsafe water to brush teeth or allow shower water to enter the mouth
- Uncooked food including seafood, shellfish, salads, vegetables, sandwiches and fruit not personally peeled
- Eating from roadside cafes and stalls

It is generally safe for athletes to consume:

- Bottled beverages from sealed containers drunk from a bottle without melted iced water on its exterior
- Drinks such as tea or coffee (without milk) served and drunk hot
- Cooked food served hot
- Fruit peeled personally
- Food from reputable hotels or restaurants, but adhering to the 'hot cooked foods' rule

Medical Support and Facilities

As complicated conditions can be experienced which require specialist management or specific attention, the availability and quality of such facilities should be investigated (Hillman 1984).

Acute appendicitis, a serious fracture or even a spinal or head injury is highly possible in a number of sports and so the training and capabilities of local medical personnel and the quality of hospitals should be known. In many instances excellent specialist assistance is available, but in less developed areas a contingency plan for evacuation to a higher level of expertise is necessary. It may be possible to stabilize the condition of the athlete and then arrange transport to more expert management, or home to the country of origin.

It is advisable to have substantial travelling medical insurance to cover injury treatment and hospitalization of touring party members and possibly a subscription to Swiss ambulance or similar for air evacuation from some areas.

Radiological and pathology investigatory facilities are available in most regions. Physical therapy equipment may be available, as part of the service supplied by event organizers to competitors, but again the quality and qualifications of such therapists should be established. If a physiotherapist forms part of the medical team, this person will either need to transport his/her own equipment, or arrange for the necessary items to be available on location from a local supplier. This may limit the amount and range of instruments and equipment available. Power sources and connections must also be checked and the necessary electrical adaptors brought if equipment is to be taken from the home country.

When a medical practitioner accompanies a group of sports persons as the sole practitioner, it is necessary to also fulfil the role of a physiotherapist; therefore, he or she must be competent to use various types of electrotherapy and to undertake taping. For some groups massage techniques should also be learnt so that pre- and post-event massage can be performed when this is part of the normal support for competitors in various types of sports or events.

Medical Assessment

Soon after team selection a full medical assessment must be made of all team members, in which current and past medical histories are taken and a full medical examination performed. The individuals in the group who are athletes also need a thorough skeletal system assessment, as no team member should be allowed to travel overseas with a chronic musculoskeletal injury. A dental examination is also an important part of these tests, as dental

problems on tour can create difficulties as well as interruption to sleep and training (Fig. 21.2).

Team officials also require careful assessment as they will frequently have arduous duties to perform over long hours and must be declared fully fit for their job. Blood tests, including a full blood count and biochemical screening, electrocardiograph and submaximal fitness test should be performed. If significant medical problems are detected, they must either receive treatment to lift them to the medical level required or withdraw from the team.

The team must also be briefed on such matters as hygiene, health hazards which may be encountered, water and food, and warnings in relation to banned drugs and medications which may be taken inadvertently. As an added precaution all team members should have any medication they are taking, even over-the-counter preparations, checked by the team doctor. It may be necessary for the medical practitioner to change some prescriptions to ensure that they are not on the banned list (Badewitz-Dodd 1992).

Immunization and Disease Prevention

Before departure the routine immune status of all athletes and officials must be established and brought up to date.

Tetanus and diphtheria vaccination is administered in childhood and a booster is recommended every 10 years. Adult diphtheria and tetanus is recommended as a booster rather than tetanus toxoid alone to confer immunity to both tetanus and diphtheria.

A *poliomyelitis* booster dose of oral trivalent vaccine, that is OPS (Sabin) is required every 10 years following the initial course of vaccine. When only a partial course has been administered the primary series should be repeated.

Smallpox vaccination has not been required since May 1980, when the World Health Organization accepted that this disease had been eradicated throughout the world.

Yellow fever vaccine is administered as a single subcutaneous injection for those travelling in parts of South America and Africa where the disease occurs. As case fatalities in this mosquito-spread disease can be as high as 50% for non-indigenous individuals exposed to it, vaccination is essential for persons travelling in endemic areas. Yellow fever vaccination can only be administered by an approved Yellow Fever Vaccination Centre so that an International Certificate of Vaccination can be filled in and validated with the Centre's stamp.

Cholera vaccine is a heat-killed vaccine which is not recommended due to its minimal efficacy and short duration of action. Careful selection of food and water in countries where cholera may occur is the best method of prevention. Cholera is endemic in Asia, Africa, the Middle East and parts of Oceania; however, not all countries follow the advice of the World Health Organization, hence travellers to cholera endemic countries may require a single cholera vaccination injection to satisfy

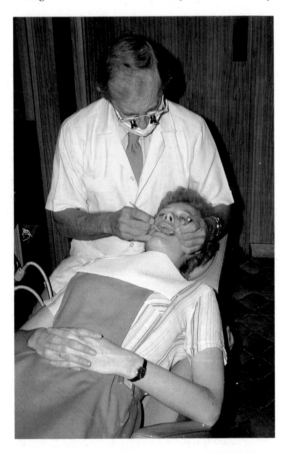

Fig. 21.2 A dental examination is an important part of the medical assessment before athletes travel overseas.

entry requirements to that country (Cook 1987). This is best administered some time before departure so that any reaction to the injection is over well before competition.

For *typhoid fever*, parenteral vaccines provide reasonable protection against light water-borne infection but not against a heavier food-borne type. As the vaccine only offers limited immunity to infection, care must be taken in the selection of food and water in countries where the disease is more common such as Asia, Africa, Latin America and the Pacific Islands. The primary immunization is by the administration of two subcutaneous injections preferably at 4–6 week intervals, or the second after not less than a 7 day interval if it needs to be given urgently before an imminent departure. A single booster is required at any time after 3 years if further exposure to the infection is likely to occur. A more recently developed oral vaccine using a live attenuate *Salmonella typhi* strain may be more effective than the parenteral form; but soon to be released is a parenteral single dose form, which gives 3 years' protection before a booster is required.

Hepatitis A is more prevalent in developing countries but even 50% of adults in Western countries have developed an immunity through prior contact with the disease. A satisfactory vaccine has been developed; however, if time does not permit its administration for satisfactory protection prior to departure, normal human immunoglobulin is recommended for persons travelling in developing countries away from main centres, where they will be consuming food and fluids from sources where hygiene is not strictly controlled. If it is administered by deep intramuscular injection with a dose to weight ratio, protection is provided for 3–6 months.

Hepatitis B, while being endemic throughout the world, is more prevalent in West Africa, South-East Asian and Pacific countries. This disease is spread by contact with any of the body fluids of an infected person or carrier, and since an effective vaccine is available, it is highly recommended for those at risk, or those in close contact with blood and other body fluids of persons who may carry the virus. While it is probably prudent for medical personnel to be vaccinated, sports persons for whom such vaccination is recommended are only those travelling frequently to, or spending long periods of time in, countries where the disease is prevalent. However, athletes who compete in body contact sports where open wounds may be experienced, or against athletes who are at risk of being in contact with the disease, should be vaccinated against hepatitis B.

Hepatitis C has a similar mode of transmission to hepatitis B, being blood borne, but has no vaccine available to protect against it. Hence the precautions against blood-borne diseases should be observed as indicated by the Australian Sports Medicine Federation (1993) Infectious Diseases Policy.

There is a potential for the transmission of *blood-borne disease* in sport, in particular hepatitis B and C and human immune deficiency virus (HIV). For transmission to occur, the virus has to pass from the body of an infected person and enter the bloodstream of an uninfected person. For this to happen the blood of a person infected with or carrying the disease, would have to contact an open breach in the epithelium or mucosa of an uninfected athlete. As well, the number of viral elements as represented by the quantity of blood in contact with the skin lesion and the concentration of viral particles in such blood, has a bearing as to whether infection will occur in the uninfected person.

As sexual transmission constitutes a considerable risk with the virus being present in the semen and vaginal fluids of infected persons, athletes should be advised to restrict their number of sexual partners and to use condoms as a means of reducing the risk of infection. The hepatitis B and C virus may also be present in tears, saliva, sweat and urine but, the concentration is such in these particular body fluids that contact with them is unlikely to cause infection.

The HIV virus does not survive long in the open but a case of seroconversion has been reported in a sportsman (Torre 1990; Torre *et al.* 1990) following infected blood coming in contact with a skin wound. It is therefore imperative that, particularly in contact sports, all measures be taken to protect against the spread of blood-borne infection. Normal social contact such as touching, shaking hands, hugging and the sharing of facilities such as change rooms,

toilets, showers and swimming pools constitute no danger of infection. However, the potential for the spread of a variety of infections makes the sharing of toothbrushes, razors, toothpaste and bucket and sponge inadvisable.

It should be stressed that the spread of blood-borne diseases is minimized for persons treating athletes by arresting the bleeding from any wound, cleaning any blood from adjacent areas, keeping any open wound covered with a suitable dressing and by wearing protective gloves.

The following precautions and management minimize the risk of transmitting blood-borne infectious disease during sports participation:

- Assume that all casualties are HIV antibody positive
- Wear protective disposable plastic or rubber gloves if in contact with athletes' blood or other body secretions
- Open cuts, abrasions and skin lesions should be covered with protective dressings before participation, particularly in contact sports
- Skin is cleaned of blood using antiseptic solution or soap and water
- All blood contaminated clothing and equipment must be replaced
- Clothing should be cleaned by soaking for half an hour in a 1 in 10 solution of household bleach or disinfectant solution, then washed in hot water
- Any equipment or dressing room surfaces contaminated by blood should be considered as potentially infectious and treated with household bleach (1 in 10 solution)
- Communal bathing in spas or baths must be discouraged
- Sharing of towels, shaving razors and drink containers must not occur and the use of the 'bucket and sponge' from player to player is no longer permitted

Persons known to be HIV positive should be discouraged from participation in body contact sports; however, they can be encouraged to undertake regular aerobic exercise such as jogging, swimming and cycling to maintain fitness and musculo-skeletal strength. They should not, however, engage

Table 21.2 Countries with malaria risk

*Afghanistan	*Ghana	*Papua New
Algeria	Guatemala	Guinea
*Angola	*Guiana-French	Paraguay
Argentina	*Guinea	*Peru
*Bangladesh	*Guinea-Bissau	*Philippines
Belize	*Guyana	*Rwanda
*Benin	Haiti	*Sao Tome &
*Bhutan	Honduras	Principe
*Bolivia	*India	*Saudi Arabia
*Botswana	*Indonesia	*Senegal
*Brazil	*Iran	*Sierra Leone
*Burkina Faso	Iraq	*Solomon
*Burma	Jordan	Islands
*Burundi	*Kenya	*Somalia
*Cambodia	*Laos	*South Africa
*Cameroon	*Liberia	*Sri Lanka
*Central African	Libyan Arab	*Sudan
Republic	Jamahiriya	*Surinam
*Chad	*Madagascar	*Swaziland
*China	*Malawi	Syria
*Colombia	*Malaysia	*Thailand
*Comoro Islands	*Mali	*Togo
*Congo	*Mauritania	Turkey (*P. vivax*
Costa Rica	Mauritius	only)
*Côte d'Ivoire	Mexico	*Uganda
Djibouti	Morocco (*P. vivax*	United Arab
Dominican	only)	Emirates
Republic	*Mozambique	*United Republic
*Ecuador	*Namibia	of Tanzania
Egypt	*Nepal	*Vanuatu
El Salvador	Nicaragua	*Venezuela
*Equatorial Guinea	*Niger	*Vietnam
*Ethiopia	*Nigeria	*Yemen
*French Guiana	*Oman	*Zaire
*Gabon	*Pakistan	*Zambia
*Gambia	*Panama	*Zimbabwe

*Countries where chloroquine resistant malaria is encountered. National Health and Medical Research Council (1993).

in strenuous training or competition beyond normal levels as this can cause immunological stress and potentially worsen their condition.

Malarial prophylaxis may be required in some countries and Table 21.2 lists the places where this may be necessary. The risk of malaria varies with the season and region in the country being visited. It may be far less a risk where residence is in an air-conditioned city hotel and when training and competition occur during the day in a city location.

Visiting the urban fringe or rural areas increases the likelihood of contracting the disease, as does the length of stay in such areas.

Malaria is spread through the bite of the female anopheline mosquito and can be contracted by transfusion with infected red blood cells. Of the four species of malaria, *Plasmodium falciparum* is the most life-threatening. Any feverish illness experienced by a traveller from a malarial area should have malaria included in the differential diagnosis.

Prophylaxis against malaria should be through a reduction in mosquito contact and chemoprophylaxis. Mosquito protection is via the use of effective mosquito nets impregnated with repellent and the use of knock-down sprays. As dark-coloured clothing, perfumes and aftershave lotion attract mosquitoes these should be avoided and light-coloured clothing, preferably covering the limbs, should be worn at and after dusk. Chemoprophylaxis requires the correct choice, as no single dosage is effective against all species and strains of malaria. Chloroquine is effective against most forms of the parasite but not chloroquine-resistant *P. falciparum* malaria. Where the latter is reported, Maloprim may be prescribed but chloroquine must also be taken. Chloroquine is still required to control *Plasmodium vivax* and *Plasmodium ovale* for which it is more effective than Maloprim. While Maloprim is more effective than chloroquine against *P. falciparum* when antifolate-resistant *P. falciparum* occurs mefloquine or doxycycline may be used.

The drugs are taken in single dose form each week commencing 1 week before entering a malarial risk area and continuing during the time of potential exposure and for 4 weeks after leaving the area (Malarial Guide-lines for Medical Practitioners 1989) with the exception of doxycycline which is taken a day before arrival and for 2 days afterwards but its use should not exceed an 8 week maximum.

No antimalarial chemoprophylactic regimen gives complete protection. *Falciparum* malaria must always be suspected if fever, with or without symptoms, develops at any time between 1 week after the first possible exposure to malaria and 2 months after the last possible exposure. Early diagnosis and the appropriate treatment determines the survival of persons with *falciparum* malaria (World Health Organization 1991). Blood samples should be taken if malaria is suspected and examined microscopically for malarial parasites. A further blood test should be repeated if the first is clear but fever persists. If facilities for blood examination are not present, three Fansidar tablets should be taken as this drug is only used for treatment and not as a prophylactic.

It must be further noted that antimalarial drugs should be taken with food and also that they have side-effects, so that they are only to be taken in areas where a malarial risk is known to exist. Chloroquine should not be taken if there is a history of generalized psoriasis and mefloquine must not be prescribed if there is a past history of allergy to this drug. Nor should maloprim or fansidar be prescribed in the case of sulfonamide sensitivity. As doxycycline may cause skin photosensitivity, it should be prescribed with caution to those likely to be exposed to prolonged direct sunlight and such persons should use strong protective sunscreens.

AIR TRAVEL

Air travel, particularly over long periods of time, can have a number of effects on passengers and it is well to be aware of these so as to reduce their symptoms.

'Jet lag' can create problems for athletes and it is the term given to the fatigue and lassitude effect experienced by travellers after long air flights (Loat & Rhodes 1989).

Associated features are sleep and eating deficiencies and reduced physical performance. A number of factors contribute to this, including the hours spent in flight and travel and the number of time zones covered.

Altitude

Owing to the high altitude of operation, aircraft cabins are pressurized. Because the cabin pressure is not that of sea level but is corrected to about 2000 m, some high-altitude effects are experienced, since the blood oxygen saturation is reduced.

Teams should be located in the non-smoking areas of international aircraft, because smoking further inhibits the oxygen-carrying capacity of the blood in aircraft, as the carbon monoxide produced from tobacco smoke binds to red blood cell haemoglobin. Hence the oxygen-carrying capacity of the blood is inhibited by the carbon monoxide inhaled from cigarette smoke and compounds the problems of the already reduced oxygen saturation through the reduced air pressure of oxygen. Thus smoking is even less advisable at altitude than at sea level and is a further argument in favour of the banning of smoking during air travel.

Dehydration

This is another contribution to jet lag and arises through the dry atmosphere of aircraft cabins. The air in the cabin is sucked in from outside and compressed. This high-altitude air is at a very low humidity and hence the air inside the aircraft is drier than usual, thereby increasing the insensible perspiration loss from the skin and through respiration during flight. Another factor which can increase dehydration is the consumption of drinks which have a dehydrating effect, for example beverages containing alcohol and caffeine such as coffee, tea and cola.

Therefore, to avoid such dehydrating effects, regular fluid consumption is required. Water, diluted cordials and fruit juices provide the best forms of fluid, as aerated drinks may cause discomfort with the expansion of intestinal gases on ascent.

Time Zone Changes

The disturbance to circadian rhythms when a number of times zones are crossed also contributes to jet lag as the 'body clock' is disturbed and sleep and wake patterns are altered. It has been suggested that it takes 1 day to regain normal body rhythm for each time zone crossed in flight. This sleep disturbance is not affected by north–south travel and east–west travel causes less disruption than that in the west–east direction.

On arrival at the destination, it is recommended that in order to resume a normal sleep pattern, one should delay retiring for bed until nightfall. A light exercise session soon after arrival is also good practice to help restore normal body function.

Travel Inertia

Being seated for long periods results in the slowing of the circulation and can produce oedema of the lower limbs from the pooling effect. This is compounded by wearing tight-fitting garments, particularly those which encircle the waist and legs.

Long periods of immobility should be avoided by taking walks around the aircraft, train or bus during transit and at any stop during the trip. Exercises which contract and relax the limb muscles and stretch various joints while seated assist in reducing pooling and encouraging the blood flow.

Upper Respiratory Tract Infection

Air travel can create complications for the athlete who has an upper respiratory tract infection because of the effect of the changes in air pressure on secretions from the nasal region. The sinus orifices or eustachian tubes can become blocked, producing sinus and middle ear complications. Decongestants should be used immediately prior to take off and descent and care taken to ensure that they are not of a kind which is a prohibited agent for a competing athlete.

Contact Lenses

A long flight, with dry air in the aircraft, can produce complications for a contact lens wearer as the lenses tend to dry out. Lens fluid should be carried in the cabin or normal glasses worn in flight.

General Guide-lines for Travelling

The following information should be adhered to by the athlete while travelling:

- Rest before setting out and avoid fatiguing pre-departure activities or festivities
- Drink copious quantities of fluid in flight and avoid aerated, alcoholic and caffeinated beverages

- Wear loose fitting garments and avoid tight-waisted or constricting clothing
- Move around on a long flight and do not sit motionless for extended periods of time
- Have a light exercise session on arrival
- Avoid going to bed on arrival during daylight hours and wait until nightfall before going to sleep

EQUIPMENT AND SUPPLIES

The range of instruments, equipment, drugs and dressings taken by the team physician will depend on the type of sports in which competitors are participating and the availability of such items at the training and competition locations being visited. As a general rule, where there is any doubt with relation to the various pharmaceutical lines which should be taken, it is wise to carry supplies which embrace the normal range of general practice, as the team physician will have more general medical conditions than injury problems to treat in most instances.

The instrument and treatment bag must contain the full range of diagnostic and treatment instruments, syringes and drugs that will normally be available for home competition. Whether additional supplies are carried will depend on the level of medical care in the locations being visited.

The range of drugs taken for use by the team doctor on tour should include:

- A range of antibiotics
- Simple analgesics, for example paracetamol, aspirin
- Hypnotics
- Anti-inflammatory tablets — a variety being advisable as many athletes will feel one particular drug suits them best
- Gastrointestinal preparations — antacids; anti-diarrhoeals, for example kaolin, loperamide, diphenoxylate; simple laxatives, for example senna fruit extract; anti-emetics, possibly an H_2 antagonist; an anti-spasmodic
- Respiratory preparations — nasal sprays; throat lozenges; gargles; bronchodilators including β_2 agonist aerosol sprays; corticosteroid bronchial

and nasal sprays; a simple cough mixture, for example senega and ammonia

- Aural drops or ointments
- Ophthalmic preparations — topical antibiotics and decongestive drops
- Antihistamines
- An antivertiginous agent
- An antimigrainous preparation without caffeine
- Oral and possibly other contraceptives
- Topical preparations — antibiotics; corticosteroids; antifungals; antiseptic solutions and creams, including some vaginal and rectal preparations
- Sunscreen agents

Drug Use in Sport

In the selection of drugs care must be taken to ensure that no proscribed preparation is included which could lead to the disqualification of a team member (Badewitz-Dodd 1992). Athletes are advised never to take an agent from a banned class and, when taking any prescribed or over-the-counter preparation, to ascertain that the medication is permitted under regulations relating to drug use in sport. Only in an extenuating medical situation or as a hospital inpatient would such variation from this policy ever occur. Team doctors should only ever prescribe permitted drugs for athletes, even out of competition, as random out of season testing may be conducted. Athletes may also retain some of the medication and use it later to control similar symptoms should they develop at the time of competition, so care must be taken not to over-prescribe.

The team doctor has a very important part to play in drugs and sport education. It is advisable to address a team before departure and again after arrival at a destination. The doctor should inspect all medication athletes have in their possession to establish whether it is safe in relation to inadvertent doping. Further, the team doctor's advice should be sought for any symptoms requiring treatment so that only permitted drugs are used. This particularly applies to over-the-counter preparations and athletes are cautioned against accepting another individual's medication for treating similar symptoms.

A detailed discussion appears in Chapter 26 which deals with doping in sport. It is very important that the team doctor be fully conversant with this information as the number of banned drugs has greatly increased during the last 10 years.

ACCOMMODATION

Comfortable accommodation and back-up services are essential if the team is to perform well. The following factors need to be attended to:

- Accommodation should be close to training and competition venues. A long trip by car or bus to such venues becomes tedious after one or two journeys and may promote boredom or even anxiety if traffic congestion jeopardizes punctual arrival for competition
- Room comfort is assisted by adequate ventilation and temperature control. Fans, heaters or extra bed covers may be required to ensure the team members' comfort
- Freedom from noise associated with traffic, neighbouring activities and other accommodated persons will assist the athlete to get adequate rest
- The doctor should have a separate room in the accommodation area in which to consult and, if not, a sleeping room to himself which is also used for consulting purposes
- The capacity to segregate team members suffering from a temporary infectious condition, such as an upper respiratory tract infection, is an advantage. The spread of such an infection through a team can be limited by having such a facility
- Room-mates must be compatible in personality and sleep patterns. If they are in different events with varying timetables, consideration needs to be given to each individual's rest and sleep routines
- The type and quality of food must be assessed and the management or kitchen staff must be consulted if it is not satisfactory. General cleanliness and hygiene should be satisfactory, with adequate bottled drinking water available in the accommodation area and transported to

athlete participation areas in situations where tap water should not be consumed

- Safety factors to be addressed are the notifying of fire escape routes to all team members, the avoidance of any unsafe areas in the locality and adherence to security advice and measures recommended by the hosting authorities. Competition and training location areas and changing rooms should be inspected to exclude any hazards. The supply of condoms to those requesting them and advice regarding safe sex practice for those who wish to engage in such practices is a team doctor's responsibility

- Entertainment for team-members relieves boredom. Away from the usual home activities there is often more leisure time to fill between training and competition commitments. Local touring and shopping can fill in some of this time but other activities need to be arranged. Playing cards, scrabble and other board games, videos, quiz competitions, reading material, etc. can be transported with the team and it is possible that table tennis and cue ball games will be available. Such occupational activities assist morale and team spirit

MALPRACTICE INSURANCE AND LICENCE TO PRACTICE

Team physicians must ensure that their medical defence insurance provides cover while abroad. North America is often excluded from policies and if travelling in this region, discussion with the relevant medical body well before departure is advisable.

As a general rule a team physician treating only team members has no obligation to seek or obtain a medical licence while abroad. However, it should be noted that such situations do not permit the dispensing of prescriptions written by the team doctor, so the assistance of a local medical practitioner will be invaluable. Temporary licences to practice may be organized for the Olympic Games on the presentation of the appropriate documentation.

REFERENCES

Australian Sports Medicine Federation (1993) *Infectious Diseases Policy,* 3rd edn. ASMF Ltd, Canberra.

Badewitz-Dodd L. (1992) *Drugs and Sport,* pp. 11–16. IMS Publishing, Sydney.

Cook I. (1987) Malaria and other 'tropical' hazards (Editorial). *Australian Family Physician* 16, 87.

Hillman R. S. (1984) Travel. In Strauss R. H. (ed.) *Sports Medicine,* pp. 492–500. W. B. Saunders Co., Philadelphia, PA.

Kulund D. N. (1988) (ed.) The athlete's physician. In *The Injured Athlete,* pp. 1–34. J. B. Lippincott Co., Philadelphia, PA.

Leach R. (1988) Medical examination of athletes. In Dirix A., Knuttgen H. G. & Tittel K. (eds) *The Olympic Book of Sports Medicine I,* pp. 572–578. Blackwell Scientific Publications, Oxford.

Loat C. E. R. & Rhodes E. C. (1989) Jet lag and human performance. *Sports Medicine* 8, 226–238.

Looke D. F. M. (1990) Traveller's diarrhoea. *Australian Family Physician* 19, 194–203.

Malarial Guidelines for Medical Practitioners (1989) National Health and Medical Research Council, Australian Government Publishing Service, Canberra, pp. 7–12, 35–41.

Murtagh J. (1987) Travelling: Preventive advice for patients. *Australian Family Physician* 16, 1617.

National Health and Medical Research Council (1993) *Malaria Prophylaxis.* NHMRC, Canberra.

Scott D. A. (1990) Norfloxacin for the prophylaxis of traveller's diarrhoea in US military personnel. *American Journal of Tropical Medicine and Hygiene* 42, 160–164.

Shephard R. J. (1988) Environmental conditions. In Dirix A., Knuttgen H. G. & Tittel K. (eds) *The Olympic Book of Sports Medicine I,* pp. 153–177. Blackwell Scientific Publications, Oxford.

Torre D. (1990) HIV disease and sport. *Lancet* 335, 1532.

Torre D., Sampietro C., Ferraro G., Zeroli C. & Speranza F. (1990) Transmission of HIV-1 infection via sports injury. *Lancet* 335, 1105.

World Health Organization (1991) *International Travel and Health,* pp. 61–73. WHO, Geneva.

Appendix A Principles and ethical guide-lines of health care for Sports Medicine — Medical Commission of the International Olympic Committee

The Medical Commission of the International Olympic Committee recommends the following ethical guide-lines for physicians who care for athletes and sportspersons (hereinafter termed athletes). These have been based on those drafted by the World Medical Association (*World Medical Journal* **28**, 83, 1981) and recognize the special circumstances in which medical care and guidance are provided for participants in sports.

1 All physicians who care for athletes have an ethical obligation to understand the specific physical and mental demands placed upon them during training for and participation in their sport(s).

2 It is recommended that undergraduate and postgraduate training in sports medicine be available to medical students and those doctors who desire or are required to provide health care for athletes.

3 When the sports participant is a child or an adolescent, the sports physician must ensure that the training and competition are appropriate for the stage of growth and development. Sports training and participation which may jeopardize the normal physical or mental development of the child or adolescent should not be permitted.

4 In sports medicine, as in all other branches of medicine, professional confidentiality must be observed. The right to privacy relating to medical advice or treatment that the athlete has received, must be protected.

5 When serving as a team physician, it is acknowledged that the sports doctor assumes a responsibility to athletes as well as team administrators and coaches. It is essential that from the outset, each athlete is informed of that responsibility and authorizes disclosure of otherwise confidential medical information but solely to specified and responsible persons and for the express purpose of determining the fitness or unfitness of that athlete to participate.

6 The sports physician must give an objective opinion on the athlete's fitness or unfitness as clearly and as precisely as possible. It is unethical for a physician with a financial investment or incentive in a team to act as team physician.

7 At sports venues it is the responsibility of the team or contest physician to determine whether an injured athlete may continue in or return to the event or game. This decision should not be delegated to other professionals or personnel. In the physician's absence these individuals must adhere strictly to the guide-lines established by the physician. In all cases, priority must be given in order to safeguard the athlete's health and safety. The outcome of the competition must never influence such decisions.

8 To enable him/her to undertake this ethical obligation, the sports physician must insist on professional autonomy over all medical decisions concerning the health, safety and legitimate interests of the athlete, none of which can be prejudiced to favour the interest of any third party whatsoever.

9 The sports physician should endeavour to keep the athlete's personal physician fully informed of relevant aspects of his or her health and treatment. When necessary, they should collaborate to ensure that the athlete does not exert himself or herself in a manner detrimental to their health and does not employ potentially harmful techniques to improve performance.

10 The sports physician should be cognizant of the contributions to athlete performance and health from other sports medicine professionals, including physical therapists, podiatrists, psychologists and sports scientists, including biochemists, biomechanists, physiologists, etc. As the person with the final responsibility for the health and well-being of the athlete, the physician should co-ordinate the respective roles of these professionals and those of appropriate medical specialists in the prevention and treatment of disease and injury from training and participation in sports.

11 The sports physician should publicly oppose and in practice refrain from using any method which has been banned by the IOC Medical Commission, is not in accord with professional ethics or which might be harmful to the athlete especially:

11.1 Procedures which artificially modify blood constituents or biochemistry.

11.2 The use of drugs or other substances whatever their nature and route of administration which artificially modify mental and physical ability to participate in sports.

11.3 Procedures used to mask pain or other protective symptoms for the express purpose of enabling the athlete to participate and thus risk aggravation of the condition, whereas in the absence of such procedures participation would be inadvisable or impossible.

11.4 Training and participating when to do so is incompatible with the preservation of the individual's fitness, health or safety.

Appendix A   continued

12 The sports physician should inform the athlete, those responsible for him or her and other interested parties of the consequences of the procedures he or she is opposing, guard against their use, enlist the support of other physicians and other organizations with similar aims, protect the athlete against any pressures which might induce him or her to use these methods and help with supervision against these procedures.

13 Physicians who advocate or utilize any of the abovementioned unethical procedures are in breach of this code of ethics and are unsuited to act or be accredited as a sports physician.

14 The sports physician must never be party to any contract which obliges them to reserve any particular form of therapy solely and exclusively for any individual or group of athletes.

15 When sports physicians accompany national teams to international competitions in other countries, they should be accorded the rights and privileges necessary to undertake their professional responsibilities to their team members while abroad.

16 It is strongly recommended that a sports physician participates in the framing of sports regulations. As an addition it can be stated that it is unwise for a team doctor to hold a number of other offices in a club, for example President, Director or selector as in so doing, he or she may be jeopardizing a truly satisfactory confidential medical communication with team members.

CHAPTER 22

CHILDREN IN SPORT

A. S. Watson

Physical growth during childhood is accompanied by hormonal changes associated with sexual maturation, the learning of basic skills, the setting of patterns of behaviour and the incorporation of social values and cultural norms. Children are structurally and physiologically different in each biological age group and, more importantly they differ from adults. Children mature at varying rates, exhibiting considerable variation within the same chronological age group. Physical activities should thus be appropriate for the stage of physical and psychological development of the individual child.

Illness or structural and developmental problems, peculiar to or first manifested in childhood, may be

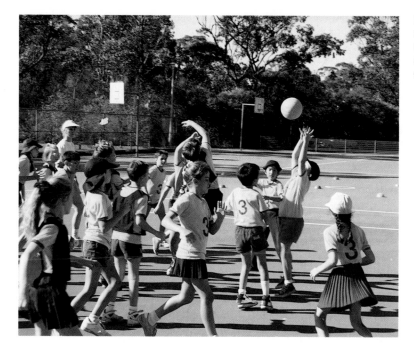

Fig. 22.1 There are no compelling reasons for segregating sporting activities by sex until approximately 14 years of age.

exacerbated by physical activity. These should be identified and considered in exercise programme design and sports selection.

Because children are largely dependent on adults to structure and supervise sporting activities and to provide models of acceptable behaviour, a special onus is placed on parents, teachers, coaches, sports administrators, sports physicians and other health professionals to be aware of the special problems posed by children's sport. All should be mindful of the child's limitations, fears, needs and wishes, to ensure that sport can be enjoyable and safe and a positive factor in the child's development.

GROWTH AND MATURATION

There is obvious marked variability in the physical growth of children of the same chronological age. In Australia the biological age variation has been demonstrated to be as much as 6 years (Russo *et al.* 1975) which is similar to that of other Western countries. For example, a rugby or basketball team of 13 year olds may contain individuals ranging in biological age from 10 to 16 years. This causes the mismatching often seen with respect to height, weight and skill development.

The average peak height velocity (PHV), or age at maximum growth rate, is 12 years for Australian girls, which is roughly 2 years earlier than for boys and is similar to other Western countries. A great deal of variability may also occur at the onset of the growth spurt in girls and boys. Girls on average are taller than boys only during the period from 11 to 14 years because of the earlier onset of the adolescent growth spurt. Girls may have greater muscular strength than boys until the age of 14–16. However, by the age of 10 years boys have significantly higher cardiovascular fitness levels, as measured by maximal oxygen uptake per kilogram of bodyweight per minute. While individual differences must be taken into account on the basis of growth and maturation, there appear to be few compelling reasons to segregate the sexes for sporting activity until approximately 14 years of age. This is when size, weight and strength begin to significantly favour the maturing boys (Fig. 22.1).

PHYSIOLOGICAL DIFFERENCES IN THE CHILD

Aerobic Power

Maximal aerobic power ($\dot{V}_{O2max}$), which is one measure of adult endurance capacity, is not significantly lower in children when taken as a function of bodyweight. Even when expressed as proportional to body segment length, which some researchers feel provides a more valid comparison, maximal aerobic power is only slightly less than in adults. The metabolic cost of walking and running, however, is distinctly higher in children than in older individuals. This may be due to a more mechanically wasteful running or walking style in smaller children. It appears that this can be affected positively by training and is one explanation for the improvement in walking and running performance when children are trained, despite the lack of a significant increase in $\dot{V}_{O2max}$.

Anaerobic Power

Anaerobic capacity of children, even when expressed per kilogram of bodyweight, is distinctly lower than in older age groups (Falk & Bar-Or 1993). This lower capacity is reflected in their ability to perform short-term all-out power output tasks and an 8 year old boy may produce only 65–70% of the mechanical power produced by a 14 year old boy. During adolescence this performance steadily improves with age, although in girls it does not appear to increase markedly beyond 11–12 years.

The utilization rate of glycogen, essential to the production of anaerobic power, is much less in the child than in the adult because the main limiting enzyme in glycolysis (phosphofructokinase) has a much lower activity in children than in adults. Similarly, children are less able to reach a low blood pH value (a measure of lactate production) during anaerobic exercise also reflecting their lower capacity for anaerobic tasks.

The Cardiovascular System

Children have a higher maximal heart rate and a lower stroke volume at rest and during exercise than adults. They appear, however, to have a better peripheral blood flow adjustment to exercise and consequently a greater arterial–venous oxygen difference. This reflects more efficient oxygen extraction by the tissues. Although arterial blood pressure particularly systolic, is relatively low in children, both at rest and during exercise, this is neither beneficial nor detrimental to endurance capacity.

The Respiratory System

Very young children have a relatively shallow breathing pattern, with a low ratio of tidal volume to vital capacity during maximal exercise. This results in a lower absorption of oxygen from the inspired air and a higher respiratory frequency, the major disadvantage being a greater oxygen cost of respiration.

Trainability

Children respond to basic conditioning or specific training regimens with improved performance but these improvements sometimes occur with very little increase in V_{O_2max}. This raises the question of whether traditional measurements such as this are applicable to children as a valid criterion of maximal aerobic power. Effectiveness of aerobic training appears to be much greater after the PHV and the trainability of aerobic power appears to be lowest 6 months before PHV in boys and coincides with PHV in girls (Bar-Or 1993a). Metabolic specialization into either an aerobic or anaerobic performer appears to begin in late puberty (Falk & Bar-Or 1993).

Exercise in Hot and Cold Environments

Children are vulnerable to temperature extremes, as small children may have a ratio of surface area to volume 30–40% higher than adults. This results in greater responses to changes in environmental temperature, losing body heat much faster than adults in cold conditions and increasing body (core) temperature much faster in hot environments.

The most efficient method for heat loss during the increased heat production of exercise is through the sweat/evaporation system. Children have a fully developed sweating apparatus by 3 years of age; however, they perspire much less than adults (Davies 1981). The child's sweating mechanism is not fully operative until after the adolescent growth spurt, therefore they are particularly susceptible to heat stress when exercising in hot environments. Heat injury may cause permanent damage to the thermoregulatory system, causing long-term heat intolerance.

The sweating/evaporation system poses other problems for children exercising in the heat, as they have a relatively low circulating blood volume and are far more prone to dangerous dehydration than are adults. Any fluid loss due to sweating must be rapidly and adequately replaced. Unfortunately, the drive of the thirst mechanism is not sufficient to replace such fluid losses (Bar-Or 1980), thus, adult supervision of immediate fluid replacement by drinking adequate amounts of water is essential to prevent dangerous dehydration or heat stress in children exercising in hot conditions.

Exercise in cold environments also presents hazards for children, as they are particularly susceptible to dangerous convective heat loss during immersion in cold water. Children, particularly those with low body fat insulation, should be carefully supervised during long-distance swimming in cold water.

Children exercising on land in cold environments should be encouraged to wear clothing in layers which may be removed or added according to the intensity of exercise and body temperature. Insulating head gear is particularly important in such circumstances, as a great deal of heat loss occurs from convex surfaces, notably the head and neck. Hypothermia may occur more rapidly on windy days due to the wind-chill factor and wind-proof clothing is particularly important for small children under such conditions.

NUTRITIONAL CONSIDERATIONS FOR THE YOUNG ATHLETE

During the adolescent growth spurt approximately 15% of adult height and 48% of skeletal mass are attained. It is important that the active adolescent's diet reflects this increased need for energy, vitamins, minerals and other nutrients. Nutritional surveys show that adolescents have irregular eating habits and often obtain a considerable amount of their nutritional intake from snacks between irregular meals, sometimes missing breakfast and lunch. Calcium, iron, zinc and Vitamins A, B_6, C and folic acid have frequently been reported as inadequate in the teenage diet. Female athletes involved in an intense exercise programme may often consume less than 60% of the minimal daily requirement of calcium and are also the group most likely to be deficient in iron (Harvey 1984).

The average amount of energy consumed by girls aged 16 years is about $10\,500$ kJ·day^{-1}, whereas males require approximately $15\,000$ kJ at this age. In endurance sports such as long-distance running, cycling or cross-country skiing, boys may have energy requirements in excess of $21\,000$ kJ·day^{-1}. Training and practice sessions often interfere with normal meals and additional meals and snacks become essential for adequate nutritional and energy intake. In these cases, sometimes a low concentration of carbohydrate may be used to supplement energy requirements in the rehydration fluid.

As dietary manipulation and nutritional status have been fully covered in Chapter 5, the reader should refer to this chapter if further information is needed for the child competing in high-level sport.

PSYCHOSOCIAL CONSIDERATIONS

Motor Learning

Physical activity at various levels of competitiveness is an important way for young children to learn about their physical and mental capabilities and their environment. The first 7 years of life are an intense period of motor learning as the majority of the motor subroutines that provide the foundation for later skilled sports performance are learned and in place by the end of this period. Increasingly complex closed skills in early childhood play, such as running, jumping, swinging, skipping and climbing, teach balance and co-ordination and enhance proprioception (position sense) and praxis (spatial awareness).

Once the basic movement patterns which co-ordinate both sides of the body and the more complex motor tasks, such as tracking objects, are

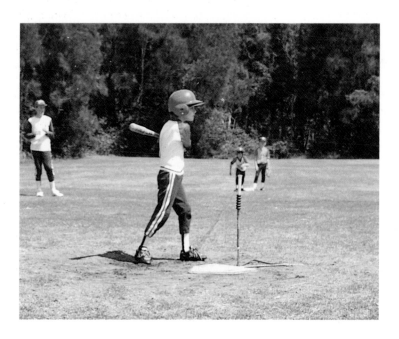

Fig. 22.2 More complex skills should be simplified so as to be appropriate for the skill level of the child. T-ball simplifies the teaching of batting skills and reduces the risk of injury by omitting pitching.

successfully mastered, attention can then be applied to focusing on external cues and variables relevant to the performance of open skills, such as avoiding collisions or evading other players. The skills of selective attention necessary for success in more complex sports are thus learned (Fig. 22.2).

Children are unable to selectively attend to movement characteristics until about 12 years of age. Children younger than 7 tend to over-exclude visual cues and may detect only a portion of the available visual information relevant to the task. Thus a 5 year old may attend only to the stance but not the body transfer when observing a baseball batter. An 11 year old in contrast may tend to over-include visual cues. For example, noticing the batter's brand of shoes as well as the correct batting position (Weiss *et al*. 1993).

Rewards of Physical Activity

Children are aware of, and actively seek, adult approval for their performances from a very early age. Between the ages of 5 and 7 they also begin to compare their physical performance with their peers. The child is becoming aware of the rewards of physical activity which include, at this stage of development, feelings of competence and mastery, experiencing personal self-esteem, engaging in enjoyable behaviour, achieving desired goals and gaining the admiration and esteem of others.

Sport versus Play

After the age of 5 children begin to organize themselves into games of greater complexity involving co-operation and competition. Formal games with rules and teams are neither common nor appropriate until age 8 or 9. In order to analyse the positive and negative effects of sporting participation, it is necessary to consider the nature of sport and identify areas where negative social pressures may apply. During early childhood, socialization starts to become important and behavioural norms begin to become established. Self-judgement, comparison of performance, frustration, aggression and certain negative aspects of sports performance become more apparent.

The continuum from unstructured play towards organized sport is characterized by the following developments:

- There is a severe reduction in spontaneity and the activity becomes less related to the specific needs or wishes of each individual player
- Formal rules become important, stressing structural roles and position relationships
- Individual liability increases with an increase in responsibility for the quality and the character of one's behaviour
- The relevance of the outcome becomes more important to the participants and spreads to non-participants as well
- The goals become diverse, complex and more related to values from outside the activity
- More time is consumed in preparation and practice
- More physical and mental effort is required beyond the limits of just recreation or a simple interest in an activity

In competitive sport, the player not only tries to obtain a set goal but also attempts to prevent the opponent from achieving his or hers. This involves direct conflict and often aggression in reducing the opponent's achievements by direct interference. Sometimes the fine line between legitimate application of aggression and skill in play, and violence, is difficult to define. It appears that the direct contact or collision sports (almost exclusively team sports), particularly those which are also classified as spectator sports and are more prone to the concepts of 'winning at all costs', can have a negative effect on children. These negative influences from parents, coaches and other adults in authority over children must be counterbalanced by positive education from those bodies who administer their sport.

Psychological Costs of Sport

One of the major negative influences in children's sport occurs when adults and children erroneously impose a professional sporting model on what should be a recreational and educational experience for children (Hodge & Tod 1993).

Studies on behaviour modelling (Bandura 1977),

strongly suggest that violence in top-level sports seen and often replayed on television, may teach or reinforce similar violent responses in the observers, particularly children. This is most likely to occur if the players involved are admired or respected and if this behaviour is not genuinely deplored by the parents or the peer group.

Another source of negative influence in children's sport is the over-emphasis on winning, which is more evident in team sports. The only fair and realistic goal for children is to apply what skill and ability they possess to the game as best they can. It is the effort and personal improvement which should be the goal. Over-emphasis on outcome rather than effort may tend to stereotype children as losers by themselves, their peer group and those in authority. Positive reinforcement of personal effort and improvement enhances feelings of self-worth and mastery. As children have no control over outcome, authority figures who attach importance to this, or even worse, punish 'unfavourable' outcomes, reinforce feelings of helplessness, negative self-esteem and deny the child enjoyment (Smith 1984). Less skilful players are often denied optimum participation by being dropped from teams or left sitting on the bench. This limits the active participation and enjoyment of the game by these members and also limits their opportunity for more skill development.

The aims of sporting involvement for children should include:

- Exposing them to a wide range of sporting experiences
- Improving their physical skills
- Improving their proprioception and selective attention (positive factors in learning generally)
- Developing positive socialization
- Fostering feelings of personal mastery and self-esteem

These aims are better achieved if children are carefully graded for sport according to their size and skill as well as by age.

The positive effects on the psychological development and socialization of the child from a well-planned and supervised competitive team sport include:

- Relatively safe training in risk-taking behaviour
- Satisfaction in achievement
- The feeling of working towards a defined goal
- Personal role definition
- The awareness of, and adherence to, rules in sports that are similar to social rules
- The importance of sharing experiences and effort with the members of the team (peer group interaction)
- The importance of respecting other competitors
- The promotion of regular, long-term physical activity to maintain physical well-being

Further, there is evidence to suggest that adolescents who are involved in sport show better academic results than those who are not and although no definite cause and effect relationship has been established, this remains one of the many aims of physical education and competitive sport.

THE IMMATURE MUSCULOSKELETAL SYSTEM

Apart from the obvious differences in size and strength, there are more subtle differences in tissue properties in children. The most obvious anatomical difference is the presence of growth cartilage in the immature skeleton. This is present in three sites: the articular surfaces; the epiphyseal (growth) plates; and the apophyseal insertions of major muscle–tendon units (Fig. 22.3).

The growing articular surface in the child's long bones is more susceptible than adult cartilage to shear, particularly at the elbow, knee and ankle joints. Blood supply to the subchondral bone in the epiphyses of these joints is critical and recurrent microtrauma may cause ischaemic necrosis of a bone resulting in osteochondritis dissecans, possible loose body formation and permanent joint damage.

The epiphyseal or growth plate is also vulnerable during vigorous sport. This is because it has the least fibrocellular cartilage matrix and the structural weakness in this area increases the susceptibility of the growth plate to slip or fracture (Salter & Harris 1963). Often, fractures through the growth plate will occur in the immature skeleton rather than ruptures of the ligaments or tendons, which would result from similar proportional stress in adults.

The ligaments and musculotendinous units elongate subsequent to long bone growth and during periods of rapid growth significant muscle tightness may develop. This increases the risk of muscle attachment (apophyseal) overuse injury and of acute avulsion. Muscle and fascial tightness during periods of rapid growth may also cause postural changes.

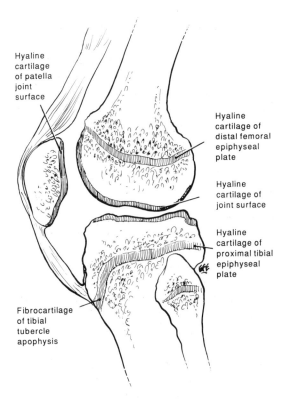

Hyaline cartilage of patella joint surface

Hyaline cartilage of distal femoral epiphyseal plate

Hyaline cartilage of joint surface

Hyaline cartilage of proximal tibial epiphyseal plate

Fibrocartilage of tibial tubercle apophysis

Fig. 22.3 Sites of growth cartilage in and around the immature knee joint.

The increased lumbar extension posture (lordosis) often seen in adolescents is due to rapid growth of the vertebral bodies anteriorly and relative tightness of the dense thoracolumbar fascia. This postural change may increase the risk of stress fracture of the posterior elements of the spine through the pars interarticularis and may also predispose to disc injury (Micheli 1983).

Effects of Exercise on the Immature Musculoskeletal System

A minimum amount of activity is necessary to support normal human growth and maintenance of skeletal tissue (Caine & Lindner 1985). Very intensive strength training by children, however, may cause growth plate injury and bony deformation (Micheli 1983), while heavy physical training, particularly when combined with a low percentage of body fat in young women, may cause a prolonged prepubertal state. This may also cause relatively longer limbs to develop during prepubertal growth because the limbs at this time grow faster than the trunk (Caine & Lindner 1985).

Children playing organized sports, particularly when they specialize early, are often subject to predictable repetitive demands, especially in activities such as throwing, pitching and bowling in cricket or in breast-stroke swimming. This may cause imbalances in strength and joint range of movement and problems such as shoulder impingement may occur as an overuse injury from muscle tendon imbalance during the growth period (Gerrard 1993).

Factors Associated with the Incidence of Sports Injuries in Children

Injury rates from children's sport are approximately 3 per 100 children per year; however, the very serious injuries only approximate 0.69 per 100 children per year (Watson 1984). Fortunately, the injury rate for children below the age of 12 is very low and it appears that sport is relatively safe for prepubertal children (Fig. 22.4). There is a sharp increase in injury rate at age 14, particularly in males, and this continues with age (Davidson *et al.* 1978; Watson 1984). The incidence of injury appears, however, to peak at about 15 years of age in females.

Watson (1984) has identified a number of factors which are believed to be of importance in children's sporting injuries and these are as follows:

- Recklessness of the injured party
- Foul or illegal play by another
- Poor playing area or equipment (facilities)

Fig. 22.4 The incidence of sports injury casualty presentations by age (adapted from Smithers & Myers 1985).

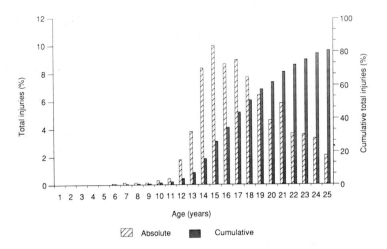

- Inappropriate body size or strength for the activity or the opposition encountered in it
- Inadequate fitness levels or postural problems
- Lack of, or defective, protective gear
- Poor footwear or sports gear
- Incomplete recovery from a previous injury
- Poor supervision or refereeing
- Lack of adequate warm-up

Various researchers place the above in differing order of importance and their relative contribution to injury is difficult to determine in most cases. Backx *et al.* (1989) suggested that an incomplete recovery from a previous injury was a factor in 30% of acute and 50% of overuse injuries.

Physical education programmes in schools account for approximately a quarter of all injuries; however,

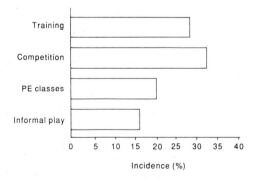

Fig. 22.5 Situations in which sports injuries occur in children (adapted from Backx *et al.* 1989).

there is a much greater incidence among boys in out-of-school sport and a large number of these occur during training (Fig. 22.5). Many overuse injuries develop during training with the high level of repetition of some activities, such as jumping to lay up in basketball, and blocking or spiking in volleyball.

Falling, often as a result of a collision, appears frequently to produce injury as can twisting or misstepping (Fig. 22.6). Such injury mechanisms may be reduced or eliminated by competent skills coaching and training.

Approximately 30% of sports injuries to children require medical attention, and 11% require hospital admission. Moreover, of those who are hospitalized, approximately 12% suffer long-term joint dysfunction or physical deformity (Tursz & Crost 1986).

A number of studies have attempted the difficult task of defining the role of skills and the performer's ability in the incidence of injury. Watson (1984) suggested that the average or above-average sportsperson was more likely to be injured than the high-level athlete, and those of below average ability were least likely to be injured.

Prevention of Injury

In order for the risks to be assessed with the objective of introducing effective preventive measures, accurate, reproducible and standardized

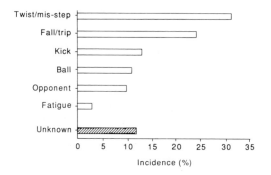

Fig. 22.6 The causes of childhood sporting injuries.

clinical research is required into the incidence of injuries in all types of childhood physical activity.

Possible preventive measures include the following:

- Rule modifications
- Equipment modification for size, strength and skill level (Fig. 22.2)
- Appropriate footwear, protective equipment and orthotic devices, if indicated
- Appropriate sports selection and grading for certain individuals
- Improvements in coaching techniques and training programmes including correct warm-up, appropriate strength and flexibility exercises and graded intensity and volume of workload

The results of research in this area and awareness programmes which highlight the severity and incidence of certain types of injuries may be enough to encourage appropriate rule and equipment changes, although this has been slow to occur. The enforcement of appropriately tested eye protection in ice hockey and squash are good examples of effective and essential benefits from sports injury research.

ACUTE SPORTING INJURIES

Many of the injuries sustained by children are similar to those seen in adults. However, because they are growing, children suffer injuries which do not occur in adults and in some cases injury patterns and principles of management differ. It is not the purpose of this chapter to present a comprehensive coverage of all the acute childhood sporting injuries, but rather to discuss those which have special implications for the young athlete, or in which the management principles differ significantly from those applicable to the adult.

Head and Neck Injuries

Serious head and neck injuries in sport are extremely rare below 11 years of age. However, there is a dramatic increase in incidence in the 15–18 year age group. It is in this group that most of the fatalities and permanent spinal cord injuries occur. Although the incidence of central nervous system injury is relatively low, amounting to 1–5% of all sports-related injuries, these account for 50–100% of the mortality (Bruce *et al*. 1984). The estimated rate of severe spinal injury in rugby is 2.74 per 100 000 players per season. The injured players are most frequently the forwards and 60% of all severe spinal injuries occur in the set or loose scrummage (Burry & Gowland 1981).

As children grow older they are less likely to complain of or report injuries, particularly if it may mean exclusion from the team. Symptoms of amnesia, altered consciousness, difficulty in concentrating, vomiting, neck pain and burning pain or 'pins and needles' in the arms, should be actively investigated by the coach, team physician or parents and always taken seriously.

The principles of assessment and management of head and neck injury are essentially the same as for adults (see Chapter 15). Particular attention should be paid to follow-up after minor head injury and to careful medical assessment prior to return to playing or training.

Preventive measures are particularly important for the child. The risk of injury in football, for example, may be reduced by adequate skills training and the use of headgear or helmets. Pre-participation screening may serve to exclude or counsel those individuals with long, thin necks and poor musculature from high-risk positions, such as the front row of a rugby scrum. Rule modifications such as reducing the scrum size, or strictly controlling the method of packing down into a scrum in junior rugby and strict refereeing control of scrums and mauls, have come about as a direct result of consultation between sports medicine professionals and the governing body of the sport. The promotion or enforcement of protective helmet use in skiing, ice hockey and American football has demonstrably reduced the risk of both open and closed head injury.

Non-physeal or Diaphyseal Fractures in Children

Immature bone is softer and less brittle than adult bone and will often withstand considerable bending before a fracture occurs, producing the incomplete or greenstick fractures seen in children. Immature bone generally has a good blood supply and heals rapidly, so children need less time in a cast, and most fractures may be treated conservatively by closed reduction. As bone remodelling in children is very active, shaft (diaphyseal) fractures may be immobilized with minor displacement. However, no angular or rotational deformity should be accepted. When open reduction is required for fractures with wide displacement, internal fixation pins and screws should be placed to avoid injury to growth plates.

Management principles and possible complications will be illustrated by discussion of supracondylar fractures of the humerus.

SUPRACONDYLAR FRACTURE OF THE ELBOW

This fracture, usually caused by a fall on the hand with the elbow flexed, occurs proximal to the condyles of the humerus. The distal fragment, with the forearm, is displaced backwards and often rotated. Urgent accurate reduction is required and a slight shift may be accepted, but a tilt or twist must be fully corrected. This can be performed closed without internal fixation; however, the pulse should be carefully monitored during and after reduction of the fracture. Injury to the brachial artery and radial nerve may occur and this risk can be reduced significantly by careful first aid with immediate immobilization. Often swelling with the elbow held flexed may cause diminished circulation to the forearm, causing serious ischaemic damage

unless detected early. Normal circulation can be restored by careful extension of the elbow until a pulse is felt, without compromising the stability of the reduced fracture.

Growth Plate Injury: Salter-Harris Lesions

ACUTE FRACTURES

Acute fractures may occur involving the growth plates at a number of sites. These have been classified by Salter and Harris (1963) into horizontal fractures (Types I and II) and vertical fractures (Types III and IV) with Type V being a compression fracture. The complication rate with respect to growth arrest is lower in the Type I fracture, which represents a horizontal displacement of the growth plate and the Type II fracture, where the fracture line leaves the growth plate and runs through the adjacent metaphysis (Fig. 22.7). Relatively higher complication rates are described in Type III and IV vertical fractures, as the joint surface is involved. Accurate anatomical reduction (complete correction of the displacement, angulation and rotation) in Type III and IV fractures is essential to prevent long-term degenerative changes in the joint and to make growth disturbance less likely. Recently, it

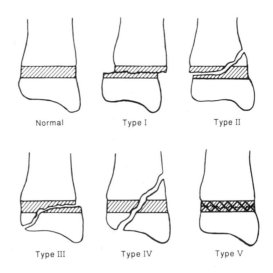

Fig. 22.7 The modified Harris-Salter classification of growth plate fractures.

has become apparent that the complication rate is determined more by the degree of initial displacement than by the Salter-Harris type of fracture (McManama 1988).

Transphyseal fracture of the head of femur

A transphyseal fracture of the femoral head (Salter-Harris Type I) may represent an acute slipped capital femoral epiphysis, which is discussed later. As such it may be associated with certain disease states such as renal osteodystrophy or hypothyroidism. Urgent anatomical reduction with internal fixation is required, as there is a high risk of avascular necrosis of the femoral head.

Fractures of the distal femoral epiphysis

Fractures of the distal femoral epiphysis are common in the young athlete in response to severe twisting

Fig. 22.8 Diagrammatic representation of valgus stress injury to an adolescent left knee. This causes a growth plate fracture rather than a tibial collateral rupture (TCL) rupture (more common in the adult). The proximal tibial growth plate is protected by the more distal TCL attachment to the tibia.

or valgus injury of the lower limb (Steiner & Grana 1988). These fractures are often difficult to diagnose and stress X-rays may be required, but closed reduction is normally successful. There is a greater than 20% incidence of subsequent significant growth disturbance, as this growth plate is responsible for 70% of the longitudinal growth of the femur. The risk of growth disturbance is greater if the amount of initial displacement is large.

Fracture of the upper tibial growth plate

The insertion of the tibial collateral ligament distal to the upper tibial growth plate tends to protect this plate from injury (Fig. 22.8). Fractures of the upper tibial growth plate, however, occasionally occur as a result of severe trauma or with avulsion of the patella tendon distally (Fig. 22.9). After closed or open reduction, if this is necessary, the knee should be immobilized in a back slab rather than a plaster cylinder and should be monitored carefully. This type of fracture is often complicated by injury to the popliteal artery or subsequent deep posterior leg compartmental pressure syndrome. Those fractures involving the articular surface (Salter-Harris Types III and IV) will frequently

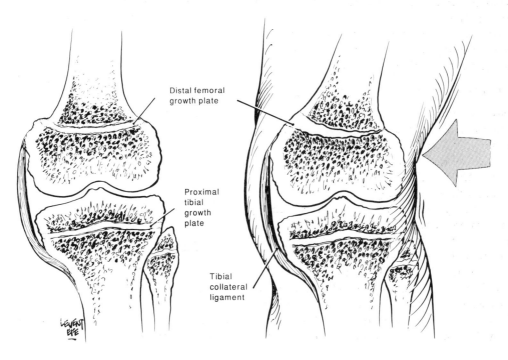

Distal femoral growth plate

Proximal tibial growth plate

Tibial collateral ligament

require open reduction and internal fixation. As the major part of longitudinal growth in the tibia occurs at this growth plate, the prognosis for subsequent growth disturbance is similar to that for the distal femoral fractures.

Avulsion fracture of the anterior cruciate ligament

Avulsion fracture of the anterior cruciate ligament (ACL) attachment to the tibial eminence of the proximal tibial epiphysis may occur in a rotational, valgus stress injury to the knee. This injury may occur in the adolescent knee rather than the more common ACL rupture in the adult. The older the child the greater is the likelihood of injury to the ACL. The knee usually becomes rapidly painful, stiff and swollen due to blood in the joint (haemarthrosis) and if the knee is aspirated to relieve pain

and to further the diagnosis, fat globules from the exposed bone marrow are seen in the aspirated blood. The dynamic extension test, Lachman test and pivot shift test will all be positive, indicating deficiency of the ACL (see Chapter 20). Successful anatomical reduction, with or without internal fixation of the avulsed fragment, is essential for the restoration of rotational knee stability.

Other avulsion fractures

Avulsion fractures may occur at the apophyseal attachments of large muscle groups in the adolescent athlete. The most common sites are the attachment of the rectus femoris muscle to the anterior inferior iliac spine (Fig. 14.9), the hamstrings to the ischial tuberosity (Fig. 14.8b), the sartorius to the anterior superior iliac spine (Fig. 14.10), the patella tendon to the tibial tuberosity, the iliopsoas tendon to the lesser trochanter and the attachment of the abdominal muscles to the iliac crest apophysis. These injuries are seen in sprinters, jumpers and football players, and occur when a sudden, violent muscular contraction causes severe pain and loss of power in the affected muscle group. Sometimes a contraction is resisted making avulsion more likely, as in a blocked kick in soccer. The attachment of the forearm flexors to the medial epicondyle at the elbow may also be avulsed in throwers. The highest incidence of such injuries is in the 14–17 year age group just prior to closure of the apophysis. The pain is often severe with local tenderness, swelling, inhibited action and pain on contraction of the involved muscle group.

Initial management involves cold therapy and support in a posture which allows relaxation of the involved muscle group. After the pain has subsided gentle limited range-of-motion exercises are allowed with no resistance. After a full range of motion is regained gentle resisted exercises are started. These may include stationary cycling, freestyle kicking with flippers, swimming or wading. When approximately 50% of the patient's strength has returned, more complex integrated movements of the whole limb may be started and sports activity such as jogging, jumping, swerving, starting and stopping, may be commenced, with gradual increases in speed and intensity. Supervised light training should only

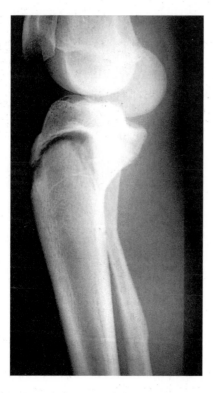

Fig. 22.9 A Harris-Salter type II fracture of the proximal tibial growth plate which occurred on take-off in a 14-year-old high jumper. It required open reduction and internal fixation using a wire to approximate the distal patellar tendon attachment to the tibial metaphysis.

be permitted after the patient returns to the full, pain-free range of movement and full strength. Occasionally, if displacement is greater than 10 mm or if a painful fibrous union or non-union occurs, internal fixation or excision of the apophysis with reattachment of the avulsed musculotendinous unit may be necessary. As these fractures nearly always occur towards the end of growth, no significant growth disturbances have been reported.

EPIPHYSIOLYSIS

Occasionally displacement may occur at a growth plate without major trauma. Epiphysiolysis or slipped epiphysis, occurs most commonly at the capital femoral epiphysis in the hip joint. The slip occurs suddenly in 30% of cases and gradually in 70% of cases and may be the result of sporting trauma, with half the cases giving a history of acute injury. There may be an underlying abnormality such as an endocrine imbalance as in hypothyroidism or renal osteodystrophy and many of these patients are obese and sexually underdeveloped. The condition is often bilateral (25%) and the capital femoral epiphysis of the other side may slip at the same time or up to 2 years later.

Epiphysiolysis is more common in boys with an average age of 15 years. In girls the average age of occurrence is 12 years and the condition rarely occurs after the onset of menstruation.

Sometimes there is groin pain, although the pain may only be felt in the thigh or knee and may settle, only to return with further sporting activity. As displacement progresses the affected leg becomes obviously shorter and externally rotated and there is a limp (Fig. 22.10). Hip abductor weakness and inhibition is a common finding, as evidenced by dipping of the other side of the pelvis when the subject stands on the affected leg (positive Trendelenburg sign). The movements of hip abduction and internal rotation are reduced proportionally to the severity of the slip.

X-ray examination shows widening of the growth plate and the epiphysis appears slipped posteriorly and inferiorly, so that a line drawn along the superior surface of the femoral neck fails to pass through the epiphysis, as in a normal hip. X-rays should be obtained of both hips because of the high incidence

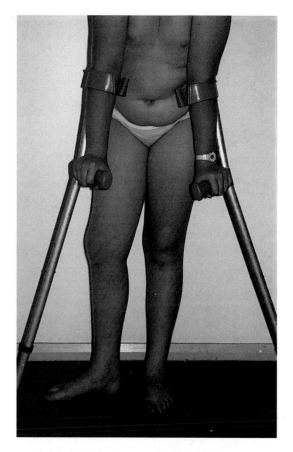

Fig. 22.10 A 12 year old girl with a slipped right capital femoral epiphysis, demonstrating the typical body type and external rotation attitude of the hip joint.

of bilateral involvement. Patients in whom this diagnosis is suspected should be sent for early orthopaedic assessment because the impending or early slip must be internally fixed before major displacement occurs. If appropriate, their endocrine and renal status should be checked.

Open reduction has a 30% complication rate. If the slip is minimal no reduction is attempted. Often it is safer to fix the head in its displaced position (Fig. 22.11) and to compensate for the displacement with an osteotomy following closure of the growth plate. The epiphysis has a precarious blood supply and if this is interrupted by severe displacement, death of the femoral head (avascular necrosis) with progressive destruction of the hip joint may occur.

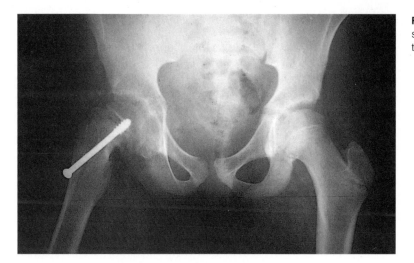

Fig. 22.11 A late epiphyseal slip stabilized by internal fixation in the same patient as Fig. 22.10.

OVERUSE INJURIES

Most individuals are much more physically active during their childhood than at any other period of their lives. Because of their size, capacity for repair and the supervision usually provided for them, overuse injuries in children mostly present early and resolve rapidly with early appropriate treatment. Competitive sport, habitually high levels of activity, peer group and other pressures, poor compliance with treatment, activity restrictions and growth, however, may complicate management.

The Osteochondroses

Children do develop some of the common adult overuse syndromes such as tendinitis and stress fractures. However, the osteochondroses, disorders of growth centres, occur as the most common

Table 22.1 Conditions in children which may present as overuse injury

Osteochondroses
Epiphysiolysis (slipped epiphysis)
Osteomyelitis, Brodie's abscess
Bone tumours, metastases
Muscle and fibrous tissue tumours
Metabolic disease (e.g. rickets)
Congenital structural problems — tarsal coalitions, mild talipes

group of overuse injuries in childhood. Other childhood conditions may also present as overuse injuries and must be excluded in the diagnostic process (Table 22.1).

The osteochondroses are self-limited, idiopathic developmental disorders of primary or secondary ossification centres. They may be classified into four categories (Pappas 1989) and may be intra- or extra-articular (Table 22.2). The frequency and severity of these conditions are determined by a number of factors including genetic predisposition and excessive activity levels. Individuals with osteochondritis are statistically more likely to develop it at more than one site.

Outcome is determined by the following:

- Stage and extent of involvement at diagnosis
- Skeletal and articular development
- Mechanical demands on the involved area
- Adequate management
- Compliance with the rehabilitation programme

TRACTION OSTEOCHONDROSIS (APOPHYSITIS)

These conditions occur commonly at the attachment of major tendons in the immature skeleton, particularly at the knee and heel.

Osgood-Schlatter's disease

Osgood-Schlatter's disease may be classified as a traction apophysitis (non-articular osteochondrosis).

Table 22.2 The osteochondroses

Classification	Name	Sites(s)
Non-articular traction (pulling)	Osgood-Schlatter's	Tibial tubercle
	Sinding-Larsen-Johansson's disease	Inferior pole of patella
	Sever's disease	Calcaneus
Articular subchondral (crushing)	Perthes' disease	Femoral head
	Kienböck's disease	Lunate (wrist)
	Köhler's disease	Navicular (mid-foot)
	Freiberg's disease	Second metatarsal head
Articular chondral (splitting)	Osteochondritis dissecans	Femoral condyle (knee)
		Capitellum (elbow)
		Talar dome (ankle)
Physeal	Scheuermann's disease	Thoracolumbar spine
	Blount's disease	Tibia (proximal)

The mechanism of injury is repetitive traction applied to the tibial tuberosity by the patellar tendon, which causes partial avulsion of the developing secondary ossification centre with repetitive healing and bone accretion. The condition is self-limited by the ossification and fusion of the tibial tubercle.

This condition is the most common specific complaint of athletes under the age of 16 years (Beovich & Fricker 1988) and appears more frequently in boys with the onset of the growth spurt, but is also seen in younger girls aged between 10 and 12 years. A high level of physical activity in such sports as football, basketball, netball or gymnastics is often implicated, and there may be a history of only one or a number of acute injury episodes. The pain is most severe after activity involving vigorous quadriceps contraction or direct local trauma to the tibial tubercle.

Examination typically reveals tender enlargement of the tibial tubercle, often with increased skin temperature over the area of tenderness and tightness of the quadriceps and hamstring muscle groups.

It is important to exclude internal derangement of the knee. Other serious conditions in this age group, such as slipped capital femoral epiphysis may present with knee pain and, because Osgood-Schlatter's disease is common, diagnosis of the latter does not necessarily exclude the former.

Radiological examination (Fig. 14.15) is often not necessary on first presentation, particularly with a typical history. It may be indicated, however, if there is a recurrence of symptoms or failure of the symptoms to subside, especially if this occurs past the age when ossification and fusion of the tibial tubercle should have been complete.

Treatment should start with a careful explanation of the nature of the injury to the athlete and the parents, emphasizing the fact that no permanent joint damage will ensue. A flexibility programme should be instituted for tight musculature, particularly the quadriceps and hamstrings, and a graded strengthening programme for the quadriceps and its synergists (calf and hamstring muscles) should be added. Initially a straight-leg-raising regimen is employed, with progression to resisted exercises such as leg presses. The strengthening programme should emphasize mainly concentric muscle contraction initially, followed by eccentric contraction. These exercises also should be graded to become progressively more specific for range, speed and eventually load.

According to symptoms, some modification should be made to sporting activity, especially running and jumping. If a definite avulsion can be demonstrated either clinically or radiologically, at least 2–3 weeks complete rest from running activity should be enforced. Cast or rigid brace immobilization is rarely necessary but may be warranted for severe cases. This should be limited to 3 weeks and must be followed up by careful, graded rehabilitation of the wasted muscles. Anatomical malalignment, particularly varus malalignment of the foot or leg, which may increase rotational stress on the quadriceps mechanism, should be treated with orthotic devices if necessary. Shock absorbing footwear may also be used to reduce the load on the quadriceps mechanism. Padded braces which include a constricting strap above and below the patella, may resist lateral movement of the patella and may also provide some protection of the tibial tubercle from direct trauma during the patient's return to sporting activity.

If objective muscle testing shows significant inhibition of the quadriceps muscle due to pain and/or weakness, the child should be excluded from contact or collision sport because of impairment of the important protective function that the quadri-

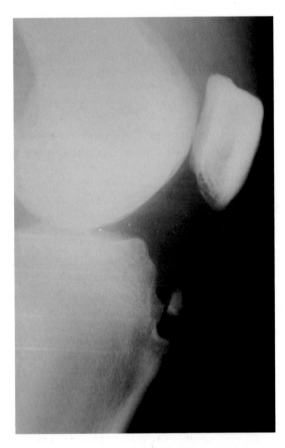

Fig. 22.12 A separate symptomatic ossicle within the patella tendon following Osgood-Schlatter's disease.

ceps have on the knee joint and the patellofemoral joint. Corticosteroid injections are contraindicated and anti-inflammatory medication is not particularly useful. Ice applications after activity and ice massage can be very effective in relieving symptoms in most cases.

In cases where separate ossicles within the patella tendon remain symptomatic following fusion of the tibial tubercle (Fig. 22.12), they should be excised along with the excision of any underlying increased prominence in the tibial tubercle.

Sinding-Larsen-Johansson's disease

A traction osteochondrosis may occur at the inferior pole of the patellar at the superior attachment of the patellar tendon (the most common site for adult patellar tendinitis). This is called Sinding-Larsen-Johansson's disease. In some cases a tear-drop-shaped patella deformity, sometimes with a separate ossicle, may persist. A frank avulsion may occur requiring rest and protection.

Sever's disease

Sever's disease (calcaneal apophysitis) is a traction apophysitis of the heel. It is common in young runners aged between 7 and 15, particularly if they are involved in the various football codes, field hockey, basketball and other games involving many sessions per week, as is often the case in this age group. Sixty per cent of these are bilateral and boys are three times more likely to develop this problem than girls (Micheli 1983).

The ununited calcaneal apophysis in children is the site of insertion of the Achilles tendon and the plantar fascia. Repetitive resisted plantar flexion in running and jumping sports causes microfractures and inflammation adjacent to the growth plate. This may be compounded by heavy heel strike, causing further trauma to the vulnerable apophysis. During rapid growth relative overgrowth of the long bones causes tightness of the gastrocnemius and soleus muscles. Varus malalignment of the leg or foot can contribute to this problem by adding shearing and torsional stress to the apophysis from compensatory increased pronation.

The pain is often worse following training (when

starting to walk after resting) and may cause the patient to limp or walk on the toes. The heel is tender over the apophysis especially laterally and tightness of the gastrocnemius/soleus muscles is usually present. Ideally there should be at least 15° of dorsiflexion available at the ankle joint with the knee extended and the subtalar joint locked (Gregg & Das 1982). What is ideal, however, depends on the range of motion requirements of the sporting activity. Weakness of the ankle dorsiflexors may be present and patients often exhibit heavy heel strike on gait analysis.

Activity modification with reduced running and jumping, limited by pain, is essential, and while active the child is encouraged always to wear shoes. These should be well constructed and well fitted with a firm heel counter (Fig. 28.15) and orthotic correction should be added if indicated. A 4 mm heel-raise, heel cup can be used if preferred.

Graded strengthening exercises for the dorsi-flexors and the intrinsic and extrinsic muscles of the foot responsible for the integrity of the longitudinal arch, should be carefully supervised. Heel raises with the knees flexed and while pushing down strongly with the toes (flexion) tend to isolate the appropriate muscles. These exercises are graded towards the range, load and speed specificity of the sporting activity and should be combined with frequent static stretching for the gastrocnemius and soleus muscles during and after activity. Dorsi-flexion night splints may be useful in some cases of severe calf muscle tightness.

X-ray examination should be saved for cases which appear to be clinically atypical and not responding to these normal measures. Such examination should exclude neoplasia, Brodie's abscess (osteomyelitis), avulsion fractures of the calcaneus and metallic foreign bodies. Fragmentation and sclerosis of the apophysis is a normal radiological appearance and is not diagnostic.

Apophysitis of the fifth metatarsal

Lateral mid-foot pain in a child or adolescent may be due to traction apophysitis of the base of the fifth metatarsal. Pain is felt on jumping or running, especially on uneven or banked surfaces or around

curves. There is marked tenderness over the styloid process at the base of the fifth metatarsal at the insertion of the peroneus brevis. Resisted eversion of the foot often reproduces the pain.

Treatment should be directed towards modification of the activities which cause pain, attention given to footwear to avoid direct frictional irritation of the styloid process (sometimes requiring padding and strapping), stretching of the peroneal muscles and carefully graded strengthening work for the evertors of the foot. Performing these exercises in plantar flexion may reduce some of the stress on the peroneus brevis initially. Cold therapy and other local modalities are also helpful in reducing the patient's symptoms.

Apophysitis of the tarsal navicular

In an older child or adolescent, focal pain and swelling may be noticed over the medial and inferior aspects of the tarsal navicular. This may be due to traction apophysitis or inflammation of an accessory navicular bone and its attachment to the main body of the navicular. The accessory bone is separated from the navicular by fibrocartilage and the inflammation is caused by traction at the attachment of tibialis posterior or by mechanical irritation of the prominence of the tubercle (or accessory navicular) by footwear. Problems related to this anomaly are worsened by hyperpronation, which lowers the arch and rolls the foot in, increasing the medial prominence, which is thus exposed to pressure from footwear. This also increases stress on the tibialis posterior, one of the major dynamic stabilizers of the longitudinal arch (Gregg & Das 1982). Radiological examination may show a prominent tubercle of the navicular or an accessory navicular bone and, if required, a computerized tomography (CT) scan allows differentiation between a stress fracture of the former and a separate ossification centre in the latter.

Oral and topical anti-inflammatory agents sometimes help relieve pain as does footwear modification and careful padding. Orthotics should be used to control excessive pronation and flexibility and strengthening exercises should be performed for tibialis posterior, tibialis anterior and the long flexors of the toes. If these more conservative measures fail, 3–4 weeks of immobilization in a short leg cast may be required. If the cast is unsuccessful, resection of the symptomatic accessory navicular or prominent tuberosity with inferior transposition of the tibialis posterior tendon is curative. Both surgical treatment and cast immobilization should be followed by a carefully graded full rehabilitation programme. Following surgery athletes normally require 6–9 months before returning to sporting activity.

Apophysitis of the medial epicondyle of the humerus

Active young throwers or tennis players often develop pain and tenderness related to apophysitis of the medial epicondyle of the humerus. The medial epicondylar apophysis is the last of the growth plates of the elbow to close and may be present up to age 18 or 19 years and therefore this condition often presents considerably later than the other forms of traction apophysitis. The use of a non-stretch circumferential arm brace over the mid-belly of the forearm flexors and the use of cold applications after playing and training may be helpful in preventing recurrence and allowing protected return to activity. Throwers or pitchers often require a 4–6 week period of gentle elbow exercises with no throwing and relative rest. Swimming and running are suggested during this period with a graded programme of progressive strengthening exercises for the triceps and wrist flexors. When throwing does resume, there should be a gradual increase in the number of repetitions and the distance thrown, starting with approximately 10 m. A similar graded programme is used for tennis players. In some cases this condition may recur with activity, even though there may have been no symptoms for 4–6 months. For this reason it is essential to enforce adequate warm-up and gradual build-up following any disruption to training and certainly at the beginning of each season.

Apophysitis at other sites

Traction apophysitis may also occur at the following sites:
- At the origin of the hamstrings at the ischial

tuberosity (in sprinters, gymnasts and aerobic dancers)
- At the origin of the sartorius at the anterior superior iliac spine
- At the origin of the rectus femoris at the anterior inferior iliac spine
- At the insertion of the iliopsoas at the lesser trochanteric apophysis (mainly in sprinters, hurdlers, jumpers and football players)
- At the insertion of the abdominal muscles to the anterior portion of the iliac crest apophysis (especially in young middle distance runners)

The same general management principles apply to all such conditions and these are as follows:

- Activity modification
- Local physical treatment
- Identification and correction (if possible) of postural problems, muscle imbalance and tightness
- Graded strengthening exercises for synergist muscles
- Graded, protected, supervised return to physical activity as allowed by symptoms

'Crushing' osteochondritis

Articular subchondral or crushing osteochondritis may occur in the femoral head, the lunate, the tarsal navicular or in the second metatarsal head. Any of these conditions may present as an overuse syndrome and may be worsened by physical activity.

Perthes' disease

Perthes' disease is one of the most common osteochondroses and is the most likely to produce poor long-term results. The usual age of onset is 4–10 years, with peak incidence at 5–6 years (Pappas 1989) and the older the child the worse the long-term prognosis. The most common symptom is a relatively painless limp which may be associated with discomfort in the groin, the anteromedial thigh, or the knee.

Examination reveals limitation of internal rotation of the affected hip, spasm on rotation of the hip in extension and the joint is often held in slight flexion and adduction. Weakness and atrophy of the muscles of the hip and thigh region occur early. The radiological appearance is often far more dramatic than the clinical picture, with increased density and flattening of the femoral capital epiphysis.

Treatment is aimed at minimizing the deformation of the femoral head and maximizing its containment within the cup of the acetabulum. Initially a period of rest and traction is useful, with gentle exercises to maintain as full a range of motion of the hip joint as possible (once the initial pain subsides). Various abduction braces may be used to maximize containment of the femoral head and weight-bearing is allowed using such devices. Despite early and effective treatment, deformity of the femoral head is often significant enough to produce later osteoarthritis in the hip joint. Return to sport is permitted once there is evidence of revascularization and healing of the femoral head as determined by clinical and radiological assessment. In some cases of more severe deformity, containment may be enhanced by an osteotomy of the femur or an innominate osteotomy of the pelvis (Apley & Solomon 1982). Counselling those with significant deformity of the hip joint to avoid physical activities involving violent twisting and changing of direction, such as in football and squash, or repetitive weight-bearing activity such as in distance running, may serve to minimize and delay the onset of osteoarthritis.

Köhler's disease

Pain in a young child on the medial aspect of the foot in the region of the tarsal navicular may be due to Köhler's disease. This is a form of osteochondritis occurring mainly in 3–7 year olds. Those afflicted are normally physically active children and boys are more commonly affected than girls. These children exhibit an abnormal gait pattern often associated with aching on the medial aspect of the foot and swelling and tenderness over the navicular bone. Radiological examination will often show slight sclerosis and irregular rarefaction of the navicular, but this appearance sometimes occurs in the normal navicular and the diagnosis must therefore be clinical.

Application of a walking cast for 6–8 weeks, followed by orthotic support, may decrease the symptomatic period to one-fifth that in the untreated. This, however, does not appear to influence favourably or otherwise the development of a normal navicular in the adult (Williams & Cowell 1981).

Freiberg's disease

Freiberg's osteochondritis is an ischaemic necrosis of the epiphysis of the second (and occasionally the third) metatarsal head. This condition occurs in adolescence, rarely before 12 years of age and is the only osteochondrosis more common in girls. It may not present until secondary degenerative changes occur in the metatarsophalangeal (MTP) joint in early adulthood. There may be pain and tenderness associated with swelling of the MTP joint. The metatarsal head becomes flattened, enlarged and migrates dorsally. The clinical diagnosis can be confirmed by X-ray examination, which shows deformation and fragmentation of the epiphysis, often with flattening of the metatarsal head (Fig. 22.13).

If Freiberg's disease is diagnosed early before closure of the growth plate, deformity and disability may be reduced by modifying physical activity to exclude running and jumping, by metatarsal neck support padding and by wearing shoes with no heel or a 'negative' heel. In unresponsive or advanced

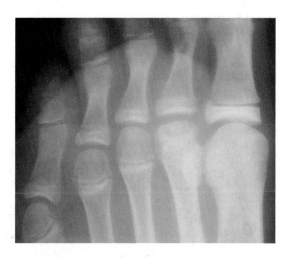

Fig. 22.13 A radiograph of Freiberg's osteochondritis of the second metatarsal head.

cases where angulation and flattening of the metatarsal head with osteophyte formation has occurred, a generous cheilectomy (capsular release with trimming of osteophytes) may return good function. If chondral damage and loose body formation has occurred, the joint requires resection arthroplasty with debridement of the metatarsal head (Sproul *et al.* 1993).

Kienböck's disease

Kienböck's disease of the wrist presents most commonly in the young adult but may occur rarely in adolescence. This condition is classified also as a crushing osteochondritis and results in avascular necrosis of the lunate bone. It may be related to a relative shortening of the ulna (compared with the radius). There is aching and stiffness in the wrist and localized tenderness over the lunate, which may be balloted between the thumb and forefinger just on the ulnar side of the centre of the wrist joint.

In early cases 'Velcro'-fastened wrist splints or strapping may be useful for controlling symptoms during physical activity and may remove or delay the need for surgical treatment.

ARTICULAR CHONDRAL OSTEOCHONDROSIS

Osteochondritis dissecans may occur as a result of repetitive sporting trauma. Major injuries or repetitive trauma cannot, however, explain all cases. Individuals with osteochondritis dissecans in one site are more likely to have it in another and this condition may in some cases be an inherited, mild form of epiphyseal dysplasia (Steiner & Grana 1988). If the osteochondral fragment becomes separated, there is a significant risk of joint dysfunction and later onset of osteoarthritis.

Frequently the patient is male, aged between 10 and 16 years, and the most common site affected is the medial femoral condyle in the knee. This condition may also affect the convex surfaces of the lateral femoral condyle, the tibial plateau of the knee, the patella, the talus in the ankle, the capitellum in the elbow, the first metatarsal head, or the head of the femur in the hip. The most common presentation is vague joint pain following activity. In later stages where there is separation of the fragment, joint effusion and mechanical symptoms such as catching or locking occur. In patients with osteochondritis dissecans of the medial femoral condyle, resisted quadriceps contraction in full knee flexion will often cause pain. This test has been called the active patellofemoral compression test (Berg 1993).

Radiological confirmation of the diagnosis is made by identification of a characteristic, demarcated area of irregular ossification, or a crescent-shaped area of translucency in the subchondral bone. Magnetic resonance imaging (MRI; Fig. 22.14) may show fluid around the fragment, suggesting that separation and displacement is imminent and technetium bone scans are useful in assessing progress. Increased isotope uptake indicates active reincorporation of the fragment and provides evidence that healing is occurring.

In contrast to juvenile osteochondritis dissecans (JOCD), patients who present with this condition after skeletal maturity have a poor prognosis. Early diagnosis allows careful follow-up and the possibility of early reduction and internal fixation of the

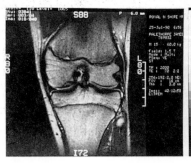 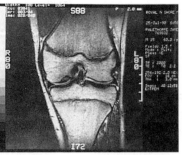

Fig. 22.14 In a T_2-weighted MRI, joint fluid appears white. Although the area of osteochondritis dissecans is well demarcated on the lateral aspect of the medial femoral condyle, no fluid can be detected around the fragment suggesting that separation is not imminent at this stage.

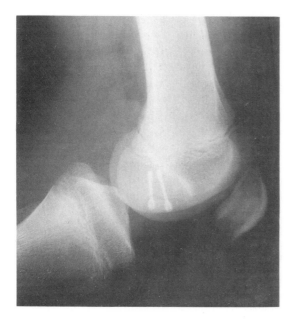

Fig. 22.15 A radiograph of osteochondritis dissecans of the medial femoral condyle of the knee of a 14 year old footballer necessitating internal fixation.

osteochondral fragment should it separate, particularly in the knee joint (Fig. 22.15). If diagnosed early, treatment can be directed at modification of sporting activity to prevent separation of the fragment. Arthroscopic drilling is advocated in some cases affecting the knee joint in an attempt to revascularize and stabilize a loose fragment.

During the time in which the fragment is judged unstable, sports involving running, jumping and rapid change of direction should be avoided. Gentle resisted exercises for the joint should be used, including non-weight-bearing activities such as swimming or paddling and later, cycling. When this condition occurs in the elbow it is wise to cease gymnastics, weight-lifting or throwing until the fragment is stabilized.

PHYSEAL OSTEOCHONDROSIS

Scheuermann's disease

Scheuermann's disease of the spine is classically described as a form of physeal osteochondrosis. This condition affects the ring apophyses of the thoracic and lumbar spine. These apophyses do not participate in the longitudinal growth of the vertebral body (as was assumed by Scheuermann) but act more like traction apophyses. Scheuermann's disease is thought to result from repetitive trauma. In the lower thoracic spine and the thoracolumbar junction this trauma is most probably a compressive force resulting in an excavation of the apophyseal region and anterior wedging of the vertebrae. In

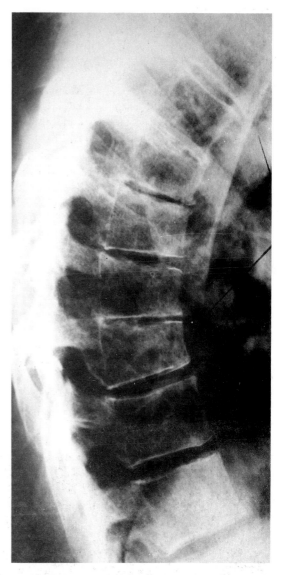

Fig. 22.16 A radiograph of Scheuermann's disease of the thoracic spine.

the lumbar spine, however, the trauma is most probably a traction force resulting in a separation of the anterior part of the ring apophysis causing a persisting apophysis or enlargement of the apophyseal region (Sward *et al.* 1993). Scheuermann's disease is often associated with an increase in the mid-thoracic kyphosis and an associated increase in lumbar lordosis. The kyphosis is usually smooth and rigid and there is often marked tightness of the thoracolumbar fascia and tightness in the hamstring muscles (Pappas 1989). This condition often presents in the physically active adolescent with thoracic or lumbar pain during or after activity.

Irregularity of the ring growth plates of the vertebral body with progressive anterior wedging may be identified on X-ray examination (Fig. 22.16).

As this condition presents most commonly during the last 2–3 years of skeletal growth, early diagnosis, significant activity modification to minimize repetitive flexion and extension of the spine and aggressive but conservative treatment are essential. If significant wedging (greater than 5°) has occurred at more than two levels, a brace producing extension of the thoracic spine and decreased lordosis in the lumbar spine may be considered. A comprehensive physiotherapy programme should be directed at minimizing tightness in the thoracolumbar fascia and hamstring muscles and strengthening abdominal muscles.

Blount's disease

A similar condition termed Blount's disease (osteochondrosis deformans tibiae) may occur in the posteromedial portion of the proximal tibial growth plate. This may result in rotation and varus deformity of the proximal tibia. Corrective osteotomy may be required in cases in which the resulting deformity is significant enough to cause mechanical problems in the lower limb.

Stress Fractures

With an increase in children's competitive sport and improvements in diagnostic methods, stress fractures are being more commonly diagnosed in adolescence. These are often related to sudden increases in training intensity and are most common in the weight-bearing long bones of the lower leg, the tarsal bones, the metatarsals, the femur, pelvic bones and vertebral bodies. Diaphyseal stress fractures may be readily diagnosed clinically or, if doubt exists, by using bone scans. Stress fractures of the growth plates have also been recorded particularly in the distal radial epiphysis of gymnasts (Markiewitz & Andrish 1992). X-ray changes include widening and haziness of the growth plate, cystic changes and a more pointed appearance of the epiphysis (Caine & Lindner 1985). Treatment involves modification of activity to within limits of pain. Few cases of growth disorder have been reported following such injuries.

Certain critical stress fractures, particularly of the femoral neck, the tarsal navicular and the pars interarticularis in the lumbar spine, require early diagnosis to prevent significant complications and may require surgical intervention. Young athletes involved in activities which cause hyperextension and often rotation of the lumbar spine such as gymnastics, diving, blocking in American football or fast-bowling in cricket, risk developing stress fractures of the pars interarticularis of the vertebrae of the lower lumbar spine (Fig. 14.25). This condition is often associated with incorrect technique and worsening lower back pain is experienced with the activity. Standing with the lumbar spine extended and laterally flexed toward the painful side with weight on the lower limb of the same side as the pain reproduces the pain. Plain X-rays are usually normal in the first stages of development. Bone scanning may assist if performed early, but to confirm the diagnosis a reverse angle CT scan is usually necessary. In cases of early bilateral pars interarticularis stress fractures with no slip, an antilordotic brace ('Boston' brace) may assist healing. In unilateral cases rest from the activity is followed by identification of the faulty technique or other factors and a full rehabilitation programme. Stress fractures are discussed in more detail in Chapters 17 and 20.

Malalignment Syndromes

Congenital musculoskeletal malformation or malalignment may produce significant problems for children involved in physical activity. Such foot and lower limb syndromes are discussed in more detail in Chapter 28; however, tarsal coalitions are dealt with in this chapter to illustrate the diagnosis and management of such problems in the adolescent athlete.

TARSAL COALITIONS

Tarsal coalitions are caused by fibrous, cartilaginous or bony fusion bars between the tarsal bones. These occur most commonly between the calcaneus and navicular and the calcaneus and talus. They are more common in males, are frequently inherited as an autosomal dominant trait (with incomplete penetrance) and therefore usually have a strong family history of similar foot pain (Olney 1992). Tarsal coalitions occur in only 1% of the general population but in approximately 40% of close relatives of those with a diagnosed tarsal coalition. They are often bilateral and are present from birth, but usually do not present until adolescence following minor trauma to the ankle or repetitive running and jumping activities. The most common symptom is chronic mid-foot pain sometimes associated with a limp. Subtalar joint motion is often significantly restricted, particularly in talocalcaneal coalitions, and is often associated with a rigid flat foot (valgus deformity). The foot may also be foreshortened and in a small number of cases there may be persistent spasm in the peroneal muscles.

Special X-ray views including a 45° oblique view (Fig. 22.17) and a weight-bearing lateral view (Fig. 22.18), may be necessary. If these show no abnormality, a CT scan or MRI may provide an accurate diagnosis.

In mild cases, with little restriction of subtalar range, orthotic control may be helpful. Short-term immobilization in a short leg walking cast for 3–6 weeks with the hindfoot in slight varus, may also be useful in reducing symptoms and allowing return to physical activity. In severe cases, early surgical excision of the bar is indicated, especially if the patient is young when symptoms develop. If the pain persists despite conservative treatment, or if muscle spasm is a problem, surgery may be curative if performed before degenerative changes occur. Possible complications include the recurrence of the bar, incisional neuromas and reflex sympathetic dystrophy (O'Neill & Micheli 1989).

CHRONIC CHILDHOOD ILLNESS AND PHYSICAL ACTIVITY

For many young athletes, involvement in sporting activity is limited by chronic health problems. Certain sporting activities may pose specific problems or risks to such individuals. An understanding of the limitations imposed by such illnesses allows the sports physician and others involved in the medical supervision of physical activity, to recommend involvement in sport and exercise while minimizing the risks and maximizing the beneficial affects of physical activity (Bar-Or 1993b).

Asthma

Virtually all young asthmatics develop exercise-induced bronchospasm (EIB) or exercise-induced asthma (EIA). EIB may also be demonstrated in a proportion of non-asthmatics with hay fever, wheezy bronchitis or cystic fibrosis. This may vary in severity from severely debilitating (during which the child may feel in danger of suffocation) to that which is detectable only by measurements of pulmonary function. This condition is under-diagnosed and often inadequately managed in children and may lead to unnecessary restrictions on exercise activity (see Chapter 28, part I).

Diabetes Mellitus

This is the most common metabolic/endocrine disease encountered in childhood. The early symptoms may be noted in relation to sporting activities and include inordinate or increasing fatigue, abnormal thirst, urinary frequency and weight loss. Considerations relevant to sport and physical activity in children with diabetes are discussed in full in Chapter 28, part III.

Cystic Fibrosis

This condition is characterized by general exocrine gland dysfunction. The most noticeable clinical manifestations include chronic recurrent sinus and respiratory tract infection and digestive tract disorders leading to malnutrition. Cystic fibrosis (CF) is the most common fatal genetic disease in childhood (1 in 2000 births) and is transmitted as an autosomal recessive trait. As carriers (heterozygotes) show no trace of the disease, the carrier state (5% of the Caucasian population) is undetectable with current technology.

Children with CF are small and frail with very low body fat and they often avoid any form of exercise. Exercise onset is associated with marked coughing and may cause bowel and bladder urgency. Exercise intensity is limited early by respiratory factors; however, there is evidence that regular exercise, if correctly supervised, may improve the quality of life, although the effect on life expectancy is unknown. Significant improvements have been identified in mucus clearance, exercise tolerance and pulmonary function.

Suggested exercise includes swimming, cycling, fast walking or jogging. Swimming appears to be of particular benefit in bronchopulmonary hygiene and may reduce the need for time-consuming chest

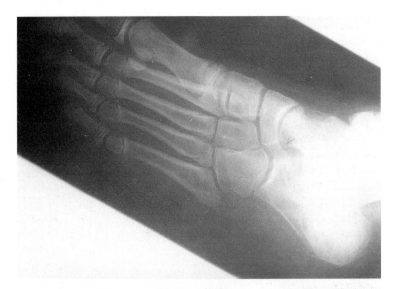

Fig. 22.17 An oblique anteroposterior view of the foot demonstrates a calcaneonavicular tarsal coalition.

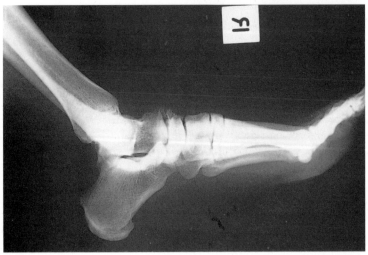

Fig. 22.18 X-ray showing marked 'beaking' of the talonavicular joint in an advanced case of tarsal coalition.

physiotherapy treatment. Patients with CF have very low body fat levels and therefore poor cold water tolerance and a high body density. The buoyancy and heat loss problems can be solved by swimming in warm water (28°C) with a flotation vest or with a wet suit to provide insulation and buoyancy. As this condition affects the sweat glands, exercise in hot environments should be approached with caution.

Epilepsy

Epileptic episodes may range from brief staring spells lasting a few seconds (*petit mal*) to complex and bizarre automatic behaviour (temporal lobe epilepsy) or severe, generalized, tonic/clonic seizures with falling, unconsciousness and a recovery phase of deep sleep (*grand mal*).

All childhood sporting activity involves some risk-taking and in children with epilepsy the risks may be increased according to the type of activity and type and control of seizures. Decisions regarding sports selection require consideration of how the seizures manifest themselves, precipitating factors, timing and frequency, the time since the last seizure, medications, the effect of medication on control, behaviour or function and the child's sporting interests. This condition is discussed more fully in Chapter 28, part II.

Children with Heart Disease

Congenital heart disease is present in five per 1000 school-aged children and one or two of these individuals will have the disease severely enough to affect their participation in sport. Rheumatic heart disease is present in one per 1000 school-aged children and in most instances the valvular damage is mild. Cardiomyopathy, myocarditis and hereditary syndromes with cardiac defects (e.g. Marfan's syndrome) are present in less than one per 1000 school-aged children. Up to 10% of adolescents may have some form of mitral valve prolapse, but as far as exercise is concerned, there is only an important lesion in approximately 1% of them. A significant rhythm disorder is present in less than one per 1000 children and congenital coronary anomalies, for example aberrant origin of the left coronary artery, occur in only two per 100 000 children. There is thus no place for routine exercise testing of children to detect heart disease or to assess the safety for exercise activities (Cumming 1993).

Cardiac conditions most commonly associated with sudden death which may occur during sport and exercise, rest or sleep include:

- Aortic stenosis
- Right to left shunts with pulmonary stenosis (tetralogy of Fallot)
- Hypertrophic obstructive cardiomyopathy
- Pulmonary hypertension of a moderate to severe degree
- Myocarditis

Conditions which have been associated with sudden unexpected death in young athletes include:

- Hypertrophic obstructive cardiomyopathy
- Aberrant left coronary artery
- Aortic dissection secondary to Marfan's syndrome
- Coronary artery disease
- Acute myocarditis
- Idiopathic long QT syndrome (Van Camp 1992)

It is possible and desirable to exclude these conditions on a comprehensive routine pre-participation health evaluation prior to involvement in competitive sporting activity and the examination is discussed later in this chapter. If cardiac abnormality is detected the child should be referred to a paediatric cardiologist with experience in managing children with heart disease in exercise situations.

Children with mild to moderate forms of congenital cardiac abnormality often have a normal myocardium and therefore the ability to compensate for the specific defect. These children can therefore tolerate exercise and sports activities and may reach adulthood without symptoms. In these children, with the exception of those with aortic stenosis, the exercise electrocardiogram (ECG) is generally normal.

ISCHAEMIC HEART DISEASE

This presents rarely in children and adolescents. However, in a child with a family history of premature atherosclerosis, serum total cholesterol, high-density lipoprotein cholesterol and triglyceride levels should be obtained. In the unlikely event that these are abnormally high, a maximum exercise stress test should be performed.

CARDIOMYOPATHIES

Hypertrophic cardiomyopathy does occur in the juvenile population and represents one of the most frequent causes of sudden, unexpected death from sport among young people, as a result of arrhythmias. These patients also have haemodynamic problems with exercise and all sports activity should be excluded in all forms of cardiomyopathy.

ARRHYTHMIAS

Various types of arrhythmias may be seen in children. In evaluating appropriate sport and physical activity in each case the following factors need to be considered (Venerando et al. 1988):

- The type and severity of any associated heart condition
- The type of arrhythmia in terms of origin, the maximum heart rate reached, the duration of the episodes accompanying symptoms and frequency of occurrence
- The responsiveness of the arrhythmia to medication
- The type and intensity of demands on the cardiovascular system required by the sporting activity

ECG with provocative tests such as sympathetic and vagal stimulation and exercise and use of Holter monitoring, are useful in determining the type of arrhythmia. Echocardiography is a reliable and non-invasive method of ruling out some cardiac abnormalities as a cause of the arrhythmias.

The most common arrhythmias in school-aged children include ectopic beats of atrial, junction or ventricular origin, paroxysmal supraventricular tachycardia (PST) and atrioventricular block. Patients should be questioned about fainting or palpitations. The use of caffeine-containing substances (such as coffee, tea and cola drinks), tobacco, alcohol and medications (especially bronchodilators), may be responsible for causing premature ventricular

contraction (PVC). Often the avoidance of such compounds will result in complete resolution of this type of arrhythmia.

Supraventricular arrhythmias, as well as PVC, are generally considered benign and of little risk to the active child if they are unifocal, infrequent and disappear with exercise, if the heart rate is greater than 140 (Strong & Steed 1984). Frequent, sporadic PVC, or those with fixed coupling may be associated with myocarditis and should be actively investigated. PST should not necessarily preclude participation in sports if control can be achieved with medication. Similarly, the Wolff-Parkinson-White syndrome should not prevent participation in competitive sport if the child is asymptomatic, well-controlled on medications and does not have anatomical heart disease.

Children with Hypertension

Arterial hypertension is sometimes encountered in children and adolescents. For children less than 10 years old upper limits of normal blood pressure are 120/80 mmHg. For adolescents 10–15 years the usual maximum values are 140/85 mmHg. Three abnormal blood pressure measurements on three separate occasions are required for the diagnosis of hypertension. It is important that advice is sought regarding diagnosis of primary or secondary causes of hypertension, before sports participation is allowed. Knowledge of present or past symptoms of heart disease and especially family history is important. Physical examination should always include palpation of femoral and radial pulses simultaneously to exclude coarctation of the aorta. A full blood count, urine analysis, serum electrolytes, blood urea nitrogen and creatinine should be performed.

Studies in adults have shown that blood pressure decreases in association with increased cardiovascular fitness. This can be achieved by moderate to intense aerobic exercise. Thus there is no reason to limit sporting activity in children with mild primary hypertension. Whether children with secondary hypertension should be allowed to participate in competitive sport is determined by the underlying disease process.

It is reasonable to perform an exercise test to assess the blood pressure and ECG response to high-intensity exercise (Strong & Steed 1984). Children or adolescents with even mild hypertension should not be encouraged to participate in primarily isometric activities such as weight-lifting, wrestling and possibly water-skiing.

Other Chronic Conditions

A well-constructed and supervised exercise programme can provide significant benefits in physical, psychological and social development for children with certain other chronic medical conditions. These conditions include: cerebral palsy, muscular dystrophy, mental retardation, anorexia nervosa, chronic renal failure, obesity, haemophilia and rheumatoid arthritis. There are also obvious benefits in the use of appropriate, modified sport and physical activity in the rehabilitation and long-term management of children disabled by head or spinal injury.

ACUTE ILLNESS AND SPORTS PARTICIPATION

Infectious Mononucleosis

This condition, commonly known as glandular fever, is an acute viral illness which is usually self-limited. Long-term complications are rare but are significant in terms of sports participation. Approximately 90% of the population have been infected by the age of 30 and peak age incidence is between 15 and 25 years. The Epstein-Barr virus is the infective agent. There is very low transmission to contacts and the incubation period is 30–50 days followed by a 3–5 day prodromal period of malaise, headache, anorexia and fatigue. This is followed by 5–15 days of fever, sore throat, painful enlarged lymph glands, profound malaise and fatigue. Diagnosis is made in most cases by the positive heterophile antibody test (Monospot).

The complication of infectious mononucleosis most relevant to sporting activity is splenic rupture, which occurs in 0.1–0.2% of all cases. A significantly enlarged spleen occurs in 40–60% of patients and

splenic rupture has been reported to occur only in spleens enlarged to two to three times their normal size. All splenic ruptures occur either during the acute phase or in early convalescence. Abdominal pain, left shoulder pain (due to diaphragmatic irritation) or pain in the scapula area, is suggestive of splenic rupture, as are the accompanying signs of shock. Confirmation can be made accurately by ultrasound scanning and if the diagnosis is missed this complication is potentially fatal.

Athletes should be prevented from returning to training for at least 4 weeks from the onset of symptoms mainly because of the risk of splenic rupture. The progress of splenic enlargement may be assessed using ultrasound, but the subjective feelings of the patient may also delay return to sporting activity. Malaise and excessive fatigue may last as long as 6 months, although some athletes seem to recover more quickly than non-athletes. A careful check should be made for possible complications prior to making a decision to return the child to sporting activity (Maki & Reich 1982). This should be done one activity at a time, monitored by parents and coach and starting with low-intensity individual sports. The child's response should be assessed before progressing to other, more strenuous activity.

Other Acute Illnesses

The presence of other forms of acute illness should also limit sports participation. Such conditions may cause fatigue, malaise, vestibular symptoms (causing problems with balance) and, if a fever is present, problems with thermoregulation (increased risk of heat stroke). Another important consideration, particularly in team sports, is the possibility of infecting other children. The risk of spreading disease to other team members may be reduced by employing the simple rules of hygiene. Towels, eating utensils and clothing should never be shared and the use of a communal wet sponge or water bottle should not be allowed.

Children with viral infections have a greatly varied infective period, from the incubation period to well after the disappearance of acute symptoms. Streptococcal infection is most communicable during the period of acute illness and gradually decreases over weeks in untreated individuals. Children may be regarded as non-infective within 48 h of treatment. *Mycoplasma pneumoniae* has an incubation period of 2–3 weeks and the affected children may be infective for some weeks or months.

Particularly in a team situation, it is essential that throat swabs and other appropriate tests be done to identify the organism. Appropriate antibiotics should only be used for proven bacterial infections, particularly those caused by β-haemolytic streptococci. If *Mycoplasma* infection is prominent in a community and cold agglutinin tests are positive, Erythromycin may be useful. Paracetamol or acetaminophen should be used for analgesia and to reduce the fever in preference to aspirin, which may cause problems in patients with infectious mononucleosis such as thrombocytopenia and splenic rupture. Of equal concern is the risk of Reye's syndrome associated with the use of salicylates (aspirin) in children with influenza.

Medications which cause drowsiness, such as antihistamines, may have a significant adverse effect on performance in school sports on return to activity and, for those athletes involved in elite competition, it is important to bear in mind that some decongestants contain banned substances. Athletes should be discouraged from using over-the-counter compounds which may contain such substances without the knowledge of the coach, team physician or treating doctor.

Rest is an important factor in recovery from viral illness and return to activity should be gradual following the resolution of symptoms. There should be frequent rest periods and work-outs should be light. A useful evaluation of return to fitness may be made by monitoring resting pulse rates and recovery after exercise. Again, the risk of infection of team-mates and other children should be carefully considered in each case (Nelson 1989).

Preventive measures against the spread of skin infections such as herpes simplex in wrestling or tinea pedis in the locker room, involve simple hygienic measures such as occlusive dressings, withdrawal from competition while infective or the wearing of shoes or socks (to prevent the spread of tinea). The risk of blood-borne disease transmission in contact sport may be minimized by immediate attention to open wounds, dressing of skin lesions, withdrawal from play and, in the case of hepatitis B, immunization should be considered.

High-level (particularly international) athletic competition does appear to adversely affect the immune system in some cases. This may lead to a higher rate of mainly viral infections. Preventive measures include the maintenance of an adequate, well-balanced diet, minimizing the impact of all types of stress (psychological, cold, heat, altitude, time zone changes and sleep deprivation) and measures to prevent exposure to pathogens and prevent cross-infection between team members (Shephard & Shek 1993).

THE PRE-PARTICIPATION HEALTH EVALUATION (PPHE)

Pre-participation screening of children before involvement in a sports or exercise programme can have an important role in injury prevention, avoidance of complications of existing disease states (caused by physical activity) and determining limitations and precautions.

A number of objectives have been identified relevant to the active child (McKeag 1989) and it is important to:

• Determine the general health of the athlete

Table 22.3 Conditions requiring further evaluation and possible disqualification from sport

Unresolved organic heart disease
Sustained hypertension with exercise
Loss of consciousness with exercise
Serious CNS trauma or surgery
History of recurrent CNS symptoms
  (unconsciousness, dizziness, seizures)
Persistent heat intolerance
Intractable orthopaedic problems
Single organ
Haemorrhagic disorders
Chronic infections
Chronic debilitating illness
Enlarged abdominal viscera
Obvious physical immaturity

Modified from Linder (1989).

- Disclose defects that may limit or increase the risks of participation
- Uncover conditions predisposing the athlete to injury
- Identify attributes in the athlete which predispose him or her to certain types of sporting activity (first stage of talent identification)
- Fulfil legal and insurance requirements for organized sports programmes

Organization

A multi-station group technique is usually effective where a team of sports medicine professionals perform and evaluate specific components of the PPHE. Having one individual perform all the measurements of one particular type improves reliability. The overall organization should be supervised preferably by a primary care sports physician with knowledge and experience in health screening for sport.

Components

A comprehensive PPHE includes completion of a history questionnaire, a comprehensive physical examination, investigations (only where indicated), evaluation and specific recommendations with regard to precautions and restrictions on involvement in various types of sport and physical activity. These recommendations should also include, if necessary, remedial exercise programmes designed to rectify problems identified during the examination and protective equipment or strapping required in individual cases.

The PPHE should be integrated into the child's continuing health care, preferably with the cooperation of the regular family physician. Ongoing educational programmes on problem detection and injury prevention should also be integrated into this programme. This education should be directed not only at the players but also at the coaches, teachers and parents.

The history form should be ideally filled out by the child and the parents together, the day or evening before the medical examination. The health history should cover current medications, allergies,

present symptoms, a system review, past history of illness, injury or operations, absence of organs such as an eye, kidney or testicle, relevant family history and the use of glasses, contact lenses, dental devices, braces or other protective devices. The history sheet should also require completion of details regarding immunizations, particularly against tetanus. This section may be required to be more comprehensive if overseas sporting travel is contemplated. The medical history should also include details of menstruation in the female. Questions regarding symptoms of potentially dangerous conditions such as chest pain, dizziness or fainting with exercise and specifically problems with heart or blood pressure should be also included. Adequate space should be allowed on the form to provide details of positive answers in the questionnaire, which should be checked by the examining physician prior to the next component of the PPHE. Most positive findings during the examination which may cause restrictions of, or disqualification from, sporting activity involve the cardiovascular system and the musculoskeletal system. Patients with symptoms of heart disease or a family history of heart disease and athletes with a previous history of neck injury, should be subject to specific careful evaluation of these problems during the examination.

A thorough cardiovascular examination should be performed, including simultaneous palpation of radial and femoral pulses, palpation of the praecordium for cardiac impulses, measurement of blood pressure and auscultation. Cardiac murmurs are the most common potentially abnormal finding (30% of athletes examined). The vast majority of these are innocent functional murmurs, normally systolic in timing, without obliteration of the first heart sound nor running through the second heart sound. Should anything in the personal history or examination suggest that the murmur detected is anything but innocent, further specialist evaluation should be organized and clearance for sporting activity delayed.

Careful examination of all joints and muscle groups to assess stability, range of motion, mechanical signs, wasting, imbalance, inflexibility or weakness should be undertaken, with particular attention to those areas noted in the history to have been previously injured or symptomatic. Examination of the respiratory and neurological systems, and of the abdomen, ears, throat and vision tests should all be performed.

Anthropometric measurements appropriate to the proposed sporting activity should also be carried out. Individuals who are unusually tall, particularly if they have a family history of Marfan's syndrome, should have a measurement of the ratio of height to arm span taken. If arm span is greater than height this may suggest that Marfan's syndrome is likely and careful examination of the eyes and cardiovascular system should be carried out as appropriate.

Laboratory investigations at this level are not often useful and findings from urinalysis rarely give additional information. Consideration should be given to iron studies, particularly in groups of more elite competitive athletes involved in endurance events. Of particular concern here is the adolescent female heavily involved in an endurance running programme, where training, menstrual and dietary factors may combine to cause iron deficiency.

Certain conditions are generally considered to require further evaluation, possible disqualification or at least careful restrictions in exercise prescription (Linder 1989; Table 22.3).

GENERAL GUIDELINES FOR SAFETY IN CHILDREN'S SPORT

The Australian Sports Medicine Federation (1988) has produced a comprehensive series of guide-lines for safety in specific children's sports. General recommendations include the following:

- Coaches should be well trained and accredited through the national accreditation system in conjunction with the appropriate sporting organization
- Adequate supervision should be provided at all times for children involved in sporting activity
- Coaching for children should emphasize enjoyment and skill development (Fig. 22.19)
- A programme should be individually tailored to the child wherever possible, taking into account physical maturation, skill level, ability to learn

new skills, enthusiasm and the presence of physical limitations, including injury
- Sporting organizations should be encouraged to assist coaches or members of the parents' support group to undertake at least a Level 1 National Sports Trainer's Course, which gives a basic grounding in sports first aid
- Children proceeding to higher levels of competition should be subject to a PPHE
- Sound preparation, learning of skills, warm-up and warm-down should be encouraged
- Flexibility appropriate to the ranges of motion required in the various joints should be achieved and maintained and stretching should be done carefully without forcing or pain
- Any complaint of pain, tenderness, limitation of movement or instability or the presence of growth disorders or illness should be assessed by the sports physician associated with the sporting body or the local medical officer. Signs of significant sporting injury relevant to the particular activities should be taught so there is a general awareness of these among the coaches, parents and participants
- Specialized medical advice should be available, particularly on menstruation problems in female athletes
- Equipment should only be used for the purpose for which it was intended. The equipment used should be well constructed, in good repair and appropriate to the size and ability of the individual athlete
- Protective devices (Fig. 22.20) such as helmets, shin pads and eye protection should be used wherever appropriate
- The complexity of the activity should be appropriate to the skill level and psychological (attentional) capacity of the children involved. This may involve rule modification in some instances as mentioned earlier
- Unsafe training and playing practices, including inappropriate, high-risk exercises and violence in contact sports, should be identified and a sound and comprehensive education programme mounted against these
- Advice and education on diet, weight control, fluid replacement, skin damage from sunburn

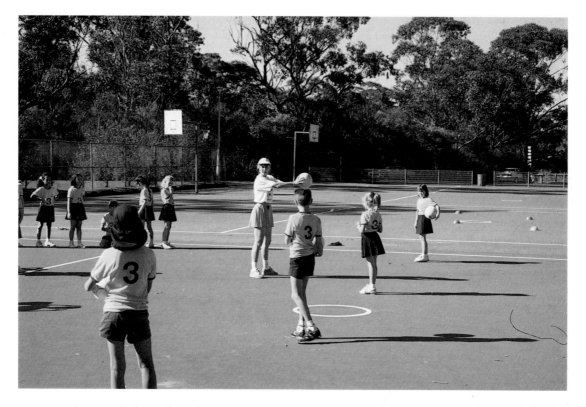

Fig. 22.19 Coaches in children's sport should concentrate on teaching simplified skills emphasizing enjoyment and ensuring equal involvement of all children.

and exercise in hot or cold environments should be available to the coaches, parents and participants
- Positive written guide-lines should be provided wherever appropriate

Parents are perhaps the most important supervisors of child physical activity and sport, particularly in the crucial early stages. Parental encouragement for the child to become involved in physical activity may be beneficial, if the right values are emphasized and the goals presented to the child are realistic and attainable in the individual case. Emphasis on outcomes (winning) should be discouraged. Parents should be supportive and

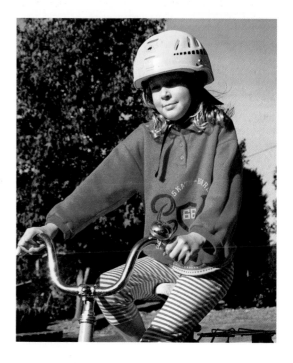

Fig. 22.20 The use of adequate, appropriate protective equipment should be actively encouraged in sport and recreation.

patient, hiding disappointment and sharing the enjoyment while promoting responsibility, adequate preparation, the use of appropriate, protective equipment and safe sporting practices in the child. In most cases it is only the parents and not the individual coaches who are aware of exactly how much physical activity the children are doing. It often thus falls to the parents to suggest to the child some rationalization of sporting activity to prevent overtraining and overuse injury.

There should be open and free communication between the parents, coach and teachers with due consideration of each other's roles and responsibilities. This should foster co-operation rather than interference (National Health and Medical Research Council 1987).

CONCLUSIONS

There will always be some risks involved with childhood sports and physical activity. Such activity can be beneficial in developing healthy life-style habits, emphasizing enjoyment and improving quality of life. Sport may prove a positive socializing influence and assist in development of physical, social and psychological skills. Appropriate structuring of the activity, general community awareness of factors relevant to injury prevention, adequate coaching, skills training and supervision and identification of risk factors and exercise prescription in individual cases, should all serve to minimize the costs and maximize the benefits to the child.

REFERENCES

Apley A. G. & Solomon L. (1982) *System of Orthopaedics and Fractures*, 6th edn, pp. 258–262. Butterworths, London.

Australian Sports Medicine Federation (1988) *Guidelines for Safety in Children's Sport*.

Backx F. J. G., Erich W. B. M., Kemper A. B. & Verbeek A. L. (1989) Sports injuries in school-aged children: An epidemiologic study. *American Journal of Sports Medicine* 17, 234–240.

Bandura A. (1977) *Social Learning Theory.* Prentice-Hall, Englewood Cliffs, NJ.

Bar-Or O. (1980) Climate and exercising children — A review. *International Journal of Sports Medicine* 1, 53.

Bar-Or O. (1993a) Importance of differences between children and adults for exercise testing and exercise prescription. In Skinner J. S. (ed.) *Exercise Testing and Prescription for Special Cases*, 2nd edn, pp. 57–74. Lea & Febiger, Philadelphia, PA.

Bar-Or O. (1993b) Effects of training on the child with a chronic disease: Beauty and the Beast? *Clinical Journal of Sport Medicine* 3, 2–5.

Beovich R. & Fricker P. (1988) Osgood-Schlatter's disease: A review of the literature and an Australian series. *Australian Journal of Science and Medicine in Sport* 20, 11–13.

Berg E. E. (1993) Adult femoral osteochondritis dissecans: Study of the patellofemoral relationship. *Clinical Journal of Sport Medicine* 3, 101–105.

Bruce D. A., Schut L. & Sutton L. N. (1984) Brain and cervical spine injuries occurring during organised sports activities in children and adolescents. *Primary Care* 11, 175–194.

Burry H. C. & Gowland H. (1981) Cervical injury in rugby football: A New Zealand survey. *British Journal of Sports Medicine* 15, 56–59.

Caine D. J. & Lindner K. J. (1985) Overuse injury of bones: The young female gymnast at risk? *Physician and Sports Medicine* 13, 51–64.

Cumming G. R. (1993) Children with heart disease. In Skinner C. S. (ed.) *Exercise Testing and Exercise Prescriptions for Special Cases*, 2nd edn, pp. 291–316. Lea & Febiger, Philadelphia, PA.

Davidson R., Kennedy M., Kennedy J. & Vanderfield G. (1978) Casualty room presentations and schoolboy rugby union. *Medical Journal of Australia* 1, 247–249.

Davies C. T. M. (1981) Thermal responses to exercise in children. *Ergonomics* 24, 55–61.

Falk B. & Bar-Or O. (1993) Longitudinal changes in peak aerobic and anaerobic mechanical power of circum-pubertal boys. *Pediatric Exercise Science* 5, 318–331.

Gerrard D. F. (1993) Overuse injury and growing bones: The young athlete at risk. *British Journal of Sports Medicine* 27, 14–18.

Gregg J. R. & Das M. (1982) Foot and ankle problems in the preadolescent and adolescent athlete. *Clinics in Sports Medicine* 1, 131–147.

Harvey J. S. (1984) Nutritional management of the adolescent athlete. *Clinics in Sports Medicine* 3, 671–678.

Hodge K. P. & Tod D. A. (1993) Ethics of childhood sport. *Sports Medicine* 15, 291–298.

Linder C. W. (1989) The preparticipation health evaluation of high school athletes. In Smith N. J. (ed.) *Common Problems in Pediatric Sports Medicine*, pp. 358–366. Yearbook Medical Publishers, Chicago, IL.

Maki D. G. & Reich R. M. (1982) Infectious mononucleosis in the athlete: Diagnosis, complications, and management. *American Journal of Sports Medicine* 10, 162–173.

Markiewitz A. D. & Andrish J. T. (1992) Hand and wrist

injuries in the preadolescent and adolescent athlete. *Clinics in Sports Medicine* 11, 203–225.

McKeag D. B. (1989) Preparticipation screening of the potential athlete. *Clinics in Sports Medicine* 8, 373–397.

McManama G. B. (1988) Ankle injuries in the young athlete. *Clinics in Sports Medicine* 7, 547–562.

Micheli L. J. (1983) Overuse injuries in children's sports: The growth factor. *Orthopedic Clinics of North America* 14, 337–360.

National Health and Medical Research Council (1987) *Children and Adolescents in Sport.* Canberra.

Nelson M. A. (1989) A young gymnast with an acute upper respiratory infection. In Smith N. J. (ed.) *Common Problems in Pediatric Sports Medicine*, pp. 204–209. Yearbook Medical Publishers, Chicago, IL.

Olney B. W. (1992) Tarsal coalition. In Drennan J. C. (ed.) *The Child's Foot and Ankle*, pp. 169–181. Raven Press, New York.

O'Neill D. & Micheli L. J. (1989) Tarsal coalition: A follow up of adolescent athletes. *American Journal of Sports Medicine* 17, 544–549.

Pappas A. M. (1989) Osteochondroses: Diseases of growth centers. *Physician and Sports Medicine* 17, 51–62.

Russo P. F., Sutton J., Lazarus L., Harvey J. & Marder K. (1975) A growth and fitness study of Sydney school children. In Collins J. K. (ed.) *Studies of the Australian Adolescent* p. 24. Cassell, Sydney.

Salter R. B. & Harris W. R. (1963) Injuries involving the epiphyseal plate. *Journal of Bone and Joint Surgery* 45, 587–622.

Shephard R. J. & Shek P. N. (1993) Athletic competition and susceptibility to infection. *Clinical Journal of Sport Medicine* 3, 75–77.

Smith R. E. (1984) The dynamics and prevention of stress-induced burnout in athletics. *Primary Care* 11, 115–127.

Smithers M. & Myers P. T. (1985) Injuries in sport: A prospective casualty study. *Medical Journal of Australia* 142, 457–461.

Sproul J., Klaaren H. & Mannarino F. (1993) Surgical treatment of Freiberg's infarction in athletes. *American Journal of Sports Medicine* 21, 381–384.

Steiner M. E. & Grana W. A. (1988) The young athlete's knee: Recent advances. *Clinics in Sports Medicine* 7, 527–546.

Strong W. B. & Steed D. (1984) Cardiovascular evaluation of the young athlete. *Primary Care* 11, 61–75.

Sward L., Hellstrom M., Jacobsson B. & Karlsson L. (1993) Vertebral ring apophysis injury in athletes. *American Journal of Sports Medicine* 21, 841–845.

Tursz A. & Crost M. (1986) Sports-related injuries in children. *American Journal of Sports Medicine* 14, 294.

Van Camp S. P. (1992) Sudden death. *Clinics in Sports Medicine* 11, 273–289.

Venerando A., Zeppilli P. & Caselli G. (1988) Cardiovascular disease. In Dirix A., Knuttgen H. G. & Tittel K. (eds) *The Olympic Book of Sports Medicine*, pp. 505–530. Blackwell Scientific Publications, Oxford.

Watson A. W. S. (1984) Sports injuries during one academic year in 6799 Irish school children. *American Journal of Sports Medicine* 12, 65–71.

Weiss R., Ebbeck V. & Wiese-Bjornstal D. M. (1993) Developmental and psychological factors related to children's observational learning of physical skills. *Pediatric Exercise Science* 5, 301–317.

Williams G. & Cowell H. (1981) Köhler's disease of the tarsal navicular. *Clinics in Orthopedics* 58, 53.

CHAPTER 23

THE FEMALE ATHLETE

R. J. Carbon

Sport and exercise have measurable health benefits and provide enjoyment, friendship and fulfilment. The benefits of physical activity, in terms of weight control, self-esteem, motor co-ordination, cardiovascular health and fitness, and integrity of bone may in fact be greater for women than for men. Regular exercise and sport for women should be promoted and encouraged.

In modern cultures, principally Christian societies, women are gradually achieving parity with men in sport. From total exclusion in the ancient Olympics, to the role of spectator in the early modern Olympics, the strength, talent and competitive prowess of women is now well recognized.

Concern over the effects of intensive training on the health, both short-term and long-term, of female athletes has created much interest and scientific research. It seems that the so-called 'curse' of our mothers and grandmothers, menstruation, is now being viewed as a necessary part of health and an asset rather than a detriment in sport and exercise. Similarly, motherhood does not diminish physical prowess and appropriate exercise can improve general well-being during pregnancy and birth.

The challenge for sports medicine and science is to ensure that female athletes can reach the peak of their physical performance while enjoying continued good health.

PHYSICAL DIFFERENCES BETWEEN THE SEXES

There are obvious anatomical and less obvious physiological differences between the sexes. These mostly favour males in sports and physical activities that require greater strength and size. However, many of the differences can be altered by physical training so that the physiological parameters of a trained woman can exceed those of a lesser trained

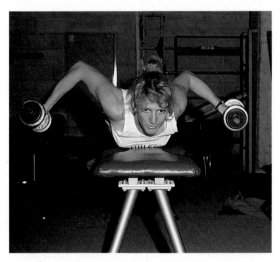

Fig. 23.1 Women can improve muscle strength with training.

man. The differences between the sexes are largely irrelevant in sport as women usually compete against their female peers.

The physical dimensions of a male are on average 7–10% greater than those of a female at maturity. There is very little difference in the size of children until puberty, when girls are temporarily taller and heavier than boys. This is due to the earlier onset of puberty in girls (9–13 years) than in boys (10–14 years) who mature later and over a longer period of time.

Under the influence of the male hormone testosterone men grow taller, with a wider shoulder girdle, narrower pelvis and longer limbs. Females through the effects of oestrogen develop narrower shoulders, a wider pelvis relative to their height and a greater 'carrying angle' of the elbow joints, which confer a mechanical disadvantage for running and throwing.

Oestrogen is also responsible for the preferential deposition of fat in the female during adolescence, while testosterone favours muscular development in males. When expressed as a percentage of their total bodyweight, adult women have approximately twice the body fat of men.

While males attain greater muscle mass and hence greater total power, muscle strength when expressed per unit of cross-sectional area is equivalent for both sexes.

Women are more flexible than men and this may be due to basal levels of the hormone relaxin, which is secreted in high concentrations during pregnancy.

Men have approximately 1 L more blood volume than women and a higher haemoglobin concentration (15.8 g·L^{-1} ± 0.9 cf. 13.9 g·L^{-1} ± 1.1). Cardiac dimensions are greater in males, with subsequent higher stroke volumes and lung volumes which exceed those of females by about 10%. Women have a slightly higher resting pulse rate, although maximal heart rate is determined by age and is equal for both sexes.

Training Capacity of Women

Much of the original research on the physical capabilities of women was performed on untrained subjects, which indicated relatively poor work capacity and in part was responsible for restrictions imposed on women's sports participation. However, women are eminently trainable and there is less difference between the physiological parameters of trained women and trained men than between the 'average' woman and man, a fact which is probably indicative of the lower levels of exercise taken by the 'average' woman.

Women can increase muscle fibre diameter and total muscle mass and strength with systematic strength training, but not to the same extent as men because of relatively lower testosterone levels. Initial gains in strength may occur without muscle size increase because of improved neuromuscular unit recruitment.

Body fat content decreases in response to training and many female endurance athletes carry considerably less body fat than many male power athletes.

Women excel in ultra-endurance events and currently hold most of the world records in long-distance swimming. The physiology of this supremacy is not well understood but may relate to improved fat metabolism, superior muscle endurance at low workloads, tolerance of temperature extremes and greater buoyancy in water.

Aerobic Fitness

The ability to transport and utilize oxygen is determined more by training and biological potential than by gender. Men and women participating in the same sport will be closer in aerobic capacity ($\dot{V}_{O_2max}$) than athletes of the same sex in different sports (Drinkwater 1988). In absolute terms men have an advantage of up to 50% and this reflects their greater mass, cardiac and blood volumes, and haemoglobin. However, when expressed as a proportion of body mass (weight), which is the usual 'load' carried in most sporting events, the difference may be as little as 10%. If body fat is eliminated and oxygen consumption is expressed per lean bodyweight, the values of elite athletes are virtually identical.

Well trained women tolerate hypoxia, high altitude and heat stress at least as well as trained men.

Injuries

It appears that women do not suffer sporting injuries more or less often than men. In an extensive review, Marti (1991) concluded that female gender is not a risk factor for injury in the habitually active. Generally, women do not participate in heavy contact sports and are therefore spared many of the traumatic injuries caused by external forces such as contusions, fractures and concussion. Injuries are hence more sport specific than sex specific.

Injury statistics and surveys are an inaccurate method of determining the true prevalence of injuries as they are subject to bias. Initial data indicating high injury rates for females, especially military recruits probably indicated low levels of strength and fitness of women at that time. More recent statistics confirm equivalent injury rates of athletes training at the same level (Drinkwater 1988).

An exception to this may be amenorrhoeic athletes who have been shown to have a high injury incidence, notably stress fractures. This is discussed further in the section on bone density.

EXERCISE AND MENSTRUAL FUNCTION

Effect of Menses on Physical Performance

Most girls and women are able to enjoy their physical activity, both recreational and competitive without any undue regard for their menstrual pattern.

It has long been recognized that menstruation itself is not a contra-indication to physical activity. Indeed, the symptoms of menstrual pain (dysmenorrhoea) and premenstrual syndrome in the form of fluid retention, breast discomfort and anxiety are minimized rather than exacerbated by regular exercise. These effects may be due to changes in central neurotransmitters such as β-endorphins and/or reduction of prostaglandins, the mediators of pain in the uterus.

Scientific studies investigating physiological parameters of exercise have failed to show any consistent changes in performance associated with the stages of the menstrual cycle. However, self-reported questionnaires indicate that many women consider they perform least well at their sport during or just before their menstrual flow begins (Puhl & Brown 1986). By contrast Olympic records have been established by women during menstruation.

There are no medical indications for a woman to cease physical activity during her menses, although any individual may wish to avoid activity because of her own specific symptoms. Swimming may pose a problem for younger girls who may be unwilling to wear tampons. This needs to be recognized by coaches and allowances made if necessary for alternative training. Pain (dysmenorrhoea) may be effectively treated by non-steroidal anti-inflammatory medication because of its antiprostaglandin action. As the cause of premenstrual symptoms remains unknown, management is difficult. Pharmacological doses of Vitamin B_6 (50–100 mg daily), progesterone in pessary form and dopamine agonists have been suggested. Care must be taken to avoid proscribed drugs such as diuretics for competitive athletes. Heavy menstrual bleeding can be controlled by the use of norethisterone 15 mg daily or by regular oral contraception, which also minimizes dysmenorrhoea. The timing of menstruation can be adjusted to suit competition by the use of single dose oral contraceptives. This is done by continuation of the medication's active hormone tablets, thus avoiding the 7 day break from hormonal control which induces a bleed. Breakthrough bleeding can occur, however, particularly on the first or second cycle of therapy. Alternatively, an earlier cycle may be shortened by ceasing medication early and then commencing a complete 3 week course of tablets to create a withdrawal bleed prior to competition.

Effect of Physical Activity on Menstrual Function

The term 'athletic amenorrhoea' has been coined to describe the cessation of menstruation some athletes experience during rigorous training and competition. Attempts to characterize these changes have led to the realization that the significance of menstrual change in athletes lies in the secondary manifestations of altered fertility and skeletal integrity.

Menstrual change may constitute a lessening of the number of menses per year — oligomenorrhoea; or complete absence of menses — amenorrhoea. Amenorrhoea may be primary, that is a delayed onset of menarche; or secondary, after menses have initially been established.

INCIDENCE OF MENSTRUAL CHANGES IN ATHLETES

The incidence of menstrual changes in athletes is difficult to ascertain because of the varying forms menstrual disturbance assumes, from a short luteal phase to amenorrhoea. Furthermore, the problem is complicated by methodological variation in research and there is no exact definition accepted by all researchers for amenorrhoea, oligomenorrhoea or even regular cycles. Similarly, different populations of athletes are not always well defined, for example anaerobic or aerobic athletes, recreational joggers or elite endurance runners. These difficulties are evidenced by the wide range of incidence reported in the literature, namely 0–100%.

The following definitions are a consensus of terms used in the literature when classifying the incidence of menstruation:

- Eumenorrhoea relates to regular menses where bleeding occurs at intervals of between 21 and 35 days (10–13 menses per year)
- Oligomenorrhoea is when menses occurs at intervals between 35 and 90 days (4–9 menses per year)
- Amenorrhoea is when no menses occurs for 3 consecutive months, or no more often than three times per year

Menstrual bleeding is an inaccurate measure of menstrual function and serial hormonal assays or measurement of basal body temperature is needed to totally define menstrual status. It is likely that a luteal phase of 10 days, as determined by basal body temperature, is necessary to determine that someone is totally eumenorrhoeic.

The definition of menstrual change is complicated further by the 'dynamic dimension' of menstruation as described by Prior (1982), whereby any individual

can fluctuate between the different stages of menstrual change from 1 month to the next.

Menstrual changes are most common in distance runners, dancers and gymnasts and less common in cyclists and swimmers. There are very few data, however, on the large numbers of girls who play court or field sports. The American College of Sports Medicine (1980) has reported that approximately one-third of competitive female long-distance runners between the ages of 12 and 45 years experience periods of amenorrhoea or oligomenorrhoea.

Statistics on recreational and anaerobic sports indicate that menstrual patterns do not differ from those of sedentary women. It is wrong to infer that all athletic activity is associated with increased incidence of menstrual disturbance or that all highly trained female athletes have altered menses.

DELAYED MENARCHE

While several studies have noted a higher incidence of either delayed menarche or subsequent menstrual irregularity in girls participating in intense physical activity prior to menarche, other researchers have found no such association (Puhl & Brown 1986). Frisch et al. (1981) proposed that in premenarche trained swimmers and runners, menarche was delayed 5 months for each year of training. However, the possibility of self-selection exists in ectomorphic long-limbed girls who naturally attain late menarche. Studies of sisters of athletes confirm a familial predisposition to late menarche, although the athletes menstruated later than their siblings (Stager & Hatler 1988).

ASSOCIATED FACTORS

Research has identified several factors which appear common to athletes who experience menstrual change with physical activity (Table 23.1).

Age

Several studies suggest that young athletes, under the age of 25, are more prone to amenorrhoea.

Prior menstrual irregularity

While the majority of research indicates that oligo/amenorrhoeic athletes are more likely to have

Table 23.1 Factors associated with menstrual change in athletes

Factors associated with menstrual regularity	Factors associated with menstrual irregularity
Maturity of reproductive axis	Youth
Established ovulatory cycles	Nulliparity (no pregnancies)
Adult age	Decreased bodyweight
Motherhood	Decreased body fat
Increased bodyweight	Low energy diet
Increased body fat	High volume, high-intensity exercise
Gradual increase in activity	Rapid increase in exercise workload
Low-intensity exercise	Psychological stress

experienced irregular menses prior to regular training, this is not a consistent finding. Bullen *et al.* (1985) recorded the onset of some form of menstrual disturbance with training in nearly all of the subjects studied, irrespective of previous menstrual history.

Nulliparity

Evidence indicates that athletes who are mothers are less likely to develop amenorrhoea than those with no history of pregnancy.

The above three factors indicate that menstrual change is less likely to occur in the presence of a mature reproductive (hypothalamic–pituitary–ovarian) axis, once ovulatory cycles have been established.

Weight loss

Menstrual change in athletes has been associated with low bodyweight, excessive weight loss with training, diminished per cent body fat and dietary inadequacies. Some studies, however, indicate comparable height, weight and weight loss in amenorrhoeic and menstrually regular runners.

Frisch and McArthur (1974) proposed the 'critical fat theory'. In this they hypothesized that 17% of body fat was necessary for menarche and maintenance of normal menses and that 22% of body fat was needed to resume menses after amenorrhoea, secondary to loss of body fat. This rigid theory has not been substantiated by subsequent research; however, it would appear that there is a threshold body fat or total body mass (weight) below which

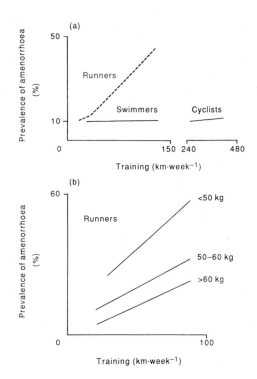

Fig. 23.2 (a) The prevalence of amenorrhoea increases linearly as training distance increases in runners ($P < 0.001$), but not in swimmers or cyclists. (b) Prevalence of amenorrhoea increases in runners as bodyweight decreases (adapted from Sanborn *et al.* 1982).

menses are affected and that this threshold is different for different individuals. This threshold may also be affected by other factors, such as activity levels (Fig. 23.2a,b).

Conflicting reports in the literature may be due

to the inadequacy of methods used for the determination of body composition and the calculation of percentage body fat (Loucks *et al.* 1984). Accurate methods of determining body composition are discussed in Chapter 1.

Diet

The effect of extreme weight loss secondary to dieting with subsequent amenorrhoea is epitomized by the condition anorexia nervosa. Anorectics, however, may also engage in regular physical activity. Eating disorders, food fads and vegetarianism are also common in athletes (Barrow & Saha 1988), although the incidence may be no greater than the general population (Weight & Noakes 1987). The relationship between eating disorders, amenorrhoea and osteoporosis has been described as the 'female athlete triad' by some authors (Nattiv *et al.* 1994). This is in recognition of the disordered behaviour of food deprivation and exercise obsession leading to amenorrhoea and low bone mass in some women. Nutritional needs of female athletes are further discussed in Chapter 5.

High-intensity exercise

An association between increased training distance of runners and the incidence of menstrual disturbance has been shown in many studies, including an almost linear relationship with amenorrhoea when the training distance rose above 30 km·week^{-1} (Sanborn *et al.* 1982).

Furthermore, athletes, including dancers, are known to resume menses during a training lay-off due to holidays or after injury, when there is no change in bodyweight.

A number of studies show no correlation between the level of exercise and menstrual change and it may be that intensity (per cent of maximal exercise sustained in training) or a rapid increase in training, rather than total distance or hours, may be more important determinants of menstrual change. Most sports with a high incidence of amenorrhoea involve aerobic rather than anaerobic training. However, this may be more related to the compounding factors of stress and low bodyweight as swimmers do not have a high incidence of menstrual distur-

bance, while gymnastics and ballet dancing, which involve high volume, short duration, predominantly anaerobic training, have some of the highest recorded levels of amenorrhoea.

Stress

While it is difficult to evaluate the role of stress, the observation that athletes have a higher incidence of amenorrhoea while participating in strenuous sports raises the possibility of a stress-related phenomenon. Women are known to experience menstrual irregularity at times of emotional stress such as bereavement or home shift, and complete gonadal atrophy has been reported in female prisoners on death row. Recent research has shown increased levels of the 'stress hormones', the corticosteroids and adrenocorticotrophic hormone (ACTH), in amenorrhoeic compared with eumenorrhoeic athletes. Reports on the psychological traits of amenorrhoeics have yielded conflicting results; one study indicating a close correlation between traits of depressive illness and anorectic behaviour in amenorrhoeics while other studies have failed to identify any particular abnormal psychological profile in amenorrhoeics (Schwartz *et al.* 1981; Gadpaille *et al.* 1987).

Neuroendocrinology of Menstrual Disturbance

Athletic amenorrhoea is characterized by hypothalamic dysfunction and as such can be described as 'hypogonadotrophic hypogonadism'; the athlete's ovaries fail to function adequately because of decreased stimulation from the pituitary trophic hormones, which in turn are dependent on hypothalamic function (Fig. 23.3).

Menstruation is dependent on accurately timed pulses of gonadotrophin-releasing hormone (GnRH) from the hypothalamus. One pulse every 60–90 min results in a steady pulsed release of follicle-stimulating hormone (FSH) and increasing pulses of luteinizing hormone (LH) from the pituitary gland throughout the first half (follicular phase) of the cycle. This culminates in a LH surge at midcycle. Appropriate oestrogen secretion and for-

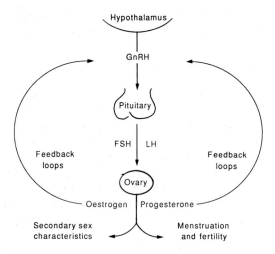

Fig. 23.3 Schema of the female reproductive axis.

mation of a follicle in the ovary is dependent on the correct ratio of FSH to LH; the LH surge resulting in ovulation. The remaining corpus luteum of the ovary secretes progesterone, and a luteal phase of at least 10 days follows in preparation for fertilization and pregnancy. Alternatively, the corpus luteum degenerates and menses ensue some 28 days after the hormonal interplay began.

The changes of athletic amenorrhoea are considered to be initially of abnormal GnRH pulse secretion, the timing of the pulse being too frequent or infrequent. Pituitary FSH secretion is diminished and the LH surge is inadequate both in intensity and duration. Ovarian function becomes depressed, with lower oestradiol (E_2) secretion and an inadequate (shorter in length with lower progesterone levels) luteal phase. Ultimately, the LH surge may become ineffective in stimulating ovulation and the anovulatory cycle becomes prolonged. Menstruation may occur episodically as shedding of the inadequately progesterone primed endometrium or as a response to infrequent ovulation. Eventually, menses may cease altogether (Fig. 23.4).

All of the above changes are reversible on the removal of the initiating stimulus. Hence an athlete may progress along the continuum in either direction depending on her level of training, weight, diet or other contributing factors at any given point in time.

Altered hypothalamic/pituitary function is not unique to female athletes, as low LH pulses and testosterone levels have been recorded in male marathon runners.

FSH, LH, E_2 and progesterone levels are typically reduced in the oligo/amenorrhoeic athlete. However, due to a wide range of 'normal' values, not all amenorrhoeics are hypo-oestrogenic.

The exact mechanism responsible for disturbance of the reproductive axis in athletes is yet to be determined. Research into the vast array of neuro-endocrinological changes with exercise is now beginning to outline possible aetiological pathways. However, there are significant difficulties in assessing the multifactorial stimuli affecting athletes under different laboratory and field environments.

Fig. 23.4 Schematic representation of the continuum of possible changes in the reproductive cycle of athletes.

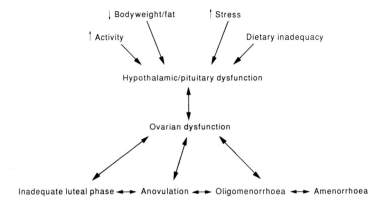

During acute exercise insulin levels decrease, while the secretion of glucagon, growth hormone, the catecholamines, the sex steroids, prolactin, dopamine and β-endorphin increase. Chronic training may modify both the basal level of circulating hormones and central transmitters, as well as the response to acute exercise. Body temperature, diurnal rhythms, eating patterns and the phases of the menstrual cycle itself also affect the hormonal response to exercise. Furthermore, it is likely that the neuroendocrine response of highly trained competitive athletes is different from that of recreational exercisers and that certain hormonal responses may be different between the sexes.

Chronic hyperprolactinaemia, as seen in pituitary tumour, is a well described cause of amenorrhoea and it has been postulated that recurrent exercise may mimic this effect. However, basal prolactin is decreased in individuals taking regular exercise.

The 'fat theory' formulated 20 years ago by Frisch and McArthur (1974) was based on a presumption of reduced formation of oestrogen (oestrone E_1) from androgens in the smaller fat stores of athletes. However, ovarian oestradiol (E_2) and not E_1 is decreased in amenorrhoeics, as aromatization of androgen to oestrone occurs readily in muscle. More recently, Brown (1992) postulates that repetitive rises in E_2 levels following exercise may diminish pituitary gonadotrophin levels through feedback mechanisms to GnRH. This effect would be increased during the luteal phase of the cycle when the increase in E_2 after exercise is greater, and subsequent disruption of the FSH/LH ratio results in an abnormal luteal phase and/or anovulation and amenorrhoea.

Increased levels of β-endorphin and dopamine, which are secreted by cells close to the GnRH cells in the hypothalamus, may inhibit GnRH secretion. This is consistent with the infusion of naloxone, an opiate antagonist, significantly increasing LH and FSH pulse amplitude in amenorrhoeic runners.

Jenkins and Grossman (1993) demonstrated a direct relationship between cortisol levels and amenorrhoea in elite athletes indicating a possible stress-related phenomenon. They also showed a positive correlation with insulin-like growth factor binding protein (IGF-I BP), which is inversely related to insulin levels, and they postulated an altered metabolic state in amenorrhoeics.

Sequelae of Menstrual Disturbance

It is a matter of contention whether athletic amenorrhoea constitutes an adaptation to exercise or a 'dysfunction' in the sense of disease. Prior (1982) argues strongly that in view of the spectrum and reversibility of menstrual changes, athletic amenorrhoea should be viewed as an adaptation. However, amenorrhoea may constitute a maladaptation as part of a global overstressing/overtraining syndrome in an athlete and there are reported similarities in the neuroendocrinology of the two states. Amenorrhoeics have increased incidence of injury and while lower fertility levels are reversible, the accompanying bone mass loss may not be. For these reasons athletes with menstrual disturbances should be counselled to remedy these changes, as athletic amenorrhoea is no longer considered a benign condition.

FERTILITY AND MENSTRUAL DISTURBANCE

Any menstrual 'cycle' that does not result in ovulation or is accompanied by an inadequate luteal phase (less than optimal for conception and implantation) will result in infertility or subfertility.

However, the majority of women in hard training do not seek conception and therefore infertility is not a problem. Furthermore, athletic amenorrhoea can be reversed by an increase in weight and/or a decrease in activity. The large numbers of highly trained athletes who now continue their career into motherhood is an indication that long-term fertility in these women is not compromised.

If an athlete is unable or unwilling to recommence ovulatory menses by changing her diet and training, ovulation can be induced with clomid if oestradiol (E_2) levels are sufficiently high. This can usually be achieved if levels exceed $150 \, pg \cdot L^{-1}$. Clomid can be administered orally for 5 days either from the fifth day of the cycle or randomly if no cycle is evident.

If E_2 is insufficient to produce ovulation, parenteral gonadotrophin administration or pulsatile injection of GnRH has been shown to result in ovulation and pregnancy. However, fetal birthweight may be reduced in underweight women in whom ovulation is artificially induced.

BONE DENSITY AND MENSTRUAL DISTURBANCE

Cann *et al.* (1984) reported decreased lumbar bone mineral density in amenorrhoeic runners and this finding has since been confirmed by several other investigators.

In 1986 Drinkwater *et al.* demonstrated that bone mineral loss in the spine is at least partly reversible when menses and reproductive hormone levels have returned to normal. However, peak bone mass may be jeopardized in prolonged amenorrhoea. These findings have important ramifications for female athletes.

Osteoporosis, or loss of bone mineral density, is now at epidemic proportions in the Western world. The clinical manifestations include an increased incidence of fractures of the skeleton (especially in the spine, wrist and hip), kyphosis of the spine secondary to spontaneous vertebral crush fractures and concomitant back pain. The condition affects one in every five women over the age of 60 years, and women are affected four times more often than men. This is because women achieve lower peak bone mass and lose bone more quickly after menopause.

DETERMINANTS OF BONE DENSITY

Bone mass in any individual is determined by genetic, hormonal and environmental factors, which are briefly outlined below:

- Genetic determination for bone mass is evidenced by the familial tendency to osteoporosis
- Hormonal determination of bone mass is complex. Androgens are responsible for increased bone mass in men, while oestrogen and probably progesterone are important factors in women
- Environmental factors include physical activity, diet and the negative effects of cigarette, caffeine and alcohol consumption. (Calcium and nutritional factors are dealt with in more detail in Chapter 5.) Physical inactivity and weightlessness (as in space flight) result in rapid bone loss and a negative calcium balance, while physical exercise is positively correlated with

increased bone density. Athletes have higher bone mass than sedentary subjects and exercise has been shown to increase bone mass in young people (Margulies *et al.* 1986). Bone cells respond to the stress of gravity and muscle contraction by increased remodelling and new bone formation. Osteoclasts resorb bone while osteoblasts lay down bone in accordance with Wolff's law whereby bone structure adapts to external physical force.

Bone mass increases rapidly during adolescence and reaches a peak in the third to fourth decade when it remains steady. With the onset of menopause and falling oestrogen levels there is a rapid bone loss of up to 4% per annum for approximately the first 5 years, after which the rate of loss slows. Oestrogen inhibits the activity of osteoclasts and as such is an 'antiresorptive' agent. Thus oestrogen deprivation increases bone resorption and decreases bone mass. An analogous situation occurs in the hypo-oestrogenic amenorrhoeic athlete who, despite the beneficial effects of high-activity levels, may suffer reduced bone mass (osteopenia). This effect is greatest in trabecular bone, which has a high turnover rate. Cortical bone is largely preserved in amenorrhoeics in response to the exercise stimulus.

With the delayed onset of menarche in many athletes, the adolescent rise in bone mass is also delayed, further jeopardizing the attainment of peak bone mass. It is the latter which is considered perhaps the most important factor in avoiding the onset of osteoporosis in later life (Fig. 23.5).

STRESS FRACTURES

Reports from military data indicate that stress fractures are more common in women than men, but this difference between the sexes is not evident in injury statistics of sporting populations. However, several studies (Lloyd *et al.* 1986; Barrow & Saha 1988) have shown an increased incidence of injury, notably stress fractures, in amenorrhoeic compared with eumenorrhoeic athletes. It has been suggested that hypo-oestrogenaemia may predispose these athletes to an inadequate bone structure resulting in more fractures. However, caution should be exercised as these results may simply be

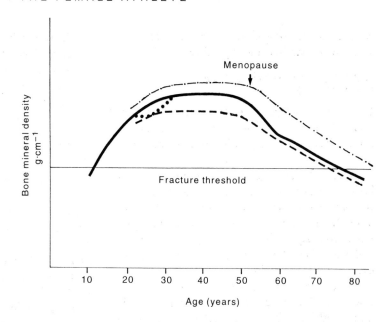

Fig. 23.5 Changes in bone mass in females with age and hypothetical changes in amenorrhoea. Hypo-oestrogenic states increase the risk of osteoporotic fractures in later life. Average bone density (——). Possible changes in bone density with regular activity: eumenorrhoea (—•—); short-term amenorrhoea (•••); long-term amenorrhoea (— —). Note: (i) the sudden decline at menopause which can be lessened by regular activity; and (ii) the fracture threshold of bone density at which fractures can occur with minimal trauma.

suggesting that female athletes who run further or exercise harder (and become amenorrhoeic) sustain more stress fractures. Stress fractures occur predominantly in weight-bearing cortical bone such as the tibia and metatarsals, but rarely in sites typical of osteoporotic fractures. Furthermore, athletes suffering stress fractures have been shown to have similar cortical and trabecular bone mass when compared with matched athletes without stress fractures, despite a significantly delayed age of menarche in the injured group (Carbon *et al.* 1990). One difficulty in understanding the relationship between bone mass, fractures and amenorrhoea are the limitations of current techniques of measurement (Ott 1994). Similarly, measurements of bone mass may not equate with bone quality or turnover, especially in the younger subject.

Certainly, the fear exists that amenorrhoeic athletes will suffer premature osteoporosis. However, one report on veteran athletes indicates that those who continue to train have normal bone mass despite episodes of oligo-amenorrhoea (Wilson *et al.* 1993).

PREVENTION AND TREATMENT OF OSTEOPOROSIS

Once established, osteoporosis may never be cured and treatment is aimed at halting or minimizing further loss. The most logical form of management is therefore prevention.

All women should be encouraged to exercise regularly throughout their lifetime, as bone mass is positively correlated with muscle strength and weight-bearing force. Research indicates that resistance training has a greater effect on bone mass than does aerobic exercise. Elderly patients demonstrate a decrease in the rate of bone loss in the majority of studies on physical activity as an intervention for osteoporosis, although this effect is not as great as that of exercise increasing bone mass in youth.

While appearing simplistic, it is known that most fractures are sustained as the result of falls, and exercise which improves mobility and postural control has a significant effect on reducing the incidence of fractures.

Adequate lifelong calcium, especially during adolescence, is important to ensure the attainment of peak bone mass. An intake of 800–1500 mg·day^{-1} of calcium is recommended for females and is discussed further in Chapter 5; however, the effect of calcium supplementation on fracture incidence remains unproven (Evans 1990).

Hormonal replacement therapy during the menopause remains controversial and one difficulty is the dilemma of deciding which women are at risk of

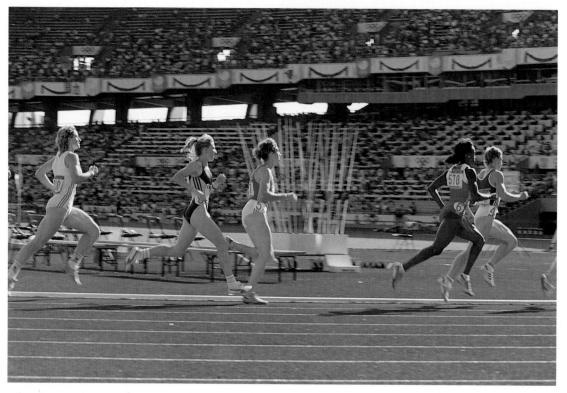

Fig. 23.6 Weight-bearing physical activity is positively correlated with increased bone mass.

sustaining fractures. Bone mass tends to be lower in Caucasian, ectomorphic, inactive women who have not had children or have not taken an oral contraceptive.

Low dose oestrogen (0.625 mg conjugated oestrogen or 10–20 μg oestradiol daily) for 3 weeks of the month combined with a progestagen (medroxyprogesterone 5 mg or levonorgesterol 30 mg daily) for the third week is a practical regimen for women with an intact uterus. It is best instituted early in the menopause to avoid the coincident phase of rapid bone loss.

Symptomatic osteoporosis may also be treated by the use of fluoride supplements, Vitamin D and calcitonin under medical supervision. Preliminary evidence indicates calcitonin and biphosphonate administration may increase bone mass.

OTHER SIDE-EFFECTS OF LOW OESTROGEN LEVELS

Post-menopausal women suffer from ischaemic heart disease at rates approaching those of their male counterparts, while menstruating women have cardioprotection as a result of their hormonal profile. Lipoprotein levels may be altered in amenorrhoea, but the long-term effects of this are not known.

Unopposed oestrogen secretions of chronic anovulation may create endometrial hyperplasia which increases the risk of endometrial carcinoma. However, athletes suffer fewer reproductive and breast cancers than the general population.

MANAGEMENT OF MENSTRUAL DISTURBANCE IN ATHLETES

Menstrual change in an athlete must never be assumed to be due to her training programme until history, examination and, if necessary, investigation confirms the diagnosis of athletic amenorrhoea. Absence of menses for 6 months or primary amenorrhoea over the age of 16 years warrants assessment and management.

A diagnosis of pregnancy should always be considered and, if appropriate, investigated from the outset. Amenorrhoea can also be part of the virilizing effects of anabolic steroids, and oral contraception may result in loss of withdrawal bleeding.

History should include the age of menarche and prior menstrual pattern in relationship to regular training programmes. Factors such as the onset of, or rapid increase in training levels, weight loss, dietary change or evidence of an eating disorder immediately preceding the onset of amenorrhoea should be sought. Other important factors include stressful events such as bereavement, home shift, or top-level sporting competition. The occurrence of stress fractures and other injuries may also be relevant.

Further history and examination should seek to exclude organic causes of amenorrhoea. The differential diagnosis includes:

- Pregnancy
- Anorexia nervosa
- Primary ovarian failure
- Hyperprolactinaemia
- Polycystic ovarian disease
- Virilizing syndromes, such as congenital adrenal hyperplasia
- Genetic or anatomical abnormalities in primary amenorrhoea
- Thyroid disease

Relevant aspects of the physical examination include:

- Height, weight, sum of skinfolds and percentage of ideal bodyweight
- Low pulse rate and body temperature, lanugo hair and parotid gland swelling may indicate an eating disorder
- Galactorrhoea from gentle compression of the nipples, which may suggest hyperprolactinaemia
- Signs of virilization include hirsutism, acne, clitoromegaly and voice change
- Signs of thyroid disease such as eye changes, tremor and elevated pulse rate
- Perineal and pelvic examination which may indicate an anatomical abnormality. A pelvic ultrasound is a valuable investigation and may be more appropriate in younger girls

If history and examination clearly indicate athletic amenorrhoea then it is reasonable to manage the athlete with minimal investigation: a low serum E_2 and normal serum prolactin is consistent with the diagnosis of athletic (hypothalamic) amenorrhoea.

Treatment of menstrual disturbance consists initially of an attempt to physiologically reverse the spectrum of change associated with hypothalamic amenorrhoea. The number of menses per year that ensure adequate bone mineralization and prevent endometrial hyperplasia is uncertain; however, at least four menses per year is advocated.

In practice an athlete with low bodyweight should be encouraged to increase her weight by at least 10% and decrease her training by a similar amount over a period of 2–3 months. Evidence suggests menses will return in the majority of athletes and this is also evident in the resumption of menses common to dancers and athletes after an enforced rest following injury.

If the athlete is unwilling to change her exercise and dietary patterns, if alteration of the possible precipitating factors does not result in the return of menses, or if history and examination indicates the possibility of other pathology, then more rigorous investigation is warranted. Tests may include:

- Serum FSH, LH, E_2, progesterone
- Serum prolactin
- Thyroid function tests
- Serum testosterone, dehydroepiandrosterone sulfate (DHEAS)
  (All the above blood tests should be taken after 24 h of rest)
- Pelvic ultrasound (it should be noted that cystic ovaries may be a non-specific finding)
- Cranial computerized tomography scan or magnetic resonance imaging for pituitary tumour
- Bone mass measurement (dual energy X-ray absorptiometry; DEXA) may be appropriate if amenorrhoea is prolonged, E_2 levels are very low or if there is concern for bone integrity

If results exclude other pathology and are consistent with hypothalamic amenorrhoea, then several options for management are open to the athlete and her clinician.

Progesterone challenge

Medroxyprogesterone 5–10 mg daily for 5–10 days may result in a withdrawal bleed indicating a sufficient oestrogen response in the endometrium. It is debatable whether this confirms sufficient endogenous oestrogen to maintain normal bone mass; however, the use of progesterone may be beneficial, as there is some evidence that it is a bone trophic hormone (Prior 1989). This regimen can be repeated every 1 or 2 months.

Hormone replacement therapy

This is similar to that described for postmenopausal management, using 0.625 mg conjugated oestrogens or 10 μg or more of oestradiol for days 1–21 of the cycle, combined with 5–10 mg medroxyprogesterone daily for days 14–21. This ensures maintenance of bone mass while not necessarily depressing the hypothalamic–pituitary axis. Alternative forms of contraception such as barrier methods are necessary, as the athlete may spontaneously ovulate while on this treatment.

Oral contraceptives

This is an option in those women who have had established regular menses at some time. Suppression of the reproductive axis is reversible and adequate oestrogen levels for bone health as well as contraception are assured.

The choice of management in any athlete should be based on her individual needs and wishes as well as on clinical indications.

CONTRACEPTION FOR ATHLETES

Data from North America indicate that athletes use barrier methods of contraception more, and the oral contraceptive pill less, than the general population (Jarrett & Spellacy 1983). Oral contraceptive pill use is more prevalent in Australia than in the United States or United Kingdom.

Barrier methods of contraception, including the condom and diaphragm have some advantages for the athlete. There is no interference with normal hormonal cycling and they are reliable when used in conjunction with spermicidal jelly. The intrauterine device may cause increased bleeding and should not be used in nulliparous women because of the risk of infection.

Avoidance of the oral contraceptive pill by athletes may be due to the fear of side-effects and a desire to avoid 'unnatural' contraception. However, modern low-dose combination pills present very few problems in terms of real health risks in the absence of cigarette smoking. Weight increase or decrease among oral contraceptive pill users is not significantly different from the rest of the population when large numbers of women are studied. Lipid profiles, and hence risk of ischaemic heart disease, are improved by oestrogen administration and made worse by progestagens; the combination of both in low dose has little overall effect. Similarly, thrombotic effects are minimized, with progestagens reducing and oestrogens increasing clotting factor activity.

The oral contraceptive increases the risk of cardiovascular disease in older, obese hypertensive women who smoke, and who are also more likely to be inactive.

The consensus of research indicates there is a reduced risk of ovarian and endometrial malignancy, while the risk of breast cancer continues to be debated. Increase in cervical neoplasia in oral contraceptive pill takers may be related to the confounding risk factors of increased sexual activity.

There is some evidence from two small prospective studies that $\dot{V}_{O2max}$ is decreased by oral contraceptive use. However, neither anaerobic performance nor aerobic endurance at 90% of $\dot{V}_{O2max}$ were affected. As the concentrations of both oestrogen and progestin components in oral contraceptives decreases, it is likely that the diminution in other side-effects is accompanied by a similar lessening of any significant implication for the exercising woman (Lebrun 1993). Certainly, many elite athletes have recorded peak performances while taking the oral contraceptive.

Less than 1% of women experience 'post pill amenorrhoea' for more than 12 months. Most of them have a prior history of irregular menses and lose substantial amounts of weight while on the pill or undertake very heavy exercise programmes (Shearman 1986). Hence athletes have a small but definite risk of prolonged amenorrhoea after oral contraceptive pill use, but this is associated with the intrinsic factors responsible for athletic amenorrhoea rather than long-term effects of the oral contraceptive pill itself. Alleviation of such factors, by an increase in weight and decrease in exercise, result in the return of menses and fertility as discussed earlier. The establishment of regular menses, at least at some time of the athlete's life, is desirable before the commencement of oral contraception.

Use of the oral contraceptive results in regular light withdrawal bleeding, the timing of which can be manipulated, if necessary, for competition. Dysmenorrhoea is lessened through the inhibition of ovulation, because prostaglandin production is decreased.

It is ironic that those athletes who may require oestrogen supplementation because of their menstrual disturbance are those who risk prolonged amenorrhoea after oral contraceptive pill use. In view of the reversibility of the latter and the increased risk associated with prolonged hypo-oestrogenaemia, oral contraceptive use may, in balance, be the preferred option for these athletes.

Progesterone-only 'mini-pills' do not reliably inhibit ovulation and allow natural hormonal cycling. Their predominant mode of action is on cervical mucus production whereby sperm motility is inhibited. Use of the mini-pill is hampered by poor cycle control and irregular bleeding in many women and efficacy requires regular precise dosage each day.

It is important for athletes to be aware that oligomenorrhoea and even amenorrhoea do not necessarily confer infertility and if pregnancy is to be reliably avoided regular contraception is always required.

EXERCISE AND PREGNANCY

In the past, socio-economic factors rather than medical science have determined the activity levels of pregnant women. However, evidence indicates that exercise is safe and probably beneficial for the majority of pregnant women.

Many athletes now train throughout their pregnancies and go on to improved sporting performances in motherhood. Ingrid Kristiansen set her best world marathon time 18 months after the birth of her first child, having trained throughout pregnancy and returned to full training by 1 month postpartum.

The reason some athletes improve performance after childbirth is not known. Physiologically, the increased blood volume and effort required to exercise at a greater bodyweight may have long-term benefits; or the psychological effects of enduring pregnancy, labour and motherhood may also be important.

Zaharieva (1972) wrote of the capabilities of Olympic athletes who became mothers:

> after childbirth Olympians . . . usually equalled and often improved on the records they achieved before pregnancy . . . The physical and functional condition is better than before. They feel physically more stable and psychically more balanced.

Exercise is contra-indicated in high-risk pregnancies and the level of activity for these women should be decided on an individual basis by their obstetrician.

Contra-indications to exercise include the following:

- Pre-eclampsia (toxaemia)
- Multiple pregnancies
- Intrauterine growth retardation
- Bleeding or premature labour
- Habitual abortion (miscarriage)

SCUBA diving should not be undertaken during pregnancy because of the possibility of gas emboli in the placental/fetal circulation and parachute jumping is similarly contra-indicated. A wetsuit should be worn during water-skiing to avoid forceful vaginal douching.

Risks of Exercise During Pregnancy

Although, traditionally, women and their doctors have always been concerned about the effect of exercise and sport on the unborn child, research has shown much of the concern to be overstated.

541

DIRECT TRAUMA

The uterus is a pelvic organ which is safe within the bony walls of the pelvis until the 12th week of pregnancy. After this the fetus is protected by the thick spongy layers of the uterus and up to a litre of amniotic fluid. Hence, fetal trauma as a result of maternal activity is very rare.

However, the combination of a shifting centre of gravity, lumbar lordosis and increasing ligamentous laxity increases the likelihood of maternal trauma in advanced pregnancy. As a consequence, sports where contact may occur, including many field and court sports, should be avoided in the third trimester (Fig. 23.7).

DECREASED UTERINE BLOOD FLOW

Animal studies have indicated that blood flow to the uterus may be reduced during exercise but

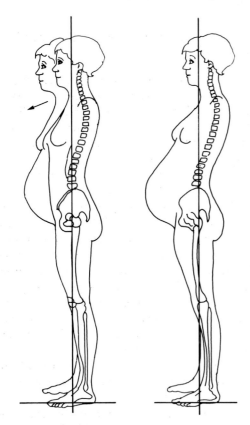

Fig. 23.7 Postural changes in advancing pregnancy. Note the increasing lumbar lordosis.

research results have been inconsistent (Wells 1985). In some studies risks to the fetus were not apparent when exercise was confined to the first half of pregnancy or if the animals were aerobically trained. Furthermore, there is evidence of a diversion of blood from the uterine muscle to the placenta as well as a compensatory increase in oxygen extraction across the uterine circulation during maternal exercise (Clapp 1978).

There have been many studies measuring human fetal response to maternal exercise, mostly involving running or cycling programmes and none of these studies has shown that the fetal outcome was adversely affected (Carbon 1988).

Because it is technically very difficult to monitor the fetus during exercise, cardiotocography is used to measure fetal heart rate immediately after maternal exercise. While some reports indicate a bradycardia or no change in fetal heart rate, most indicate a short period of fetal tachycardia after maternal exercise. Collings and Curet (1985) suggest this may be due to increased fetal arousal, placental transfer of catecholamines, increased fetal temperature or a reduction in uterine blood flow. Their study concluded 'neonatal findings provided further evidence that quantitated maternal exercise up to 70% maximal capacity does not interfere with normal fetal growth and development'.

There is evidence that continued daily endurance training near to delivery, along with poor maternal weight gain, is associated with low birthweight. Consequently, attention should be paid to good nutrition and training should probably be limited to alternate days in the third trimester (Bell *et al.* 1995).

Because of the risks of decreased uterine blood flow, maternal exercise to exhaustion should be discouraged; however, studies of maternal exercise at 90–100% $\dot{V}_{O_2max}$ have failed to report any deleterious effect on the fetus (Artal *et al.* 1986).

HYPERTHERMIA

There is an increased incidence of neural tube defects in the offspring of pregnant animals who have been artificially heated to core body temperatures over 39°C for several days. Similarly, 10% of women who delivered anencephalic babies gave a history of febrile illness or sauna bathing in early pregnancy (Miller *et al.* 1978). These reports have caused concern regarding the possibility of fetal damage secondary to hyperthermia during exercise in early pregnancy.

Recent research, however, indicates that the rise in rectal temperature of pregnant women is less than their preconceptual rise during treadmill exercise, suggesting an increased efficiency of heat dissipation during pregnancy (Clapp *et al.* 1987). Although this is an area requiring further research, as yet there are no reports in the literature of fetal malformation attributable to hyperthermia during maternal exercise. It should be remembered that dehydration increases the risk of diminished uterine blood flow and hyperthermia and must be avoided by pregnant women during exercise.

Childbearing Potential of Athletes

The childbearing potential of female athletes has been doubted by some sections of the medical profession in the past. Obstetricians feared that the 'narrow pelvis' and well developed perineal musculature of trained women resulted in more difficult deliveries.

Research findings over the past three decades, however, indicate that there is probably no statistically significant difference between the length or complication rates of labour in exercising or sedentary women (Carbon 1988). Furthermore, pH measurements of umbilical blood taken at the time of delivery indicate that fit women and their babies tolerate the rigours of labour better than unfit women (Erkkola & Rauramo 1976).

While there have been some reports of exercise being associated with increased uterine muscle activity, there is no direct evidence that exercise initiates preterm labour in a normal pregnancy.

Effect of Pregnancy on Exercise

Many pregnant women have completed marathons, one being 6 months pregnant in the 1984 US Olympic trials. However, it is well documented that the majority of women spontaneously decrease their level of activity in the third trimester of pregnancy as a result of increasing size with postural and cardiovascular changes. It is now known that some pregnant women are capable of manifesting a training effect (decreased exercising pulse rate and increased stroke volume) through pregnancy and into the postpartum period. However, a rise in resting pulse rate and limitation of venous return imposed by the developing uterus on the abdominal vena cava may limit cardiac reserve in late pregnancy. Venous pooling in the legs may result in hypotension if exercise is abruptly stopped in late pregnancy. Exercise in the supine position further limits venous return and should be avoided.

There is a suggestion that the increased blood volume and pulmonary alkalosis of early pregnancy may, in fact, improve aerobic performance. This has been supported by press reports that some athletes may actually seek pregnancy to improve their athletic performance.

Guide-lines for the Care of Pregnant Athletes

Women who wish to continue their exercise programmes into pregnancy need empathic medical personnel able to guide them through to delivery. Provided there is no indication of fetal or maternal compromise, there is no valid reason to discourage a woman from enjoying exercise. Swimming, cycling and low-impact aerobic dance are appropriate activities in advancing pregnancy.

The American College of Obstetrics and Gynecology (1985) has published guide-lines for exercise in pregnancy targeted at the general population; however, they are probably too conservative for fit athletes. The Australian Sports Medicine Federation (1994) has recently published guide-lines on pregnancy and collision sports for women.

The following is an outline of appropriate medical care for women who exercise while pregnant. Medical practitioners should:

- Ensure that the pregnancy is not high risk and that the athlete does not have a poor obstetric history
- Ascertain the preconceptual level of fitness and expertise and explain that this should not be exceeded during pregnancy

- Ensure that the pregnant athlete attends regularly for antenatal assessment. In particular maternal weight gain must be monitored as well as checking that fetal size and movements are appropriate for the stage of pregnancy

The pregnant athlete should be counselled to:

- Avoid exercise to exhaustion — she should be able to converse during prolonged exercise
- Avoid exercise in the heat — especially in early pregnancy
- Drink sufficient fluid
- Begin and finish exercise gradually, that is 'warm up' and 'warm down'
- Beware of signs to stop exercise, such as pain or bleeding
- Exercise regularly to maintain fitness rather than in spasmodic arduous bouts
- Be prepared to reduce exercise levels at least in the third trimester

GENDER VERIFICATION

Separate competitions have been an accepted part of sporting history because of the inherent anatomical and physiological differences between the sexes.

It is interesting to note that the first 'sex testing' took place in the original Olympic Games where male competitors competed naked to prove their masculinity as no women were allowed in the sporting arena.

During the modern era of sport, increasing numbers of women have competed in world championship events and the Olympic Games with steadily improving performances. During the 1950s and 1960s it became evident that some female competitors could emulate their male counterparts by using exogenous androgens (anabolic steroids), and this led to the need for drug testing procedures at major sporting events. Furthermore, it was feared that male competitors might masquerade as women. Alternatively, an individual who was psychosocially female but with increased androgenicity due to a chromosomal or endocrinological defect, may hold an unfair physical advantage over other female competitors. In order to protect all competitors, major sporting bodies decided that individuals who

wished to compete as women would be required to pass a 'Femininity Test' before they could compete.

Dr Hay of the International Olympic Committee (IOC) in his address to the International Amateur Athletics Federation (IAAF) Medical Congress in 1985 stated that:

> The femininity control would eliminate the cases in which a genetic alteration gives the competitor registered as a female anatomical advantages of masculinization due to the abnormal differentiation of the embryonic gonads. The reason the IOC and the international sports federations separate events by sex is not on account of social status but for an equal opportunity for every participant.

The IOC decided in 1964 to form a medical commission to police the use of drugs and femininity controls in future Olympic Games. In the 1966 European Track and Field Championships in Budapest full visual examination of all female competitors was introduced. Such an examination is an ordeal for many women and is no longer used as a screening method.

The IOC established its rules and procedures governing femininity controls in the 1968 (Mexico City) Games and these rules embraced the following principles (Hay 1988):

- The investigation of the femininity of women participating in the Olympic Games is to ensure that the athletes are competing on an equal basis, considering their physical status
- Absolute secrecy is maintained in cases where results disqualify participation, so as not to provoke any possible social and psychological disturbances to the individuals concerned
- Ease of test performance

Testing Procedures

The buccal smear test is currently considered by the IOC as the least offensive, easiest to administer and cheapest method of screening available. In practice, cells are scraped off the buccal mucosa (inside of the cheek) with a spatula, smeared on a glass slide, fixed, stained and examined under a microscope. The nuclear chromosomes may be assessed in a variety of specific techniques: from

1968 to 1988 the Barr body test was used and at the 1992 Olympics this was changed to the polymerase chain reaction (PCR) test. Such tests are based on the detection of the normal human sex chromosomes: designated as XX for women and XY for men. In women, one X chromosome is inactivated and can be detected as a Barr body (Fig. 23.8), a darkly staining chromatin body at the inner surface of the nuclear membrane. Twenty-five per cent of cells must carry a Barr body for the test to be deemed positive for female chromosomes. The PCR detects the SRY locus of the Y chromosome, which is the DNA sequence for testes determination and hence is positive in men.

If any abnormality is detected on screening, a blood test for karyotyping is performed. Athletes are subject to a clinical gynaecological and musculo-skeletal examination to detect cases in which a genetic disorder gives any masculine anatomical physical development, allowing an advantage to the athlete in performance. This examination is performed by a female Genetics Specialist of the Medical Services of the Organizing Committee who with a member of the IOC Medical Commission and the Medical Officer of the athlete's National Olympic Committee submit the results in the strictest confidence to the IOC Medical Commission, which decides whether the athlete can compete. The IOC will accept her withdrawal for 'personal reasons' and will ensure absolute secrecy in the case (Hay 1988).

The IOC is proud of its 25 year record of total secrecy and absence of media leaks during the time it has been conducting femininity tests. Other instances, however, have become public. Eva Klobukowska, Olympic gold medallist in 1964, was banned from competition after failing a 'chromosome test' at the Women's European Athletics Cup in 1967, despite having been passed by a medical examination in Budapest in 1966 (Dyer 1982). Such incidents are a clear indication of the need for professional confidentiality.

However, the secrecy of the IOC and other sporting bodies, as well as the testing procedures themselves, have also invoked criticism from some scientific and medical experts. De la Chappelle (1988) considers the Barr chromatin test totally unsuitable and states that it 'detects 10% or less of those individuals who are female in appearance but male in muscle strength'.

The problem inherent in the use of laboratory analysis of gender is the fact that genetic chromatin does not have a one to one relationship with physical and sexual manifestation in the individual. Nor are the tests involved always 100% accurate. The Barr test requires considerable operator expertise while the PCR is very sensitive, even to any male cells which may be inadvertently left on laboratory equipment.

Abnormal Sexual Development

There are many different forms of abnormal sexual development where genetic and phenotypic manifestations are not identical; only the more common are presented here.

XO, Turner's syndrome, fails the Barr test as there is only one X chromosome, but passes the PCR test. Male individuals with the XXY Klinefelter's syndrome pass the Barr test but not the PCR. Genetic mosaics occur where different cells have different sex chromosomes, XX, XY or combinations thereof which lead to variable sexual expression. When detected by screening these

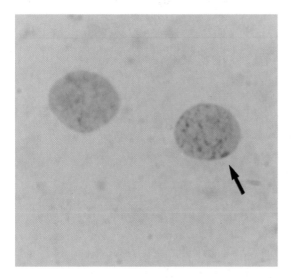

Fig. 23.8 The cell on the right demonstrates a Barr body.

women may have masculine physical characteristics which would preclude them from participation under the IOC rules.

There is a reported incidence of 1 in 20 000 individuals who are totally male in appearance and strength but who possess XX sex chromatin and hence pass both screening tests. XY gonadal dysgenesis results in a phenotypic female with bilateral streak gonads. The dysgenic testes may produce significant amounts of testosterone, and virilization may be evident at birth or puberty. Once detected by Barr or PCR testing, a clinical decision must determine suitability for competition.

Androgen insensitivity syndromes

The best known of these is testicular feminization which is an hereditary condition. An XY individual in whom there is end organ insensitivity to testosterone develops as a female, with what appears to be normal secondary sex characteristics. However, the person bears intra-abdominal atrophic testes, no ovaries and a vagina which ends in a blind pit. There is no physical advantage in sport because

there is no masculinization of the musculoskeletal system and such a person will pass a clinical examination as a phenotypic female and be allowed to compete. However, she would fail both the Barr and PCR tests.

Adrenogenital syndrome (congenital adrenal hyperplasia)

Steroid biosynthesis in the adrenal gland, under the control of trophic hormones from the pituitary gland, results in the production of the corticoid hormones, as well as oestrogen and testosterone in differing amounts for each sex. Enzyme deficiencies at each step of the biosynthetic pathway have been described. They may occur in males or females and are transmitted as autosomal recessive characteristics with variable expression. The most common form of congenital adrenal hyperplasia is the 21-hydroxylase deficiency, with an estimated incidence of 1:300–1000 in its mildest form in some communities. Because cortisol cannot be produced in normal amounts there is loss of the normal negative feedback loop to the pituitary and subsequent increased ACTH secretion results in adrenal stimulation. Furthermore, there is a 'damming up' effect of steroids preceding the block and hence increased formation of the androgen DHEAS and, perhaps, testosterone (Figs 23.9 and 23.10). In untreated

Fig. 23.9 Steroid biosynthesis in the adrenal gland indicating enzyme block in congenital adrenal hyperplasia at 21-hydroxylase.

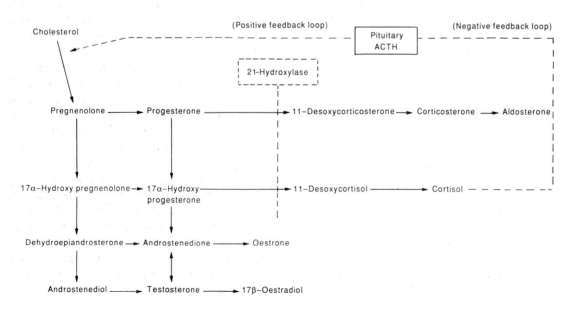

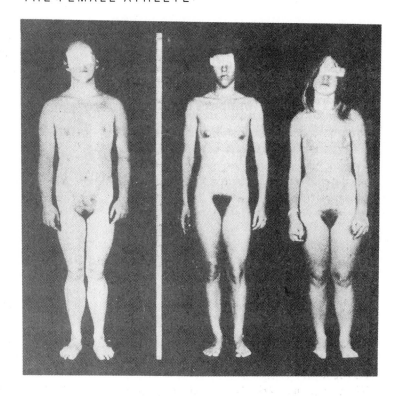

Fig. 23.10 Pubertal girls with congenital adrenal hyperplasia. Treatment commenced at age 16 years for the girl on the left, age 9 years for the girl in the centre and age 4 years for the girl on the right (New *et al.* 1983; with permission).

women there is early epiphyseal closure, short stature at maturity, increased muscle bulk and clitoromegaly. In milder forms the only manifestation may be increased muscular strength in a woman who is likely to be a good athlete (de la Chappelle 1988). These women pass the Barr and PCR screening tests and are allowed to compete.

There are several cases of men who have undergone sex change operations and have wanted to compete as women. They have had variable success in convincing sporting associations of their femininity. Such individuals would not pass laboratory screening tests as they have male (XY) genotype.

Recent Developments in Gender Verification

The IOC and other major sporting bodies are well aware of the difficulty of sex testing. In deference to athletes the IOC Medical Commission is resistant to calls for physical examination as a screening procedure. However, in response to directives from its medical advisers, the IAAF reverted to a pro-

cedure of physical examination for the 1991 World Championships. This was not universally accepted by the athletes and medical staff and, as it is now considered 'extremely unlikely' that a man would masquerade as a woman, the IAAF stopped formal gender screening in 1992 (Simpson *et al.* 1993). However, the Athletic Federation 'retains the option to investigate individual exceptional cases'.

Certainly, in view of the known inadequacies of the screening tests, no sporting organization should conduct testing without the necessary medical and administrative expertise to assure all athletes complete accuracy and confidentiality of their results.

Many female athletes are tall, well muscled, perhaps somewhat hirsute or amenorrhoeic and, when confronted with a test of their sexual identity, may hold real fears of the outcome. The simplicity and non-threatening nature of the buccal smear, as well as the intent to stop men competing against women, should be explained when the tests are first mentioned. Medical personnel can allay unnecessary fears and stress on athletes at a time when they are preparing for major competition.

CONCLUSIONS

Women continue to enjoy physical activity in increasing numbers and are steadily achieving higher levels of performance. While there are specific health issues relating to their unique reproductive function, the health benefits of regular exercise far outweigh any currently known negative effects.

REFERENCES

American College of Obstetrics and Gynecology (1985) *Exercise During Pregnancy and the Postnatal Period.* AGOC Home Exercise Programs, Washington DC.

American College of Sports Medicine (1980) Opinion Statement on the Participation of the Female Athlete in Long-distance Running. *Sports Medical Bulletin* 15, 1, 4, 5.

Artal R., Wiswell R., Romen Y. & Dorey F. (1986) Pulmonary responses to exercise in pregnancy. *American Journal of Obstetrics and Gynecology* 154, 378–383.

Australian Sports Medicine Federation (1994) Participation of the pregnant athlete in contact and collision sports. *Women in Sport Committee, Canberra.*

Barrow G. W. & Saha S. (1988) Menstrual irregularity and stress fractures in collegiate female distance runners. *American Journal of Sports Medicine* 16, 209–216.

Bell R., Palma S. & Lumley J. (1995) The effect of vigorous exercise during pregnancy on birthweight. *Australian and New Zealand Journal of Obstetrics and Gynaecology* 35, 46–51.

Brown W. J. (1992) Oestradiol response to exercise 'through the ages'. *Australian Journal of Science and Medicine in Sport* 24, 18–24.

Bullen B. A., Skrinar G. S., Beitins I. Z., Mering G. von, Turnbull B. A. & McArthur J. W. (1985) Induction of menstrual disorders by strenuous exercise in untrained women. *New England Journal of Medicine* 312, 1349–1353.

Cann C. E., Martin M. C., Genant H. K. & Jaffe R. B. (1984) Decreased spinal mineral content in amenorrheic women. *Journal of the American Medical Association* 251, 626–629.

Carbon R. (1988) Exercise and pregnancy. *Excel* 5, 6–10.

Carbon R., Sambrook P. N., Deakin V. *et al.* (1990) Bone density of elite female athletes with stress fractures. *Medical Journal of Australia* 153, 373–376.

Clapp J. F. (1978) The relationship between blood flow and oxygen uptake in the uterine and umbilical circulations. *American Journal of Obstetrics and Gynecology* 132, 410–413.

Clapp J. F., Wesley M. & Sleemaker R. H. (1987) Thermoregulatory and metabolic responses to jogging prior to and during pregnancy. *Medicine and Science in Sport and Exercise* 19, 124–130.

Collings C. & Curet L. B. (1985) Fetal heart rate response to maternal exercise. *American Journal of Obstetrics and Gynecology* 151, 448–450.

De la Chappelle A. (1988) Why sex chromatin should be abandoned as a screening method for 'gender verification' of female athletes. *Sports Medicine in Track and Field Athletics, Proceedings of the Second IAAF Medical Congress, Canberra, Australia,* pp. 45–48. Marshallarts Printing Services, UK.

Drinkwater B. (1988) Training of female athletes. In Dirix A., Knuttgen H. G. & Tittel (eds) *The Olympic Book of Sports Medicine I,* pp. 309–327. Blackwell Scientific Publications, Oxford.

Drinkwater B., Nelson K., Ott S. & Chesnut C. H. (1986) Bone mineral density after resumption of menses in amenorrhoeic athletes. *Journal of the American Medical Association* 256, 380–382.

Dyer K. F. (1982) *Challenging the Men. Women in Sport,* p. 65. University of Queensland Press, Brisbane.

Erkkola R. & Rauramo L. (1976) Correlation of maternal physical fitness during pregnancy with maternal and fetal pH and lactic acid at delivery. *Acta Obstetrica et Gynecologica Scandinavica* 55, 441–446.

Evans R. A. (1990) Calcium and osteoporosis. *Medical Journal of Australia* 152, 431–433.

Frisch R. E. & McArthur J. W. (1974) Menstrual cycles: Fatness as a determinant of minimum weight for height necessary for their maintenance or onset. *Science* 185, 949–950.

Frisch R. E., Gotz-Welbergen A., McArthur J. W. *et al.* (1981) Delayed menarche and amenorrhoea of college athletes in relation to age of onset of training. *Journal of the American Medical Association* 246, 1559.

Gadpaille W. J., Sanborn C. F. & Wagner W. W. (1987) Athletic amenorrhoea, major affective disorders and eating disorders. *American Journal of Psychiatry* 144, 939–942.

Hay E. (1988) Femininity controls in the Olympic Games. Sports Medicine in Track and Field Athletes. *Proceedings of the Second IAAF Medical Congress, Canberra, Australia,* pp. 49–52. Marshallarts Printing Services, UK.

Jarrett J. C. & Spellacy W. N. (1983) Contraception practices of female runners. *Fertility and Sterility* 139, 374–375.

Jenkins P. J. & Grossman A. (1993) The control of the gonadotrophin releasing hormone pulse generator in relation to opioid and nutritional cues. *Human Reproduction* 8, 154–161.

Lebrun C. M. (1993) Effect of the different phases of the menstrual cycle and oral contraceptives on athletic performance. *Sports Medicine* 16, 400–430.

Lloyd T., Triantafyllou S. J., Baker E. R. *et al.* (1986) Women athletes with menstrual irregularity have increased musculoskeletal injuries. *Medicine and Science in Sport and Exercise* 18, 374–379.

Loucks A. B., Horvath S. M. & Freedson P. S. (1984)

Menstrual status and validation of body fat prediction in athletes. *Human Biology* 56, 383–392.

Margulies J. Y., Simkin A. & Leichter I. (1986) Effect of intense physical activity on the bone mineral content in the lower limbs of young adults. *Journal of Bone and Joint Surgery* 68, 1090–1093.

Marti B. (1991) Health effects of recreational running in women: Some epidemiological and preventive aspects. *Sports Medicine* 11, 20–51.

Miller P., Smith D. W. & Shepard T. N. (1978) Maternal hyperthermia as a possible cause of anencephaly. *Lancet* 519–521.

Nattiv A., Agostini R., Drinkwater B. & Yeager K. K. (1994) The female athlete triad: The inter-relatedness of disordered eating, amenorrhoea and osteoporosis. *Clinics in Sports Medicine* 13, 405–418.

New M. I., Dupont B., Grumbach K. & Levine L. S. (1983) Congenital adrenal hyperplasia and related conditions. In Stanbury J. B., Wyngaarden J. B., Fredrichson D. S., Goldstein J. L. & Brown M. S. (eds) *The Metabolic Basis of Inherited Disease*, p. 984. McGraw-Hill Book Co., New York.

Ott S. M. (1994) Bone mass measurements: Reasons to be cautious. *British Medical Journal* 308, 931–932.

Prior J. C. (1982) Endocrine 'conditioning' with endurance training: A preliminary review. *Canadian Journal of Applied Sport Science* 7, 148–157.

Prior J. C. (1989) Trabecular bone loss is associated with abnormal luteal phase length: Endogenous progesterone deficiency may be a risk factor for osteoporosis. *International Proceedings Journal* 1, 70–73.

Puhl J. C. & Brown C. H. (eds) (1986) *The Menstrual Cycle and Physical Activity*. Human Kinetics Publishers, Champaign, IL.

Sanborn C. F., Martin B. J. & Wagner W. W. (1982) Is athletic amenorrhea specific to runners? *American Journal of Obstetrics and Gynecology* 143, 859–861.

Schwartz B., Cumming D. C., Riordan E., Sely M., Yen S. S. C. & Rebar R. W. (1981) Exercise-associated amenorrhoea: A distinct entity. *American Journal of Obstetrics and Gynecology* 141, 662–670.

Shearman R. P. (1986) Oral contraception agents. *Medical Journal of Australia* 144, 201–205.

Simpson J. L., Ljungqvist A., de la Chappelle A. *et al.* (1993) Gender verification in competitive sports. *Sports Medicine* 16, 305–315.

Stager J. M. & Hatler L. K. (1988) Menarche of athletes: The influence of genetics and prepubertal training. *Medicine and Science in Sport and Exercise* 204, 369–373.

Weight L. M. & Noakes T. D. (1987) Is running an analog of anorexia? A survey of the incidence of eating disorders in female distance runners. *Medicine and Science in Sport and Exercise* 19, 213–217.

Wells C. C. (1985) *Women, Sport and Performance. A Physiologic Perspective.* Human Kinetics Publishers, Champaign, IL.

Wilson J. H., Harries M. G., Reeve J. (1993) Bone mineral density in premenopausal veteran athletes and the influence of menstrual irregularity (Abstr.). *Clinical Science* 86, 2.

Zaharieva E. (1972) Olympic participation by women. Effects on pregnancy and childbirth. *Journal of the American Medical Association* 221, 992–995.

CHAPTER 24

THE DISABLED ATHLETE

K. E. Fallon

HISTORICAL PERSPECTIVE

Before the 1940s many of the disabled, especially those with spinal injuries, were relatively neglected. A comfortable and convenient placement was found for them and they were forgotten. It was felt that little could be done for these unfortunate people and sooner or later many succumbed to infection or other complications. Early sports participation by the disabled was by individual initiative. For example, Lord Byron in the 1800s, despite a congenital lower limb deformity, became proficient in rowing, swimming and boxing. The earliest amputee race recorded was between two one-legged amputees, each with a wooden leg, at Newmarket in England in 1880 (Guttman 1977). Karoly Tacacazs, Olympic gold medallist in pistol shooting in 1948 and 1952, lost his normally dominant right arm in 1938 and performed from that time on with his retrained left arm.

Formal sports organizations for the disabled are over 100 years old, with a sports club for the deaf being founded in Germany in 1880. In the United Kingdom the Disabled Drivers' Motor Club was founded in 1922 and the British Society of One-armed Golfers developed in 1932. In 1924 the first World Games for the Deaf were conducted in Paris.

The Second World War, with its large numbers of disabled ex-servicemen, provided a great impetus for rehabilitation programmes, which included games as a component of their therapy. Sir Ludwig Guttman opened a spinal injuries centre at Stoke Mandeville in England in 1944 and his theories pertaining to sport as an overall training method for the neuromuscular system and as a natural way to prevent boredom during rehabilitation, led to the first great leap forward in disabled sport.

Following successful experiments with punchball exercises, darts, rope climbing and snooker, Guttman introduced wheelchair polo as the first competitive team sport for paraplegics. Badminton, archery, table tennis and basketball soon followed and in 1948 the first Games for the paralysed were held, with 16 competitors participating.

The development of international competition for the disabled is briefly outlined below:

- 1949 — First World Winter Games for the Deaf in Austria
- 1957 — First Australian team at Stoke Mandeville Games
- 1960 — First Disabled Olympics, Rome; 21 countries participating
- 1962 — At the instigation of Sir George Bedbrook — First Commonwealth Paraplegic Games in Perth, Australia
- 1968 — International Special Olympics founded
- 1976 — Disabled Olympics, first including blind and amputee athletes
- 1984 — Wheelchair Olympics, New York, 3000 competitors taking part
- 1984 — Los Angeles Able-bodied Olympics

with demonstration sports, for example women's 800 m and men's 1500 m wheelchair competitions

- 1984 — First wheelchair athlete to appear in an able-bodied Olympics; Neroli Fairhall, representing New Zealand, placed 38th in Women's Archery event

The history of sports medicine for disabled athletes commenced with Guttman's clinical observations in the 1940s; however, it is only since the late 1970s that significant sports medicine–sports science data have been collected on the disabled. The physiology of the paraplegic is well documented as are the biomechanics of wheelchair propulsion; however, research is still lacking on the specific sports medicine problems of many disabled groups. This important data base will only grow with increased involvement of sports medicine and science personnel who are prepared to carry out further research in the field.

DISABLED GROUPS TO BE CONSIDERED

This chapter will attempt to summarize the currently available data on the following groups:

- The spinal cord injured
- The wheelchair athlete
- The mentally handicapped — the Special Olympics
- The blind
- The amputee
- The deaf
- Those athletes with cerebral palsy
- 'Les autres'

AVAILABLE SPORTS

With some specific restrictions relating only to special groups, the disabled are currently involved in virtually every sport available to the able-bodied athlete.

Track and field events, basketball, shooting, archery, table tennis, lawn bowls, swimming and weight-lifting are the sports most commonly associated with the disabled. However, they now involve themselves in sports which are considered high risk for even the able-bodied athlete, such as downhill snow skiing, rock climbing, SCUBA diving, sky diving, car racing, motor cross and water-skiing.

THE PROBLEMS OF A SEDENTARY EXISTENCE

The able-bodied and the disabled person are both at risk of medical complications related to a sedentary existence. These include obesity, osteoporosis, ischaemic heart disease, hypertension, blood lipid abnormalities and non-insulin-dependent diabetes mellitus.

Regular exercise is associated with a general feeling of well-being in the normal population. It is used as a treatment modality for non-specific psychosocial stress and it has been shown to produce transient reductions in somatic tension and subjective anxiety. Further, it has been shown to ameliorate the symptoms of clinically diagnosed depression. It is clear that the adoption of an active life-style including regular exercise and sports participation has value for the able-bodied person, but it would seem that its benefits may be even more valuable for the disabled individual.

THE SPINAL CORD INJURED: THE WHEELCHAIR ATHLETE

Pathophysiology

When the spinal cord is damaged there is a loss of motor and sensory function below the level of the spinal cord lesion. The extent of the motor and sensory loss depends upon this level as well as upon the degree of damage of the spinal cord. Quadriplegia at the level of the cervical region and spastic paraplegia at the thoracic region may result. At the level of the lumbar spine flaccid paralysis occurs due to injury of the cauda equina. Paraplegia is defined as complete paralysis of both lower limbs and paraparesis as incomplete paralysis of both lower limbs. The term quadriplegia or tetraplegia is used to describe paralysis of all four limbs and quadriparesis as incomplete paralysis of all four limbs.

Between 40 and 50% of spinal cord injuries are attributed to motor vehicle accidents. Falls, which are the second most common cause, account for perhaps 25%, followed by sports injuries, such as those resulting from diving into swimming pools and rivers. Not all spinal cord injuries are caused by trauma: non-traumatic causes include tumours, multiple sclerosis, disc protrusions, transverse myelitis and infective and vascular lesions. Peak incidence of paraplegia in both males and females occurs between the ages of 15 and 25 years. Quadriplegia in males most commonly has its onset at age 15–35, or above 55 years of age in traumatically induced cases and males are four to five times more likely to be affected than females.

Neurological Disability

Neurological disability can be divided into three areas: motor loss, sensory loss and disruption to autonomic control.

MOTOR LOSS

The level of dysfunction is related to the level of spinal cord trauma. A complete lesion of the cord above C3 results in paralysis of most of the skeletal muscles of the body. The diaphragm is innervated by nerves arising from C3 to C5 and a lesion at or above C3 causes inability to breathe and is usually fatal. The upper extremity is innervated from levels C5 to T1 and upper arm innervation involves C5–C8. The forearm involves C6–C8 and the hand C7–T1.

The intercostal and thoracic muscles are innervated from levels T2 to T8 and the abdominal muscles from T7 to T12. The lower extremity is innervated from levels L2 to S2, the upper leg muscles from L2 to S2, the lower leg muscles from L4 to S2 and the foot from L4 to S2. Lesions above C5 lead to complete quadriplegia, whereas a lesion above L2 will produce paraplegia (Fig. 24.1).

SENSORY LOSS

Skeletal muscle paralysis is accompanied by loss of sensation from the areas of the body innervated by the relevant sensory nerves. While appreciation of sensory information at the cortical level is lost,

local spinal cord reflexes usually remain intact. These reflexes, however, are released from inhibitory signals derived from the now isolated upper CNS levels. This leads to hypersensitivity of α motor neurons which directly drive muscle contraction, leading to uncontrolled and often prolonged or repetitive muscle contractions.

LOSS OF AUTONOMIC CONTROL

The autonomic nervous system may also be disrupted following spinal cord injury. Parasympathetic outflow is divided into two sections. The cranial outflow, arising in the mid-brain and medulla, regulates cardiac and gastrointestinal activity, while the sacral parasympathetic outflow, arising between levels L5 and S5, regulates function of the rectum and bladder. Disruption to the sacral portion of the parasympathetic outflow leads to loss of control of bladder and bowel sphincter function.

A disturbance of the sympathetic outflow is especially relevant to the wheelchair athlete, as an intact sympathetic nervous system is vital to high-level exercise performance. A number of important cardiovascular adjustments to exercise, including increases in heart rate, blood pressure and myocardial contractility, as well as vasoconstriction in inactive tissues, are under sympathetic control, where outflow arises between spinal cord levels T1 and L2 (Glaser 1985).

Special Medical Consequences of Inactivity in the Wheelchair Athlete

Early studies of para- and quadriplegics revealed a 1 year mortality approaching 80% (Shephard 1988). The most common cause of death was renal failure or septicaemia following an ascending infection (Bean 1988). Recent improvements in survival rates are related to the development of spinal injury units, increased research emphasis on the spinal injured, the development of antibiotics and increased emphasis on rehabilitation. Reduction in early mortality has resulted in a life expectancy for the spinal cord injured approaching or equal to that among the general population. Difference in prognosis is related to sepsis in the urinary or respiratory tracts, other renal disease, gastrointestinal compli-

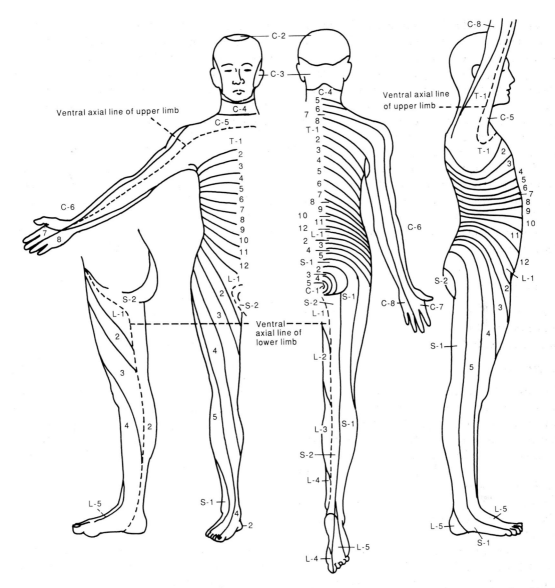

Fig. 24.1 The cutaneous distribution of spinal nerves and dermatomes.

cations and, most importantly, cardiovascular disease. Cardiovascular mortality in the spinal injured appears to be somewhat greater than that in the general population aged 20–44 and this appears to be directly related to low levels of physical activity. Obesity is common among the spinal injured and is related to a decrease in basal metabolic rate, a decrease in activity and in lean body mass and an associated increase in body fat. Low levels of high density lipoprotein cholesterol have also been found in the spinal cord injured.

Hypertension is the most common type of cardiovascular disease in the paraplegic and the reason for its increased incidence is unclear (Shephard 1988). Poor nutritional practices and cigarette smoking may also contribute to the high incidence of coronary heart disease in the spinal injured.

Low levels of activity have been found to be

correlated with the development of osteoporosis in the able-bodied, so the spinal cord injured patient is also at high risk for osteoporosis. Loss of bone mineral in this group involves the whole skeleton in the early months following injury and later becomes maximal in the areas of bone below the level of the injury. Osteoporosis leads to three major problems in the spinal cord injured. The first of these is a high risk of spontaneous or stress fractures related to muscular spasms, stretching during rehabilitation programmes and transfers from bed to wheelchair, etc. A second problem is heterotrophic ossification, an unusual form of extra-articular new bone formation of uncertain aetiology. The para-articular ossification occurs commonly around the hip and elbow joints. Ossification may be severe, leading to pseudo-ankylosis of the affected joints. The large degree of bone mineral loss leads to an increased serum calcium concentration, which increases the risk of the third consequence of osteoporosis, the formation of renal calculi. High serum calcium leads to high levels of calcium in the urine and the development of renal and bladder calculi. Apart from causing pain and potential obstruction, renal calculi also predispose the bladder to infections, which are already a significant problem in patients who have lost parasympathetic control of the urinary system.

In summary, the low levels of physical activity in the paraplegic predispose them to:

- An increased risk of cardiovascular disease by unfavourable modification of risk factors
- The development of diabetes and other medical problems associated with obesity and
- The development of osteoporosis and renal calculi

Wheelchair Exercise Physiology: Physiological Characteristics of the Paraplegic

CARDIAC FUNCTION

As previously noted, spinal cord lesions above the level of T1 lead to a lack of sympathetic cardiac innervation and the maximum heart rate is decreased. It is generally found to be between 110 and 130 beats·min^{-1}, the level being determined by the intrinsic sinoatrial rhythm (Hoffman 1986). There is a decrease in stroke volume, a 25% decrease in resting cardiac output and a 32% decrease in maximum cardiac output. Maximum cardiac output is found to be approximately 70% of that of the able-bodied and is related to a loss of chronotropic reserve and a decrease in stroke volume. These determinants of cardiac output are restricted by a loss of catecholamine response to exercise and a lack of exercise related increase in venous return. There is no increase in leg vascular tone in response to exercise with lesions above T7 and an irregular response occurring for lesions between T7 and T10 (Hoffman 1986). This leads to venous pooling and a consequent lack of increase in cardiac preload with exercise. With high-level cord lesions, augmentation of venous return may be lost due to ineffectiveness of the thoracic pump mechanism.

Loss of sympathetic regulation in exercising muscle may lead to inappropriate muscle blood flow. Loss of exercise-induced vasoconstriction in inactive tissues such as the splanchnic bed may also disturb appropriate distribution of cardiac output.

Consequent upon these effects, the maximum oxygen uptake ($\dot{V}_{O_2max}$) of the quadriplegic or paraplegic is often lower than that of the similarly trained or untrained able-bodied person. Sedentary subjects with thoracic or lumbar spinal cord lesions typically exhibit a $\dot{V}_{O_2max}$ between 20 and 30 mL·kg^{-1}·min^{-1}. The lower the spinal cord injury, the higher the $\dot{V}_{O_2max}$, most difference being noted between category 1 (complete or incomplete quadriplegia) and category 2–5 injuries (cord lesions below T1). Spinal cord injured females typically have a $\dot{V}_{O_2max}$ 25–35% lower than males, compared with a 15–20% difference in the able-bodied.

A diminution of $\dot{V}_{O_2max}$ of 3 mL·kg^{-1}·min^{-1} per decade is found in paraplegics, compared with a decrement of 4 mL·kg^{-1}·min^{-1} per decade in the able-bodied (Hoffman 1986).

Respiratory function in the spinally injured is limited depending upon the level of lesion. A lesion at the C3–C4 level paralyses the phrenic nerve and therefore the diaphragm and such a lesion at C3 or above is incompatible with unsupported life. The intercostal muscles are innervated from levels T1 to T11 and the abdominal muscles from levels T7 to L4. A decrease in vital capacity is noted with the ascending level of the lesion. Reduced capacity for ventilation appears not to limit exercise capacity in quadriplegics but it may be a limiting factor in highly trained paraplegics. The effect of a spinal cord injury on body composition is controversial, some studies noting normal levels of body fat and body mass, other studies suggesting decreases in lean body mass accompanied by increases in body fat and extracellular fluid volume (Shephard 1988).

The Effects of Training

Training is important for the spinal cord injured patient. It may prevent the medical consequences of inactivity, aid in psychological rehabilitation, allow greater levels of mobility with lower cardiovascular stress and lead to more effective rehabilitation.

The spinal cord injured patient depends on arm exercise for his or her mobility and arm exercise has been shown to be more stressful to the cardiovascular system than leg exercise (Glaser 1985). This is most likely due to the small muscle mass of the arm as training of the upper limb muscles leads to the utilization of a smaller percentage of maximum effort for any particular activity. It should be noted that such training will attenuate this increased cardiovascular stress. At an equivalent maximal power output a greater metabolic demand in arm exercise is shown via higher lactate levels and $\% \dot{V}_{O2max}$ requirement. At equivalent submaximal levels, increased stress in arm activity is denoted by a higher heart rate, total peripheral resistance, systemic blood pressure, stroke work and ventilation. Arm exercise is associated with a lower stroke volume and lower cardiac output when compared with leg work (Glaser 1985). This is related to an increased afterload and a decreased end-diastolic volume consequent upon low or inadequate venous return. Arm exercise through its production of a higher rate-pressure product at a given workload is more likely to induce symptoms of ischaemic heart disease and therefore limit mobility and rehabilitation in this population, which is already predisposed to such problems.

Controversy exists as to the site of production of the training effects. It is generally agreed that a central training effect will not occur in quadriplegics and there is conflicting evidence for a central training effect following arm training in paraplegics. Peripheral intramuscular adaptations appear to be the most important effects to be found in the spinal cord injured following training. An increase in mechanical efficiency is most often noted in the early phases of wheelchair use and after changes in characteristics of wheelchair design or operation.

The following changes in physiological parameters have been noted after various training regimens:

- Peak $\dot{V}_{O2max}$ increases of between 0 and 60%. The average increase is approximately 20% following 4–20 weeks of training (Hoffman 1986). This is consistent with the training response of the able-bodied
- Average increases of 30% in maximum power output; increases of 30–40% in physical work capacity
- At submaximal levels of activity there are decreases in heart rate % $\dot{V}_{O2max}$ requirement, serum lactate, ventilation and respiratory quotient (RQ)
- Maximal exercise data following training have also reported increases in ventilatory volumes and serum lactate levels
- An increase in cardiac output has been found and probably relates to an increase in stroke volume, which is related to a decrease in afterload, consequent upon a lower blood pressure rise during submaximal exercise. The dependence on increases in cardiac output for increases in $\dot{V}_{O2max}$ is illustrated by the fact that in some studies no change in $(a-v)O_2$ difference has been found following training in paraplegics. Training leads to a reduction in ventilatory fatigue due to increases in the strength and endurance of the respiratory muscles. The abovementioned training effects have been demonstrated by programmes of intermittent and continuous activity and have also been noted following both wheelchair and arm ergometry training
- Decreases in body fat and increases in high density lipoprotein cholesterol have been found following various training regimens

Despite the fact that muscle strength and endurance are important in wheelchair locomotion, particularly in overcoming difficulties of terrain, hills and transfers, few studies in the area of muscle strength have been published. The following is a summary of the research which is currently available:

- Grip strength in the wheelchair user appears to be only slightly greater than that of the able-bodied person (Gass & Camp 1979). This may reflect the fact that fast wheelchair operation does not require gripping
- General hypertrophy of the upper arm muscles has been noted in wheelchair athletes
- On isokinetic testing, 10–57% increases in peak moment, peak power and average power in the arms have been found following training (Davis et al. 1986)
- 20–100% increases in shoulder abduction torque have been found (Shephard 1988)
- Increased elbow isokinetic strength has been demonstrated in wheelchair swimmers (Shephard 1988)
- Similar to findings in the able-bodied, short-term (8 weeks) forearm cranking training produces increases in strength but little change in muscle dimensions, highlighting the importance of neural mechanisms in early strength gains
- Aerobic and anaerobic enzyme levels per unit of muscle mass have been shown to be low, normal or above normal in various groups of well-trained wheelchair athletes
- Arm ergometer training of unspecified duration has been shown to lead to an 80% increase in muscular endurance (Davis et al. 1981)

In an effort to produce a more effective form of cardiovascular training for spinal cord injured individuals, electrically induced contractions of the paralysed leg muscles have been used (Figoni 1992). The advantages of this technique include the recruitment of a large muscle mass, return of function of the leg muscle pump and a consequent increased possibility of an aerobic training effect. Improved exercise performance was found following electrical stimulation using leg cycle ergometry, with varying effects on peak heart rate, stroke volume, cardiac output and total peripheral resistance being reported (Regnarsson 1988). To date, no training studies involving combined arm and leg (hybrid) exercise have been published.

Efficiency

The efficiency of wheelchair locomotion has been estimated to be approximately 5%. This is compared with 7–10% for wheelchair ergometry, the higher figure occurring at higher power outputs, 20% for walking and up to 18% for forearm cranking (Glaser 1985). Inefficiency in wheelchair propulsion has been related to several factors including arm position, synchronization of arm movements, increase in static work related to stabilization of the trunk and an increased concentration of fast twitch muscle fibres in upper body muscles.

Gains in the efficiency of wheelchair propulsion may be possible through the following:

- A learning effect
- Smaller diameter hand rims which have been shown to produce lower cardiovascular stress
- Gearing systems for wheelchairs
- Arm crank propulsion which at a given power output produces a lower $\dot{V}_{O_2max}$, ventilation, heart rate, cardiac output and blood pressure when compared with hand rim propulsion

Characteristics of the Elite Wheelchair Athlete

Elite wheelchair athletes are able to develop higher cardiac outputs than their untrained counterparts. As previously mentioned this is mainly dependent on an increase in stroke volume. Increases in arteriovenous differences and therefore increased oxygen extraction are controversial areas at the present time. In the paraplegic, $\dot{V}_{O_2max}$ levels greater than 40 mL·min⁻¹·kg⁻¹ are commonly found (Hoffman 1986), the highest so far reported being 49 mL·min⁻¹·kg⁻¹ in a T12 paraplegic wheelchair racer (Gass & Camp 1979). Among paraplegics, track athletes commonly demonstrate a $\dot{V}_{O_2max}$ in the range of 35–40, swimming athletes in the range of 30–40, and athletes in skilled sports average about 25 mL·kg^{-1}·min^{-1} (Cameron 1977). $\dot{V}_{O2max}$ in a quadriplegic wheelchair athlete at the Olympic level was 15.9 mL·min^{-1}·kg^{-1}. Cross-sectional studies comparing wheelchair athletes with their inactive counterparts have shown a 57% greater maximum power output, 44% greater peak $\dot{V}_{O2max}$ and 53% greater minute volume (Shephard 1988).

In common with able-bodied runners, wheelchair athletes tested on a treadmill over a 5 km distance showed that performance correlated with $\dot{V}_{O2max}$, a percentage of sustainable $\dot{V}_{O2max}$ and onset of blood lactate accumulation equal to 4 mmol·L^{-1}. In wheelchair marathoners operating at race pace compared with able-bodied runners, the RQ is higher, indicating increased anaerobic activity. The wheelchair marathoner uses a higher percentage of available $\dot{V}_{O2max}$ and a higher percentage of heart rate maximum than his able-bodied counterpart. The elite wheelchair athlete demonstrates a larger vital capacity and maximum ventilation compared with his sedentary counterpart. Wheelchair athletes also tend to have lower percentages of body fat.

Training Principles for the Wheelchair Athlete

GUIDE-LINES FOR TRAINING

Standard guide-lines for exercise training involve recommendations for frequency, intensity, duration and mode of exercise. Similar guide-lines to those used for the able-bodied can be applied to the spinal cord injured. For the latter, the American College of Sports Medicine guide-lines need to be modified only in that the appropriate heart rate is lower, at 50–70% heart rate maximum.

Because the arm muscles are smaller than the leg muscles which are typically used by the able-bodied in endurance activities, there is a narrower margin between an effective training stimulus and over-training in the spinal cord injured. Studies of heart rate response indicate that swimming and long-

Fig. 24.2 A wheelchair athlete undergoing a $\dot{V}_{O2max}$ test. (Courtesy of West Australian Disabled Sports Association Inc.)

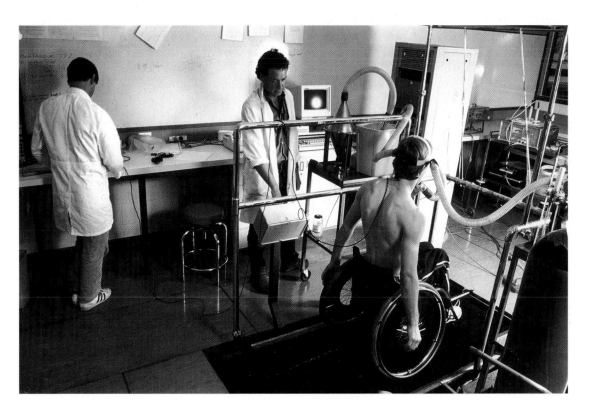

distance wheelchair racing training are modes of exercise likely to satisfy the above guide-lines. Wheelchair soccer, basketball and arm ergometer training have also been shown to induce a training effect. Functional electrical stimulation, that is electrical stimulation to intact motor neurons or motor points on muscle to produce contraction, has been shown to increase muscle strength and endurance by local muscle adaptations and to increase local bone density (Rugnarsson 1988). This adjunctive form of therapy is used acutely following spinal cord injury to minimize initial muscle wasting. It is also useful in increasing exercise capacity of partially paralysed muscle groups. Use of such stimulation of leg muscles in association with modified bicycle ergometers has been shown to induce significant cardiovascular stress, which is sufficient to induce central cardiovascular training responses in quadriplegics and paraplegics. The combination of voluntary arm ergometer and induced cycling leads to higher peak, and higher ventilation, heart rate and cardiac output and lower total peripheral resistance than during either exercise modality used alone (Glaser 1989). Functional electrical stimulation can also produce a positive calcium balance useful in the prevention of osteoporosis.

EXERCISE TESTING

Exercise testing to measure the physiological effects of training has been conducted using various systems including:

- Arm crank ergometers
- Wheelchair ergometers, which have the advantage of task specificity
- Free wheeling, for example, the 12 min distance covered test
- Wheelchair operation on a treadmill (Fig. 24.2)
- Wheelchair operation on rollers

The arm crank ergometer, while being less task specific than the wheelchair ergometer, has greater mechanical efficiency; some studies suggest up to 18%. At a particular submaximal exercise level, heart rate, cardiac output, blood pressure, minute ventilation, serum lactate, $\dot{V}_{O2max}$ and respiratory exchange ratio are lower. The rate-pressure product, otherwise known as the double product, is also lower. Higher peak heart rate, peak blood lactate and peak power outputs occur with the arm crank ergometer (Shephard 1988). Overall, arm cranking induces a lower metabolic and circulatory stress.

Factors favouring performance on the arm ergometer include the following

- The use of neural pathways adapted to asynchronous movement
- Less requirement for isometric muscle activity used for trunk stabilization
- Improved gearing ratios
- Different mode of torque transmission, for example, handle versus rim pressure
- The ability to push and pull

Arm ergometry testing is generally limited by local fatigue and pain rather than central cardiovascular factors. Because of the small muscle mass used, the maximum aerobic power of arm work is generally 60–80% that of leg work. This difference decreases as the specificity of the activity increases.

For upper extremity work there is a fairly consistent relationship between power output and $\dot{V}_{O2max}$. A good correlation exists between power output and $\dot{V}_{O2max}$ in paraplegics using both wheelchair and arm ergometers. In quadriplegics there is no significant correlation between power output and $\dot{V}_{O2max}$ (Hoffman 1986). Various regression equations relating $\dot{V}_{O2max}$ and submaximal arm ergometry are currently being investigated.

In stress testing for diagnosis of ischaemic heart disease, the procedure should follow standard guide-lines for the able-bodied and should include history, physical examination and resting electrocardiogram. The stress test itself must be conducted with the following in mind. The disabled population may be at a higher risk of coronary artery disease, therefore they may exhibit abnormal circulatory responses. Autonomic dysfunction, as related to sympathetic outflow deficiency, may be present. Blood pressure responses, in particular, may be unusual. High-level spinal injured patients may, through a fall in total peripheral resistance, exhibit a fall in blood pressure with increasing intensity of exercise. The classical pain of angina may be absent in quadriplegics as the cardiac afferents enter the spinal cord at upper thoracic levels.

In summary, spinal cord injured patients are at a higher risk of contracting medical problems which relate closely to their sedentary life-style than are their able-bodied counterparts. Maintenance of fitness and the consequent metabolic and physiological changes are extremely important in this group.

Wheelchair Sports Injuries: Prevention and Management

The field of sports medicine witnessed an explosion in popularity among physicians during the exercise boom of the early 1970s. Since that time, many of the able-bodied sports have had their medical problems investigated in great detail. This has not been the case for sports-related problems of the wheelchair athlete and the total amount of information available in the medical literature on injuries sustained by these athletes is remarkably small. The most quoted study (Curtis 1982), surveyed over 1200 athletes in regional wheelchair competitions during the 1981 athletic season and her research indicated that the average wheelchair athlete of

both sexes participates in sports approximately 4 days per week. There was a wide variation in the number of hours spent training per week, with mean values about 6–10 h. A large proportion of the athletes (69%) reported using protective equipment in an effort to minimize the risk of sport-related injury, while 72% of the subjects had contracted at least one sport-related injury. The incidence of the 10 most common wheelchair sports injuries is shown in Table 24.1.

Table 24.1 The 10 most common wheelchair sports injuries

Injury	Percentage of all injuries reported
Soft tissue injuries (includes sprains, strains, muscle pulls, tendinitis, bursitis)	33%
Blisters	18%
Lacerations/abrasions/cuts (includes skin infections)	17%
Decubitus/pressure areas	7%
Arthritis/joint disorders	5%
Fractures	5%
Hand weakness/numbness	5%
Temperature regulation disorders (hypo- or hyperthermia)	3%
Head injury/concussion	2%
Dental injury	1%

Curtis (1982).

Fig. 24.3 The injury risk of high participation sports for the disabled (Curtis 1982).

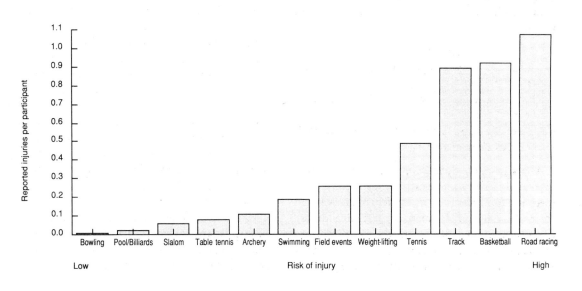

Table 24.2 Wheelchair sports associated with the greatest number of injuries

Sport	No. of injuries reported	Percentage of all injuries reported
Track	93	26%
Basketball	84	24%
Road racing	77	22%
Tennis	20	6%
Field events	15	4%
Swimming	13	4%

Curtis (1982).

In the above study the sports leading to the highest number of injuries were track and field, basketball and road racing, while tennis, field events, weight-lifting and sledding produced considerably fewer injuries (Table 24.2).

An analysis of injury risk of a number of wheelchair sports is summarized in Fig. 24.3.

The risk of sport-related injury increases with the number of sports involved and with an increase in the number of hours spent in training. Medical problems encountered during training in a rehabilitation unit environment have been outlined by Nilsen et al. (1985), as they performed a retrospective study of patients with complete spinal cord injury at spinal level C7 or below. The patients participated in a training programme for an average duration of 25 days, the activities including weight-lifting, pulking (snow skiing in a sitting position) swimming, volleyball and callisthenics. A total of 11 955 training hours were studied and during this period 30 patients developed complications, 53% being strains and sprains, 17% pressure sores and 27% urinary tract infections. Training was intense and involved 3.5 h per day, 6 days per week. The sprains and strains were felt to be associated with the initiation of training and too rapid an increase in activity level. Of the 16 patients in the strain and sprain category, 12 had pain related to the shoulder, four being specifically diagnosed as being either supraspinatus or bicipital tendinitis and the other eight having non-specific shoulder pain. Three patients reported elbow and arm pain; one described as epicondylitis, one tendinitis (site not specified) and one non-specific muscular pain. The overall incidence of complications during training was 2.51 per 1000 training hours, which is a low risk compared with any able-bodied sportsperson. The low rate of injury was attributed to the presence of highly skilled instructors, close medical supervision, attention to the technical details of the skills used, submaximal levels of training and variation in training routines.

THE SHOULDER

Despite the importance of shoulder function in wheelchair locomotion, very few papers have been published which are specifically related to the shoulder problems of the wheelchair athlete.

A study by Nicholls et al. (1979) looking at a non-athletic population, found that 51% of their group reported having suffered from pain in or around the shoulder. The frequency of the pain and its duration increased with time since the onset of disability and the tendency for pain to become bilateral was noted. Unfortunately, this study failed to address the specific pathology involved in the production of shoulder pain.

Shoulder injuries common in the wheelchair athlete include tendinitis of the long head of the biceps, inflammation of the rotator cuff tendons, subdeltoid bursitis and capsular tears and muscle strains from the throwing sports. Fractures of the clavicle and acromioclavicular joint separations are related mainly to falls from the wheelchair but only occur occasionally. There is, however, a high risk of deltoid muscle strain if the wheel rims of the chair are not positioned close to the body.

In view of the dependence of the wheelchair athlete on normal shoulder function for locomotion, it is difficult for the sports medicine physician to include rest as a treatment modality for shoulder problems and prevention strategies need to be devised. These include strengthening of the shoulder stabilizers, adequate training in correct technique, gradual progression of training loads, adequate warm-up, cool-down and stretching procedures, equipment modification and early reporting and treatment of shoulder pain. Specific treatment procedures include relative rest, ice and anti-inflammatory medication. Physiotherapy modalities and rehabilitation for shoulder problems in the wheel-chair athlete are similar to those of the able-bodied and are described in detail in Chapter 13.

THE UPPER BACK

The most commonly reported upper back problem is muscular pain and spasm. This is related to overuse during maintenance of trunk stability or the presence of poor posture. Postural correction, gradually increased training load and specific strengthening exercises for the upper dorsal area are recommended.

Blistering of the skin is not uncommon at the top of the seat post on the back of the wheelchair and prevention is achieved by the athlete wearing a shirt, while at the same time padding the back of the chair where necessary.

THE ELBOW AND FOREARM

Problems in this region sporadically described in the literature include lateral and medial epicondylitis, tendinitis of the flexors and extensors of the wrist and tendinitis at the insertion of the triceps and of the biceps brachii.

Most of the disorders involving this area have been found in weight-lifters performing the bench press. Because disabled athletes start this lift from the 'down position' in contrast to the starting 'up position' in the able-bodied competitor, it is thought that in starting from zero acceleration more stress is placed on the lifting muscles.

The inner aspects of the upper arms are common sites for abrasions and bruises and often contact tyres of racing wheelchairs, particularly on the down stroke. The wearing of clothing on the upper arms or the use of tube socks in that area, combined with changing the camber (i.e. the angle of the wheels) decreases the risk of these injuries.

THE WRIST

The common problems encountered at the wrist in the wheelchair athlete are lacerations, abrasions and carpal tunnel syndrome.

Carpal tunnel syndrome involves an entrapment neuropathy of the median nerve in the carpal tunnel at the wrist joint (see Chapter 19). This most commonly follows overuse of the wrist, particularly with repeated flexion and gripping movements of the hand. This syndrome in paraplegics has been specifically studied by Aljure *et al.* (1986) who found that 40% of subjects had clinical signs and symptoms. Further, electrophysiological evidence of carpal tunnel syndrome was noted in 63% of athletes. Coincidentally, ulnar neuropathy at the elbow joint occurred in 40% of the cases and the incidence of these complications appeared to be related to the duration of the spinal cord injury and an incidence of 90% was noted at 30 years after injury. Increased use of the hands and direct pressure over the carpal tunnel from use of the heel of the hand in wheelchair propulsion were postulated as aetiological factors. In view of the high incidence of subclinical evidence of carpal tunnel syndrome, it was recommended that median and ulnar nerve function be tested during the first 5 years following injury and re-evaluated periodically after that time. Preventive measures include the use of padded push rims on the wheel chair, the use of gloves and padding over the wrist and heel of the hand and early intervention at the onset of symptoms. Management is essentially similar to that of the able-bodied and includes rest, use of ice, non-steroidal anti-inflammatory drugs, resting splints, cortico-steroid injections and possibly surgery.

THE HANDS AND FINGERS

Skin abrasions and lacerations, particularly of the knuckles, avulsion of the nails and finger injuries related to the catching of fingers in the spokes of the wheelchair are common. Preventive measures include the use of gloves, taping, padded push rims, plastic wheel covers, the removal of brakes and filing or covering of sharp edges on the wheelchair (Magnus 1987).

THE BUTTOCKS

The occurrence of pressure areas and decubitus ulcers is the major problem in this region. Poor circulation, pressure from prolonged sitting and shear forces transmitted from upper body movements lead to abrasions and ulcerations. The use of track wheelchairs with knees held higher than the buttocks may also contribute to this problem. These wheelchairs are used primarily to increase

Table 24.3 The anatomical requirements necessary for the competitive wheelchair stroke

Joint	Action	Muscles
Drive phase		
Shoulder	Abduction	Medial deltoid
	Flexion	Anterior deltoid
	Depression	Trapezius
Elbow	Extension	Triceps brachii
Wrist	Flexion — ulnar deviation	Wrist flexors
Recovery phase		
Shoulder	Abduction	Medial deltoid
	Extension	Posterior deltoid
	Elevation	Trapezius
Elbow	Flexion	Biceps brachii
Wrist	Extension — radial deviation	Wrist extensors

Davis *et al.* (1988).

Table 24.4 Strength training exercises for the wheelchair athlete

Joint	Exercise	Muscle
Shoulder	Bench press	Pectoralis major
	Seated	Deltoid
	Military press	Pectoralis major
		Triceps brachii
	Dips	Deltoid
		Triceps brachii
	Chin-ups	Latissimus dorsi
		Biceps brachii
	Flys	Deltoid
		Pectoralis major
	Lateral pulldown	Latissimus dorsi
		Posterior deltoid
		Biceps brachii
	Upright rowing	Deltoid
		Trapezius
		Biceps brachii
Elbow	Olympic curls	Biceps brachii
	Elbow extension	Triceps brachii
Wrist	Wrist curls (4 directions)	Wrist flexors and extensors

Davis *et al.* (1988).

efficiency during racing and to decrease the risk of injury to the feet.

In summary, the majority of injuries to wheelchair athletes involve overuse, sudden strain or tearing and problems with equipment. As in the able-bodied, the principles of training are important for prevention and these include adequate warm-up and cool-down, stretching, progressive increase in training load, specific strengthening for involved muscle groups, attention to technique, equipment safety and its modification.

With these factors in mind, Table 24.3 is a summary of the joints, joint actions and muscle groups involved during the drive and recovery phases of the competitive wheelchair stroke (Davis *et al.* 1988).

For optimum performance and injury prevention the wheelchair athlete should specifically train those muscles mentioned in Table 24.3. Flexibility, strength, power and endurance capabilities should receive equal attention and Table 24.4 details specific exercises for the development of the muscles involved. The use of free weights and exercise machines, for example Nautilus, Universal, Polaris, Keiser, etc., is very appropriate for the wheelchair athlete.

Recommended weight-training regimens for the short or middle distance wheelchair racer include the principles of high intensity and overload. The athlete should work at approximately 75% of his or her maximum, with three to four sets of four to six repetitions. The endurance wheelchair athlete should emphasize high-repetition programmes and an intensity of 50–60% of maximum with 10–12 repetitions in three to four sets would be appropriate (Davis *et al.* 1988).

Wheelchair Design

Modification of wheelchair design is important for both performance and safety. One of the earliest and most obvious changes in wheelchair design was to decrease the weight of the chair. Standard old style chairs weighed approximately 20 kg, with newer models weighing closer to 10 kg and racing models as low as 6–7 kg (Fig. 24.4). Custom-made, individualized wheelchairs, while being more ex-

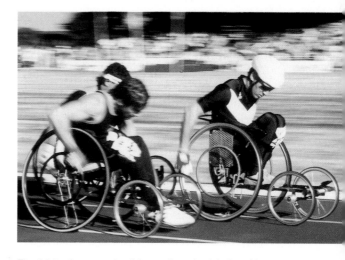

Fig. 24.4 An example of two racing wheelchairs with one athlete using the 'knees-up' position.

pensive, are seen now as more appropriate than standard models. Some chairs permit relief of pressure on the ischial tuberosities by increasing the load carried on the posterior aspects of the thigh.

Straps can be incorporated into the wheelchair to increase stability and to prevent the feet from falling off the front of the chair and becoming injured. Improved cushioning devices are continually being developed and plastic wheel guard covers are used to prevent an athlete's fingers from catching in the spokes of the wheel.

'Wheeley' bars, that is small wheeled stops attached to the rear of the wheel chair frame, can prevent tipping over in various sports, particularly basketball (Bloomquist 1986). Padded push rims are used to decrease the risk of carpal tunnel syndrome and cambered wheels prevent abrasions to the inner aspects of the upper arms and allow for greater lateral stability of the chair. Changeable drive ratios similar to gears on an ordinary bicycle are available for the competitive wheelchair. Variations in the size of the push rims allow for greater chair acceleration. The compensator, a control apparatus between the two front wheels that improves balance on inclines and curves and allows the racer to sit further forward in the chair, leading to improved acceleration and faster starts. Design changes which allow a combination of asynchronous force application and higher drive ratios may lead to a reduction in metabolic and cardiopulmonary stresses produced by wheelchair operation.

Specific Problems of the Wheelchair Athlete

HEAT AND COLD STRESS

Hypothermia

The wheelchair athlete is at a greater risk of developing excessively low body temperatures than the able-bodied athlete, especially at the end of an event when heat production decreases dramatically. The able-bodied response may include shivering but following spinal cord injury, shivering will not occur below the level of the lesion. Despite this the skin continues to be covered with sweat, is vasodilated and heat loss may continue for a considerable period. Wet clothing may contribute to further evaporation and an increased cooling effect. Because of the inability to shiver, the use of standard aluminium foil blankets for rewarming is inappropriate. Wet clothing should be removed immediately and replaced by multiple layers of dry clothing. The limbs can then be wrapped in plastic if the temperature warrants such an action or a warm shower immediately after an event may also be appropriate. In warming body parts below the level of the spinal cord lesion, care must be taken to avoid burning the athlete. In alpine sports, such as snow skiing, the paralysed parts of the body need to be heavily insulated in thermal pants and frequent examinations should be carried out to detect early signs of injury due to the cold environment.

Hyperthermia

The risk of heat stress injury such as cramps, heat exhaustion and heat stroke is greater in the disabled athlete than in the able-bodied, the risk being highest for the long-distance wheelchair racer. With a pushing efficiency of only 7–8% it has been estimated that the wheelchair athlete incurs the same net energy cost and the same heat production levels as the able-bodied runner. With efficient heat loss mechanisms, body core temperature rises $0.5°C$ for every 100 W of power output, 1000 W power output leading to a body temperature of approximately 41°C. The less efficient heat dissipation mechanism of the wheelchair athlete increases both the extent and rate of overheating.

Dehydration also exacerbates the problem, leading to decreased sweating related to lower cardiac output and consequent lower skin blood flow.

The disadvantages of the paraplegic are twofold. Because sweating may be deficient below the level of the spinal cord injury (due to loss of cholinergic sympathetic nervous system output), the athlete has to rely on an evaporative heat loss from the arms and trunk alone. Second, vasomotor paralysis and loss of the lower limb muscle pump lead to venous pooling in the lower limbs and a state of relative hypovolaemia and in this situation dehydration poses a greater threat to the wheelchair athlete. The usual preventive measures against hyperthermia are also relevant, including maintenance of correct hydration, acclimatization, training, clothing considerations, awareness of environmental conditions and avoidance of factors predisposing to heat injury.

These include obesity, alcohol consumption and the use of various drugs, extremes of age, chronic physical illness and intercurrent febrile conditions.

Gass et al. (1988) recently identified a potential problem in the assessment of hyperthermia in the spinal injured as they concluded that rectal temperature measurement may underestimate core temperature. Underestimation was greater in the highly endurance trained and in those with lesions at lower spinal levels.

PROBLEMS RELATED TO EXCESSIVE PRESSURE

The wheelchair athlete will encounter three specific skin problems which relate to excessive pressure and shear forces. These are blisters, calluses and pressure ulcers, which are dealt with below (see Fig. 24.5):

- Blisters. A blister is a fluid-filled sac situated between the epidermal and dermal layers of the skin. Mechanical friction and shear stress leads to the disruption of the epidermal–dermal junction and local cellular damage results in

Fig. 24.5 In games such as wheelchair basketball, various problems can occur which relate to excessive pressure and shear forces on the body. (Courtesy of West Australian Disabled Sports Association Inc.)

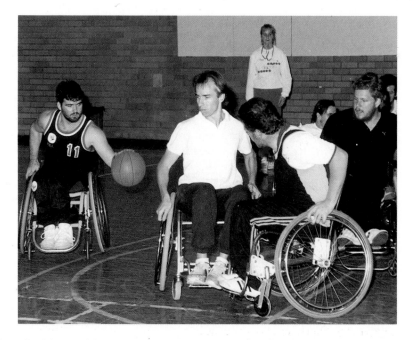

fluid accumulation. In the wheelchair athlete blisters most commonly occur on the hands and fingers. Prevention includes the use of various padding materials, modification to wheelchair prominences, taping of fingers and the wearing of gloves. Control of local moisture by the use of absorbent materials or frequent glove or clothing changes and gradual increases in training are also important. In areas known to be susceptible to blistering, skin hardening may be achieved by the application of tincture of benzoin daily for 7–10 days. Early recognition of 'hot spots' and areas of erythema followed by early intervention will prevent the formation of a full-blown blister. For the management of blisters the reader is referred to Chapter 13.

- Callus. A callus is a localized area of thickened skin resulting from chronic pressure, friction and shear applied to the skin, especially over a bony prominence. Calluses are particularly common over the hypothenar eminence of the hand and over the volar aspects of the fingers of the wheelchair athlete. Calluses are sometimes uncomfortable but the major problem associated with them is the formation of a deep blister under the callus. Treatment involves pressure

relief, which may require a change of technique or the use of local padding. Application of a softening cream containing urea or salicylic acid may be beneficial. Light abrasion with a pumice stone or sand paper if used early may prevent the accumulation of thickened skin. Treatment may also involve paring of the callus after soaking in a warm antiseptic solution.

- Decubitus ulcers. Decubitus ulcers or pressure sores were once a major problem for the bed or wheelchair ridden patient. The ulcers most commonly occur in the ischial region and are the result of the patient sitting for too long in one position without relieving the weight on the buttocks. Occasionally, a sitting pressure sore can also develop over the tip of a prominent coccyx. The sports physician requires a knowledge of the early signs of excessive pressure and may be called upon to treat the consequences of neglected pressure areas. Excessive pressure leads to obstruction of capillary flow, local ischaemia, accumulation of metabolic products, small vessel thrombosis and local cell necrosis.

The first sign of excessive pressure is an ill-defined area of reactive hyperaemia most commonly occurring over a bony prominence, usually the ischial tuberosities, but also over the heels or toes of the sitting wheelchair athlete. Should a Grade 1 lesion go unnoticed, a break or blister occurs in the epidermis accompanied by local erythema and induration. This Grade 2 lesion is potentially reversible.

Grade 3 lesions are characterized by surface ulceration. However, this surface ulceration generally represents only the 'tip of the iceberg' and is underlined by deeper ischaemia and cell necrosis. Deep ulceration can occur through the whole thickness of the skin down to the fascial or bone level. In sports participation friction and shear are commonly added to normal pressure and lead to these lesions.

Several factors, some of which are potentially correctable or reversible, lead to an increased risk of pressure ulceration. These conditions affect cellular metabolism and include anaemia, occlusive vascular disease, diabetes, local oedema, negative nitrogen balance consequent upon poor nutrition, increasing age, immobilization, excessive moisture, heat, lack of sensation and local skin lesions including bruises, pimples and boils.

Prevention of decubitus ulcers, which often need prolonged periods of hospitalization for cure, involves modification of the abovementioned factors. Correct skin care is important, with repeated observation, cleansing and local hygiene measures. Changes in position and pressure relief can be simply performed by lifting the subject off the wheelchair seat as frequently as possible even for as little as 10–20 s every 10–20 min. Transfer techniques for the wheelchair-bound should include direct lifting rather than dragging, to avoid abrasion of compromised skin areas. Early attention to this problem is vital, as the management of established pressure areas may involve specialist consultation, hospital admission and perhaps even skin grafting procedures.

URINARY PROBLEMS

Just as the sports physician performs many general medical services for able-bodied athletes, he or she may be called upon to perform similar duties for the disabled. A knowledge of the physiology of the urinary tract in the spinal cord injured is important, as a significant number of the medical problems of this group relate to this area.

Normal bladder reflexes are controlled by the reflex voiding centre located at the sacral 2, 3 and 4 levels of the spinal cord. These areas of the spinal cord lie opposite the first lumbar vertebra. In a spinal cord injury above the reflex voiding centre, or above L1 if a fracture is the cause of the spinal cord lesion, the bladder spinal reflexes are intact leading to a reflex or upper motor neuron bladder disturbance. Patients with this level of lesion are able to establish automatic or reflex micturition. The bladder may empty automatically or a reflex contraction may be produced by tapping over the bladder. Following this, gentle pressure in the suprapubic area leads to the attainment of a low residual volume. A low residual volume accompanied by a high fluid intake, with a large urinary output, decreases the risk of urinary tract infection. Some type of incontinence appliance is required in this situation.

If reflex micturition cannot be established, intermittent self-catheterization four times a day and a restriction of fluid intake to avoid bladder overfilling is appropriate. If the patient cannot self-catheterize, an indwelling catheter may be required.

With a fracture at or below L1, or with damage to the reflex voiding centre, the bladder reflexes are lost and the external sphincter is flaccid. Micturition occurs by the use of the Valsalva manoeuvre or manual expression through suprapubic pressure. An incontinence appliance is particularly appropriate for these patients during sports activities which often lead to an increase in intra-abdominal pressure.

Renal calculi occur more frequently in the athlete with a spinal cord injury. This is related to osteoporosis, hypercalcaemia and hypercalciuria. Management includes a large fluid throughput, a low calcium diet and a diet with normal protein content. This may be a problem for weight-lifters who often believe that high protein diets are important for strength gains. Ammonium chloride can be used to decrease stone formation, but some studies have suggested that the use of acidifying agents can impair performance even in short-term events.

The management of urinary tract infection in

these patients differs somewhat from that of the able-bodied population. Should the patient be symptomless and be known to have persistent bacteriuria, no treatment is required as long as no vesico-ureteric reflux is present. If the patient is symptomless but is known to have normally sterile urine and infection is noted on urine culture, treatment with antibiotics is appropriate. If the patient has systemic symptoms and an accompanying urinary tract infection, treatment with antibiotics is mandatory (Bean 1988).

AUTONOMIC DYSREFLEXIA

Autonomic dysreflexia is most often a problem in quadriplegics and high-level paraplegics and may be relevant to sports performance. A painful stimulus occurring in an area that has no residual sensation, for example, a distended bowel or bladder, renal colic, pressure sores, sports injury or simply an ingrown toenail, will lead to sensory impulses that may enter the cord below the transection. The sympathetic nervous system may react to local spinal reflexes, producing an outflow discharge leading to vasoconstriction, sweating and pilo-erection. Significant hypertension may be produced, the patient complaining of a headache, excessive sweating and appearing pale. The blood pressure elevation may take on the proportions of a hypertensive crisis and may require management with vasodilators including clonidine, labetalol or diazoxide.

CONCLUSIONS

Until recently, the sports medicine community has had little involvement with the wheelchair athlete. While much is known about the physiological responses of the spinal cord injured to exercise, specific studies of sports injuries are rare. It has been demonstrated that close monitoring of wheelchair athletes during training decreases the incidence of injury. It therefore behoves the sports medicine doctor to become increasingly involved with the wheelchair athlete as, currently, minor problems are ignored or not treated and may progress to serious injuries or chronic disorders. The wheelchair athlete also needs to be educated in injury prevention and the early management of sports injuries.

The role of the sports physician lies in pre-participation examinations, medical classification of athletes, prevention and management of injury, education of disabled athletes, research into the nature and treatment of their injuries and in encouraging the spinally injured to involve themselves in sport and exercise opportunities.

THE ATHLETE WITH AN INTELLECTUAL DISABILITY

There are two main organizations involved with athletes who have an intellectual disability:

- INAS-FMH (International Sports Federation for Persons with an Intellectual Disability)
- Special Olympics Foundation

INAS-FMH is a founding member of the International Paralympic Committee and as such facilitates inclusion of athletes at an elite level. The affiliated Australian organization is AUSRAPID (Australian Sport and Recreation Association for Persons with an Intellectual Disability). This organization liaises with national sporting bodies to encourage the integration of athletes through sport

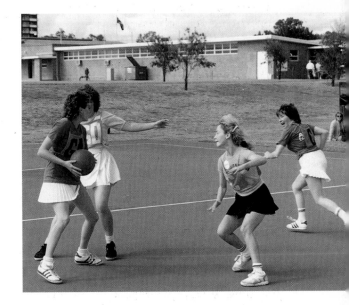

Fig. 24.6 Mentally handicapped athletes participating in a netball game. (Courtesy of West Australian Disabled Sports Association Inc.)

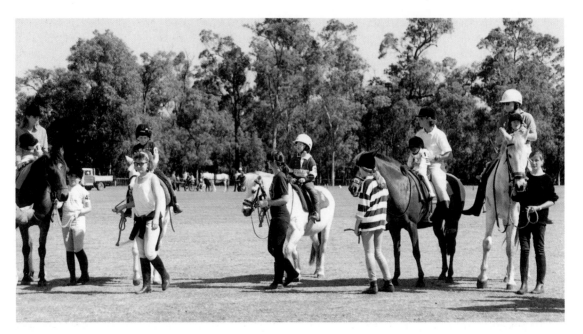

Fig. 24.7 Mentally handicapped children taking part in equestrian activities.

and recreation at local, state, national and international levels. In July 1968 the first international Special Olympics were held in Chicago. The current Special Olympics now involves more than 1 million athletes from 60 countries. Their programme includes track and field athletics, basketball, bowling, gymnastics, floor and poly hockey, figure and speed skating, downhill and cross-country skiing, soccer, softball and volleyball. The most recent demonstration sports at the Special Olympics include canoeing, cycling, equestrian events, racquet sports, roller-skating and weight-lifting. Entry into the Special Olympics programme is restricted to mentally retarded individuals aged 8 years and over.

Athletes with an intellectual disability first competed in the Paralympics in Madrid in 1992, in parallel with the Barcelona Olympics. Events included track and field, swimming, basketball (men and women), futsal (indoor soccer) and table tennis. These athletes were able to achieve high levels of performance as is shown by the following:

- World record, men, 100 m, athletics, 11.31 s
- World record, men, javelin, 51.52 m
- World record, men, 50 m freestyle, 27.68 s

Before the establishment of the Special Olympics very few opportunities for recreation and competition for the mentally retarded existed. Approximately 45% of all mentally retarded children received no physical education and only 25% experienced as much as 60 min of organized recreation per week. Fortunately, however, this situation has changed considerably in recent times (Figs 24.6 and 24.7).

The mentally retarded, prior to systematic training, are often not as physically fit as their counterparts in the general population, therefore a pre-participation evaluation is of special significance for them. Current recommendations include a full physical examination every 2 years with a yearly health evaluation. This involves specific examinations of recently injured body parts or of systems involved in recent significant illnesses. The Special Olympics Foundation requires each athlete participating in the Special Olympics sponsored competition to have a current certificate of fitness to compete.

Approximately 75% of mentally retarded individuals have one or more associated medical disorders. Fifteen to 20% of athletes at any Special Olympics event will have trisomy 21 (Down syndrome) and approximately 12–15% of this group have atlanto-axial instability. This disorder is characterized by excessive movement at the level of C 1–2 and ligamentous and muscle laxity often leads to malalignment. In this disorder, neck flexion is the movement most likely to lead to subluxation and cord trauma and medical evaluation includes cervical spine X-rays with views in full flexion and extension.

The sports which are contra-indicated in the athlete with atlanto-axial instability are gymnastics, diving, high jump, pentathlon, butterfly stroke in swimming, soccer and other activities that place pressure on the head and neck. Training procedures involving forced flexion of the neck should also be avoided.

An estimated 50% of Down syndrome athletes have a congenital heart defect, common specific problems being large cushion septal defects and tetralogy of Fallot. The suitability of these patients for competition depends on the specific cardiac defect and exercise testing is recommended for this group before they participate in cardiovascular endurance events.

Epilepsy is common in the mentally retarded, with various studies indicating an incidence between 14 and 46% in this population. The majority of the affected athletes will use anticonvulsant medication and Chapter 28 should be studied for further details. A thorough knowledge of the athlete's history, including fit frequency and control, type of seizure, medication levels and compliance and sports participation will be required for decisions regarding the safety of participation for the athlete. Comprehensive knowledge of anticonvulsant medication and the management of convulsions is mandatory for the physician responsible for the care of the mentally retarded athlete.

Dietary disorders, including poor eating habits and obesity are very prevalent in the mentally retarded population. In view of the detrimental effects of obesity and incorrect nutrition on performance, counselling in these areas is likely to be part of the role of the sports medicine physician.

Irrespective of age group, mentally retarded persons usually have cardiovascular fitness levels from 20 to 40% lower than those individuals in the general population (Fernall et al. 1988). A training study of adolescents failed to demonstrate significant improvements in cardiovascular fitness following a cycling programme; however, the small sample size could have affected the findings. On the other hand cardiovascular fitness in adults has been shown to improve following a training programme (Compton et al. 1989).

Specific Problems of Competition

A study by Bedo (1976) compiled data on the pre-existing conditions of athletes participating in the 1975 Special Olympics. It was found that 8.7% of participants had pre-existing conditions. The most common were found to be seizures (predominantly grand mal and petit mal) and heart disease (mostly congenital). Diabetes mellitus, diabetes insipidus, hernia, blindness and obesity were less common pre-existing conditions. A significant number also reported drug allergies, one-third of these being to penicillin.

A review of two studies published on injury incidence during Special Olympics competition (Bedo 1976; Birrer 1984) reveals the following injuries in decreasing level of incidence: abrasions, contusions, blisters, sprains, lacerations, cramps, head injury and fractures. In order of decreasing frequency, the most common general medical conditions encountered were ear, nose and throat conditions, exhaustion (usually related to heat stress), upper respiratory tract infection, gastroenteritis, conjunctivitis, non-traumatic headache, convulsions, sunburn, otitis media, insect bite and ocular foreign body. Each study, which has been carried out at the Special Olympics events, makes particular mention of heat-related problems and the provision and liberal use of sunscreen is of importance to these athletes. An adequate fluid intake, shelter from the sun and cooling procedures are also necessary and it is important that heat-related disorders should be emphasized at all medical briefings. A recent study (McCormick et al. 1990) reported that Down syndrome athletes were 3.2 times more likely to encounter a medical problem during a Special Olympics event than other Special Olympics athletes. They also noted that the overall relative risk of injury at Special Olympics is 0.4

injuries per 1000 participant hours, indicating a low risk of participation. It has been demonstrated that it is safe for mentally retarded athletes to participate in competitive sports and that they require at least the same levels of care and support as able-bodied athletes.

THE AMPUTEE ATHLETE

The amputee athlete usually participates in sport with or without a prosthesis, or in a wheelchair. Grading or classification systems are based on double or single amputations above or below the knee or elbow.

Apart from the previously noted medical and psychological benefits of sports participation, sport may help to prevent atrophy of the stump muscles, improve circulation of the stump and strengthen the remaining muscles in the affected limbs.

The majority of problems encountered in the amputee athlete include musculoskeletal problems proximal to the stump, problems with stump fitting, friction-related disorders and infection of the stump itself.

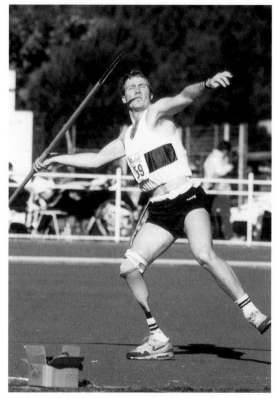

Fig. 24.8 Repetitive ground impact may loosen alignment settings leading to prosthetic foot and ankle malalignment.

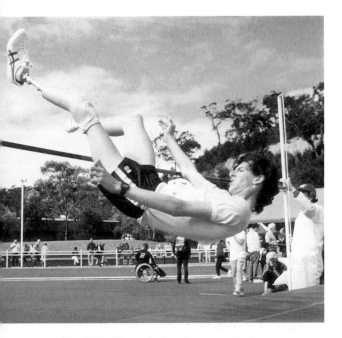

Fig. 24.9 Care must be taken to avoid stress on the stump and the joint proximal to the prosthesis.

Alignment of the prosthesis requires constant monitoring and repetitive ground impact may loosen alignment settings leading to prosthetic foot and ankle malalignment (Fig. 24.8). Some concern has been voiced in the literature over the stress and strain on the stump and the joint proximal to the prosthesis (Fig. 24.9). Studies conducted in non-athletes have indicated an increased incidence of osteo-arthritis in joints proximal to the prosthesis. Increased ground impact, ground reaction force and stance phase loading occur on the side requiring the prosthesis.

Back pain is not uncommon in the amputee athlete. This may be related to the increased ground reaction force transmitted through the prosthesis or to a 'short leg' syndrome. Some prostheses are specifically shorter than on the normal side, to facilitate ground clearance during the swing phase of gait.

The amputee is commonly involved in various sports including swimming, track and field athletics, weight-lifting, volleyball, table tennis, lawn bowls and archery. As yet no specific data are available on sports medicine concerns in the amputee athlete in these events.

The most studied sport involving amputees is alpine skiing (McCormick 1985). The majority of amputee skiers use a tritrack system involving a single ski and two outrigger ski poles. Amputations above the ankle usually do not allow the skier to wear a weight-bearing prosthesis as there is insufficient control of the ski on the weak side. If a skier wearing such a prosthesis were to fall, a significant stump injury could occur. The outrigger injury is specific to handicapped skiers and occurs as the sharp metal edges of the outrigger ski poles contact the skin, leading to lacerations.

Retropatellar pain is one of the common limiting factors in the alpine skier's performance. Preventive measures include isometric quadriceps strengthening exercises, skiing in a relatively upright position, limitation of quick, high-speed turns, rest periods between runs, avoidance of steep or mogulled terrain and early presentation of injury. Quadriceps fatigue is a common problem usually related to long downhill runs with prolonged knee flexion. Other common problems include fractures to the lower limb, contusions and lacerations.

Cold injury to the stump is not uncommon and this problem is related to poor circulation. The use of woollen stump socks or a stump shell is highly recommended.

The incidence of skiing-related injuries in the handicapped is approximately equal to that of the able-bodied skier. Such injuries can be prevented by attention to equipment, including bindings, use of shorter skis, training in the disposal of the outrigger ski poles during a fall, pre-season training and avoidance of fatigue.

The next most common alpine sport for the disabled is sit-skiing. Sit-skiing has been designed for skiers whose leg strength and co-ordination is insufficient to support upright skiing and is most often performed by the paraplegic. The ski is a modified sled with a leg cover, roll-bars, an evacuation system and runners which, like skis, may be sharpened or waxed. Stabilization of the ski is by the use of hand picks.

Sit-skiing injuries have been the subject of some research which has reported that sit-skiers are eight times more likely to sustain an injury than disabled skiers who do not use the sit-ski. The upper body sustains the majority of sit-ski injuries and shoulder injuries include contusions and dislocations, mostly occurring when the skier rolls the ski. Deltoid strain is usually related to steering the ski with hand picks. Several head injuries have also been reported and the wearing of helmets is necessary. Use of the ski pick is associated with 'skier's thumb' which is a rupture of the ulnar collateral ligament of the thumb or a fracture at the base of the thumb. Prevention is by holding the hand pick with the thumb on the same side of the grip as the fingers. In view of the low position of sit-skiing, protective goggles are recommended.

Pressure sores and heat loss may also be a problem and their management is discussed in the section of this chapter concerning paraplegics.

THE CEREBRAL PALSIED ATHLETE

There is a paucity of published data concerning sports-related problems and injuries in the athlete with cerebral palsy; however, an awareness of the pathophysiology of this condition and the problems associated with cerebral palsy will aid the sports medicine physician in the general medical care of these athletes.

Cerebral palsy is a group of disorders of impaired brain and motor function which onset before or at birth, or during the first years of life and the condition has multiple aetiologies. The most obvious manifestation is impaired function of the voluntary musculature. Classification of the cerebral palsied is based on motor deficit and is classified as follows:

- Class 1. Spastic type (50–70%). Characteristic features include exaggerated stretch reflexes, hypertonia, muscle weakness and jerky and uncertain muscle movement. The most common posture involves inward rotation of the legs, flexed elbows, wrists and fingers and poor posture due to spasticity of the antigravity muscles

- Class 2. Choreoathetosis (10–20%). This is most often associated with the spastic type. Characteristically uncontrollable, jerky, irregular twisting movement of the limbs occur which interfere with normal movements
- Class 3. Ataxic (1–5%). This group is characterized by poor balance, unsteady gait, poor hand–eye co-ordination and decreased kinaesthetic awareness
- Class 4. Hypotonic (uncommon). This group is characterized by failure of muscle response to volitional command

A large proportion of cerebral palsied athletes have associated problems, and 88% have three or more disabilities.

Common associated disabilities are:

- Convulsions. These occur in 60% of the cerebral palsied population and in 30% of athletes in this group
- Visual defects, occur in 21–58% of the overall cerebral palsied population and 25% of these occur in athletes with this problem

Fig. 24.10 A blind cyclist racing in a tandem event. (Courtesy of West Australian Disabled Sports Association Inc.)

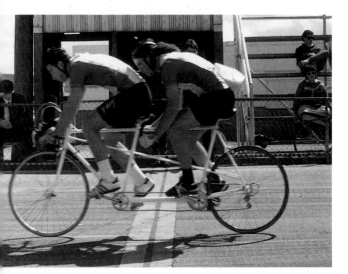

- Deafness occurs in 20–25% of the cerebral palsied, and in 12% of cerebral palsied athletes
- Intellectual disability is prevalent in approximately 45% of the cerebral palsied population but only 10–15% of cerebral palsied athletes have this handicap
- Perceptual and visuomotor problems (learning disabilities) are found in 60% of cerebral palsied athletes. These disabilities create various problems with relation to competition. Such things as maintaining position on the field of play and staying in lanes while competing in events create coaching and officiating problems

It also should be remembered that half the cerebral palsied athletes compete in wheelchairs.

The first comprehensive study of injuries sustained by the cerebral palsy athlete during competition was conducted at the 1988 Seoul Paralympics (Richter *et al.* 1992). Of the 45 injuries or illnesses reported in a total of 75 US athletes, 42% were not directly related to sport, 40% were sustained during training and 18% occurred during competition. Of the above, 26% were illnesses, mainly involving infection of the upper respiratory tract. The majority of the injuries were strains (59%), the remainder being predominantly abrasions and contusions. All of the injuries were considered to be minor, the most frequently injured areas being shoulders (16%), and low back, neck, upper arm and knees (8% each).

THE BLIND ATHLETE

The degree of blindness for participation in sporting activity has been defined as a visual acuity of 6/60 or less.

A large range of sports including track and field events, skiing, golf, swimming, rowing (in pairs), cycling (in pairs) (Fig. 24.10), sky-diving (in a group) and adapted events such as beep-ball, a form of baseball with the ball emitting a sound, are available to the blind athlete.

Performances of the legally blind include qualification for the able-bodied US wrestling team, water-skiing across the English channel, gold medals in the able-bodied 200 m and 400 m events at World

Masters games, completion of the Ironman Triathlon in Hawaii and sub-par golf rounds. Moreover, in July 1981 five blind climbers and an amputee, an epileptic and two deaf hikers reached the 4390 m peak of Mt Rainier in the United States.

The only specific sports medicine problem for the blind is related to falls. Falls on the outstretched upper limb are not uncommon, leading to the same types of fractures and soft tissue injuries as in the able-bodied sportsperson. Sprains of the knee and ankle ligaments are also not uncommon.

In the only published study concerning injuries sustained by blind athletes during national level competition (Ferrara *et al.* 1992), 53% of injuries were to the lower extremity, predominantly involving the ankle and lower leg. In the upper body 31% of the injuries involved the upper limb and half of these were related to the shoulder region. The rest were sustained in the neck and spine (7.6%), trunk (5.6%) and head and face (2.8%). As is the case in many similar studies, an exact diagnosis for each injury was not recorded.

THE DEAF ATHLETE

The deaf athlete has received little specific attention from the sports medicine community.

Major dangers for the deaf athlete arise from a lack of audible warnings and potential slowness in communication. Apart from serious trauma consequent upon these problems, there is little evidence to suggest that the injuries sustained by the deaf differ significantly from those of the able-bodied.

'LES AUTRES' ATHLETES

'Les autres', the French term for 'the others' is used in sport terminology to denote other locomotor disabilities. The types of disabilities encompassed by this classification include:

- Dwarfism, otherwise defined as short stature, the most common disorder in this group being the chondrodystrophies
- Congenital disorders of bones and connective tissue. For example, osteogenesis imperfecta, an inherited condition characterized by multiple fractures of abnormally soft and brittle bones and Ehlers-Danlos syndrome, a disorder of collagen predisposing to joint hypermobility and dislocations, looseness of skin, slow wound healing and blood vessel fragility
- Athrogryphosis multiplex congenita — a congenital disorder associated with multiple joint contractures
- Limb deficiencies, including absence of arms or legs, or absence of the middle segment of a limb, but with intact proximal and distal portions
- Anisomelia — a condition of asymmetry between limbs (eligibility for participation in disabled sports requires at least 7 cm asymmetry for most sports and 10 cm asymmetry for swimming)
- Ankylosis, arthrodesis or arthritis of major joints
- Conditions characterized by muscle weakness related to peripheral nerve damage, including Guillain-Barré syndrome
- Muscular dystrophies
- Multiple sclerosis
- Friedrich's ataxia

Currently, no definite data are available on sport-related problems in these athletes.

CLASSIFICATION

The classification of disabled athletes, aimed at providing fairness in competition, is the subject of continual controversy. Part of the role of the sports physician treating the disabled athlete is to have a sound working knowledge of the various disability classifications which can be obtained from the disabled sports associations who administer each group (Sherrill 1986).

PSYCHOSOCIAL ASPECTS OF SPORT FOR THE DISABLED

Common problems for the disabled include stereotyping, stigmatization, difficulty with education and employment, and problems with interpersonal relationships. These often lead to feelings of inferiority, depression, personality changes, poor socialization and isolation, negative life-style choices including the use of nicotine, alcohol and recreational drugs, and negative attitudes towards physical activity.

Clinical studies, particularly with paraplegics, reveal a decrease in subjective and objective disturbance of psychological function among those participating in sport. Findings included decreased scores for anxiety, phobia, obsession, somatization and depression (Monnazzi 1982).

Sport has many psychological advantages for the disabled because it is an enjoyable way to exercise and helps to alleviate the boredom of rehabilitation. It allows voluntary choice, personal decision-making and increased opportunities for diversion and fun. It permits the disabled to regain contact with the normal world and to facilitate social reintegration. The disabled athlete may well be able to train and in some cases compete with normal athletes. Feelings of inferiority decrease and there are increased opportunities, options and experiences available to the disabled so that their self-esteem increases. The disabled may gain the respect of the able-bodied community and an increased acceptance of themselves as a result of sports participation, thereby aiding them in their fight against prejudice and stigmatization. The disabled athlete may be perceived as a specialized athlete and no longer as a paraplegic, cerebral palsied or blind person.

The psychological and physical benefits of sport and exercise participation for the disabled are therefore significant. The rehabilitation specialist, sports medicine physician and general practitioner should all be involved in encouraging the disabled person to participate in some type of sporting activity.

REFERENCES

Aljure J., Eltorai I., Bradley W. E., Lin J. E. & Johnson B. (1986) Carpal tunnel syndrome in paraplegic patients. *Paraplegia* 23, 182–186.

Bean A. (1988) Paraplegia and tetraplegia in general practice. *Patient Management* 12, 109–126.

Bedo A. V. (1976) Special Olympics athletes face special medical needs. *Physician and Sportsmedicine* 4, 51–56.

Birrer R. B. (1984) The Special Olympics: An injury overview. *Physician and Sportsmedicine* 12, 95–97.

Bloomquist L. E. (1986) Injuries to athletes with physical disabilities: Prevention implications. *Physician and Sportsmedicine* 14, 97–105.

Cameron B. J., Ward G. R. & Wicks J. R. (1977) Relationship of type of training to maximum oxygen uptake and upper limb strength in male paraplegic athletes. *Medicine and Science in Sports* 9, 58.

Compton D. M., Eisenman P. A. & Henderson H. L. (1989) Exercise and fitness for persons with disabilities. *Sports Medicine* 7, 150–162.

Curtis K. A. (1982) Wheelchair sports medicine — Part 4 Athletic injuries. *Sports and Spokes* **February**, 21–24.

Davis G. M., Shephard R. J. & Jackson R. W. (1981) Cardio-respiratory fitness and muscular strength in the lower-limb disabled. *Canadian Journal of Applied Sport Science* 6, 159–165.

Davis G. M., Tupling S. J. & Shephard R. J. (1986) Dynamic strength and physical activity in wheelchair users. In Sherrill C. (ed.) *Sports and Disabled Athletes*, pp. 139–146. Human Kinetics Publishers, Champaign, IL.

Davis R., Ferrara M. & Byrnes D. (1988) The competitive wheelchair stroke. *NSCA Journal* 10, 4–10.

Fernall B., Tymeson G. T. & Webster G. E. (1988) Cardiovascular fitness of mentally retarded individuals. *Adapted Physical Activity Quarterly* 5, 12–28.

Ferrara M. S., Buckley W. E., Cairbe McCann B., Limbird T. J., Powell J. W. & Robl R. (1992) The injury experience of the competitive athlete with a disability: Prevention implications. *Medicine and Science in Sports and Exercise* 24, 184–188.

Figoni S. F. (1992) Exercise response and quadriplegia. *Medicine and Science in Sports and Exercise* 25, 433–441.

Gass G. C. & Camp E. M. (1979) Physiological characteristics of trained Australian paraplegic and tetraplegic subjects. *Medicine and Science in Sports* 11, 256–259.

Gass G. C., Camp E. M., Nadel E.R., Gwinn T. H. & Engel P. (1988) Rectal and rectal vs. esophageal temperatures in paraplegic men during prolonged exercise. *Journal of Applied Physiology* 64, 2265–2271.

Glaser R. M. (1985) Exercise and locomotion for the spinal cord injured. *Exercise and Sports Science Reviews* 13, 263–303.

Glaser R. M. (1989) Arm exercise training for wheelchair users. *Medicine and Science in Sports and Exercise* 21 (Supplement), S149–157.

Guttman L. (1977) *Textbook of Sport for the Disabled*. University of Queensland Press, St Lucia, Qld.

Hoffman M. D. (1986) Cardiorespiratory fitness and training in quadriplegics and paraplegics. *Sports Medicine* 3, 312–330.

Mangus B. C. (1987) Sports injuries, the disabled athlete and the athletic trainer. *Athletic Training* 22, 305–310.

McCormick D. P. (1985) Injuries in handicapped Alpine ski racers. *Physician and Sportsmedicine* 13, 93–97.

McCormick D. P., Niebuhr V. N. & Risser W. L. (1990)

Injury and illness surveillance at local Special Olympic Games. *British Journal of Sports Medicine* **24**, 221–223.

Monnazzi G. (1982) Paraplegics and sports: A psychological survey. *International Journal of Sports Psychology* **13**, 85–95.

Nichols P. J. R., Norman P. A. & Ennis J. R. (1979) Wheelchair user's shoulder? *Scandinavian Journal of Rehabilitation Medicine* **11**, 29–32.

Nilsen R., Nygaard P. & Bjorholt P. G. (1985) Complications that may occur in those with spinal cord injuries who participate in sport. *Paraplegia* **23**, 152–158.

Richter K. J., Hyman S. C., Mushett C. A., Ellenberg M. R. & Ferrara M. J. (1992) Injuries in world class cerebral palsy athletes of the 1988 South Korea Paralympics. *Journal of Osteopathic Sports Medicine* **5**, 15–18.

Rugnarsson K. T. (1988) Physiologic effect of functional electrical stimulation-induced exercises in spinal cord injured individuals. *Clinical Orthopaedics and Related Research* **233**, 53–63.

Sherrill C. (ed.) (1986) *Sport and Disabled Athletes*, pp. 269–275. Human Kinetics Publishers Champaign, IL.

Shephard R. J. (1988) Sports medicine and the wheelchair athlete. *Sports Medicine* **4**, 226–247.

CHAPTER 25

MEDICAL CONSIDERATIONS IN AQUATIC SPORTS

J. J. Kellett

As a medium for activity, water has its own distinct pleasures as is evidenced by the variety of activities and the number of people of all ages who choose aquatic pursuits for both competitive and recreational purposes. Water also has unique physical properties which give rise to a number of medical conditions quite distinct from those occurring with land-based activities.

This chapter deals with some of the common medical problems related to sport and exercise in water and includes the following topics.

- Decompression sickness
- Arterial gas embolism
- Barotrauma
- Hypothermia
- Near drowning
- Nitrogen narcosis
- Breath-hold diving
- Medical conditions of swimming
- Marine bites or stings

DECOMPRESSION SICKNESS

Decompression sickness (DCS) is a term used to encompass a multitude of signs and symptoms, which may involve virtually any of the organ systems and have as a common aetiology the formation of nitrogen bubbles in either the body's tissues or blood (Gorman 1989).

As the name implies, bubble formation occurs as a result of the decrease in pressure which accompanies ascent from a dive. DCS may occur at any time from the beginning of ascent, but is usually apparent within the first 24 h following ascent (Thomas & McKenzie 1981).

According to Henry's law[1] the amount of nitrogen in the blood is proportional to the pressure of nitrogen in contact with the blood which, in turn, is proportional to the water depth. The amount of nitrogen dissolved in various tissues of the body depends also on the duration of exposure to that pressure and to the nature of the body tissue involved. The rate of nitrogen pressure equilibration depends on the affinity of the tissue for nitrogen and on the blood flow to that particular organ (Thomas & McKenzie 1981). Consequently, equilibration occurs more rapidly in some tissues than in others. In the nervous system the myelin of the nerve sheath has a particularly high affinity for nitrogen and the brain has a high blood flow. This combination makes the nervous system highly susceptible to DCS.

These factors of pressure magnitude, or depth, and duration of exposure are combined in the form of decompression tables which guide divers on the rate of ascent following dives. Controlled ascent rates allow equilibration of nitrogen pressures and

---

[1] The amount of gas dissolved in a liquid at a given temperature is directly proportional to the partial pressure of that gas in contact with the liquid.

thereby prevent bubble formation. In the tables the term 'no decompression limit' allows dives of certain depths and duration without requiring staged ascent to prevent DCS (Kindwall & Strauss 1991). Studies have shown that nitrogen bubble formation occurs in most dives deeper than 7 m without causing any symptoms (Gorman 1989). Presumably, such bubbles do not reach a volume sufficient to cause symptoms, or they are filtered out of the blood in the lungs (Gorman 1989).

By definition, symptoms and signs of DCS may arise at any time from the onset of decompression, that is from the beginning of ascent. Approximately 80% of signs or symptoms are present on surfacing and 95% are evident within 4 h of surfacing. Almost all attacks of DCS occur within 24 h of the dive. There is a tendency for more severe symptoms to develop early and any such development should be treated urgently as DCS until proven otherwise. Almost any organ system may be involved and frequently combinations of systems are affected with a high proportion of nervous system involvement. Edmonds *et al.* (1992) indicate that non-specific generalized symptoms such as weakness, apathy, tiredness or malaise may be the most common presentation of DCS. Table 25.1 outlines some of the signs and symptoms that may result from DCS.

DCS is a medical emergency because appropriate early treatment may completely reverse established signs and symptoms. Conversely, any delay in treatment may result in permanent deficit; therefore experienced medical assistance is vital. Nevertheless, as dramatic recoveries have been recorded after delays of up to 9 days before treatment was instituted (Jerrard 1992), a delay of some days is no contra-indication to definitive (recompression) therapy. Immediate first aid may be limited by circumstances to the provision of oxygen and the management of acute complications such as cardiac arrest.

The cornerstone of definitive treatment of DCS is recompression (Gorman 1989), which brings about the reversal of bubble formation. In the majority of cases this will require transfer to a centre where a suitable recompression facility is available. However, because commercial aircraft are pressurized to the

equivalent of approximately 1000–2000 m above sea level (Thomas & McKenzie 1981), such transport may result in a worsening of signs and symptoms because of further decompression. Transport must therefore be by aircraft pressurized to sea level, with the plane flying no more than 300 m above the sea, or via a transportable recompression chamber.

During transport 100% oxygen should be administered via a sealed mask (Neuman 1987), but in order to prevent the development of oxygen toxicity, a 5 min break for air breathing every 30 min is necessary. Pure oxygen, in contrast to air, results in an increase in the nitrogen pressure gradient from the body's tissues to the lungs and consequently promotes more rapid elimination of nitrogen. Increased oxygen delivery to the already damaged tissues may minimize further damage and during transport accurate records of oxygen administration should be maintained.

Longer dives accompanied by cold exposure result in the suppression of antidiuretic hormone release (Neuman 1987), causing blood volume depletion and haemoconcentration. Empirical evidence has demonstrated that oral or intravenous fluid replacement decreases the likelihood of morbidity or mortality and it appears that the severity of DCS correlates with the patient's haematocrit, which is a measure of blood concentration.

A chest X-ray prior to recompression is recommended to exclude a pneumothorax which could develop into a tension pneumothorax. This is the progressive accumulation of air outside the lung but within the thorax which compresses the lung tissue.

Strict adherence to decompression tables during diving greatly reduces the risk of DCS, but does not guarantee immunity. Multiple ascents during a single dive and diving on several consecutive days may increase the risk of developing DCS. Other factors contributing to an increased likelihood of DCS include poor physical fitness, obesity, heavy exertion, dehydration and hypothermia (Edmonds *et al.* 1992). Divers are also advised against flying shortly after diving, because of the enhanced decompression effect of altitude. Flying should therefore be postponed at least 4 h after a 'no decom-

Table 25.1 Decompression sickness: signs and symptoms

Signs and symptoms	Notes
Central nervous system	
Spinal cord	
Back pain which may radiate to the abdomen	The nervous system is involved in at least 80% of cases
Numbness and paraesthesiae ('pins and needles')	of DCS (especially thoracic spinal cord)
Loss of control of bladder, bowels	Any nervous system involvement may lead to
	permanent neurological damage
	Nervous system involvement may be precipitated by
	brief deep dives and may have a rapid onset
Cerebral	
Visual disturbance ('double vision', 'blind spots')	
Hemiplegia (paralysis of one side of the body)	
Loss of consciousness	
Difficulty with speech	
Headache	
Confusion	
Staggering, ataxia, incoordination	
Tremor	
Convulsions	
Personality or behavioural changes	
Skeletal system	
Joint pains	Joint pain is often preceded by a feeling of numbness or
	discomfort
	The glenohumeral (shoulder) joint is most frequently
	involved
	Affected joints are often held in a bent position for
	comfort ('the bends')
Cardiovascular–respiratory system	
Dyspnoea (difficulty breathing) ⎫	Dyspnoea, chest pain and cough may be due to
Chest pain ⎬ 'the	obstruction of the pulmonary artery by nitrogen bubbles
Cough ⎭ chokes'	Air embolism is due to bubbles passing through the
Myocardial infarct ('heart attack')	pulmonary blood vessels or through cardiac shunts to
Cardiac arrest	the left side of the heart and then to the arterial
Air embolism (air bubbles obstructing	circulation
blood vessels)	
Skin	
Pruritus (itch)	A 'marbled' skin rash indicates serious DCS
Measles-like rash	
Bluish 'marbling' appearance of skin	
Gastrointestinal system	
Anorexia (loss of appetite)	
Nausea and vomiting	
Haematemesis (vomiting blood)	
Abdominal cramps	
Diarrhoea which may contain blood	
Blood	
Disturbances of coagulation (clotting) .	Disorders of coagulation include thrombocytopenia (low
	platelet count), platelet aggregation and endothelial cell
	damage (lining blood vessels)

pression limit' dive and for 24 h after a dive requiring decompression.

After an episode of DCS, repeated examination of the affected organ systems is necessary. For example, a neurological examination of the central nervous system (CNS) and investigations such as an electroencephalogram, computerized tomography (CT) or magnetic resonance imaging (MRI) may be necessary. The clinical examination, however, is often more sensitive than a CT or MRI scan (Edmonds *et al.* 1992).

Any long-term sequelae of DCS must preclude further diving. Even when signs and symptoms resolve completely, diving should still be avoided for a minimum of 4 weeks. Although there are no data to indicate an increased risk of a second attack of DCS in this situation, a conservative approach to diving is advised because of the poor response to treatment of any second attack (Gorman 1989).

ARTERIAL GAS EMBOLISM

Arterial gas embolism (AGE) is largely due to pulmonary overdistension due to descent while breath holding. This increase in pulmonary pressure results in alveolar rupture with escape of air into the pulmonary vein to the left side of the heart and systemic circulation as emboli, which may obstruct arterial circulation. The presence of congenital arteriovenous communications such as patent ductus arteriosus and septal defects are other mechanisms by which gas bubbles that form move readily in the venous circulation and gain entry to the systemic circulation. Such venous bubbles are normally filtered out during passage through the pulmonary circulation.

The symptoms of AGE include loss of consciousness, seizures, paralysis, aphasia, visual disturbances and paraesthesia. The brain is much more frequently involved with AGE because of the upright position of most divers on the ascent and the tendency for bubbles to rise within the circulation. The spinal cord and the coronary circulation are much less frequently involved. AGE causes symptoms which are more immediate in onset. Virtually 100% occur within 10 min of surfacing and frequently follow rapid uncontrolled ascent (Edmonds *et al.* 1992).

AGE is neither time nor depth dependent and frequently may occur after brief and shallow dives (Greer & Massey 1992).

Again, recompression is the essential element in treating AGE.

BAROTRAUMA

Barotrauma describes the damage to various bodily tissues which results from pressure imbalances between gas spaces in the body and adjacent body tissues or fluids. Barotrauma of the ear is the most common injury affecting divers.

With changes in depth and consequently pressure, the volume of gases in the body changes correspondingly (Fig. 25.1). This volume change occurs with both descent (volume decrease) and ascent (volume increase) by the diver. With descent and decreasing gas volume, the term 'squeeze' is used to describe the effects of barotrauma. 'Squeeze' occurs where a gas space exists which does not completely collapse and where there is a pressure difference between that gas space and the ambient pressure. Tissues lining the gas spaces, such as the middle ear chamber, may swell and if blood vessels are present they may rupture and bleed in an attempt to equalize pressure.

Haemorrhage into the air space may ease the severe pain that accompanies squeeze. Table 25.2 details the more common forms of barotrauma of descent.

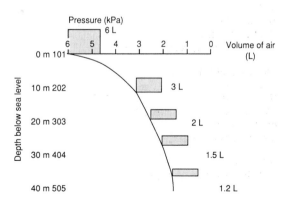

Fig. 25.1 The pressure–depth–volume relationship.

Table 25.2 Barotrauma of descent

	Pathology	Symptoms and signs	Treatment	Notes
Middle ear squeeze	Haemorrhage into middle ear/ear drum Tympanic membrane (ear-drum) rupture/ stretch Disruption of ossicles (small bones of middle ear)	Increasing pain with depth Conductive hearing loss Vertigo (dizziness) Tympanic membrane rupture Bleeding from nose/ mouth	Decongestants ± antibiotics Rupture requires ear, nose and throat specialist review	Eustachian tube dysfunction (inability to equalize pressure between middle ear and pharynx) Most frequent diving injury Often occurs in first 10 m of dive Check ability to equalize pressure before diving Tympanic membrane rupture usually heals in 2 days−8 weeks or surgery may be indicated
Inner ear	Rupture of round or oval window Perilymph fistula	Tinnitus (ringing in ears) Vertigo Nystagmus (spontaneous eye flickering) Hearing loss	Specialist review if vertigo or hearing loss persists beyond 3 days	Prohibit further diving
External auditory canal Sinuses	Wax or ear-plugs may create an enclosed gas space Haemorrhage into sinuses	Ear pain Difficulty 'clearing' ears on descent Severe shooting or stabbing pain Bloody nasal discharge	Remove obstruction Decongestants ± antibiotics Surgery to correct any deformities obstructing sinus passages	Frontal sinuses are particularly susceptible Associated with sinusitis rhinitis, hay fever, nasal polyps, upper respiratory tract infection (URTI) No diving with URTI Don't use topical decongestants prophylactically

Barotrauma of ascent ('reverse squeeze') occurs when the normal expansion of gases with ascent is prevented, usually due to some mechanical obstruction leading to a progressive increase in pressure in the enclosed gas space as ascent proceeds. Table 25.3 outlines the features of the more common forms of barotrauma of ascent.

HYPOTHERMIA

Hypothermia is defined as a core (rectal) temperature, which is less than 35°C. It may be precipitated suddenly by cold water immersion or over a period of time by exposure to cold temperatures.

The body temperature is maintained within quite narrow limits by regulation of heat production and dissipation by the hypothalamus, which responds to blood and skin temperature sensors. Within the body, uniformity of temperature does not occur, largely because of variations in blood flow. For example, at a comfortable overall body temperature the oral temperature is 37°C, the rectal temperature 38°C and the skin temperature may be 32.8°C. In addition there is a normal diurnal (daily) variation

Table 25.3   Barotrauma of ascent

	Pathology	Symptoms	Treatment	Notes
Ear	Upper respiratory tract infection → blockage of eustachian tube with ascent Damage to tympanic membrane Damage to middle ear ossicles	Vertigo (dizziness) Deafness after diving Pain with ascent	Decongestants ±antibiotics	May be difficulty equalizing with descent
Teeth	Gas expansion in decayed tooth	Toothache with ascent Dental review	Analgesia	May follow dental barotrauma of descent with bleeding into tooth air-space
Pulmonary overinflation syndromes				
Local injury	Overdistension causing localized damage to lung tissue	Haemoptysis (coughing blood)	Resolves spontaneously	May be small pleural effusion (fluid between layers lining the lung) on chest X-ray
Interstitial emphysema	Alveolar (air-sac) rupture resulting in air into tissues outside lung Air may spread along tissue planes, for example to skin	Dyspnoea (breathlessness) Dysphagia (difficulty with swallowing) Voice change Subcutaneous emphysema (air bubbles under skin)	No specific treatment	Relatively common May be associated with air embolism (air bubbles in blood vessels)
Pneumothorax	Alveolar rupture into pleural cavity (space between layers lining lung and inner chest) may produce partial lung collapse	Sudden one-sided chest pain Dyspnoea cyanosis (purple discoloration of tongue and lips)	Intercostal catheter drain if sufficiently large	Expansion pneumothorax may expand with ascent and worsen symptoms X-ray necessary to diagnose
Air embolism	Alveolar rupture allowing air to enter pulmonary vein and then to heart and via arteries to organs	Virtually any organ may be involved depending on where air bubbles lodge Nervous system frequently affected	Head down position 100% oxygen recompression	Associated with panic breath-holding Second commonest cause of death in SCUBA diving

of approximately 1°C from the early morning to the evening.

Heat production within the body occurs as a consequence of the metabolic processes of various organs, the metabolism of food, and of muscular work including shivering. Muscular activity functions at approximately 25% efficiency, with the other 75% of energy being generated as heat, which assists in maintaining body temperature in cold weather, or which must be dissipated in hot weather. Heat loss occurs by a combination of conduction, convection, radiation and evaporation, the last being vital during land exercise but of little significance in water. Water is a much more efficient

(25-fold) conductor of heat in comparison with air (Lin 1988). It thus becomes the major contributor to heat loss during cold water immersion, by increasing both conductive and convective heat loss dramatically. The increase in ventilation which occurs with cold water immersion also results in a two- to three-fold increase in heat loss via the respiratory tract.

A simple equation controls body temperature: when heat loss exceeds heat production, a fall in body temperature occurs. Basal metabolic rate (BMR) in humans is approximately 209 kJ·m^{-2} surface area·h^{-1}, but this is decreased significantly by cold exposure. For example, at 28°C body temperature, BMR decreases to approximately 50% of normal (Sarnaik & Vohra 1986), compounding the rate of temperature decrease. The rate of body cooling in water depends on:

- The temperature of the water
- The rate of movement of the water
- The degree of insulation (fat, clothing) about the immersed body
- Body size (surface area–weight ratio) and posture in the water
- Sex and age (the young and the old are more rapidly affected)
- Activity level of the person in the water

Body movement, either by voluntary activity or by shivering, increases the rate of heat production significantly, that is up to 15-fold by exercise and five-fold by shivering, for short periods of time. However, with exercise, the increased surface area exposed and the increased blood flow to the muscles and skin, causes an increased convective heat loss to the water and a net overall heat loss. In other words, more heat is lost from the body than is generated by the exercise. In fact exercise may cause a heat loss of 30–50% higher than occurs if one remains motionless in the water. Heat loss can therefore be minimized by moving as little as practicable and by exposing the minimal body surface area to the water by assuming the 'tuck' position, or huddling if in a group. All ocean temperatures are less than 35°C, so all bodies will lose some heat to the surrounding water. Insulation is essential when swimming for prolonged periods of time if the ocean temperature is less than 30°C.

Clinical effects of hypothermia include:

- Numbness, pallor, cyanosis (purple discoloration)
- Shivering, loss of body co-ordination
- Weakness, confusion, apathy
- Loss of consciousness (at a body temperature of 27°C)
- Gradual decrease in heart rate, pulse pressure and cardiac output

In the treatment of hypothermia the victim must first be removed from the water, all cold wet clothing must be taken off and the skin thoroughly dried. The individual must be moved away from any cool draughts and warm clothing or body heat from normothermic people must be provided as soon as possible. When available, a water bath for 10 min at a temperature of 36°C which is then brought gradually to 40°C, then to 44°C is recommended until the rectal temperature is above 33°C (Thomas & McKenzie 1981). Contrary to popular belief, alcohol should be avoided because the resultant peripheral vasodilation (opening of skin blood vessels) results in increased heat loss from the body.

NEAR DROWNING

Near drowning refers to the survival of an individual following asphyxia from submersion. In approximately 85% of incidents of drowning, water is inhaled into the lungs (aspirated) and in the other 15% contraction of the vocal cords (laryngospasm) prevents aspiration (Sarnaik & Vohra 1986). This latter phenomenon is sometimes referred to as 'dry drowning'. Near drowning or drowning may follow loss of consciousness from other causes such as air bubbles in blood vessels (air embolism), but drowning as such is the commonest cause of death among SCUBA divers.

The major effects of near drowning are:

- Hypoxia (lack of oxygen to body organs). This is particularly important with regard to the heart and brain, as lack of oxygen to the brain for more than 5 min typically results in irreversible brain damage. Exceptions, however, do occur, particularly involving young children suffering very cold water immersion. Lack of oxygen to the organs occurs as a consequence of the lungs filling with aspirated water and/or oedema of lung tissues, which prevents the transfer of oxygen to the blood. Cardiac complications, including cardiac arrest, may occur

- Acidosis of the blood occurs as a consequence of oxygen lack; this produces anaerobic metabolism and the build-up of lactic acid or metabolic acidosis. Failure of the lungs to remove carbon dioxide causes a build-up of carbonic acid in the blood called respiratory acidosis and this interferes with the efficient functioning of many enzyme systems throughout the body
- Salt water aspiration results in the osmotic transfer of serum from the blood into the lungs, thereby concentrating the remaining blood constituents
- Pulmonary oedema (swelling of lung tissues) results from the acute inflammatory response to inhaled water

Although it is suggested that there is a difference between salt water and fresh water drowning and near drowning, there is little significant difference in terms of either mechanism of injury or survival. Theoretical differences between the two are related to the fact that fresh water is less concentrated than, or hypotonic to, blood and when it is aspirated it diffuses across the pulmonary membrane into the more concentrated blood. This causes an increased blood volume, decreased electrolyte (sodium, potassium, chloride) concentration and breakdown of red blood cells (haemolysis). By contrast, the concentration of sea water is three to four times that of blood and results in a net transfer of fluid into the lungs and thereby an increased concentration of the blood.

However, among survivors of fresh water and salt water near drownings, the differences do not appear to be significant. Fresh water aspiration may also disrupt the surfactant system lining the lung membranes, resulting in lung collapse, whereas the surfactant remains functional in salt water aspiration. Both salt and fresh water aspiration produce

pulmonary capillary damage, resulting in a leakage of protein into the lung and pulmonary oedema (inflammatory fluid) up to several hours after an episode of near drowning.

A common sequence of immersion, breath-hold breakpoint, swallowing water, vomiting and aspiration of water or vomitus may lead to the complication of chemical or bacterial pneumonia. Survivors therefore need to be hospitalized following any near drowning episode.

Young children may survive longer than anticipated because of the phenomenon known as the mammalian diving reflex, which is an oxygen-saving mechanism strongly developed in diving mammals such as seals. This reflex conserves oxygen by redistributing blood flow to the vital organs, that is the heart, brain and lungs, while markedly decreasing blood flow to the gastrointestinal tract, the skin, muscles and other less important organs. However, as well as its beneficial preservative effect, the associated diminished heart rate may lead rescuers to misinterpret these signs as evidence of death, so they may not proceed with resuscitation measures.

Clinical signs of near drowning include coughing, cyanosis (bluish discoloration of skin), foaming at the mouth and, not infrequently, cardiopulmonary arrest with cessation of heart beat and breathing. By contrast, the victim may appear well initially and then deteriorate — a phenomenon referred to as 'secondary drowning'.

The important effects of near drowning are in the CNS and the cardiovascular system (CVS). CNS effects are largely determined by the degree and duration of hypoxaemia or low blood oxygen level, although water temperature and age of the victim may significantly, and sometimes dramatically, modify the clinical consequences. Surprisingly, restoration of circulation may produce a transient vasodilation, widespread hypotension and decreased blood flow to the brain. Further CNS damage may therefore paradoxically occur after resuscitation. This phenomenon is referred to as 'post-hypoxic cerebral hypoperfusion'.

Hypoxaemia (low blood oxygen) and acidosis of the blood may result in profound cardiovascular dysfunction, complicated by dysrhythmias, cardiogenic shock or cardiac arrest.

Table 25.4 Medical examination of SCUBA divers

	Essential requirements	Contra-indications	Comments
Ears	Intact tympanic membrane (ear-drum) Ability to equalize middle ear pressure with pharyngeal pressure	Current tympanic membrane perforation or ventilation tubes (grommets) Acute or chronic otitis media (middle ear infection) Chronic otitis externa (outer ear infection) Menière's disease; vertigo	Movement of the tympanic membrane should be visualized A tympanogram may be necessary Well healed or repaired tympanic membrane perforations — may dive if tympanic membrane is mobile and adequate eustachian tube function is present Impacted cerumen (wax) must be removed Ear, nose and throat specialist assessment after surgery, for example if mastoidectomy is necessary
Nose and sinuses	Patent nasal airways Absence of symptoms	Any obstruction which affects pressure equalization with face mask, middle ear or paranasal sinuses Acute or chronic infection	Obstruction, for example polyps, deviated septum oedematous nasal mucosa may be corrected A patient with a chronic need for oral or topical decongestants antihistamines or steroids needs thorough assessment before clearing to dive
Oral and dental	Ability to wear mouthpiece Absence of dental caries		Dental caries, loose teeth require dental review before diving
Respiratory system	Patent airways Absence of lung scarring	Active asthma History of spontaneous pneumothorax History of obstructive airways disease Active pulmonary infection	A chest X-ray is desirable for all divers and mandatory for smokers Previous thoracotomy may result in local air trapping Uncertain history of 'asthma' requires further investigation
Cardiovascular system	Adequate fitness	History of recent myocardial infarct or current angina Major congenital heart disease, for example cyanotic heart disease Aortic stenosis Certain arrhythmias, for example complete heart block, fixed second degree heart block, paroxysmal atrial tachycardia	Mitral value prolapse without arrhythmias may be permitted to dive Murmurs may need further assessment to determine haemodynamic significance Hypertension without complications may be permitted to dive

Table 25.4 continued

	Essential requirements	Contra-indications	Comments
Central nervous system	Sufficiently intelligent to comprehend the importance of diving safety measures	Epilepsy Cerebrovascular accident Residual deficit after decompression sickness	An epileptic free from seizures for 10 years without therapy may dive pending a review by a neurologist and stress EEG Specialist neurologist review after severe head injury is necessary before diving
Miscellaneous		Abdominal hernia Active hepatitis, colitis, diverticulitis, pancreatitis Diabetes mellitus requiring insulin	Return to diving 3 months after surgery is usually permissible Non-insulin-dependent diabetes assessed on the degree of control Obesity: weight loss and fitness programme and reassess

In the management of near drowning, it is important that a suspected long submersion and asphyxia should not preclude full resuscitative measures, particularly with infants and cold water immersion. However, all patients surviving a near drowning must be transported to a hospital even if apparently well, because of the risk of delayed complications such as 'secondary drowning' or pneumonia.

First aid includes cardiopulmonary resuscitation where indicated and inhaled oxygen in high concentration. Where available, the use of intravenous bicarbonate (1 mEq·kg^{-1} bodyweight) is recommended to reduce the effect of acidosis of the blood.

MEDICAL EXAMINATION OF SCUBA DIVERS

Medical assessment of individuals prior to SCUBA (self-contained underwater breathing apparatus) diving should follow the standard format. This includes checking medical and surgical history, knowledge of any medications previously or currently taken, relevant review of body systems and a physical examination and further investigations where indicated. In both the history and the examination, special emphasis is placed on those body systems relevant to the assessment of suitability for diving, in particular the ears, nose and respiratory systems and CVS and CNS.

An assessment of general fitness and of swimming fitness in older individuals is important and depends on a reliable history from the prospective diver.

Significant and common conditions which are likely to appear in the conduct of a SCUBA medical examination are listed in Table 25.4. Conditions not listed should be assessed on their merits or a specialist's opinion sought.

NITROGEN NARCOSIS

At atmospheric pressure, nitrogen is an inert gas which comprises approximately 79% of air, but at pressure above approximately 1 kPa, nitrogen has an increasingly depressant effect on the CNS. Though individual variations occur, progressive impairment of CNS function occurs at depths greater than 30 m. At a depth of approximately 55 m, divers have a questionable ability to perform reliably and diving on air at depths below 60 m is generally considered unsafe. At depths greater than 90 m unconsciousness may develop and for safety's sake SCUBA diving should be restricted to depths not deeper than 40 m.

In general the effects of increasing nitrogen pressure on the CNS are said to mimic the effects of alcohol or anaesthetic gases. The exact mechanism of the effect is unknown, but according to Henry's law, is related to the increasing quantities of nitrogen dissolved in the blood at increasing depth. Early symptoms of nitrogen narcosis include a feeling of light-headedness, a tendency to laugh, poor concentration and a short attention span. At greater depths more life-threatening behaviour such as impairment of judgement and ability to calculate, poor memory and impaired motor performance may occur, at times with fatal consequences.

Such signs and symptoms usually become apparent after a few minutes at a particular depth. These symptoms remain stable at that depth and resolve rapidly with ascent to lower nitrogen pressures. Some tolerance may develop with longer duration or repeated exposures to a given depth; however, cold, fatigue and anxiety may provoke symptoms at a shallower depth than normal.

Treatment of nitrogen narcosis involves restraining the affected person and helping him or her to ascend slowly. Beginners are strongly advised not to descend below 30 or 40 m when using compressed air. Divers who must descend beyond these depths may use an alternative inert gas such as helium, which is effective though expensive.

BREATH-HOLD DIVING

Most readers of this book have at some time participated in a contest of underwater swimming for distance, as it seems to be an innate part of our competitive nature to want to test this capacity. In general the practice by itself is quite safe provided it is not preceded by a period of hyperventilation. Hyperventilation can greatly prolong breath-holding time, but it is an extremely dangerous practice, which may have fatal consequences.

The urge to breathe (physiological breath-hold breakpoint) becomes overwhelming when the pressure of carbon dioxide in the arterial blood (Pa_{CO_2}) reaches 47–48 mmHg. By hyperventilating before a breath-hold the pressure of carbon dioxide in the lung alveoli and of the arterial blood may be lowered significantly, thereby allowing a longer period of time before the breakpoint is reached. The level of consciousness, however, is controlled by the pressure of oxygen in the arterial blood (Pa_{O_2}) so that

following hyperventilation the Pa_{O_2} may drop below this level, causing loss of consciousness before the breakpoint is reached. When breath-holding is combined with vigorous activity, the Pa_{O_2} will drop more rapidly as the muscles utilize the limited oxygen stores.

The combination of hyperventilation prior to diving and vigorous activity while breath-holding is potentiated dramatically if the subject is diving for depth rather than distance. During ascent, even without further activity, the Pa_{O_2} will decrease as ascent progresses. A Pa_{O_2} of 100 mmHg at 10 m becomes 50 mmHg at the surface, purely because of natural decompression (Kindwall & Strauss 1991).

Therefore to avoid hyperventilation complications, breath-hold diving should not be preceded by more than three breaths.

MARINE BITES OR STINGS

Shark Attack

Though spectacularly reported, shark attacks are relatively infrequent. They seem to be more common, however, in water that is not meshed, when silt is present in the water, or at dusk when sharks tend to feed. Sharks may also be attracted by splashing swim-fins or the struggling of a speared fish. They may cause extensive injuries to humans and, to prevent blood loss, pressure or tourniquets must be applied in the water, and immediate removal from the water is a high priority. Experience shows that the survival rate of shark attack victims is much higher if the patient is resuscitated at the site of the attack and medical help sent for, rather than if attempts are made to transport the victim to hospital.

Sea Wasp or Box Jellyfish (*Chironex fleckeri*)

The sea wasp (Fig. 25.2) is found in northern Australian waters from November to May. The sting to swimmers occurs when they come in contact with long tentacles which discharge stinging cells (nematocysts) into the victim's skin. The victim may experience excruciating pain on contact and

Fig. 25.2 Sea wasps which inhabit the waters of northern Australia.

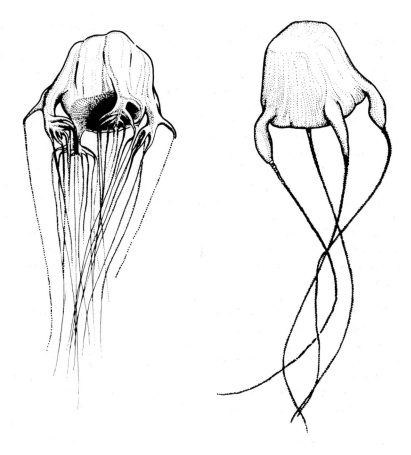

death may occur rapidly as a result of the release of a toxin into the circulation. Treatment of attacks consists of resuscitation after removal from the water. Vinegar, if available is the most effective way to disarm nematocysts and the tentacles should be removed by scraping with a knife or piece of wood. Rubbing the affected area with sand is not advised, as it may cause the nematocysts to discharge. A firm compression bandage must be placed over the affected areas or limbs and urgent medical assistance sought. Fortunately, an antivenene is now available.

Sea Anemones

Though not fatal, the sea anemone also causes pain by contact of nematocyst-laden tentacles with the skin. Vinegar is the most effective treatment to deactivate the nematocysts.

Blue-Ringed Octopus (*Hapa lochaena, H. maculosa*)

The blue-ringed octopus is found in rock pools at the beach and derives its name from the fact that it displays bluish rings if disturbed. This animal carries a toxin in its salivary glands, which it may inject with a bite that may be almost painless. The toxin can produce weakness progressing to paralysis, difficulty in breathing, choking and nausea and collapse may soon follow. Immediate treatment is resuscitation and immobilization of the bite area, with the application of a compression bandage and early transport to a medical facility.

Stonefish

Stonefish are usually found in shallow salty areas and are well camouflaged with a number of spines capable of injecting a toxin into the foot if someone stands on them, with immediate and intense pain. Occasionally in children, shock, respiratory failure and coma may develop.

Immediate treatment includes soaking the limb in hot water if possible. A compression bandage should be applied, followed by local anaesthetic infiltration around the wound and, if necessary, intramuscular injections of analgesics. A stonefish antivenene is available but should only be used if accurate identification is confirmed.

Sea Snakes

Sea snakes are highly venomous but rarely bite and tend to be inquisitive rather than aggressive. Symptoms which may develop approximately 20 min following a bite include stiffness and weakness, aching, muscular contraction and progressive paralysis. More severe developments such as respiratory arrest may also ensue.

Treatment is similar to that for land snakes and includes a compression bandage to the wounded limb, patient immobilization and washing of the surface of the wound. An antivenene is now available.

MEDICAL CONDITIONS OF SWIMMERS

Otitis Externa

The commonest problem of swimmers and divers is infection of the outer ear canal (otitis externa). The condition is more likely to occur if some or all of a number of contributing factors are present:

- Contaminated swimming water
- Continually moist outer ear canal
- The use of implements to clean or dry the ear or to remove wax
- Associated medical conditions such as eczema, diabetes, etc.

A common symptom associated with early infection is itch, which tends to provoke the response of scratching in the ear with implements, thereby compounding the problem. Subsequently, pain, tenderness and discharge develop and hearing may later be affected if debris occludes the canal.

Examination of the ear shows swelling, debris, redness in the canal and tenderness if the ear is manipulated. Occasionally, lymph nodes may be felt behind and in front of the ear. Fungus infections may, however, only cause itching and a sensation of fullness in the ear.

Treatment involves the avoidance of further swimming and other moisture into the ear and any self-treatment such as putting objects into the ear should be avoided. Careful cleaning of the ear is the most important aspect of treatment and one which is often neglected. This may be done by direct swabbing, irrigation or suction depending on the severity of pain and equipment available; however, a swab should be taken from the ear before treatment to identify the offending organisms. Antibiotic/corticosteroid medication in the form of drops, ointment or a wick can be inserted into the canal. Analgesics are usually necessary and if there is severe pain, narcotics may be administered. Frequent follow-up is necessary to monitor progress and the severity of pain and to repeat cleaning procedures where necessary.

Recurrent infections are best prevented by the use of ear plugs and a bathing cap as well as prophylactic antiseptic ear drops such as acetic acid/alcohol or commercial preparations such as 'Aqua-ear'.

Middle Ear Ventilation Tubes (Grommets)

The presence of these tubes through the tympanic membrane (ear-drum) precludes SCUBA diving and springboard or platform diving, but the consensus of opinion is that swimming is permissible. However, antiseptic ear-drops, such as acetic acid, used before and after swimming, combined with ear-plugs, are advisable.

Tympanic Membrane Perforations

These injuries may occur with sudden increases in pressure either in the outer ear, such as in diving from a board or platform, from a water-skiing fall, or during SCUBA diving with failure to equalize pressures across the ear-drum.

The majority of these injuries will heal spontaneously with time, though larger perforations need monitoring by an otologist. Antibiotic prophylaxis may be necessary, particularly if the perforation occurred in contaminated water. A well healed perforation with a mobile drum does not necessarily preclude further SCUBA diving, although thorough specialist assessment is necessary.

Outer Ear Exostoses

Occasionally, swimmers, particularly those who swim frequently in cold water, may develop bony outgrowths in the outer ear canal. These are probably a reactive change and are of no concern unless the canal is completely or almost completely occluded, in which case hearing may be affected, or problems with air entrapment with SCUBA diving may occur.

Epilepsy

The question of whether children with epilepsy should be permitted to swim depends to a large degree on the control of seizures with medication. If the child has not had any seizures for a year, swimming under adult supervision may be permitted. The practice of hyperventilation before breath-hold diving, which is dangerous even for non-epileptics, is especially contra-indicated in epileptics since it may in itself precipitate a seizure. Most studies indicate that the risk of epilepsy causing drowning is quite small and that an attack is more likely to occur in the bath tub at home than during swimming. See Chapter 28 Part II for more detailed information about epilepsy and activity.

CONCLUSIONS

Aquatic activities differ in many ways from land sports, not least because of the relatively high potential for serious injury or fatality that may occur in SCUBA diving, breath-hold diving or from marine bites. As with most potentially dangerous activities, the risks can be minimized by education, preparation and training. It is hoped that this chapter may make the reader aware of some of the more common and serious conditions that accompany water sports, as well as providing guide-lines for managing those conditions when they do arise.

REFERENCES

Edmonds G., Lowry C. & Pennefather J. (1992) *Diving and Subaquatic Medicine*, 3rd edn, pp. 159–197. Butterworth-Heinemann, Sydney.

Gorman D. F. (1989) Decompression sickness and arterial gas embolism in sports SCUBA divers. *Sports Medicine* 8, 32–42.

Greer H. D. & Massey E. W. (1992) Neurologic injury from undersea diving. *Neurologic Clinics* 10, 1031–1045.

Jerrard D. A. (1992) Diving medicine. *Emergency Medical Clinics North America* 10, 329–338.

Kindwall E. P. & Strauss R. H. (1991) Medical aspects of SCUBA and breath-hold diving. In Strauss R. (ed.) *Sports Medicine*, 2nd edn, pp. 409–430. W. B. Saunders, Sydney.

Lin Y-G. (1988) Applied physiology of diving. *Sports Medicine* 5, 41–56.

Neuman T. S. (1987) Diving medicine. *Clinics in Sports Medicine* 6, 647–661.

Sarnaik A. P. & Vohra M. P. (1986) Near-drowning: Fresh, salt and cold water immersion. *Clinics in Sports Medicine* 5, 33–46.

Thomas R. & McKenzie B. (1981) *The Diver's Medical Companion*. The Diving Medical Centre, Sydney.

CHAPTER 26

DOPING

K. D. Fitch and S. P. Haynes

The term 'doping' implies the enhancement of performance in sport by the use of chemical agents. Doping contravenes the ethics of both sport and medical science. The problem of drug misuse in society is widespread and sport is also affected as athletes strive to win because of the various rewards offered to them in modern sport.

The evolution of anti-doping strategies can be demonstrated by listing recent key events, with particular reference to the International Olympic Committee (IOC), which was the first body to conduct an organized campaign against doping in sport.

The IOC Medical Commission's definition of doping is based on the banning of various pharmacological classes of agents. Unless specifically indicated all substances belonging to the banned classes (including veterinary products) may not be used for medical treatment even if not listed as examples. The term 'and related substances' is used to describe drugs which are related by their pharmacological actions and/or their chemical structures.

In January 1994, almost every country and international sports federation agreed to adhere to the IOC list of banned categories of drugs. Table 26.1 highlights these events.

DOPING CLASSES AND METHODS

The five *classes* of doping agents are as follows:

- Stimulants

- Narcotic analgesics
- Anabolic agents
- Diuretics
- Peptide and glycoprotein hormones and analogues

The doping *methods* include:

- Blood doping
- Pharmacological, chemical and physical manipulation

In addition, the IOC lists classes of drugs subject to certain *restrictions*. These are as follows:

- Alcohol
- Marijuana
- Local anaesthetics
- Corticosteroids
- Beta-blockers

Figure 26.1 provides a schema of the 'sites of action' of the respective classes of drugs or agents listed (International Olympic Committee 1994).

Doping Classes

STIMULANTS

This group comprises the broad range of sympathomimetic amines (including *amphetamines* and *ephedrines*) as well as *caffeine* and *cocaine*.

Amphetamines produce their effect by the indirect release of adrenaline and noradrenaline from the adrenal medulla and from noradrenergic nerve

Table 26.1 A chronology of highlights concerning anti-doping activities

1960	Danish cyclist Knut Jensen died at the 1960 Olympic Games in Rome. Amphetamines were found at the autopsy
1967	The IOC banned the use of pharmaceutical agents which were intended to improve athletic performance and established the IOC Medical Commission
1968	Doping control was initiated at the 1968 Olympic Games. Central nervous system stimulants and narcotics tested only
1972	At the Munich Olympic Games seven athletes, including four medallists, were banned
1975	Androgenic anabolic steroids were banned
1976	Eight athletes at the Montreal Olympics were banned for anabolic steroid use
1983	Caffeine and testosterone were added to the banned list
1985	Beta-blockers, diuretics and corticosteroids were added to the banned list
1986	Blood doping was banned
1987	Out-of-competition, unannounced testing was instituted
1988	Peptide hormones, including growth hormone, were banned
1990	Erythropoietin was banned
1992	β-agonists including clenbuterol banned as anabolic agents
1993	Beta-blockers banned only in those sports in which performance may be increased
1994	β_3-agonists banned
	Blood testing introduced into Winter Olympic Games (cross-country skiing events only)
	All but three International Federations agree to use the IOC doping list and penalties

terminals. They have been used in the treatment of obesity, chronic fatigue, depression, narcolepsy and hyperkinesis, although use in the latter two conditions only is acceptable medical therapy. In sport, amphetamines mask fatigue, maintain or improve alertness and possibly contribute towards competitiveness and aggression.

Side-effects of these stimulants include anxiety, tachycardia, palpitations, cardiac arrhythmias, tremor, insomnia, sweating, vertigo and hypertension. Because judgement is impaired, athletes may exercise despite the presence of significantly increased blood lactate levels. Psychological and physical dependence develop with long-term use.

Amphetamine abuse leading to death is well recognized and has been attributed to hyperthermia, heat stroke, hypertensive crisis, or cardiac arrhythmia with myocardial infarction.

Ephedrine was formerly used for asthma, respiratory tract and sinus congestion, allergic conditions and nocturnal enuresis. Its mode of action is the same as for the *amphetamines*, but with fewer central effects, and similar side-effects. The use of *ephedrine* is now considered obsolete but *pseudoephedrine*, *phenylpropanolamine* and other derivatives are still widely used as decongestants. Permitted alternatives to these banned decongestants include the *imidazole* group and *phenylephrine* used topically, for they have a local effect on mucous membranes only.

The β_2-agonists which are widely used and effective in the treatment of asthma and exercise-induced asthma are classified as both stimulants and anabolic agents. When taken by mouth these drugs have powerful stimulatory and anabolic effects. However, when administered by inhalation no anabolic effects have been observed. All β_2-agonists are banned by the oral route and by injection. Currently, only *salbutamol* and *terbutaline* are permitted but only by inhalation. Physicians wishing to administer either drug during competitions should notify the relevant medical authority.

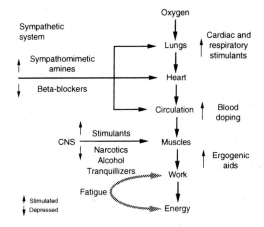

Fig. 26.1 A schema of the 'sites of action' of various drugs.

Caffeine is a methyl-xanthine derivative and is a constituent of coffee, tea, cola drinks, chocolate and many analgesic and migraine preparations. It is known to assist in reducing fatigue, has diuretic properties, stimulates cardiac and skeletal muscle and relaxes smooth muscle (Van Handel 1983). Endurance performance has been demonstrated to be greatly enhanced by caffeine ingestion, probably via a glycogen sparing effect, whereby free fatty acids are mobilized from triglycerides and used as substrates for energy (Graham & Spriet 1991). Caffeine has a stimulatory effect by blocking inhibitory adenosine receptors in the central nervous system, by increasing cyclic adenosine monophosphate activity and by increasing muscle cell membrane permeability to calcium ions thereby improving contractibility.

Side-effects of caffeine include tremor, palpitations, restlessness, anxiety, headache, irritability, diuresis and gastrointestinal symptoms. Caffeine is banned by the IOC because of its stimulant effects, but a level of caffeine of 12 mg$\cdot$L^{-1} must be obtained in the urine to be deemed positive. Table 26.2 lists the stimulants banned by the IOC.

NARCOTIC ANALGESICS

This group of drugs includes derivatives of the Asian poppy, the opiates and their related compounds, including *morphine*. They reduce moderate to severe pain and they are known for their capacity to produce dependence and addiction. They have major side-effects including respiratory depression, which may be fatal. They are banned because of

Table 26.2 Stimulants banned by the IOC

Amiphenazole	Fencamfamine
Amphetamines	Mesocarb
Amineptine	Pentylentetrazol
Caffeine*	Pipradol
Cocaine	Salbutamol†
Ephedrines	Terbutaline†
	And related substances

*Caffeine >12 mg$\cdot$L^{-1} of urine
(Note: Caffeine: 100–150 mg per cup of coffee; 30–45 mg per cup of tea; 45–65 mg per cup of cola.)
†Permitted by inhaler only and must be declared to the relevant medical authority.

Table 26.3 Narcotic analgesics banned by the IOC

Dextromoramide	Morphine
Dextropropoxyphen	Pentazocine
Diamorphine (heroin)	Pethidine
Methadone	And related substances

their ergogenic effect (masking pain and inducing euphoria) and because of the World Health Organization recommendations restricting the use and movement of these drugs internationally.

Alternatives to narcotic analgesics include non-steroidal anti-inflammatory medications, which have analgesic properties. These are not banned and include the propionic acid derivatives, the indoles and salicylates.

Codeine, dihydrocodeine, pholcodine and *dextromethorphan* are not banned. *Diphenoxylate* is permitted for the management of diarrhoea.

Table 26.3 lists the narcotic analgesics banned by the IOC.

ANABOLIC AGENTS

Androgenic anabolic steroids (for brevity termed anabolic steroids) are the most commonly identified group of drugs in positive drug tests and include those chemicals which are related in structure and activity to the male sex hormone testosterone. Figure 26.2 illustrates some examples of this group.

Testosterone produces the secondary sex characteristics of males and affects the development of the skin, hair, voice and sex organs as well as increased growth of bone and muscle during puberty. Synthetic analogues of testosterone attempt to maximize the anabolic properties of testosterone while minimizing the side-effects. Synthesis of testosterone analogues can be achieved by alkylation at the C_{17} α-portion, by esterification of the C_{17} β-hydroxyl group, and by modification of the ring structure (at C_1 in most cases, but also at C_2, C_9 and C_{11}). Each of these processes produces particular characteristics of hepatotoxicity, fat-solubility and efficacy (or otherwise) of oral and injectable preparations. For example, C_{17} alkylated derivatives such as *oxandrolone* and *stanozolol* are resistant to degradation and are hepatotoxic; the C_{17} esters such as testosterone enanthate and nandrolone

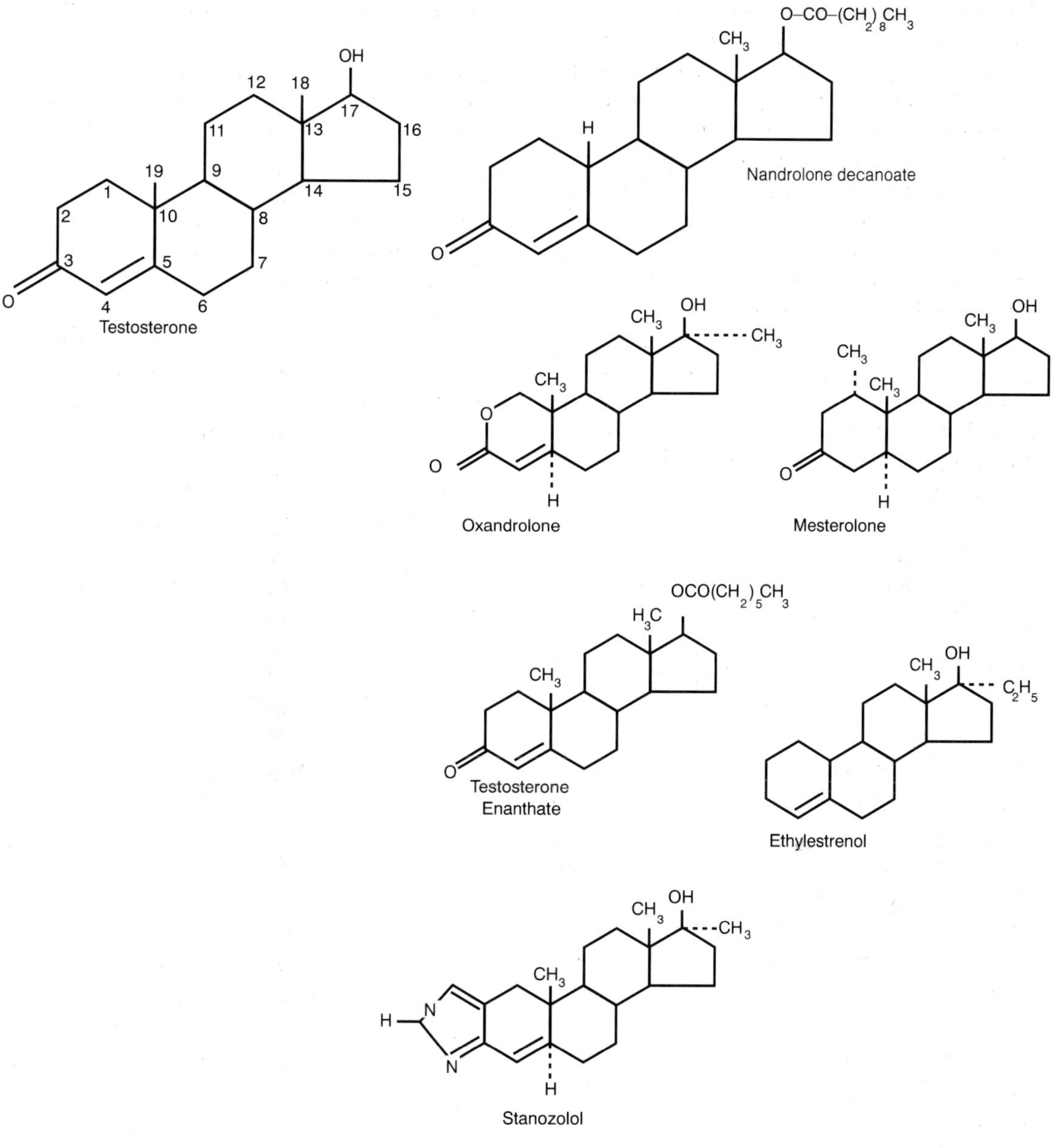

Fig. 26.2 The chemical structure of various anabolic steroids.

decanoate are highly lipid soluble and need to be injected; and C_1 methyl derivatives, such as *methenolone* and *mesterolone* are oral preparations.

Athletes using anabolic steroids are alleged to recover more quickly from hard training sessions and can therefore train at a higher intensity and more often than those individuals who are not using them. Athletes who rely on strength and power in their performances are the ones who appear to obtain the greatest benefit.

Three mechanisms for the actions of anabolic steroids in increasing muscle strength have been proposed. They are:

593

- An increase in protein synthesis in muscle as a direct action of the anabolic steroid
- Blocking of the catabolic effect of glucocorticoids after exercise, by increasing the amount of anabolic hormone available
- Steroid-induced enhancement of aggressive

behaviour that promotes a greater quantity and quality of weight-training (American College of Sports Medicine 1984)

The side-effects of anabolic steroids are listed in Table 26.4 and include many permanent, unpredictable and serious conditions.

These side-effects are compounded by the trend to cycle dosage regimens over a period of 1–4 months with a gradual increase in dosage followed by gradual reduction, and then usually a break for a few weeks or months before repeating the regimen. 'Stacking', a term indicating the concurrent use of combinations of oral and injectable preparations during the cycle, provides very large doses of anabolic steroids and further compounds the risk. In addition, some athletes take sedatives and tranquillizers to counter the anxiety and aggression or other effects of anabolic steroids. Self-injecting anabolic steroids with shared needles has resulted in the catastrophic transmission of the human immunodeficiency virus (HIV) and the hepatitis B virus (Sklarek *et al.* 1984). There is increasing evidence that physical and psychological dependence on anabolic steroids may develop in a proportion of users. Indeed this category of drugs does fulfil many of the criteria for drug dependence as defined by the American Psychiatric Association (Brower 1993).

Table 26.4 The side-effects of anabolic steroids

Psychological changes	Euphoria, mania, depression, psychosis, impulsive and aggressive behaviour, drug dependence
Metabolic changes	Salt and water retention
Hormonal effects	Gynaecomastia Testicular atrophy Decreased spermatogenesis Changes in libido Prostatic hypertrophy Decreased follicle-stimulating hormone and luteinizing hormone levels
Skin and hair changes	Acne Alopecia
Tendon	Tendinitis Rupture — partial and complete
Blood lipid alteration	Increased triglycerides Increased low-density lipoprotein cholesterol Decreased high-density lipoprotein cholesterol
Cardiovascular effects	Hypertension Atherogenesis Sudden death
Kidney tumours	Wilms' tumour
Liver	Elevated transaminases Cholestatic jaundice Peliosis hepatitis Hepatoma Carcinoma
Additionally in females	Virilizing effects Menstrual disturbances Infertility Breast atrophy Clitoral hypertrophy Hirsutism
In children	Premature epiphyseal closure Premature virilization

Table 26.5 Anabolic steroids banned by the IOC

Clostebol	Nandrolone
Fluoxymesterone	Oxandrolone
Metandienone	Stanozolol
Metenolone	Testosterone* And related substances

*Testosterone. The presence of a testosterone to epitestosterone ratio greater than six in the urine of a competitor constitutes an offence unless there is evidence that this ratio is due to a physiological or pathological condition (e.g. low epitestosterone excretion, production of androgen by a tumour, enzyme deficiency). However, before a decision is made to consider the athlete positive or negative, the results of previous tests, subsequent tests and any endocrine investigations shall be reviewed. In the event that previous tests are not available, the athlete should be tested unannounced at least monthly for 3 months.

It should be stated that the use of anabolic steroids by athletes to gain an unfair advantage is contrary to the ethical principles of athletic competition and is to be deplored. In addition, many countries have now listed anabolic steroids as controlled substances and therefore subject to legal restrictions. Examples of anabolic steroids are contained in Table 26.5.

Recent research has revealed that chronic use of anabolic steroids can result in the suppression of endogenous production of testosterone. This in turn is accompanied by reduced levels of the urinary androgens, androsterone and etiocholanolone. Estimation of these steroids is described as 'steroid profiling' and can be utilized to refute a denial by an athlete that he/she has ever used anabolic steroids, or if abnormally low, to target such athletes for future tests when out of competition (Fig. 26.3).

Recently, bodybuilders and power athletes have sought to benefit from the anabolic effects of β-agonist drugs. *Clenbuterol*, a long-acting preparation which is mainly used as a 're-partitioning' agent to increase muscle and reduce fat in cattle, sheep and pigs prior to sale for meat (Yang & McElligott

1989) has been widely used. Two of the five positive doping cases at the Barcelona Olympic Games were athletes in field events who had taken *clenbuterol*. Long-acting *salbutamol* has been demonstrated to rapidly and significantly increase strength of muscles in non-athletes who did not undertake any exercise training (Martineau *et al.* 1992). *Clenbuterol* was banned by the IOC in 1992 and all oral and injectable β_2-agonists were specifically banned as anabolic agents in 1994. β_3-agonists, which are to be marketed commercially as anti-obesity agents, are also likely to be banned because of their presumed anabolic effects.

DIURETICS

Table 26.6 lists examples of diuretics which are banned. These drugs promote water and electrolyte (particularly sodium) loss from the body by action at various sites in the kidney. The medical indications for their use include hypertension, congestive cardiac failure and some renal conditions (including renal failure). Side-effects include electrolyte depletion (hyponatraemia, hypokalaemia) and dehydration. Diuretics should only be used under medical supervision.

Diuretics are used by athletes to reduce weight quickly in sports where weight restrictions apply and to dilute the concentration in urine of banned substances in an attempt to evade detection. The risks of rapid weight loss equal the risks of dehydration, as cramps and muscle strains are common and suboptimal performance is usually evident. Severe fluid and electrolyte loss is also accompanied by a grave risk of cardiac arrhythmia. Moreover, the manipulation of bodyweight by dehydration is deemed unethical and in sports involving weight divisions or classes, athletes may be required to provide urine samples at the time of the weigh-in.

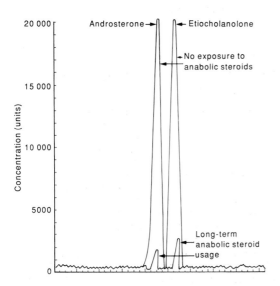

Fig. 26.3 Modification of endogenous androgenic steroids by long-term use of synthetic anabolic steroids (schematic representation of urinary chromatogram).

Table 26.6 Diuretics banned by the IOC

Acetazolamide	Mannitol
Bumetanide	Mersalyl
Chlortalidone	Spironolactone
Ethacrynic acid	Triamterene
Furosemide	And related substances
Hydrochlorothiazide	

PEPTIDE AND GLYCOPROTEIN HORMONES AND ANALOGUES

Human chorionic gonadotrophin (hCG) is a hormone produced in pregnancy which promotes fetal growth. It is known that the administration of this substance and others with similar effects increases the rate of production of androgenic steroids in males and is considered equivalent to the exogenous administration of testosterone. The use of these substances is therefore banned.

Athletes sometimes use hCG as an injectable preparation, often with other anabolic agents such as anabolic steroids and human growth hormone (hGH). The rationale for the use of hCG includes the belief that the testosterone/epitestosterone ratio, used in dope testing to determine a positive test, is normalized. Some athletes also believe that hCG prevents testicular atrophy, which is a possible consequence of ingesting anabolic steroids.

Corticotrophin (adrenocorticotrophic hormone, ACTH) is a polypeptide hormone produced by the anterior lobe of the pituitary gland which stimulates the production of corticosteroids from the adrenal cortex. Injectable synthetic forms are available which have a role in clinical medicine, especially in the area of adrenal disorders. Some athletes have misused ACTH to increase blood levels of endogenous corticosteroids and for the associated euphoric effect. ACTH is banned on the grounds that it has the same effect as oral, intramuscular or intravenous preparations of corticosteroids. Further discussion of corticosteroids and their use can be found later in this chapter.

hGH, or somatotrophin, is produced by the anterior lobe of the pituitary gland and its release is regulated by two other hormones, growth hormone releasing hormone (GHRH) and somatostatin (SS). hGH release produces somatomedins or insulin-like growth factors from the liver and other tissues. These somatomedins provide a feedback control mechanism for hGH release by stimulating SS and inhibiting GHRH (see Fig. 26.4).

hGH is an anabolic agent in that it promotes amino acid transport and protein synthesis, increases lean bodyweight and cellular growth, accelerates linear bone growth and promotes lipolysis. It has a diabetogenic effect by inducing hyperglycaemia from hepatic glycogen stores and by blocking glucose uptake into peripheral tissues such as muscle (an 'anti-insulin' effect). hGH stimulates osteogenesis and erythropoiesis, increases renal blood flow, glomerular filtration rate and tubular reabsorption of phosphate. hGH administered to hGH-deficient children normalizes their decreased number of muscle cells.

Secretion of hGH in normal people (Haynes 1986) is triggered by hypoglycaemia, amino acid infusion (notably L-arginine, histidine and phenylalanine), slow wave sleep, stress, exercise, pain, noradrenaline, serotonin, glucagon, prostaglandins, L-dopa, clonidine, beta-blockers, and bromocriptine. Excess hGH production is responsible for acromegaly and gigantism (post-dating and pre-dating epiphyseal closure, respectively). In these clinical situations, articular cartilage hypertrophies and then degenerates, muscle strengthens and then weakens and male acromegalics are usually impotent.

hGH was originally isolated from pituitary glands of cadavers but discovery of the slow virus responsible for Kreutzfeldt-Jacob disease encouraged the development of hGH production by recombinant techniques, using bacterium *Escherichia coli*. Recombinant hGH (rhGH) is used in the treatment of

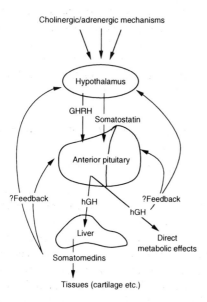

Fig. 26.4 The control of human growth hormone (hGH) secretion.

hGH deficiency in children of short stature and also in Turner's syndrome (chromosomal XO). Athletes are misusing rhGH because of its anabolic effect. It is often used with anabolic steroids. The IOC has banned its use on the grounds of ethics in competition and because of the potential for serious side-effects, such as cardiomyopathy, hypertension, diabetes mellitus and acromegaly.

Erythropoietin (EPO) is a recent addition to the list of banned substances. It is a polypeptide produced in the kidney, which stimulates red blood cell production in response to stimuli such as blood loss, altitude and hypoxia. *Recombinant EPO* (rEPO) is now freely available commercially and is administered to correct the anaemia secondary to renal failure. Side-effects of EPO include hypertension, electrolyte abnormalities, seizures, thrombosis and bone pain. rEPO has been demonstrated to be as effective as blood doping in the improvement of endurance capacity and $\dot{V}_{O2max}$ (Ekblom & Berglund 1991). Although at present there is no definitive test for its use as a doping agent, artificial elevation of red blood cell concentration constitutes doping, as there are benefits to endurance performance. The benefits of increased red blood cell concentration are discussed later in this chapter when blood doping is considered.

Doping Methods

BLOOD DOPING

Blood doping is an ergogenic procedure wherein normovolaemic erythrocythaemia (an increased concentration of red blood cells) is induced by way of reinfusion of the athlete's own blood (autologous infusion) or by transfusing cross-matched blood from another donor (homologous infusion). The result is an increased oxygen-carrying capacity of the blood (Ca_{O2}, arterial oxygen concentration) so that during peak exercise, the delivery of oxygen to the skeletal muscle is enhanced and maximal oxygen uptake ($\dot{V}_{O2max}$) and endurance capacity are improved.

In medical practice the most common indications for red blood cell transfusion are acute blood loss and severe anaemia.

Blood doping in sport contravenes the ethics of medicine and of sport. There are also the risks of blood transfusion side-effects, including allergic rashes and fevers, acute haemolysis (red cell breakdown) with inherent risk to the kidneys, transmission of viruses such as hepatitis B and HIV and fluid overload. Blood doping may also induce a hyperviscosity syndrome, leading to intravascular clotting, heart failure and death.

Therefore blood doping is banned as an ergogenic aid. Blood testing was introduced in 1989 by the FIS (Federation Internationale de Ski) in cross-country events and by the IAAF in 1993 in four Grand Prix meetings in Europe. The IOC approved blood testing in cross-country skiing events at the 1994 Lillehammer Olympic Winter Games. No problems have been encountered and acceptance by athletes has been excellent. At the current state of research only the detection of homologous blood transfusion can be proved (Fagerhol & Heier 1993).

PHARMACOLOGICAL, CHEMICAL AND PHYSICAL MANIPULATION

The use of substances and of methods which alter the integrity and validity of urine samples in doping control are also banned. Such methods include the use of catheters and other devices to substitute urine and agents such as *probenecid* to diminish the renal secretion of banned substances. The administration of epitestosterone, an inert anabolic steroid but taken to normalize the testosterone/epitestosterone ratio, is also banned. Urinary concentrations of epitestosterone greater than $200 \, mg \cdot mL^{-1}$ require further investigation.

Classes of Drugs Subject to Certain Restrictions

ALCOHOL, MARIJUANA AND SEDATIVES

Alcohol adversely affects reaction time, hand–eye co-ordination, accuracy, balance and complex co-ordination. It certainly does not improve, and may even decrease, strength, power, local muscular endurance, speed and cardiovascular endurance. Alcohol can also induce pathological changes in the heart, liver, neural tissue and muscle which may be fatal. Some athletes ingest alcohol to relax and to boost confidence, in the hope of improving their performance, particularly in shooting events. Alcohol is not prohibited but may be tested (by breathalyser) if requested by any international federation. Marijuana is also used as a relaxing agent and its use may be restricted by an international federation.

LOCAL ANAESTHETICS

Injectable local anaesthetics are permitted under the following conditions:

- Bupivacaine, lignocaine, mepivacaine, procaine but not cocaine, may be used. In conjunction with local anaesthetics, vasoconstrictor agents (e.g. adrenaline) are permitted
- Only local or intra-articular injections may be administered
- Local anaesthetics are permitted in competition only when medically justified (the details including diagnosis, dose and route of administration must be submitted in writing to the relevant medical authority)

CORTICOSTEROIDS

Chapter 13 discusses the pharmacology of corticosteroids. These agents are used in medicine as anti-inflammatory preparations and in the management of adrenal insufficiency, and are available in oral, injectable and topical forms. Systemic corticosteroids produce euphoria and a range of other side-effects, and their use requires medical supervision. These side-effects include adrenal suppression, sodium and water retention, decreased immune function, skin changes, osteoporosis and avascular necrosis of bone, notably the head of the femur.

Since 1975, the IOC has restricted the use of corticosteroids by athletes and they are banned except for topical use (aural, ophthalmological and dermatological conditions), inhalation therapy (asthma and allergic rhinitis) and local, intralesional or intra-articular injections. Because of a great and unexplained increase in the use of inhaled corticosteroids by cross-country skiers, in 1993 the IOC introduced the requirement of notification of use of these agents. A doctor who administers corticosteroids by local or intra-articular injection or by inhalation to an athlete may be required to notify the relevant medical authority and should provide the competitor with a certificate containing the details of any injection.

BETA-BLOCKERS

Adrenergic receptors are classified into α- and β-receptors. β-receptors are either β_1, found in cardiac tissue, adipose tissue and kidneys, or β_2, found in smooth muscle, glands, blood vessels, liver and bronchi. Beta-blockers prevent the effects of the β-receptors. Table 26.7 lists beta-blockers which are prescribed to treat hypertension, angina, cardiac arrhythmias, migraine, anxiety, thyrotoxicosis, glaucoma and hypertrophic subaortic stenosis. Beta-blockers usually produce little or no effect in sprint events, weight-lifting or isometric exercise (Rusko *et al.* 1980).

Table 26.7 Beta-blockers banned by the IOC

Acebutolol	Nadolol
Alprenolol	Oxyprenolol
Atenolol	Propranolol
Labetolol	Sotalol
Metoprolol	And related substances

During submaximal exercise in healthy subjects, however, beta-blockers can decrease heart rate, systolic blood pressure and cardiac output and increase the arteriovenous oxygen difference. Endurance events necessitate prolonged periods of high cardiac output and depend on the availability of metabolic substrates. Beta-blockers therefore interfere with performance in these events via the beta-blockade of glycogenolysis, lipolysis and gluconeogenesis.

Beta-blockers have been misused in shooting sports to control tremor (via blockade of β_2 receptors in muscle spindles and extrafusal fibres) and to reduce the heart rate to permit shots to be fired between heart beats. The anti-anxiety effect is the reason beta-blockers are banned in sports such as ski jumping and bobsleigh. In 1993 the IOC recommended that beta-blockers be banned only in sports in which performance may be enhanced.

These include archery, bobsleigh, diving, freestyle skiing, luge, modern pentathlon and ski jumping.

PERMITTED USE OF BANNED DRUGS

It is inevitable that on occasions an athlete will have an undeniable justification to take a drug in the banned classes of the IOC. Since 1992, the IOC Medical Commission has had a small subcommittee which examines such applications and recommends approval or regulation of such applications. The principles involved are that the athlete would:

- Experience significant impairment of health and performance if the drug was withheld
- Obtain no enhancement of performance from taking the banned drug; the sport involved may need to be considered
- Not be denied the drug if he or she was not a competing athlete

A number of countries including Australia, Finland, Norway and the USA also have a mechanism to permit the medical use of a banned drug in exceptional circumstances. To assist doctors to identify which drugs are permitted or banned in sport, in 1990 an Australian publication *Drugs and Sport* categorized every pharmaceutical product listed in Australia as either permitted or banned (Badewitz-Dodd 1992). *Drugs and Sport* has been regularly updated and other countries have followed Australia's lead and produced their own publication.

DOPING CONTROL

Selection of Athletes

Athletes are liable to be drug tested either at competitions, or during training, which is termed 'out of competition testing'. The latter targets illicit use of anabolic steroids and peptide and glycoprotein hormones and such tests are customarily unannounced or undertaken with minimal notice. Several international sports federations have the authority to perform unannounced tests using 'flying squads'. At competitions, individual place-getters are usually tested but in team events, players are selected by a random draw. Athletes may be tested on more than one occasion in a season or in a major competition.

Sample Taking

Strict rules are applied immediately an athlete is notified that he or she has been selected for a drug test after competition. The athlete is chaperoned by an official until urine samples have been obtained, identified, coded and sealed. A team official, coach or a doctor may accompany the athlete who signs appropriate documents to confirm that no irregularities have occurred during the sampling process, copies of these documents being provided to the athlete. Urine samples A and B (divided by the athlete prior to sealing) are then delivered under secure protection to an accredited laboratory.

If an athlete refuses to provide a urine sample, he or she should be warned of the consequences, as a refusal is a serious offence and usually incurs the same penalty as a positive test.

Sample Analysis

The urine sample is analysed as soon as possible after its arrival at the laboratory, and analysis follows well established methods approved by the IOC Medical Commission. Should analysis of the first sample indicate the presence of a banned substance, the second sample is analysed after prescribed procedures of notification have been completed.

Detection of Banned Substances

Analysis of urine samples is highly technical, complex and accurate. Gas chromatography or high-pressure liquid chromatography and mass spectrometer methods are used to identify the 'fingerprint' of the individual compound and are highly specific.

Testing for naturally occurring substances such as testosterone, hCG, EPO, hGH and autologous blood transfusions constitute the greater challenges. While some progress has been made with testosterone and hCG, a number of groups of scientists are currently engaged in research to develop methods to identify doping by rEPO, rhGH and autologous blood.

Testing is expensive and becoming more so as new substances are added to the list of banned substances. However, the protection of the athlete and of fair competition justify this cost.

THE ROLE OF THE TEAM PHYSICIAN

Before and during competition, the team physician should personally review all medication carried by or used by athletes in his or her care and all medications used should be recorded. Athletes must be briefed thoroughly on the philosophy behind doping control, the procedures involved in drug testing and those medications on the banned list. In particular, attention should be paid to warning athletes about the risks of ingesting over-the-counter preparations which may contain banned substances, notably pseudoephedrine.

CONCLUSIONS

There is a need for further research into physiological and psychological training programmes which contribute to improved performance and which demonstrate the possibility of achieving one's 'ultimate performance' without recourse to unethical ergogenic aids. Drug education programmes must also be developed and directed at athletes, coaches, doctors and administrators, so as to inform them of the serious side-effects of many drugs and to promote a commitment to the principles of fair competition. More experience with blood testing will provide an additional method to identify athletes who seek to cheat by pharmacological means. However, it must be stressed that urinalysis will remain the principal method of detection of drugs at least until the twenty-first century.

REFERENCES

American College of Sports Medicine (1984) *Position Statement on the Use of Anabolic–Androgenic Steroids in Sports.* American College of Sports Medicine, Indianapolis, MN.

Badewitz-Dodd L. (ed.) (1992) *Drugs and Sport.* IMS Publishing, Sydney.

Brower K. J. (1993) Anabolic steroids: Potential for physical and psychological dependence. In Yesalis C. E. (ed.) *Anabolic Steroids in Sport and Exercise*, pp. 195–209. Human Kinetics Publishers, Champaign, IL.

Ekblom B. & Berglund B. (1991) Effect of erythropoietin administration on maximal aerobic power. *Scandinavian Journal of Medicine and Science in Sports* 1, 88–93.

Fagerhol M. & Heier H. E. (1994) Detection of transfused allogenic blood. In Hemmersbach P. & Birkeland K. T. (eds) *Blood Samples in Doping Control*, pp. 161–162. On Demand Publishing, Oslo.

Graham T. E. & Spriet L. L. (1991) Performance and metabolic responses to a high caffeine dose during prolonged exercise. *Journal of Applied Physiology* 71, 2292–2298.

Haynes S. P. (1986) Growth hormone. *Australian Journal of Science and Medicine in Sport* 18, 3–15.

International Olympic Committee, Medical Commission. Definition of Doping and List of Doping Classes and Methods, September 1994.

Martineau L., Horan M. A., Rothwell N. J. & Little R. A. (1992) Salbutamol, a β_2-adrenoceptor agonist increases muscle strength in young men. *Clinical Science* 83, 615–621.

Rusko H., Kartola H., Luhtanen P., Pulli M., Videman T. & Viitasalo J. T. (1980) Effect of beta-blockers on performances requiring force, velocity, coordination and/or anaerobic metabolism. *Journal of Sports Medicine and Physical Fitness* 20, 139–144.

Sklarek H. M., Mantovani R. D., Erens E., Heisler D., Niederman M. S. & Fein A. M. (1984) AIDS in a bodybuilder using anabolic steroids. *New England Journal of Medicine* 311, 1701.

Van Handel P. (1983) Caffeine. In Williams M. H. (ed.) *Ergogenic Aids in Sports*, pp. 128–163. Human Kinetics Publishers, Champaign, IL.

Yang Y. T. & McElligott M. A. (1989) Multiple actions of β-adrenergic agonists on skeletal muscle and adipose tissue. *Biochemistry Journal* 261, 1–10.

CHAPTER 27

EXERCISE AND IMMUNITY

D. B. Pyne, A. B. Gray and W. A. McDonald

Interest in the relationship between exercise and immunity has been generated in medical, scientific and sporting communities. It is often claimed that elite athletes experience a greater incidence of illness and infection during periods of prolonged or intense training, yet paradoxically, physically active members of the general public who undertake regular bouts of moderately intense physical activity contend that they feel healthier and suffer fewer illnesses. The underlying interest for the athlete is to maintain good health and performance levels during regular training and competition. Scientific interest in the field has increased significantly over the last 5 years. It is timely that we examine the relationship between exercise and immunity, as the area can be confusing to medical practitioners and sports scientists and has potential applications to both the sporting and general communities.

It is important to note that the degree and consequences of exercise-induced changes in immune function seen in otherwise healthy athletes, are normally less than those seen in classical immunodeficiencies or immunological diseases such as rheumatoid arthritis or insulin-dependent diabetes mellitus. The concern for athletes, coaches and sports medicine practitioners is that the intensive and prolonged exercise and training programmes undertaken by some athletes may increase the risk of illness and infection. In sport, the most prevalent infections, such as the common cold or the range of viral illnesses, may compromise an athlete's ability to train and compete at his or her normal level. By studying the relationship between exercise and immunity, it is possible to formulate some training and life-style recommendations which may reduce the incidence of illness.

However, resistance to infection is not the only area where study of the immune system may be beneficial. Because the immune system plays an integral role in tissue repair, immune research may guide us to a better understanding of the effects of tissue damage and, perhaps, the process of overtraining. Study of this nature may also establish whether physical activity can play a beneficial part in the management of disease states.

This chapter outlines the components and organization of the immune system, examines the effects of acute exercise and prolonged training, reviews the infections commonly seen in athletes, provides some discussion on research into a range of daily influences on immunity and makes a number of practical suggestions to minimize the risk of illness interrupting training or competition.

OVERVIEW OF THE IMMUNE SYSTEM

While the immune system is a complex organization of physical, cellular and soluble components, its importance in protecting the body against illness and infection is understood intuitively. The following discussion is presented as a basic guide to understanding the means by which an athlete's immune system deals with the common viral and bacterial infections of the upper respiratory and gastrointestinal tracts.

The immune system undergoes a co-ordinated sequence of steps in response to various challenges, from the initial mobilization of immune cells and soluble factors (such as complement and antibodies), to the elimination of foreign material, the repair of damaged tissues (discussed in Chapter 12), and ultimately, restoration of physiological and immune health. These challenges can be categorized as either extrinsic or intrinsic in nature (Fig. 27.1). The extrinsic challenges include the classical pathogenic agents such as viruses, bacteria, parasites and fungi,

Fig. 27.1 The human immune system (cellular and soluble components) and physical barriers providing host defence against extrinsic and intrinsic challenges.

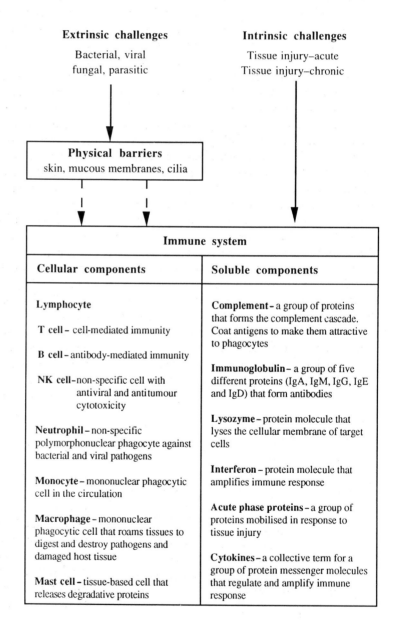

Extrinsic challenges
Bacterial, viral
fungal, parasitic

Intrinsic challenges
Tissue injury–acute
Tissue injury–chronic

Physical barriers
skin, mucous membranes, cilia

Immune system

Cellular components	Soluble components
Lymphocyte **T cell** – cell-mediated immunity **B cell** – antibody-mediated immunity **NK cell** – non-specific cell with antiviral and antitumour cytotoxicity **Neutrophil** – non-specific polymorphonuclear phagocyte against bacterial and viral pathogens **Monocyte** – mononuclear phagocytic cell in the circulation **Macrophage** – mononuclear phagocytic cell that roams tissues to digest and destroy pathogens and damaged host tissue **Mast cell** – tissue-based cell that releases degradative proteins	**Complement** – a group of proteins that forms the complement cascade. Coat antigens to make them attractive to phagocytes **Immunoglobulin** – a group of five different proteins (IgA, IgM, IgG, IgE and IgD) that form antibodies **Lysozyme** – protein molecule that lyses the cellular membrane of target cells **Interferon** – protein molecule that amplifies immune response **Acute phase proteins** – a group of proteins mobilised in response to tissue injury **Cytokines** – a collective term for a group of protein messenger molecules that regulate and amplify immune response

which are present in both the general community and specific sporting environments, such as changing rooms and competitive arenas. Intrinsic challenge relates to direct tissue damage or injury sustained through either acute (sudden onset) or chronic (gradual onset) means. Injuries of both types are commonly observed in recreational and elite athletes and, depending on the severity, initiate a variable inflammatory and immunological response.

The physical barriers of host defence include the skin, the mucous membrane lining the mouth and nose, and the mucus and cilia lining the respiratory tract. These barriers provide an initial mechanical line of defence against pathogenic agents.

The cellular and soluble immune system is categorized into non-specific (innate) and specific (acquired) divisions (Table 27.1). The non-specific immune system consists of phagocytic and natural killer (NK) cells, and a number of soluble factors in the circulation, which collectively provide an immediate response to bacterial, viral, fungal and parasitic attack. These components do not require prior contact with an infectious agent and therefore act as a first line of defence. The process of phagocytosis involves the engulfment of pathogenic agents and the release of toxic molecules which degrade and eliminate those molecules targeted for destruction. NK cells, which kill tumour cells and those infected by viruses, are a subclass of lymphocytes that do not require antigen–antibody interaction to exert their cytotoxic effects.

The specific system consists of lymphocyte cells (T cells [thymus derived], which form cell-mediated immunity and B cells [bone marrow derived], which contribute to antibody-mediated immunity) and soluble factors (immunoglobulins), which target specific infectious agents. In contrast to non-specific immunity, the specific defence mechanism is activated after an initial exposure to an antigen. The process of producing antibodies to combat previously unencountered foreign agents normally requires about 72 h. The simultaneous production of memory cells (specialized T cells) greatly enhances the rate of this process upon any subsequent re-exposure to the same foreign agent. Non-specific and specific elements work in concert to eliminate pathogenic agents.

Immunoglobulins are a group of glycoprotein molecules in serum and mucosal fluids, which carry antibody activity and are produced by plasma cells (originating from B lymphocytes). There are five classes of immunoglobulins termed immunoglobulin A (IgA), M (IgM), G (IgG), D (IgD) and E (IgE). IgA, the principal immunoglobulin in mucosal fluids, is known to inhibit the attachment and colonization of micro-organisms to host tissues, and to neutralize viruses. Given that the most common route of entry into the body for viral agents responsible for upper respiratory tract infections (URTI) is through the nose and mouth, the IgA dissolved in the mucosal fluids (e.g. saliva) lining these areas, constitutes the primary defence mechanism against these particular agents. This is achieved by the IgA molecule coating the infectious agent. For this reason, secretory IgA has been the most frequently studied immunoglobulin in relation to acute submaximal and maximal exercise and prolonged training.

SPECIFIC IMMUNE RESPONSES

Specific immune responses are categorized as either antibody-mediated immunity or cell-mediated immunity and form a central part of the body's host defence against infection. A description of these mechanisms is critical to a basic understanding of the immune system, of how specific antibodies are produced for each specific foreign antigen and for evaluating the effects of exercise and training on different aspects of immunity.

Table 27.1 Division of the human immune system into non-specific and specific host defence

Host defence	Cellular components	Soluble components
Non-specific (innate)	Neutrophils	Acute phase proteins
	Eosinophils	Complement
	Basophils	Lysozyme
	Macrophages	Interferon
	NK cells	Cytokines
Specific (acquired)	T lymphocytes B lymphocytes	Immunoglobulins

Antibody-mediated (Humoral) Immunity

Antibody-mediated (humoral) immunity involves the production of specific antibodies (immuno-globulins) which attack and neutralize an antigen (a target molecule from an infectious agent), or coat a microbe in such a way that makes it attractive to scavenger white cells such as macrophages or neutrophils. The lymphocytes responsible for this humoral immunity largely reside in the primary lymphoid organs: the thymus gland and bone marrow. After leaving these organs, the lympho-cytes travel in the circulation before reaching one of the secondary lymphoid organs: the lymph nodes, spleen, tonsils, gut or skin (Fig. 27.2). Following injury or infection, activated lympho-cytes leave the lymph nodes and travel through the lymphatic system until they enter the bloodstream.

Only 2–5% of the total lymphocyte population is normally present in the circulation; thus most of the specific immune reactions take place either in the lymph nodes or at the site of infection.

The antibody-mediated process involves a sequence of co-ordinated steps to eliminate patho-genic agents (Fig. 27.3). Professional phagocytes roam the circulation (monocytes) and tissues (macro-phages), where they ingest antigens and fragment them into antigenic peptides. These peptides are joined to major histocompatibility complex (MHC) molecules located on the phagocyte cell membrane and displayed for recognition by T-lymphocyte cells bearing the appropriate receptor for the antigenic peptide. Binding to the MHC–peptide complex causes the lymphocyte to activate, divide and release lymphokines (immunomodulatory messenger molecules), which mobilize other elements of the immune system. Among the cells

Fig. 27.2 The lymphatic system showing the primary lymphoid organs (bone marrow and thymus) and the secondary lymphoid organs (spleen, tonsils and lymph nodes): LV = lymphatic vessels.

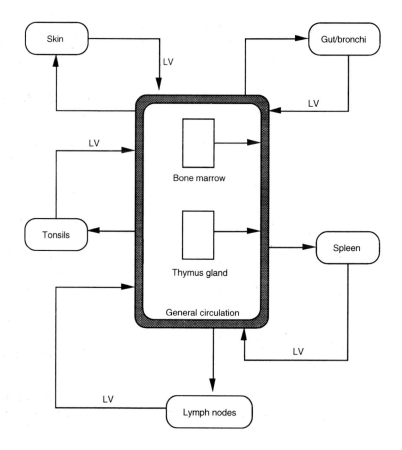

that respond to these signals are the B lymphocytes, which also bear receptor molecules of a single specificity on their surface. The B cells are activated and divide — in a process known as clonal expansion — and eventually differentiate into plasma cells which secrete antibodies (immunoglobulins). These antibodies are essentially soluble forms of the B-cell receptor. Antibody synthesis can occur at an astonishing rate with a single cell able to produce more than 10 million antibodies in an hour. The antibodies bind to the specific antigens and facilitate

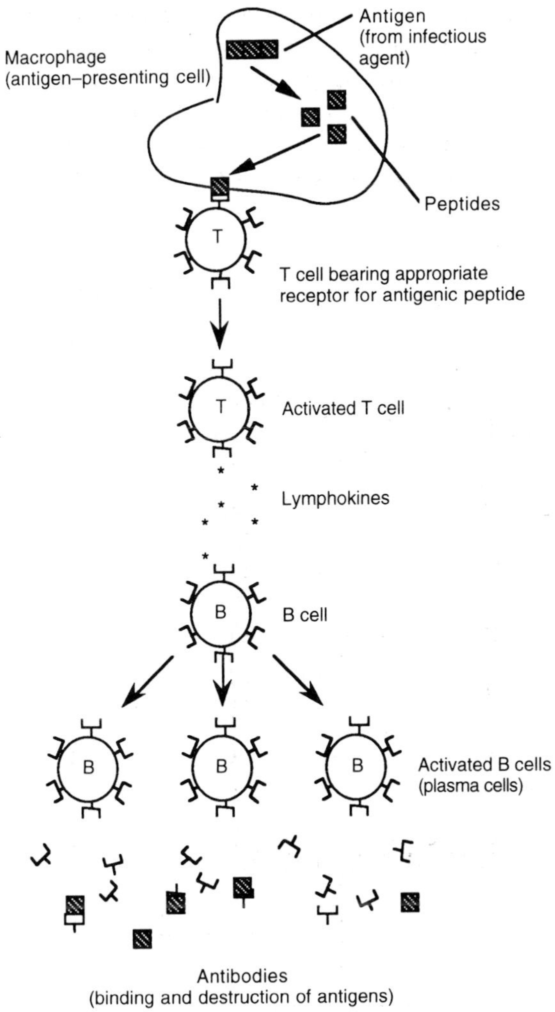

Fig. 27.3 The development of antibody-mediated immunity.

their destruction by complement proteins or by presentation to scavenger cells.

Cell-mediated Immunity

There are situations where antibodies alone cannot fully protect host tissues from infectious attack. In these cases, cell-mediated or antibody-independent immunity, involving a number of specialized T lymphocytes, is mobilized to assist the immune response. T cells consist of at least three subpopulations: T-helper (CD4), T-suppressor (CD8) and cytotoxic T cells — the CD or 'cluster designation' number refers to the internationally accepted nomenclature for classifying immune cells. T-helper cells recognize the MHC–antigen complex on macrophages and produce large amounts of lymphokines to accelerate the division of T cells and mobilize other immune cells and inflammatory mediators. T-suppressor cells help to keep these reactions under control. Cytotoxic T cells produce proteolytic enzymes (perforins) which literally punch holes in cells targeted for destruction and secrete chemicals which kill infected cells.

FACTORS AFFECTING THE ATHLETE'S IMMUNE SYSTEM

It is generally accepted that physiological, psychological and environmental factors can affect the immune system (Fig. 27.4). These factors may independently, and perhaps collectively, influence aspects of immunity and ultimately alter the risk of illness or infection. The cumulative nature of physical and psychological stress is highlighted by research showing that athletes in heavy training or preparing for major national competition experience significant changes in both mood state (Verde *et al.* 1992) and immune parameters (Nieman *et al.* 1990; Mackinnon 1992; Pyne *et al.* 1995).

Physiological Factors

Acute physical stress in various forms — surgery, space flight, burns, tissue damage — is known to influence a variety of immune responses. Exercise is known to elicit similar physiological and immuno-

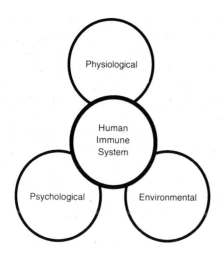

Fig. 27.4 Potential interaction of physiological, psychological and environmental factors on the immune system.

logical responses, leading to the suggestion that exercise-immune interactions can be viewed as a subset of stress immunology (Hoffman-Goetz & Pedersen 1994). The physiological mechanisms responsible for exercise-induced changes in immune cell distribution and function are influenced significantly by elevations in the plasma concentration of immunomodulatory catecholamine (e.g. adrenaline, noradrenaline) and glucocorticoid (e.g. cortisol) hormones. Intense exercise above a threshold of 60% of maximal oxygen uptake generally activates both the sympatho-adrenal and pituitary–adrenocortical endocrine systems, leading to an increase in the plasma concentrations of these immunomodulatory hormones (Smith & Weidemann 1990; Hoffman-Goetz & Pedersen 1994). The availability of substrates (principally glucose and glutamine) and nutrients (vitamins and minerals) also influences immune cell function.

The age-related decline in immune function is well documented, with several studies demonstrating an increased incidence of viral syndromes, infectious diseases, autoimmune disorders and cancers in the elderly. The T-cell population is the most affected immune component with involution of the thymus gland a major cause of immunosenescence (Mazzeo & Nasrullah 1992). The extent to which regular physical activity may ameliorate the age-related

decline in immunocompetence is not clear. Although immunosenescence is unlikely to be significant in younger athletes, future clinical studies may establish more definitive guide-lines for the prescription of exercise programmes in older population groups such as masters and veteran athletes and previously sedentary elderly individuals.

The Effects of Acute Exercise and Long-term Training

The effects of exercise and training on immune function and resistance to infection in athletes are the main focus of this chapter. With the many conflicting views expressed within the literature, coaches and athletes have looked to the scientific and medical communities for clear direction in these matters, yet the scientists and doctors themselves are still uncertain. While some researchers and commentators have implicated excessive and strenuous training with fatigue, overtraining, suppressed immunity and an increased risk of illness (Watson & Eisinger 1992; Nieman 1993), others contend that the human immune system can usually tolerate the substantial stress of training and competition (Shephard et al. 1991; Verde et al. 1992; Cannon 1993).

Careful examination of the relevant studies suggests that, in normal circumstances, the immune system in highly trained and healthy individuals experiences only temporary and minor fluctuations in response to the demands of exercise and training. Where excessive and prolonged training leads to an overtrained state, or significant psychological stress is experienced during competition, or an athlete is exposed to the potentially debilitating effects of overseas travel, foreign food and lower hygiene standards, the risk of illness and infection may be increased. In summary, the effects of exercise and training on the immune system may also depend on a number of other factors besides exercise, which vary according to each athlete's individual circumstances.

SHORT-TERM (ACUTE) EFFECTS OF EXERCISE

Studies examining the effects of exercise and training on the immune system have measured changes in the distribution (i.e. the concentration) and/or the functional activity of immune cells within the circulation. While most immune cells in the body normally reside within bone marrow, lymphoid tissue and skeletal muscle, it is relatively impractical to sample from these locations, and blood testing is the most popular method to assist the diagnostic process. Some of the tests on immune parameters are undertaken with whole blood samples whereas other techniques require the separation and isolation of individual cell types. The assumption made in these experiments is that *in vitro* measurements conducted in the test-tube are representative of the responses which occur *in vivo* (within the tissues and circulation).

The volume of literature on exercise and the immune system has increased greatly in the last 5 years. There has been a large number of studies which have examined the acute or short-term effects of single bouts of exercise. Much of this work has confirmed the notion that moderately intense exercise is immunopotentiating or beneficial to immune cell function, yet high-intensity exercise appears to be immunosuppressive. These findings have led to the so-called paradox between exercise intensity and immune cell function and a number of researchers have proposed models to explain these experimental observations (Smith & Weidemann 1990; Cannon 1993; Nieman 1993).

While research has generally supported this paradox, it should be noted that most of the changes in immune cell distribution and function in response to acute exercise are mild and transient, i.e. immune cell function is only moderately affected and normal or pre-exercise functional levels are generally restored in a few hours. Cannon (1993) suggests that many of the reports of fluctuations in immunity with exercise may be attributable to normal temporal (circadian and seasonal) variability in immune function. Verde *et al.* (1992), in a study of highly-trained distance runners in heavy training, reached a similar view, by concluding that minor and transient changes in immune function may represent a biological warning that training is becoming excessive, but that these changes have only a limited significance for overall immune function.

Analysis of the relevant studies reveals that both cellular and soluble components of the immune system can be influenced by exercise. Interested readers are directed to review articles which have examined studies on exercise and the immune system in detail (Shephard *et al.* 1991; Watson & Eisinger 1992; Cannon 1993; Nieman 1993; Hoffman-Goetz & Pedersen 1994). Interpretation of the findings is complicated by the large variation in exercise protocols and the wide range of immune parameters measured. Despite these methodological limitations, there are a number of general observations that can be made (Table 27.2).

LONG-TERM (CHRONIC) EFFECTS OF TRAINING

In contrast to the large number of studies examining the acute effects of exercise on immune function, there have been relatively few well-designed longi-

Table 27.2 Summary of research findings on the effects of acute bouts of exercise on immune cell distribution and function

Most studies have examined the effects of exercise intensity on immunity — there have been very few studies which have addressed directly the effects of the duration, frequency and type of exercise.

The intensity of exercise appears to elicit more potent effects on the immune system than does the duration of exercise.

There is a paradoxical influence of exercise intensity where moderate exercise generally elicits beneficial changes in immune cell function while intense exercise is largely immunosuppressive.

The leucocytosis (i.e. an increase in the concentration of circulating leucocytes) after exercise is characterized by an immediate lymphocytosis (which may be mediated by adrenaline) and a delayed granulocytosis (mediated by cortisol).

Changes in the concentration and functional activity of immune cells are generally transient, with baseline values normally restored within 24 h.

Serum and secretory immunoglobulin levels may decrease in response to acute exercise stress and long-term training.

Most of these studies have been laboratory-based and additional field-based studies of responses to training and competition are warranted.

tudinal studies on the effects of long-term training. Do the cumulative effects of repeated bouts of exercise result in prolonged perturbations in immune cell function (instead of the mild and transitory effects observed with acute exercise)? If long-term perturbations are evident, are these related to an increased risk of illness and infection? Other studies have addressed the question of whether prolonged moderately intense training enhances immunity and leads to fewer illnesses.

Peters and Bateman (1983) studied 150 runners who competed in a 56 km ultra-marathon race and found that the incidence of respiratory infection in the first 14 days following the race was significantly greater in those runners who had the most intensive pre-race training programmes and who ran the fastest times. Nieman et al. (1990) studied 2311 male and female runners in the 1987 Los Angeles Marathon by questionnaire on infectious episodes, training data and marathon participation. The results showed that runners covering long distances (>97 km per week) experienced a greater risk of an infectious episode during heavy training or following a marathon, than did low mileage runners (<32 km per week). Heath et al. (1991) in a 12 month study of the daily training logs of 530 male and female runners found that running distance covered was a significant risk factor for URTI. Verde et al. (1992) showed that 3 weeks of heavy training, by well-trained male runners, led to a decrease in the ability of lymphocytes to respond to stimulation. Collectively, these studies suggest that athletes undertaking intensive and/or prolonged training programmes may experience some suppression of immune function and an increased risk of an infectious episode.

The research group of Nieman and co-workers has conducted a number of studies examining the potential benefits of moderate exercise. They showed that 6–15 weeks of brisk walking is associated with increased NK cell activity, increased serum immunoglobulin levels and fewer days with URTI symptoms (Nieman et al. 1991). These positive benefits were confirmed by Nehlsen-Cannarella et al. (1991) who reported that moderate exercise (45 min of walking at 60% of maximal oxygen uptake $\dot{V}_{O_{2max}}$) led to transient increases in serum immuno-

globulin levels. In a study of physical activity and immune function in elderly women, highly conditioned individuals had superior NK and T-cell function when compared with their sedentary counterparts (Nieman et al. 1993). These data confirm the notion that moderate exercise is beneficial to immunity and health.

Fitness Level

A number of studies have examined the immunological consequences of exercise in individuals of different fitness levels. In a well-executed study, MacNeil et al. (1991) investigated the effects of four different exercise intensities on lymphocyte proliferative capacity in three experimental groups of male subjects (low, medium and high fitness, $n = 8$ in each case). They found that all exercise regimens resulted in a consistent depression of proliferative capacity, which occurred irrespective of the subject's fitness level. Hack et al. (1992) showed no difference in aspects of neutrophil function in either sedentary control or well-trained male subjects ($n = 10$ runners and $n = 10$ triathletes). However, Smith et al. (1990) found that neutrophils isolated from highly trained male cyclists prior to exercise, exhibited a significantly reduced ability to produce bactericidal reactive oxygen species in response to an exogenous challenge, compared with the same cells isolated from sedentary individuals. Collectively, the conflicting results of these studies suggest that discrete aspects of immune cell function in some athletes may be impaired compared with sedentary individuals. The clinical significance of these observations has not yet been clearly established.

Diet

While there has been extensive interest in the dietary supplementation of vitamins and minerals for the maintenance of good health and sporting performance, the relationship between nutrition, immune function and exercise performance in elite athletes has received only sparse attention. While immune function can be affected significantly by deficiencies in key nutrients or by excessive intake of some vitamins and minerals, most of the studies have been directed primarily at individuals suffering from malnutrition. Watson *et al.* (1987) examined the effect of Vitamin E and C supplementation on the immune system in athletes. Subjects were divided into two groups — either physically fit or sedentary — and given 400 IU of Vitamin E and 500 mg of Vitamin C daily for 30 days. Physically fit subjects exhibited a significant increase in the concentration of T-lymphocyte cells with supplementation, whereas the sedentary individuals did not. Peters *et al.* (1993) showed that daily supplementation with 600 mg of Vitamin C reduced the incidence of symptoms of URTI in 92 male runners after participation in an ultra-marathon running race. Zinc is also known to influence immune cell function (dosage: 50 mg Zn for 6 days) and may offer some protection against oxidative damage (Singh *et al.* 1994).

There has also been interest in the importance of the amino acid glutamine in maintaining immune function. Glutamine is metabolized as a fuel source at a high rate by immune cells. Parry-Billings *et al.* (1992) proposed that an exercise-induced reduction in the plasma concentration of glutamine may compromise lymphocyte function. Forty elite British athletes (runners, swimmers and rowers) were exercised to exhaustion and the effects of glutamine supplementation on lymphocyte proliferation were measured. While oral supplementation of glutamine prevented the plasma concentration of glutamine decreasing in these athletes, there was no change in lymphocyte proliferation in response to stimulation *in vitro*. More research into the relationship between glutamine and immune fuction during prolonged training may provide further evidence of the potential benefits of amino acid supplementation.

Iron has long been identified as a factor critical to performance in events requiring largely aerobic metabolism (Clement & Sawchuk 1988). Iron is an essential component of haemoglobin, myoglobin and cytochromes, which are ultimately responsible for the process of respiration and the production of chemical energy within cells. The role for iron in immune function has been recognized only recently (Brock 1992). Reduced iron levels have been shown to result in impaired immune function, specifically in relation to lymphocyte proliferation, NK cell activity and bactericidal activity of neutrophils (Chandra 1991). Lymphocytes have a mandatory requirement for iron before they proliferate. In light of this information, it is possible that athletes, particularly those involved in endurance sports, may be at increased risk of infection because of a reduced iron status. At present, no study has directly examined the link between iron levels and infection rate in elite athletes.

Psychological Factors

The behavioural and medical sciences have documented many studies showing a strong relationship between psychological status and aspects of immunity. Studies have revealed that individuals suffering from psychological stress associated with bereavement, sleep deprivation or university examinations, have shown disturbances in immune cell function. In relation to athletic training, the most commonly used psychological instrument to assess psychological stress has been the Profile of Mood States (POMS; refer to Chapter 8, The Individual Athlete). Verde *et al.* (1992) reported that the POMS was the best single marker of disturbed function, indicating increased fatigue and decreased vigour in highly trained runners. The psychological pressures experienced prior to and during competition can be intense, and a number of researchers have suggested that these stressors may have a cumulative immunosuppressive effect (Mackinnon 1992). Elite athletes competing in major international competition may perform under significant psychological and emotional stress, and in combination with physical stress, may be more at risk of immunosuppression and overtraining or fatigue states. Continued stress and the chronic overtraining syndrome is characterized by anxiety, depression, chronic fatigue, loss of appetite, poor sleep pattern, weight loss, decreased libido, anger and immunosuppression.

Environmental Factors

The effects of a number of environmental conditions on the immune system have been investigated.

There are no studies which have specifically examined these factors with athletes and sports directly, and consequently team physicians must apply the findings of general scientific and medical research. Athletes are often required to share accommodation, dining facilities, transport, changing rooms and crowded sporting venues, all of which offer an opportunity for the transmission of infectious agents (McLatchie 1993). In these circumstances, members of a sporting team may be more at risk than a competitor in an individual sport, with infectious agents being transferred by direct physical contact (e.g. in sports such as football), airborne droplets or blood-borne transmission. However, there are also instances where competitors in individual sports may be exposed to an increased risk of infection, e.g. in aquatic sports where 'swimmer's ear' (otitis externa) is common. Attention to organization and planning by team officials may limit the impact of these environmental factors.

Environmental conditions such as ambient temperature and wind chill factor may also affect immunity. The evidence is conflicting, with some studies showing no effects, but others reporting a deleterious effect on immunity of low ambient temperature and elevated wind chill (Cannon 1993). It is thought that the increased ventilation rates associated with exercise in cold conditions may offer a mechanism for an increased risk of URTI (Cannon 1993). The effect of airborne pollutants on the immune system is unclear. Nitrogen dioxide appears to exert only a marginal effect on lymphocyte subsets in the circulation and in the bronchial fluid of subjects undertaking moderately intense cycle ergometry for 15 min (Rubinstein et al. 1991).

Overseas travel presents special problems for athletes and is discussed in detail in Chapter 6 (Environmental Stress) and Chapter 7 (The Team Physician). The debilitating effects of jet lag, and the associated changes of climate, foreign foods, customs and languages, are well known to experienced athletes. Gastrointestinal problems are commonly experienced during travel abroad, and while it is widely accepted that such problems are a result of contact with unfamiliar pathogens, one may speculate on the added risk imparted by stress-induced immunosuppression. Personal hygiene should be stressed by washing hands before eating, strict non-sharing of water bottles and avoiding local water supplies in high-risk areas by drinking and brushing teeth with bottled water only. Prophylactic intervention with a low-dose broad-spectrum antibiotic has proved to be successful in limiting illness among Australian sporting teams travelling overseas.

PRACTICAL CONSIDERATIONS

Infections in Sport

The majority of the illnesses sustained in the athletic or sporting setting are mild and self-limiting viral infections of the upper respiratory tract (Table 27.3). A number of recent prospective and retrospective epidemiological studies have indicated that athletes in training have an increased risk of infection compared with individuals undertaking moderate recreational activity programmes, and that URTI and gastrointestinal tract infection are the most common illnesses reported by athletes (Brenner et al. 1994).

URTI fall into several clinical syndromes depending upon the part of the system affected. The most common URTI is the so-called 'common cold' with acute coryza, sore throat, cough, fatigue, malaise and fever. Irrespective of the clinical syndrome presented, approximately 75% of URTI are caused by viruses. Epidemiological studies have

Table 27.3 Infections frequently presented to a sports medicine clinic*

Upper respiratory tract viral infections/'colds'
Gastroenteritis (viral, 'traveller's diarrhoea' (*Escherichia coli*) or 'food poisoning' by other non-coliform bacterial infection)
Septic cuts and abrasions
Tinea or fungal dermatoses (e.g. 'athlete's foot')
Bacterial skin infections (staphylococcal, streptococcal)
Glandular fever (infectious mononucleosis)
Viral skin infections ('herpes gladiatorum' or 'scrum pox')
Chronic fatigue syndrome (possibly postviral)

*Department of Sports Medicine, Australian Institute of Sport, unpublished data.

shown that most young and otherwise healthy adults experience between one and six infections per year, with the average being 1.5–2 episodes per year (Berglund & Hemmingson 1990). Heath *et al.* (1992) report that the risk of respiratory infection decreases as children mature into young adults, before a later increase as subjects age. Apart from the physiological effects of exercise and training *per se* it is known that environmental factors such as the season (respiratory infections are more prevalent in the winter months) and training in an aquatic medium also influence the frequency of URTI (Seyfried *et al.* 1985).

Gastrointestinal infections may be either bacterial, viral or protozoan. The pathogens may be water-borne or passed on by the faecal–oral route of contamination. Gastrointestinal tract infections are common in athletes travelling to new environs, especially in regions which have poor sanitation, low standards of living and inadequate hygiene.

Skin infections may be caused by several types of infectious agents. These may be viral (e.g. herpes), bacterial (e.g. streptococcal) or fungal (e.g. tinea) in origin (McLatchie 1993; Brenner *et al.* 1994). Skin infections may develop through direct contact with other competitors and are facilitated by excessive exposure to ultraviolet radiation, sweating and skin friction (Sharp *et al.* 1988). These conditions are evident in both indoor and outdoor sports. Common bacterial infections in athletes include impetigo and folliculitis caused by *Staphylococcus aureus*. Common viral infections include the herpes simplex virus (HSV), which elicits the characteristic burning and itching sensations at the site of infection. HSV infection in different sports has led to the coining of colourful terms such as 'herpes gladiatorum' in wrestling and 'herpes rugbeiorum' in football, and even the more colloquial 'scrum pox'. In these sports, transmission of the HSV occurs by direct physical contact with infected individuals. Common fungal infections such as tinea pedis ('athlete's foot') and tinea cruris ('jock itch') are often transmitted in the wet surrounds of showers and changing rooms.

These illnesses may be of only minor concern to the health of normal healthy individuals, but the disruptive effects on training and especially on competition performance may be of great concern to both amateur and elite athletes. While the effects of the common infections are generally mild and short-lived, it is known that aerobic power, isometric strength and isokinetic strength of athletes are all adversely affected during acute infectious illnesses (Friman 1977). In addition to acute illnesses, there has been considerable interest in postviral and chronic fatigue syndromes, which are often associated with substantial and long-term performance decrements and perturbations in immune function. These can be debilitating syndromes and often require months or years for full recovery.

Clinical Considerations

In assessing an infected athlete, it is important to differentiate between anatomically localized infections (including the common cold and URTI) and systemic infection. Systemic symptoms and signs such as fever, myalgia, arthralgia, malaise, elevated resting heart rate, fatigue, generalized lymphadenopathy or organomegaly (especially the spleen and liver) indicate a more serious infection and a greater need for rest from exercise as part of treatment.

Initial assessment of the athlete with an infection involves a thorough history and examination. Particular note should be taken of recent training and the ability to perform as an athlete. Implicit in this is the understanding that the more seriously affected the athlete is by his or her illness, the more the training demands need to be reduced and the longer the recovery will take. The effect of illness on performance can be used as a benchmark to monitor recovery with appropriate treatment. The assessment may include blood tests and microbiological evaluation.

Blood evaluation usually commences with a full blood count (FBC) which provides a quantitative assessment of the concentration of erythrocytes (red blood cells), leucocytes (total white blood cells) and leucocyte subclasses, particularly lymphocytes, granulocytes and monocytes. The erythrocyte sedimentation rate (ESR) is another clinically useful test which can indicate the severity of illness. C-

Table 27.4 Normal ranges for the circulating concentration of leucocytes and lymphocyte subsets. Each cell type is expressed as a percentage of the total leucocyte population or as a percentage of the circulating lymphocyte subpopulation (indicated by *)

Cell type	Normal range ($\times 10^9 \cdot L^{-1}$)	Percentage %	Cluster designation (CD) classification
Leucocytes	4.0–11.0	–	–
Granulocytes	2.5–7.5	40–75	CD16
Monocytes	0.2–0.8	2–10	CD14
Lymphocytes	1.2–3.5	20–50	see below
T cells	0.8–2.8	65–79*	CD3
T helper	0.4–1.9	35–55*	CD4
T suppressor	0.2–0.6	29–40*	CD8
T-helper/T-suppressor ratio	0.9–2.5	–	CD4/CD8
B cells	0.1–0.5	5–15*	CD19
NK cells	0.1–0.5	9–21*	CD16/CD56

reactive protein, an acute phase reactant released during infection and tissue injury, can also be measured. Serological tests, which detect specific antibodies, may also be useful in the assessment of viral illnesses. Immunophenotyping of lymphocyte subsets has been greatly enhanced by the application of flow cytometry, which enables the distribution and characteristics of individual cells to be assessed (Table 27.4).

More specialized assessment of immune status may include lymphocyte function (proliferative response to mitogenic stimulation), enumeration of serum and salivary immunoglobulin (enzyme-linked immunoassay and rate nephelometry), NK cell function (^{51}Cr release assay), phagocytosis (uptake of fluorescent latex beads) and neutrophil function (activity of the oxidative burst). Such assessments are usually reserved for those with severe or recurrent infection or other signs of immune system dysfunction. Given that acute exercise influences the distribution and functional activity of immune parameters, clinicians are advised to ensure that athletes rest for at least 6 and preferably 24 h before blood sampling.

Management is guided by clinical assessment and follows traditional lines for viral and bacterial infections, respectively (Eichner 1993). Athletes warrant special consideration in respect to their training demands. In minor infections, where there are no obvious systemic effects, i.e. normal pulse rate and the absence of fever, normal sporting activity may be undertaken. In serious infections, with raised pulse rate, fever and organomegaly, exercise should be prohibited until the fever has settled and organs are returning to normal. The amount of *time off training* varies according to the disease process and the individual, and may range from a few days to several months. Between these two extremes, activity is modified according to the severity of the symptoms.

The timing of the *return to training* after infection is indicated by the resting pulse rate approaching normal, the absence of fever and a definite improvement in symptoms. Given that moderate intensity aerobic exercise is immuno-enhancing, this type of training is recommended in the earlier stages. However, one needs to be flexible during this period, and any signs of a 'flare of symptoms', especially a raised resting pulse rate, fever, myalgia or lassitude, usually indicate that further time off training is required. The workload can be increased as the athlete shows improved ability to cope with increasing volume and intensity. It should be anticipated that this process normally takes a few days with minor illness, but in more severe illnesses the return to full training may take weeks.

To assist the treatment and management process the recommendations outlined in Table 27.5 have been proposed as guide-lines, but a medical opinion should always be sought if a coach or athlete is in doubt. It is important not to underestimate the risks that are present with more severe infections

Table 27.5 Guide-lines for the cessation and resumption of training for athletes suffering a minor or major illness

	Minor illness	Major illness
Symptoms	Mild fatigue Sore throat Mild headache 'Runny nose' Sneezing	Severe headache or pain Severe fatigue Fever Myalgia (aching muscles) Arthralgia (aching joints) Diarrhoea Vomiting
Action	Restrict training to intensity only, if necessary	Cessation of training until systemic symptoms subside
Resumption of training	Graded return to full training in 1–3 days	Graded return to full training in days to weeks

(Friman & Ilback 1992). Particular caution is required for athletes or individuals suffering, or possibly suffering, myocarditis (inflammation of the heart muscle) or when recovering from infectious mononucleosis (glandular fever) with splenomegaly, to cite two examples. In these circumstances, continued exercise may augment the severity of the disease (Brenner *et al.* 1994) and a conservative and graded return to full training and ongoing medical assessment is essential.

Role of the Immune System in Tissue Repair

It is evident that mobilization and activation of immune cells is triggered by the release of chemotactic signals from damaged muscle and connective tissue, and/or the effects of an exercise-induced leucocytosis and associated elevation in the concentrations of immunomodulatory hormones. Exercise-induced tissue damage elicits a co-ordinated sequence of inflammatory and immunological events leading to removal of injured tissue, promotion of growth and repair, and ultimately restoration of normal physiological function. The sequence of physiological responses to specific tissue pathology is discussed in detail in Chapter 12. Continued physical activity in the presence of tissue injury may be detrimental in the long term and the clinical application is that the rehabilitation of athletes

should not exacerbate or prolong the immunological and inflammatory response. A premature return to intensive training may interfere with the inflammatory and regenerative process and facilitate more severe pathophysiological consequences such as chronic inflammation.

SUMMARY AND RECOMMENDATIONS

Based on the available scientific literature, Table 27.6 presents a number of practical recommendations for coaches, team managers, medical personnel and athletes, which may reduce the incidence, duration and/or severity of illnesses and infections. Again most of these recommendations are derived from general scientific and medical studies, and clinical experience, as there are no sports-specific studies which have examined these specific questions. Attention to detail in planning in both team and individual sports should reduce significantly the risk of illness and disruption to training and competition performance. Coaches

Table 27.6 Guide-lines for coaches, managers, physicians and athletes to minimize the risk of illness and infection in training and competition

Check immunization status of athletes and officials prior to overseas travel
Ensure appropriate scheduling of quality and recovery training sessions
Avoid high-intensity workouts immediately before competition
Implement stress management techniques
Provide comfortable and quiet accommodation for adequate sleep
Provide an adequate diet with hygienic food and drink preparation
Ensure that warm and adequate clothing is available and worn where appropriate
Ensure appropriate personal hygiene
Avoid confined and crowded public places and contact with infected individuals
Isolate infected athletes from other team members
Provide immediate treatment for players with open wounds or profuse bleeding to prevent blood-borne transmission of infectious agents
Always seek appropriate medical treatment where necessary

and team managers should ensure that all team members take personal responsibility for their training and preparation. It should be emphasized that even the best precautions may not prevent an episode of illness or infection.

One of the important considerations for maintaining optimal health and performance of athletes is the planning of a balanced and periodized training programme which allows recovery from training efforts. The process of periodizing the volume and intensity of training was popularized in the 1970s and 1980s. While there is only limited research which directly examines the effects of periodized training on aspects of health and immunity, it is thought that appropriate planning reduces the risk of compromising health and performance. There has been considerable effort in identifying the factors which may contribute to overtraining and fatigue states, and these are also relevant to the maintenance of a healthy immune system (Fry *et al.* 1991). The connection between overtraining and the risk of illness and infection is being examined by several research groups. Considerations in the planning of training programmes to reduce the risk of overtraining and immunosuppression have been discussed previously (Pyne & Gray 1994).

CONCLUSIONS

The immune system is a complex network of physical, cellular and soluble components which give rise to the specific and non-specific reactions of the host defence against infection. Physiological, psychological and behavioural factors may influence immunity independently, and perhaps collectively. Acute bouts of exercise elicit mild and transient alterations in the distribution and functional activity of immune cells. Exercise appears to influence immune cell function in an intensity-dependent manner with moderately intense exercise ($<60\%$ $\dot{V}_{O_2max}$) considered to be immunopotentiating, while intense exercise ($>60\%$ $\dot{V}_{O_2}$) is potentially immunosuppressive. The limited experimental evidence available on the effects of prolonged training on the immune system suggests that elite athletes may, in some circumstances, experience suppression in some immune parameters. Research is currently examining whether these changes are clinically significant.

There are a number of practical recommendations which can be implemented by coaches and officials to minimize the risk of athletes contracting common upper respiratory tract, gastrointestinal tract and skin infections. Practical guide-lines have been suggested for the management of athletes with such an illness or infection. For mild illnesses, training may be continued at a moderate intensity. In more severe illnesses, a complete rest from training is recommended until symptoms and fever subside. A graded and conservative return to full training under medical supervision is strongly recommended.

REFERENCES

Berglund B. & Hemmingson P. (1990) Infectious disease in elite cross-country skiers: A one-year incidence study. *Clinical Sports Medicine* 2, 19–23.

Brenner I. K., Shek P. N. & Shephard R. J. (1994) Infection in athletes. *Sports Medicine* 17, 86–107.

Brock J. H. (1992) Iron and the immune system. In Lauffer R. B. (ed.) *Iron and Human Disease*, pp. 161–178. CRC Press, Boca Raton, FL.

Cannon J. G. (1993) Exercise and resistance to infection. *Journal of Applied Physiology* 74, 973–980.

Chandra R. K. (1991) 1990 McCollum Award Lecture. Nutrition and immunity: Lessons from the past and new insights into the future. *American Journal of Clinical Nutrition* 53, 1087–1101.

Clement D. B. & Sawchuk L. L. (1988) Iron status and sports performance. *Sports Medicine* 1, 65–74.

Eichner E. R. (1993) Infection, immunity and exercise — What to tell patients. *Physician and Sportsmedicine* 21, 125–135.

Friman G. (1977) Effect of acute infectious disease on isometric muscle strength. *Scandinavian Journal of Clinical Laboratory Investigation* 37, 303–308.

Friman G. & Ilback N-G. (1992) Exercise and infection — interaction, risks and benefits. *Scandinavian Journal of Medicine and Science in Sports* 2, 177–189.

Fry R., Morton A. R. & Keast D. (1991) Overtraining in athletes — An update. *Sports Medicine* 12, 32–65.

Hack V., Strobel G., Rau J. P. & Weicker H. (1992) The effect of maximal exercise on the activity of neutrophil granulocytes in highly trained athletes in a moderate training period. *European Journal of Applied Physiology* 65, 520–524.

Heath G. W., Ford E. S., Craven T. E., Macera C. A., Jackson K. L. & Pate R. R. (1991) Exercise and the incidence of upper respiratory tract infections. *Medicine and Science in Sports and Exercise* 23, 152–157.

Heath G. W., Macera C. A. & Nieman D. C. (1992) Exercise and upper respiratory tract infections. Is there a relationship? *Sports Medicine* 14, 353–365.

Hoffman-Goetz L. & Pedersen B. K. (1994) Exercise and the immune system: A model of the stress response. *Immunology Today* 15, 382–387.

Mackinnon L. T. (1992) *Exercise and Immunology: Current Issues in Exercise Science Series*, Monograph No. 2. Human Kinetics Publishers, Champaign, IL.

McLatchie G. R. (1993) Infections in sport. In McLatchie G. R. (ed.) *Essentials of Sports Medicine*, pp. 112–125. Churchill Livingstone, Edinburgh.

MacNeil B., Hoffman-Goetz L., Kendall A., Houston M. & Arumugan Y. (1991) Lymphocyte proliferative responses after exercise in men: Fitness, intensity and duration effects. *Journal of Applied Physiology* 70, 179–185.

Mazzeo R. S. & Nasrullah I. (1992) Exercise and age-related decline in immune functions. In Watson R. R. & Eisinger M. (eds) *Exercise and Disease*, pp. 160–178. CRC Press, Boca Raton, FL.

Nehlsen-Cannarella S. L., Nieman D. C. & Jessen, J. (1991) The effects of acute moderate exercise on lymphocyte function and serum immunoglobulin levels. *International Journal of Sports Medicine* 12, 291–398.

Nieman D. C. (1993) Exercise and upper respiratory tract infection. *Sports Medicine Training and Rehabilitation* 4, 1–14.

Nieman D. C., Johansen L. M., Lee J. W. & Arabatzis K. (1990) Infectious episodes in runners before and after the Los Angeles Marathon. *Journal of Sports Medicine and Physical Fitness* 30, 316–328.

Nieman D. C., Nehlsen-Cannarella S. L., Markoff P. A. *et al.* (1991) The effects of moderate exercise training on natural killer cells and acute upper respiratory tract infections. *International Journal of Sports Medicine* 11, 467–473.

Nieman D. C., Henson D. A., Gusewitch G., Warren B. J., Dotson R. C., Butterworth D. E. & Nehlsen-Cannarella S. L. (1993) Physical activity and immune function in elderly women. *Medicine and Science in Sports and Exercise* 25, 823–831.

Parry-Billings M., Budgett R., Koutedakis Y. *et al.* (1992) Plasma amino acid concentrations in the overtraining syndrome: Possible effects of the immune system. *Medicine and Science in Sports and Exercise* 24, 1353–1358.

Peters E. M. & Bateman E. B. (1983) Ultramarathon running and upper respiratory tract infections. An epidemiological survey. *South African Medical Journal* 64, 582–584.

Peters E. M., Goetzsche J. M., Grobbelaar B. & Noakes T. D. (1993) Vitamin C supplementation reduces the incidence of postrace symptoms of upper-respiratory tract infection in ultramarathoners. *American Journal of Clinical Nutrition* 57, 170–174.

Pyne D. B., Baker M. S., Telford R. D. & Weidemann M. J. (1995) Effects of an intensive 12-wk training program by elite swimmers on neutrophil oxidative activity. *Medicine and Science in Sports and Exercise* 27, 536–542.

Pyne D. B. & Gray A. B. (1994) *Exercise and the Immune System*. State of the Art Review No. 36. Australian Sports Commission, Canberra.

Rubenstein I., Reiss T. F., Bigby B. G., Stites D. P. & Boushey H. A. (1991) Effects of 0.60 PPM nitrogen dioxide on circulating and bronchoalveolar lavage lymphocytes phenotypes in healthy subjects. *Environmental Research* 55, 18–30.

Rubenstein I., Reiss T. F., Bigby B. G., Stites D. P. & Boushey H.A. (1991) Effects of 0.60 PPM nitrogen dioxide on circulating and bronchoalveolar lavage lymphocytes phenotypes in healthy subjects. *Environmental Research* 55, 18–30.

Seyfried P. L., Tobin R. S., Brown N. E. & Ness P. F. (1985) A prospective study of swimming related illness. I. Swimming associated health risk. *American Journal of Public Health* 75, 1068–1070.

Sharp J. C. M., Girdwood R. W. A., Watt B., Walker E. & Fagan K. E. (1988) Infections in sport. *British Journal of Sports Medicine* 22, 117–121.

Shephard R. J., Verde T. J., Thomas S. G. & Shek P. (1991) Physical activity and the immune system. *Canadian Journal of Sports Sciences* 16, 163–185.

Singh A., Failla M. L. & Deuster P. A. (1994) Exercise-induced changes in immune function: Effects of zinc supplementation. *Journal of Applied Physiology* 76, 2298–2303.

Smith J. A. & Weidemann M. J. (1990) The exercise and immunity paradox: A neuro-endocrine/cytokine hypothesis. *Medical Science Research* 18, 749–753.

Verde T. J., Thomas S. G. & Shephard R. J. (1992) Potential markers of heavy training in highly trained distance runners. *British Journal of Sports Medicine* 26, 167–175.

Watson R. R. & Eisinger M. (1992) *Exercise and Disease*. CRC Press, Boca Raton, FL.

Watson R. R., Benedict J., Mayberry J. C. & Moriguchi S. (1987) Vitamin C and E supplementation and cellular immune functions in men. *Annals of the New York Academy of Sciences* 498, 530.

CHAPTER 28

SPECIAL MEDICAL CONSIDERATIONS

PART I

ASTHMA

A. R. Morton

Almost 1.5 million Australians are asthmatic (McLennon 1992) with the disease more prevalent among those aged between 5 and 14 years. At least 10% of Australian adults and 20% of the children have a history of current asthma while about 30% will exhibit asthma-type symptoms at some time during their lives (National Asthma Campaign 1993). Asthma is more common in boys than girls (ratio of 1.6:1.0), but more common in older women than in older men, indicating a greater remission rate among the boys. Asthma affects all races and the first episode may occur at any age.

Asthma has a significant mortality throughout life. This rate in many countries appeared to peak in the mid-1960s and then declined steadily for the next 10 years. However, by 1984 the death rate had increased in many countries, including Australia, New Zealand, England, Wales and the United States. By 1991 the Australian death rate commenced a downward trend again (National Asthma Campaign 1993).

PATHOPHYSIOLOGY

Asthma is defined as a disease involving airways inflammation, which is characterized by airways hyperresponsiveness and attacks of reversible airways obstruction (National Asthma Campaign 1993). The diversity of a person's asthma can vary from infrequent episodes of mild wheezing or breath-lessness through to frequent serious life-threatening bouts of airways obstruction.

Since the airways of the asthmatic are abnormally sensitive (twitchy), they over-react to common items in the environment and to other precipitating factors. These include infection, irritating dusts, air pollutants, exposure to allergens (such as pollens, house dust, animal hair and specific foods), psychological stress and trigger mechanisms such as laughter, changes in temperature and physical exertion. The response to precipitating factors varies among asthmatics and even in the same asthmatic at different times. Almost all asthmatics will have bronchoconstriction provoked by exercise. However, individuals vary greatly in this response, from those who develop exertional asthma rarely, to others who in the absence of pharmacological protection, become symptomatic every time they exercise.

The hypersensitive airways respond to the precipitating factors by narrowing as a result of one or more of the following: spasm of the bronchial smooth muscle, inflammation characterized by mucosal oedema, an increased mucus secretion from the goblet cells in an attempt to 'wash away' the irritation, cell infiltration and epithelial desquamation.

The narrowed airways result in an increased airways resistance, which may necessitate recruitment of accessory respiratory muscles in order to maintain a now noisy bronchial airflow or wheeze. The bronchial constriction and mucosal oedema serve to increase the unfavourable transmural pressure gradient of the intrathoracic airways, so that small airways closure may occur. This results in 'air trapping', which causes hyperinflation of the lungs because of the inability to exhale completely, an increase in both residual and functional residual volume and a decrease in the vital capacity of the lungs. If the asthma attack is mild or even moderate it may cause little inconvenience at rest. However, when even moderate exertion is attempted severe respiratory difficulty may be experienced. This breathing discomfort may be accompanied by insufficient alveolar ventilation and a drop in the oxygen saturation level of the arterial blood. In the laboratory the severity of asthma is assessed by measurement of either peak expiratory flow rate (PEFR), forced expiratory volume in the first second (FEV_1) or the forced expiratory volume per cent ($FEV_1\%$). These values are compared with normal values or against the person's own scores obtained when bronchodilated.

EXERCISE-INDUCED ASTHMA

Physical exertion can be a trigger factor to induce asthma. When this occurs it is referred to as exercise-induced asthma (EIA), which can be defined as a clinical syndrome characterized by a transient narrowing of the airways following moderate to severe exercise. Occasionally, exercise is apparently the only stimulus that provokes asthma.

When exercise provokes an episode of asthma the changes in lung function follow a typical pattern. Shortly after the activity is commenced some degree of bronchodilation often occurs, followed later by bronchoconstriction. Bronchodilation may be due to the release of catecholamines, a reduction in the normal vagal tone, an increase in the mean alveolar volume causing a mechanical expansion of the airways and/or an improvement in airways conductance due to re-opening of collapsed airways. These changes result in an initial increase in FEV_1 or PEFR, which may either persist for the duration of the exercise period (subject B, Fig. 28.1) or may be reduced to below the pre-exercise level during the latter stages of the exercise (subject A, Fig. 28.1).

After the cessation of exercise, FEV_1 and PEFR drop by at least 15% of the pre-exercise value, reaching their lowest point about 3–10 min post-exercise.

The FEV_1 and PEFR then gradually and spontaneously return towards the pre-exercise level, generally exhibiting recovery in about 60 min (Fig. 28.1). Some asthmatics do not recover spontaneously and may require medication to reverse the EIA.

Fig. 28.1 Typical changes in PEFR following exercise in asthmatic and non-asthmatic subjects.

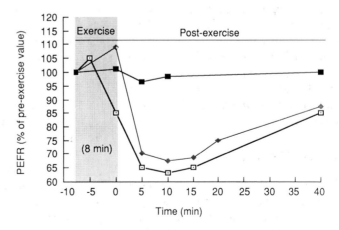

- ■ Non-asthmatic
- ◆ Asthmatic subject B
- □ Asthmatic subject A

An exercise challenge which produces these post-exercise changes in lung volumes may be utilized to confirm the tendency of EIA, to determine the asthmagenicity of different types of exercise, to study the effect of environmental conditions on the development of EIA and to examine the protective effects of pre-exercise medications.

Although non-asthmatics may show a slight increase in FEV_1 or PEFR immediately after exercise, followed by a slight reduction, these changes are seldom significant (Fig. 28.1). The minimum post-exercise decrease necessary for the diagnosis of EIA is 15%. Morton and Fitch (1993) classified a fall of 15–29% as mild EIA; 30–44% as moderate; and greater than 45% as severe EIA.

Another post-exercise response which is demonstrated by some asthmatics, primarily children, is a second or late reaction which may not develop until 3–4 h after the exercise challenge and may take a further 3–9 h to peak (Fig. 28.2). This late response may be the result of an inflammatory reaction due to mediators such as neutrophil chemotactic factor (Lee et al. 1983).

Following an episode of EIA, about 40–50% of asthmatics demonstrate a refractory period, during which a second bout of exercise will result in a bronchoconstrictive response which is substantially less than the initial episode of EIA. This refractoriness usually lasts about 60 min (Edmunds et al. 1978).

CAUSES OF EXERCISE-INDUCED ASTHMA

Despite extensive research efforts over the past 50 years the cause of EIA is still unknown. Currently, the best hypothesis is that EIA is caused by the release of a bronchoconstrictor substance, probably in response to the changes in osmolarity of the periciliary fluid. This change occurs as a result of the loss of fluid from the airways during the conditioning of the inspired air (Anderson 1984; Hahn et al. 1984).

Even when dry air at 0°C is inspired through the nose it is 'conditioned' so that by the time it reaches the delicate alveolar membrane it has been warmed to 37°C and is completely saturated with water vapour. Exposure to cold dry air can damage this delicate tissue. Most of this air-conditioning occurs in the nose, pharynx and the first 10 generations of the bronchi. Some athletes have ventilation rates exceeding 200 L·min⁻¹ during maximal exercise and this places extreme stress on the air-conditioning function, especially since the size of the nares limits the average nasal air flow to about 75–80 L·min⁻¹ with values as high as 120 L·min⁻¹ recorded. This saturation of alveolar air occurs by absorbing water from the airways during its passage from the nose to the alveolar regions. This 'dries' the airways thus concentrating the ions in the periciliary fluid.

Fig. 28.2 Typical PEFR changes in those exhibiting a late phase response.

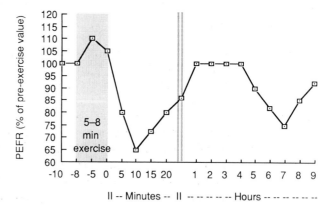

An elegant model of the pathways involved in EIA has been proposed by Godfrey and Bar-Yishay (1993). In this model they suggest that exercise results in hyperpnoea which may have a direct triggering effect. It may also increase sympathetic activity and cause the release of prostaglandins, which will provide a fast and slow protective effect, respectively. The hyperpnoea, influenced by climatic conditions, results in the drying and cooling of the airways which invokes the release of bronchoconstrictor mediators. The model indicates that the severity of the ensuing EIA is modified by the current level of bronchial reactivity which is determined by the levels of allergens, air pollution and recent infection.

The bronchoactive mediators may include histamine, leukotrienes or prostaglandins released from the mast and/or epithelial cells. They may act directly on smooth muscle, stimulate irritant receptors, which in turn cause bronchoconstriction via vagal influences, and/or produce an inflammatory reaction via constituents such as neutrophil chemotactic factor. Cooling of the airways may enhance the response to water loss.

FACTORS MODIFYING THE RESPONSE TO EXERCISE

Early studies indicated that the mode, duration, intensity, type of exercise loading, the environmental conditions and pharmacological intervention could all modify the asthmatic response to a bout of exercise.

Types of Exercise

When selecting the mode of exercise for asthmatics it must be noted that there is a degree of specificity of exercise as far as the provocation of EIA is concerned. Some activities induce greater bronchoconstriction than others (Jones et al. 1962; Morton et al. 1981). Running is the exercise most provocative of asthma, while swimming and walking are least likely to induce an attack. Cycling and kayaking are less asthmagenic than running, but greater than swimming or walking.

Duration of Exercise

When the intensity of exercise is kept constant, the severity of the post-exercise bronchoconstriction increases with the duration of exercise up to about 8 min duration after which it appears to plateau (Morton et al. 1983).

Intensity of Exercise

Silverman and Anderson (1972) have shown that if the duration of exercise is held constant, there will be an increase in post-exercise bronchoconstriction with an increase in work intensity. The maximum effect was obtained at an exercise intensity requiring 65–75% of one's maximal oxygen consumption (about 75–85% of predicted maximal heart rate).

Type of Exercise Loading

Games and activities utilizing intermittent periods of intense exercise followed by brief rest periods, such as the various codes of football, squash and tennis, are preferable to activities requiring continuous work, such as cross-country or marathon running.

Environmental Conditions

Inhalation of cold and/or dry air during exercise have both been shown to enhance the severity of post-exercise airways constriction. However, recent research has indicated that when the water content of inspired air was held constant, varying the temperature by as much as 25 °C had no significant effect on EIA and breathing hot humid air significantly inhibited EIA. Thus, water loss and not simply cooling of the airways due to heat loss appears more important in EIA and the mechanism may be related to changes in osmolarity of the fluid lining the respiratory tract (Hahn et al. 1984). The effects of changing the osmolarity of the periciliary fluid was demonstrated by Schoeffel et al. (1981) who showed that increasing or decreasing the osmolarity by inhaling hypertonic or hypotonic salt solutions could provoke asthma.

This respiratory water loss may account for much of the variability in the exercise response as far as specificity, intensity and duration are concerned, but it does not appear to explain all aspects of it. It may help to explain the lower asthmagenicity of swimming, when highly saturated air is inhaled from above the surface of the water, but it does not appear to provide the whole answer. Inbar *et al.* (1980) showed that when asthmatics breathed dry air during swimming they had smaller reductions in lung function than after running, with similar air inspirate and at equivalent levels of ventilation. Furthermore, breathing dry air during swimming at a given metabolic rate provided lung function changes which were not significantly different to those obtained while inhaling moist air under identical conditions.

Noviski *et al.* (1987) observed also that even if the amount of heat and water loss was held constant, exercise of high intensity almost doubled the severity of EIA when compared with that provoked by low-intensity exercise.

Other environmental factors which have been shown to influence the severity of EIA include the levels of air pollution and allergens. There is an increase in the severity of EIA to the same level of exercise following allergen provocation (Mussaffi *et al.* 1986).

VALUE OF CHRONIC AEROBIC EXERCISE (TRAINING)

It is not surprising that young asthmatics who experience EIA following physical activity attempt to avoid vigorous exercise. This avoidance tends to lead to low fitness levels, poor physique, chest deformity and a severe lack of motor skills. It may also be accompanied by psychological problems from a poor self-image. Such asthmatics may also suffer socially and emotionally as a result of poor peer group acceptance through failure to participate in regular childhood and/or adolescent activities. Frequent absences from school may also result in poor academic achievement. The physiological benefits which are derived from regular and frequent aerobic exercise at a moderate to heavy intensity benefit the asthmatic and the non-asthmatic alike.

However, the asthmatic obtains additional value from a more efficient respiratory system, including a decrease in the ventilation required to perform a given level of work, increased maximum attainable ventilation rate, reduced residual volume due to less air trapping and a more efficient pattern of ventilation.

All of the above training-induced changes result in the asthmatic being able to perform a given task with a smaller disturbance of his internal environment. This means that the aerobically trained asthmatic can cope better than the untrained individual with the same degree of mild or moderate airways obstruction.

Research has also indicated that an increase in aerobic fitness increases the tolerance and threshold levels of asthmatics so that a higher level of provocation is required to produce symptoms. It has been shown to decrease both absenteeism as a result of asthma and medication requirements.

It is possible that psychological and sociological benefits of increased aerobic fitness with the resulting improvement in self-image and the greater recognition and acceptance by both peer groups and parents help to remove the 'cripple' stigma from which many asthmatics suffer. It is important that young asthmatics realize that, with dedication and application, most can compete quite well with their non-asthmatic peers, provided that adequate training and pre-event medication programmes are followed. Asthmatics have even demonstrated the ability to reach top international competition standards in almost all sports. In the five Olympiads between 1976 and 1992, Australia has been represented by 1080 sports persons. Of these, 98 (9.1%) have been asthmatic. Thirty-four (11.7%) of the 1992 Olympic team were asthmatic and they competed in nine of the 25 events Australia entered. Olympic Gold medals have been won by asthmatics on the Australian team in Melbourne (1956), Rome (1960), Tokyo (1964), Mexico City (1968), Moscow (1980), Seoul (1988) and Barcelona (1992). Of the 597 US athletes participating in the 1984 Summer Olympic Games, 67 (11.2%) suffered from EIA and these athletes won 41 medals (15 gold, 20 silver and six bronze; Voy 1986). In 1989 an asthmatic cyclist (Rod Evans) reduced the 'around Australia'

(14 800 km) cycling record from 80 to 50 days. This endurance feat was more impressive when it is realized that the previous record was set by four elite Danish cyclists riding as a team, while Evans rode alone.

Therefore, even though exercise can induce asthma, sports and regular physical activity are accepted components in the total management of asthma.

A disturbing feature of exercising vigorously in very cold environments has recently been reported. Larsson *et al.* (1993) have shown that asthma, asthma-like symptoms and bronchial hyperresponsiveness is much more common among cross-country skiers than in the general population and non-skiers. They have suggested that this is most probably due to the breathing of large volumes of cold air during training and competition.

ASSESSMENT OF ASTHMA

Many asthmatics do not subjectively evaluate their asthmatic symptoms very accurately. As a result they are often unaware of the degree of existing airways obstruction, or in many cases, the severity of its change from day to day.

This is especially true when symptoms develop slowly over a number of days. In these circumstances, asthma may progress to a dangerous level before subjective assessment forces the patient to seek medical help. On occasions this delay has proved fatal.

All asthmatics who are classified as moderate or severe, should be encouraged to purchase one of the inexpensive airflow meters which are available for home use. These should be used in the morning and the evening before and after the bronchodilator (if used) and the scores plotted in a log-book. Asthmatics with a flow meter variability of 10–20%, 20–30% and greater than 30% are classified as having mild, moderate or severe asthma, respectively. Despite a recent study (Sly *et al.* 1994) which showed some inexpensive peak flow meters to be inaccurate and unreliable, the use of these instruments is still recommended with the added precaution that they be used as a guide and not relied on exclusively for assessment.

MANAGEMENT OF EXERCISE-INDUCED ASTHMA

To minimize the incidence and severity of EIA it is necessary, first, to maximize the control of a person's chronic asthma. This may necessitate a variety of measures, physical, immunological and pharmacological. It is now recommended that physicians construct an individual 'asthma management plan' for each of their patients to maximize the control of their chronic asthma (Woolcock *et al.* 1989; National Asthma Campaign 1993). If their chronic asthma is not adequately controlled it is extremely difficult to control their EIA and often severe bouts of EIA are an indication of undertreated asthma. This asthma management plan, which aims at confirming the diagnosis, abolishing symptoms and maximizing lung function, can be summarized under the following procedural steps.

Asthma Management Plan

1 Assess severity of asthma.
2 Achieve best lung function.
3 Maintain best lung function; avoid trigger factors.
4 Maintain best lung function, with optimal medication.
5 Develop an action plan to allow early recognition of deterioration and the appropriate response.
6 Educate and review regularly.

In addition, it has also been recommended (Morton & Fitch 1992) that the personal physician also develop an 'EIA Management Plan' to minimize the individual's EIA. This plan, summarized under the following seven procedural steps, should also be prepared in writing for the patient.

Exercise-Induced Asthma Management Plan

1 Follow general asthma management plan (as outlined above).
2 Determine pre-exercise medication to prevent EIA.
3 Predetermine when to avoid or cease physical exertion.

Table 28.1 Drugs used for treating asthma: Effectiveness and legal status for competition

Medication	Route of administration	Effectiveness in EIA	Legal or banned	Prophylaxis (P)* or bronchodilator (B)
Khellin derivatives				
Sodium cromoglycate	Aerosol	Good	Legal	P
Nedocromil sodium	Aerosol	Good	Legal	P
β₂-agonists				
Salbutamol	Aerosol	Excellent	Legal	B
	Rotocap	Excellent	Legal	B
	Oral	Good	Banned	B
Terbutaline	Aerosol	Excellent	Legal	B
	Turbuhaler	Excellent	Legal	B
	Oral	Good	Banned	B
Salmeterol	Aerosol	Excellent	Banned	B
Orciprenaline	Aerosol	Excellent	Banned	B
Formoterol	Aerosol	Excellent	Banned	B
Methylxanthines				
Theophylline	Oral	Good	Legal	B
Aminophylline	Oral	Good	Legal	B
Belladonna alkaloids				
Ipratropium bromide	Aerosol	Fair	Legal	B
Glucocorticosteroids				
Beclomethasone diproprionate	Aerosol	Uncertain	Legal	P
Budesonide	Turbuhaler	Uncertain	Legal	P
Prednisone	Oral	Uncertain	Banned	P

*Note Ps are often referred to as 'PREVENTERS' while Bs are referred to as 'RELIEVERS'.

4 Have available medication to reverse EIA should it develop.
5 Achieve and maintain satisfactory aerobic fitness
6 Understand techniques to minimize EIA.
7 Know which drugs are permitted in international sporting competition.

A recent paper (Morton & Fitch 1992) has reviewed the pharmacological agents available to treat asthmatics with special emphasis on those that can prevent EIA. Cromoglycate, theophylline and corticosteroids (aerosol and oral) are valuable drugs to attain and maintain satisfactory control of asthma. However, to achieve control over one's asthma, inhaled corticosteroids and/or inhaled cromoglycate, particularly in children, have become the drugs of choice for the first-line defence. Advice concerning the avoidance of 'trigger factors' will assist to reduce the risk of all episodes of broncho-constriction. It is a wise precaution for physicians

to periodically check that the asthmatic is employing the correct technique of administering aerosol medications as approximately 50% of children and 30% of adults use metered dose inhalers incorrectly.

Once the patient's asthma is controlled so that airways inflammation is reduced, by inhaled cortico-steroids or cromoglycate, the exercise response will be minimized and the amount of pre-exercise preventive medication required may be reduced or, in some cases, eliminated. The majority of asth-matics, however, require pre-exercise medication to permit participation in physical recreation and competitive sport with the minimum of respiratory disadvantage.

The asthmatic needs to be aware of the preventive benefits of the various drugs to inhibit EIA and the

Fig. 28.3 A flow diagram for the prevention of exercise-induced asthma.

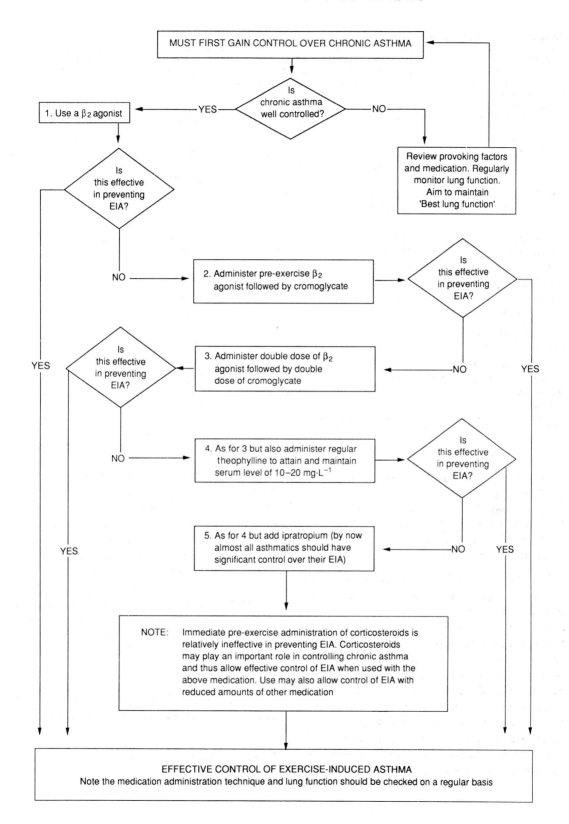

MUST FIRST GAIN CONTROL OVER CHRONIC ASTHMA

Is chronic asthma well controlled?

1. Use a β_2 agonist — YES

NO

Review provoking factors and medication. Regularly monitor lung function. Aim to maintain 'Best lung function'

Is this effective in preventing EIA?

NO

2. Administer pre-exercise β_2 agonist followed by cromoglycate

Is this effective in preventing EIA?

NO — YES

Is this effective in preventing EIA?

3. Administer double dose of β_2 agonist followed by double dose of cromoglycate

NO — YES

YES

NO

4. As for 3 but also administer regular theophylline to attain and maintain serum level of 10–20 mg·L^{-1}

Is this effective in preventing EIA?

NO — YES

YES

NO

5. As for 4 but add ipratropium (by now almost all asthmatics should have significant control over their EIA)

NO — YES

NOTE: Immediate pre-exercise administration of corticosteroids is relatively ineffective in preventing EIA. Corticosteroids may play an important role in controlling chronic asthma and thus allow effective control of EIA when used with the above medication. Use may also allow control of EIA with reduced amounts of other medication

EFFECTIVE CONTROL OF EXERCISE-INDUCED ASTHMA
Note the medication administration technique and lung function should be checked on a regular basis

most effective pharmacological agents in reversing bronchoconstriction should it supervene during exercise. Should the asthmatic reach national or international competition standards, then he or she, together with the coach and team physician, must know which medications are permitted and which are considered illegal if used during sporting competitions (Table 28.1).

When attempting to block EIA, the drugs of choice are the β_2-agonists. (Medications are listed by classification and generic names in Table 28.1.) Only salbutamol and terbutaline, by inhalation, are acceptable for use during international sporting competition. The short-acting β_2-agonists, for example salbutamol and terbutaline have a rapid action (60 s) and are effective over a relatively long duration (about 2 h) while the long-acting β_2-agonists, for example formoterol and salmeterol, may provide up to 12 h of protection. It is recommended that these be administered by inhalation 5–10 min before commencing exercise. For the athlete who may be subjected to sport drug testing it is essential that salbutamol or terbutaline, by inhalation only, be prescribed. Oral β_2-agonists have been classified as anabolic agents and are banned (see Chapter 26).

If administration of the β_2-agonist does not successfully block EIA then a combination of these drugs with sodium cromoglycate using single or even double doses of each, or with sodium cromoglycate and theophylline should be tried in that order (Fig. 28.3). If the asthmatic regularly exhibits the second late response to exercise and since β_2-agonist will be ineffective against the second phase, this person should use a combination of the β_2-agonist and sodium cromoglycate. Theophylline is administered orally and should achieve serum levels of 10–20 $\mu g \cdot mL^{-1}$ to ensure a therapeutic effect. Sodium cromoglycate and theophylline are approximately equal in their protection against EIA but inferior to β_2-agonists. While cromoglycate is virtually free of side-effects, theophylline can cause nausea, vomiting and gastro-oesophageal reflux, though sustained release preparations of theophylline are better tolerated (Table 28.1).

For subjects who still experience EIA, aerosol ipratropium bromide may be added to the medi-cation regimen. Aerosol ipratropium bromide is a belladonna alkaloid, which is a useful bronchodilator for patients who cannot tolerate or do not respond to β_2-adrenoceptor stimulants.

Glucocorticoids, both oral and aerosol, are excellent drugs to stabilize asthma, but have little effect if administered just before exercise to prevent EIA.

It must be remembered that for medication such as sodium cromoglycate and aerosol corticosteroid to be fully effective, they must be distributed to the deeper regions of the lungs. Therefore for regular or pre-event medication, the patient who is wheezing will require a β_2-agonist before administration of these other pharmacological agents.

The use of 'spacer' devices can increase the efficacy of medication administered via a metered dose inhaler (MDI) by increasing its deposition in the lungs. This is particularly important for those who have difficulty in co-ordinating the actuation and inhalation. The use of a spacer may also minimize the systemic side-effects and, in the case of inhaled corticosteroids, reduce the incidence of mouth and throat *Candida* (National Asthma Campaign 1993).

Whenever drug combinations are required, the β_2-agonist should always be administered first, since the resultant bronchodilation will then permit a more effective distribution of the cromoglycate or corticosteroid throughout the airways.

REVERSING EXERCISE-INDUCED ASTHMA

Should EIA occur during the game or activity, the aerosol β_2-agonists are the best means of reversing the bronchoconstriction. Sodium cromoglycate has little bronchodilator activity and is not effective once EIA has supervened. It is recommended, therefore, that asthmatics take a β_2-agonist aerosol spray to all training sessions and competitions.

PRESCRIBING EXERCISE FOR THE ASTHMATIC

The majority of asthmatics can, with the benefit of pre-exercise medication, participate equally with non-asthmatics of similar size, skill and fitness level. As the training programme for a top-level performer in a given sport is the same regardless of whether he is asthmatic or non-asthmatic, only a general aerobic fitness programme will be outlined here.

Warm-up

All training sessions and games should be preceded by a warm-up, which continues at least until mild sweating occurs. Even though there have been contradictory findings regarding the value of the warm-up in influencing the normal bronchial response to exercise in the asthmatic, the general benefits of warm-up still apply to the asthmatic.

The warm-up should consist of rhythmic low-level activity such as walking progressing to jogging, etc. This should be followed by some light flexibility exercise for most muscle groups, with a special emphasis on those muscles involved in the specific activity or event. A period of strengthening exercises for the same muscles can also be included.

An early warm-up session may also be used to produce a refractory period at the time of the event.

The Aerobic Segment

Exercise should begin at a low level of intensity and gradually increase in severity as the fitness level improves. The aim should be to stress the system without straining it. The activity should utilize large muscle groups in a rhythmic fashion such as in walking, jogging, running, cycling and various endurance game activities. The intensity should be such that it exceeds the threshold required for cardiorespiratory improvement, thus an intensity of 50–85% of one's maximal oxygen consumption ($\dot{V}_{O_2max}$) or 65–90% of maximal heart rate is recommended.

Duration

Each session should last between 15 and 60 min. The very unfit may need to limit sessions to 15 min initially, but should aim to increase the duration to a minimum of 30 min.

Frequency

Research has indicated that exercise three to five times per week is adequate. Greater improvement can be gained with more frequent sessions, but the increase in improvement is small in relation to the increase in time expenditure.

Exercise Loading

If the asthmatic is very unfit, the programme should commence with continuous walking, as this exercise has a low asthmagenicity and prepares the muscles for future higher intensity exercise. As the fitness level improves, especially in the musculoskeletal system, one can increase the intensity by progressing to low-level interval training consisting of walking and jogging. One then progresses to high-intensity exercise, using training intervals of 10–30 s followed by 30–90 s rest periods.

If the asthmatic gets more enjoyment from fartlek or cross-country type running, then he or she can usually pursue these activities successfully with adequate medication. Many team sports are ideal, as they require an intermittent pattern of energy expenditure.

Mode

Regular or frequent participation in fitness programmes relies on the participant gaining an adequate level of enjoyment from the activity involved. For this reason the activities in which the asthmatic shows most interest should be prescribed. One must attempt to influence asthmatics to select activities that are aerobic (to stress the cardiorespiratory system) and if possible have them spend some period of their childhood involved in swimming training. Not only is swimming less asthmagenic, but it has a very positive influence on increasing heart and lung volumes.

Asthmatics who are unwilling to use, or who do not obtain full protection from, pre-exercise medication should select those physical activities with low asthmagenicity, such as swimming and walking, or perform the activity using an intermittent work/rest regimen.

Warm-down

Every training session or game should be followed by a warm-down (or cool-down) segment. This can be accomplished by continuing light rhythmic activities such as walking until the heart rate returns to within about 20 beats·min^{-1} of the pre-exercise level. The warm-down segment should conclude with a repetition of the flexibility exercise regimen performed during warm-up.

WHEN TO AVOID OR CEASE EXERTION

If the asthmatic has taken the prescribed pre-exercise medication and is still exhibiting broncho-constriction, it is unwise to attempt vigorous exercise. Although some asthmatics find that exercise dilates the airways and improves breathing, the majority develop increased bronchoconstriction. Wheezing schoolchildren presenting to physical education class or sport should be excused for that session.

The asthmatic should cease participating in a game or vigorous exercise session if EIA develops during the activity. If inhalation of a β_2-agonist reverses the bronchoconstriction the asthmatic can resume the exercise or sporting event. If it is not successful he/she should refrain from further participation.

Performing vigorous activity while bronchoconstricted can lead to a severe drop in the oxygen saturation level of the arterial blood, carbon dioxide accumulation and hyperinflation of the lungs with an increased residual volume. This results in severe dyspnoea and general discomfort, possible worsening of the bronchoconstriction and fatigue of the respiratory muscles.

If the asthmatic regularly measures the PEFR and is thus aware of his/her normal unobstructed level, a peak flow measure made at the time of concern can be a good guide to the advisability of continuing activity. It should be at least 80% of his/her 'best' value. The availability of inexpensive peak flow meters means that school physical education departments and individual asthmatics can afford their own instruments and have them available for such use.

TRAINING FOR COMPETITIVE SPORT

The fitness requirements of the sport or event apply equally to the asthmatic and the non-asthmatic; however, the asthmatic should place particular emphasis on the pre- and early season increase in aerobic capacity.

The asthmatic should seek and follow a doctor's advice concerning pre-event medication and have a bronchodilator spray always available at games and training sessions. This aerosol should be used during workouts whenever early symptoms such as tightness in the chest, followed by dry cough, shortness of breath and/or wheeze are experienced. This will usually allow the training session to be completed even if the severity has to be reduced.

Those asthmatics who regularly experience a refractory period after a bout of EIA and who recover rapidly from it (within 30 min) should experiment with a thorough and vigorous warm-up well before the game or event is due to start. If this produces mild EIA it may then provide protection during the game or event, in which case it could be used before all subsequent games.

Asthmatics training for general fitness or for a competitive sport may find it beneficial to train while wearing a face mask (Anderson 1986). These masks increase the temperature of the inspired air, thus reducing the likelihood of EIA and are especially useful during cold weather. There are also a number of 'cold air breathing aids' on the market. These are placed in the mouth like a SCUBA mouthpiece and contain a hydrophilic fibre batting that develops heat-exchange characteristics as moisture condenses on it. It also conserves water and provides a warm, moist inspirate and the manufacturers claim that it will reduce the incidence and severity of EIA. They are, of course, impractical for use in most instances during competition itself.

If possible, asthmatics should select the time of training to coincide with minimal daily asthmagenicity. For instance, they should not train early in the morning or in the evening if the weather is cold and should refrain from training when pollens, dust or air pollution levels are high. Under certain of these conditions it is unwise for asthmatics to exercise outside of air-conditioned premises.

CONCLUSIONS

The response of asthmatics to exercise is extremely variable from person to person and to some extent, even for the same person at different times. However, as a general rule, asthmatics should participate in regular exercise and sports programmes with a minimum of restrictions. To maximize the level of participation they should use suitable pre-exercise medication in the form of aerosol β_2-agonists and/or sodium cromoglycate and if EIA does occur, it may be reversed by an aerosol β_2-agonist. If required, inhaled corticosteroid is the drug of choice to control chronic asthma. The success of asthmatics at the highest levels of sport is testimony to the benefits of exercise in overcoming their disability and a stimulus for others to include physical activity and sports in their daily lives.

REFERENCES

Anderson S. D. (1984) Is there a unifying hypothesis for exercise-induced asthma. *Journal of Clinical Immunology* 73, 660–665.

Anderson S. D. (1986) EIA: New thinking and current management. *Journal of Respiratory Disease* 7, 48–61.

Edmunds A. T., Tooley M. & Godfrey S. (1978) The refractory period after exercise-induced asthma: Its duration and relation to the severity of exercise. *American Review of Respiratory Disease* 117, 247–254.

Godfrey S. & Bar-Yishay E. (1993) Exercise-induced asthma revisited. *Respiratory Medicine* 87, 331–344.

Hahn A., Anderson S. D., Morton A. R., Black J. L. & Fitch K. D. (1984) A re-interpretation of the effect of temperature and water content of the inspired air in exercise-induced asthma. *American Review of Respiratory Disease* 130, 575–579.

Inbar O., Dotan R., Dlin R. N., Nueman I. & Bar-Or O. (1980) Breathing dry or humid air and exercise-induced asthma during swimming. *European Journal of Applied Physiology* 44, 43–50.

Jones R. S., Buston M. H. & Wharton M. J. (1962) The effect of exercise on ventilatory function in the child with asthma. *British Journal of Diseases of the Chest* 56, 78–86.

Larsson K., Ohlsen P., Larsson L., Lalmberg P., Rydstrom P-O. & Ulriksen H. (1993) High prevalence of asthma in cross country skiers, *British Medical Journal* 307, 1326–1329.

Lee T. H., Nagakura J., Papageorgiou N., Iikura Y. & Kay A. B. (1983) Exercise-induced late asthmatic reactions with neutrophil chemotactic activity. *New England Journal of Medicine* 308, 1502–1505.

McLennon W. (1992) *1989–90 National Health Status Indicators Australia.* Australian Bureau of Statistics, Catalogue No. 4370.0.

Morton A. R. & Fitch K. D. (1992) Asthmatic drugs and competitive sport: An update. *Sports Medicine* 14, 228–242.

Morton A. R. & Fitch K. D. (1993) Asthma. In Skinner J. S. (ed.) *Exercise Testing and Exercise Prescription for Special Cases: Theoretical Basis and Clinical Application,* pp. 211–227, 2nd edn. Lea & Febiger, Philadelphia, PA.

Morton A. R., Fitch K. D. & Hahn A. G. (1981) Physical activity and the asthmatic. *Physician and Sports Medicine* 9, 50–64.

Morton A. R., Lawrence S. R., Fitch K. D. & Hahn A. G. (1983) Duration of exercise in the provocation of exercise-induced asthma. *Annals of Allergy* 51, 530–534.

Mussaffi H., Springer C. & Godfrey S. (1986) Increased bronchial responsiveness to exercise and histamine after allergen challenge in asthmatic children. *Journal of Allergy and Clinical Immunology* 77, 48–52.

National Asthma Campaign (1993) *Asthma Management Handbook 1993.* National Asthma Campaign Ltd, Melbourne, pp. 1–64.

Novinski N., Bar-Yishay E., Gur I. & Godfrey S. (1987) Exercise intensity determines and climatic conditions modify the severity of exercise-induced asthma. *American Review of Respiratory Disease* 136, 592–594.

Schoeffel R. E., Anderson S. D. & Altounyan R. E. (1981) Bronchial hyperreactivity response to inhalation of ultrasonically nebulised solutions of distilled water and saline. *British Medical Journal* 283, 1285–1287.

Silverman M. & Anderson S. D. (1972) Standardisation of exercise tests in asthmatic children. *Archives of Disease in Childhood* 47, 882–889.

Sly P. D., Cahill P., Willet K. & Burton P. (1994) Accuracy of mini peak flow meters in indicating changes in lung function in children with asthma. *British Medical Journal* 308, 572–574.

Voy R. (1986) The US Olympic Committee experience with exercise-induced bronchospasm 1984. *Medicine and Science in Sports and Exercise* 18, 328–330.

Woolcock A. J., Rubinfeld A. R., Seale J. P. *et al.* (1989) Asthma Management Plan. *Medical Journal of Australia* 151, 650–653.

PART II

EPILEPSY

R. A. Reid

Epilepsy is a group of disorders characterized by chronic, recurrent seizures (Hutchinson & Frith 1989). Isolated, non-recurrent seizures such as generalized tonic–clonic seizures in normal people caused by significant sleep deprivation are not included in this classification.

Many epileptics will want to play sport and epilepsy should not bar them from participating, although common sense is required when counselling them with respect to their preferred sport and their personal aspirations.

There are various types of epilepsy despite the fact that they are often classified together and any label will be misleading in 85% of cases because of individual variation.

Approximately seven in 1000 people have some sort of seizure disorder at some time in their life, although this figure may be as high as 2% of the population (G. Danta personal communication).

CLASSIFICATION OF EPILEPSY

Partial or Focal Seizures

This type of seizure is nearly always due to some local structural abnormality and is classified as follows:

SIMPLE PARTIAL SEIZURES

These normally occur in one area, but can spread from the affected area to involve other ipsilateral body parts (Jacksonian march). There is no alteration of consciousness and an electroencephalogram

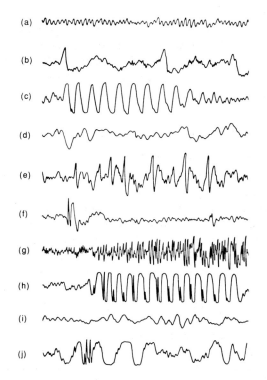

Fig. 28.4 Examples of EEG types and features (*Note*: Figs reduced by a factor of 2.5). (a) Normal, 10 per second activity. (b) Single spike waves. (c) Regular slow waves, three per second (interictal, *petit mal*).
(d) Random slow waves. (e) Spikes and poly-spike waves. (f) Spike and wave discharge. (g) Tonic–clonic seizure, onset. (h) Absence seizure, three per second spike and wave discharge. (i) Normal 5 year old, slow waves with six to nine per second activity. (j) Hypsarrhythmia in a 5 year old. High voltage irregular slow wave activity with spike seizure discharge.

(EEG) will show spike activity intra-ictally and often interictally (Fig. 28.4b).

COMPLEX PARTIAL SEIZURES

These are episodic changes in behaviour, associated with loss of contact with the environment. The first sign may be an aura, which is often a sensory hallucination. An EEG will show spikes or slow waves unilaterally or bilaterally (Fig. 28.4d), mainly in the temporal or frontotemporal regions, both intra- and interictally. Special electrodes are sometimes needed (nasopharyngeal, sphenoidal and deep electrodes) to confirm the diagnosis.

SECONDARY GENERALIZATION OF PARTIAL SEIZURES

Simple or complex partial seizures may progress, a few seconds or minutes later, to a generalized and often convulsive seizure. These patients often have post-ictal focal neurological deficits (Todd's paralysis) and post-ictal amnesia.

Primary Generalized Seizures

TONIC–CLONIC SEIZURES

This is the most common type of epileptic seizure seen clinically and is characterized by the onset of a sudden loss of consciousness and tonus. Opisthotonus may be apparent, followed by a period of clonic movements, which may be very violent. A period of relaxation is followed by confusion, which may last for some minutes. Up until the time of unconsciousness there will be no respiration, which may cause problems of oxygenation. During a seizure, urinary and faecal incontinence often occur and there may be tongue-biting.

After recovery there is a period of disorientation, which is often accompanied by post-ictal amnesia, headache and drowsiness and these patients may not feel normal for a number of days afterwards.

EEG findings are those of spikes and slow waves during the ictal period (Fig. 28.4g) and interictally there may be poly-spike or spike waves (Fig. 28.4e) and sharp and slow wave discharges. However, the interictal EEG may be normal.

TONIC SEIZURES

These are less common and of shorter duration than the tonic–clonic type of seizure. Otherwise they are similar, albeit without a period of clonus.

ABSENCE SEIZURES

These seizures may last seconds and are typified by a sudden cessation of conscious activity in which there will often be a minor motor manifestation. There is a rapid return to normal and no post-ictal confusion. They appear in children of 6–14 years and if very frequent may cause learning difficulties. The EEG is pathognomonic during seizures, with synchronous 3 Hz spike and wave discharges (Fig. 28.4c,h). The EEG is unremarkable interictally.

Absence seizures are very responsive to anticonvulsive therapy.

ATYPICAL ABSENCE SEIZURES

This type commonly coexists with other forms of seizures but not with tonic–clonic. They are often found in children with underlying neurological abnormalities and are usually very resistant to medication. The intra-ictal EEG shows a 2–4 Hz spike and wave discharge and the interictal EEG often shows a poorly developed background with spike and poly-spike activity (Fig. 28.4e).

MYOCLONIC SEIZURES

These are sudden, brief, single or repetitive muscle contractions in one part of the body or over the entire body. There is no loss of consciousness. The EEG will show poly-spike and wave (Fig. 28.4f) activity both inter- and intra-ictally and these seizures are often associated with other medical conditions. Readers are referred to relevant neurological texts for further discussion of these seizures.

ATONIC SEIZURES

This type of seizure often involves a brief loss of consciousness associated with a loss of postural tone, perhaps resulting in a fall. They are often associated with other forms of epilepsy and the EEG shows poly-spikes and slow waves (Fig. 28.4d,e).

INFANTILE SPASMS (HYPSARRHYTHMIAS)

These rare seizures normally come on in the first 12 months of life and have a poor prognosis, with 90% of children showing some form of mental retardation. An EEG will show a 'disorganized background', with random high voltage slow waves and spike and burst suppression (hypsarrhythmia; Fig. 28.4i,j).

Recurrent Patterns

SPORADIC SEIZURES

These seizures may occur months or years apart, posing problems of diagnosis, counselling and management.

CYCLIC SEIZURES

The most common of these is catamenial and is associated with menses, though other forms may occur.

REFLEX SEIZURES

These are seizures triggered by a specific stimulus. A photic stimulus is the most common, with 8–12 flashes per second being the most common frequency of seizure production (α rhythm frequency). A pattern of sound (musicogenic) or other stimulus may cause fits in people with reflex epilepsy.

Status Epilepticus

Prolonged or repetitive seizures without a period of recovery are described as status epilepticus and are classified as follows:

- Tonic–clonic seizures may be life-threatening, as there is no respiration during the time of the seizure
- With absence status and non-convulsive status the condition is often unrecognized, as there is no loss of consciousness
- Epilepsia partialis continua is status epilepticus of partial seizures

Evaluation of Seizures

HISTORY

In order to evaluate a patient presenting with a history of one or more seizures, the doctor must know their medical history. This includes a description of the seizure(s), their frequency, mode and speed of onset, presence or absence of an aura, state of consciousness, presence of motor activity, presence of pallor or cyanosis, duration, post-ictal headache or confusion, injuries sustained, incontinence, speed of recovery and post-ictal neurological deficit. Additional problems such as febrile convulsions, previous meningitis/encephalitis, significant head injuries, drug use/abuse (withdrawal fits), previous metabolic problems and any family history of epilepsy should also be known.

EXAMINATION

An examination may provide evidence of cranial trauma and/or an intracranial lesion, or possibly some specific cause of the seizure.

SPECIAL INVESTIGATIONS

Additional investigations which may prove useful will include:

- EEG. This may help define the type of epilepsy. Focal abnormalities may show and an EEG may prove useful as a 'baseline', for example monitoring of a child with absence of seizures. A sleeping EEG or sleep-deprivation EEG may also be useful in some cases and a 24 h EEG monitoring or concurrent video/EEG monitoring are sometimes used for difficult cases
- Computerized tomography (CT). For partial seizures or adult-onset seizures, this will be useful in detecting any mass lesion within the skull or increased intracranial pressure
- Lumbar puncture. If meningitis/encephalitis is suspected, a lumbar puncture should be performed
- Magnetic resonance imaging (MRI). This may be useful in detecting lesions which may not be apparent by other forms of imaging
- Blood tests. These may be useful to exclude or confirm hypoglycaemia, hypo- or hypernatraemia, hypo- or hypercalcaemia, thyrotoxicosis, renal or hepatic failure and occasionally acute intermittent porphyria and lead or arsenic poisoning

Differential Diagnosis

The differential diagnosis includes vasovagal attacks, cardiogenic syncope, transient ischaemic episodes, migraines and psychogenic seizures (psychomotor variance/hysterical seizures). Exclusion of these may require an electrocardiograph, 24 h Holter monitoring, cerebral angiography or saline provocation tests.

Management of Epilepsy

GENERAL CONSIDERATIONS

Comprehensive management of epilepsy includes the elimination or treatment of the causes of the seizures, the suppression of seizures and dealing with the psychosocial consequences of epilepsy and its treatment. This is of greater importance in sports people as the effect upon the athlete and their team-mates must also be considered.

COUNSELLING THE EPILEPTIC

Counselling may be the most important part of the treatment of epileptic athletes and should include:

- Discussion of the nature of the problem
- The effect that sports in which they may wish to participate have on them
- A referral to an epilepsy organization who can assist them
- Encouragement to maintain an independent life-style where practicable

A thorough understanding of any sport or activity contemplated by the epileptic is required and modification of an activity may be needed to make the activity safe, though few activities will require total exclusion.

Realistic goals and aspirations need to be set for the epileptic and a balance needs to be reached between possible decreases in self-esteem and the potential risks of an increased number of seizures and decreased safety. First aid procedures should be discussed with the patient, close relatives and the coach.

NON-PHARMACOLOGICAL TREATMENT

Factors which decrease the seizure threshold should be modified where possible. These include alcohol intake, sleep deprivation, hyperventilation, stress, other drugs and photic and other sensory stimuli in patients with reflex epilepsy. Alcohol is common in the sporting environment and should be used with caution because of its effect on the liver.

PHARMACOLOGICAL TREATMENT

Pharmacological suppression of seizures is designed to protect the patient while not interfering with normal cognitive function or producing harmful side-effects. New medications are continually being produced for the control of epilepsy. Many of them are 'designer-drugs' which have been developed as knowledge of some of the underlying factors causing seizures become known with research. Major changes in the way epileptics are treated — with more effective control and fewer side-effects — are likely to occur in the near future. Current research is based on the balance between glutamate (an excitatory neurotransmitter) and GABA (gamma amino butyric acid — an inhibitory neurotransmitter). Many of the newer medications are GABA analogues (GABA Pentin) or are GABA-transaminase inhibitors (Sabril [Vigabatrin], Lamictal [Lamotrigine]). At present, they seem to be better for partial seizures or as adjunctive medication in epilepsy that is not well controlled.

Monotherapy within the therapeutic range is the treatment of choice. There are groups of drugs which are used for different seizure types, although currently there seems little difference between the drugs within each group. Refer to Table 28.2 for a summary of recommended therapy.

It is important to monitor the blood levels of any anti-epileptic medication (except sodium valproate) and this should be checked four to five half-lives after the medication is started. In the blood, most anti-epileptic medications are protein-bound, but it is the unbound 'free' drug which is associated with seizure control. When prescribing for epileptics, it is necessary to understand that many anticonvulsant drugs interact with other drugs. As a consequence, serum levels of anti-epileptic drugs may be either increased or reduced. In addition, the efficacy of other drugs can be impaired or at times enhanced when administered concomitantly with anticonvulsants.

The greatest pharmacological problem with seizure control is compliance and flights across time zones may pose a problem even for stable epileptics because of the difficulty in timing the medication to maintain a therapeutic level. Two watches should be used so that compliance can be

Table 28.2 Recommended pharmacotherapy

	Type of epilepsy	First-line therapy	Second-line therapy
Group 1	Tonic–clonic	Carbamazepine	Primidone
	Partial	Vigabatrin	Lamotrizine
		Phenytoin	Phenobarbitone
	Partial with secondary generalization	Sodium valproate	Vigabatrin
Group 2	Absence	Sodium valproate	Ethosuximide
			Clonazepam
Group 3	Atonic	Sodium valproate	Clonazepam
	Tonic	Phenytoin	

maintained for 'short' trips (3 weeks or less). A gradual change, however, may be needed if the trip is longer or permanent.

Anti-epileptic medications are not banned for international competition, except in those sports which ban the use of sedatives, such as the modern pentathlon.

CARBAMAZEPINE ('TEGRETOL', 'TERIL')

This is well tolerated in the long-term; however, there is some initial drowsiness but little effect on cognitive function. Hepatic enzyme induction is almost universal and a number of drugs including erythromycin can increase plasma levels of carbamazepine.

PHENYTOIN ('DILANTIN')

This causes little disturbance of concentration and cognitive impairment is uncommon, particularly in children. However, gum hypertrophy and hirsutism are common side-effects. A long half-life means a once daily dosage is suitable, but small changes in dose may produce large changes in the blood level around the therapeutic range. Many drugs interact with phenytoin either increasing or reducing serum levels. Antibiotics such as trimethoprim, co-trimoxazole and chloramphenicol may increase blood levels as a result of competition for protein binding sites in the blood and phenytoin may be used intravenously for the treatment of status epilepticus.

SODIUM VALPROATE ('EPILIM', 'VALPRO')

There is little cognitive impairment with sodium valproate and it is the drug of choice in children with absence and myoclonic seizures. There may be sedation initially and side-effects such as nausea and vomiting can be decreased by the use of enteric-coated tablets twice daily with food. Blood levels have little relationship to either efficacy or toxicity and so are not monitored. Clinical monitoring must be used and serial EEG can be used for children with absence seizures.

LAMOTRIGINE ('LAMICTAL')

Currently, this is an 'add-on' medication used in partial epilepsy which is not well controlled with other drugs. It also has an effect on tonic–clonic seizures. It may become first-line treatment for partial epilepsy in the future (Harden 1994).

VIGABATRIN ('SABRIL')

This irreversible inhibitor of GABA transaminase is used as adjunctive therapy in patients with poorly controlled epilepsy. Because of behavioural changes which may follow the use of Vigabatrin, it is not recommended for patients with a history of or susceptibility to psychotic episodes (Harden 1994).

GABAPENTIN

This is a GABA analogue which is effective as adjunctive therapy in refractory partial seizures and secondary generalized seizures.

PHENOBARBITONE

Although in most instances this is a second-line drug, it is the treatment of choice for febrile convulsions. It causes a depression of cognitive function and sedation is common. Children and the elderly, however, may become hyperactive or hyperirritable while on it. It may be used intravenously in status epilepticus.

PRIMIDONE ('MYSOLINE')

This second-line drug is metabolized to phenobarbitone and phenylethylmalonamide. It may be useful in difficult cases, especially with partial seizures.

CLOBAZAM ('FRISIUM')

This is a benzodiazepine to which about one-third of patients develop tolerance and withdrawal seizures are common. It is the treatment of choice in catamenial seizures, where it is used for 10 days about the time of the menses. Clobazam is also effective in the treatment of partial seizures.

ETHOSUXIMIDE ('ZARONTIN')

Ethosuximide is a valuable drug to control absence seizures especially in children.

CLONAZEPAM ('RIVOTRIL')

This benzodiazepine is used for absence seizures, but is of little use in children, as behavioural disorders are common. Tolerance may develop, as for clobazam.

NEUROSURGICAL TREATMENT

This may be considered if a lesion is found, or in some cases of complex partial seizures (Hutchinson & Frith 1989) where one temporal lobe is found to have a lesion and the other side is normal.

CONCOMITANT ORAL CONTRACEPTIVE THERAPY

Hepatic enzyme induction by anticonvulsive therapy increases breakdown of oral contraceptives and therefore increases the risk of pregnancy in female athletes. A higher dose oral contraceptive may be needed or another form of contraception used.

PREGNANCY

There is an increased incidence of seizures during pregnancy and a decrease in serum levels of anticonvulsant drugs. Carbamazepine and phenobarbitone are probably the safest anticonvulsants to use in pregnancy (Hutchinson & Frith 1989). Sodium valproate should be avoided in women likely to become pregnant (Hutchinson & Frith 1989).

WITHDRAWAL OF ANTICONVULSANT

Of those who are seizure-free on medication, 50% will be seizure-free after the medication is stopped. The greatest chance of this occurs:

- When there has been a 3–4 year seizure-free period on a single medication
- When there were few seizures before control
- When there is a normal neurological examination
- When there is a normal EEG at the end of the therapeutic period (Hutchinson & Frith 1989)

There is an increased recurrence in those who have had partial seizures or where there is an underlying structural brain disease.

Medication should not be stopped suddenly but should be slowly tapered over a period of 6–12 months. An abnormal EEG is not a contra-indication to a trial of withdrawing therapy in this manner.

DOES 'CONTROL' EXIST?

It is variously reported that 55–80% of epileptics can be controlled on monotherapy and in fact most epileptics are well-controlled and can lead a relatively 'normal' life. Epileptics who are more difficult to control often have other neurological problems. Approximately 5% of epileptics who are being poorly controlled are mentally defective.

EFFECT ON SPORTS PERFORMANCE

Epilepsy

Epilepsy *per se* should not be a reason to exclude participation in sports. Common sense, however, would indicate that some sports are more dangerous for epileptics than others (American Academy of Pediatrics 1983; O'Donohoe 1983; Cowart 1986; Couch 1987). With proper medical management, good seizure control and proper supervision, there should be few exclusions.

There is no effect on the individual's physiological performance by epilepsy, although epileptics may not feel 'normal' for a few hours or days after a major motor seizure (Cowart 1986). It may be wise to restrict activities during this time, but this should not exclude epileptics from participating in sport or recreation.

Anticonvulsant Therapy

Anticonvulsant drugs do not blunt physiological responses to exercise. In high doses, however, some drugs decrease cognitive function and co-ordination, but these effects are generally minimal at therapeutic levels on monotherapy. Phenytoin has the least such effects at therapeutic levels, whereas sodium valproate and carbamazepine have more. Phenobarbitone and primidone may have significant effects at or even below therapeutic levels.

Regardless of whether there are objective or subjective effects while on anticonvulsant therapy, most patients feel better after cessation of treatment.

IMPACT OF SPORTS ON EPILEPSY

There is no change in the frequency or severity of seizures or the amount of anticonvulsant medication required in active compared with inactive epileptics (Cowart 1986). Seizure-type discharges are decreased during and after activity and there are fewer seizures during mental or physical activity in comparison with rest periods (Cowart 1986; Couch 1987). This may be because of behavioural changes, sensory inhibition or metabolic changes. Stress, hyperventilation and exhaustion may all trigger seizures (O'Donohoe 1983; Cowart 1986). Hyperventilation causes a respiratory alkalosis and a decrease of blood flow to the brain, which increases absence seizures in susceptible athletes.

Sports may be associated with an increase in metabolism of anticonvulsant drugs (Cowart 1986), but this is not widely reported as a problem. In general, it seems that sports have a positive effect on epilepsy.

PSYCHOSOCIAL CONSIDERATIONS

Parents who witness their child's convulsions often fear for the child's life (O'Donohoe 1983), although unexplained death in epileptics is uncommon: approximately 1:1000 of the total epileptic population. Restriction of activity because of this parental fear is likely to cause psychosocial damage and longer-term problems for epileptics, such as lack of self-confidence, poor self-esteem and lack of interpersonal skills (American Academy of Pediatrics 1983; O'Donohoe 1983).

The development of a positive self-image in the epileptic child is very important and sports activity may be a major factor in achieving this. A patient's physical life-style will be determined to some extent by sports activity as a child (American Academy of Pediatrics 1983; Cowart 1986) and this is probably the most important area in the management of epileptics. The negative consequences of lack of self-confidence and interpersonal skills may have wide-ranging physical, social and economic effects for the epileptic adult who has not learned the above skills during their formative years.

Some athletes who develop epilepsy will have many of the doubts that the parents of an epileptic child have. They will often feel like dropping out of sport and be depressed over the possible effects it will have on their future performance. However, most epileptics will be able to return to their sport once their condition is stabilized.

RECOMMENDATIONS

General

Recommendations and advice as to how the person can cope while playing sport need to be given on an individual basis. It would be unfortunate to exclude a sport or activity which is not affected by a person's seizure disorder and there may be little or no need to restrict activity of people with only sleep-related seizures.

Some authors (Van Linschoten et al. 1990) have noted that the risk of relapse after 2 years seizure-free is the same as that for a first seizure.

Medical guidelines for driving licenses (e.g. Australian Association of Neurologists' Advisory Committee 1988) may be used as a basis of recommendations for sports and various physical activities, as driving a motor vehicle encompasses many of the potential problems of sports and other activities.

Sports and activities which may require some restriction are those associated with high levels of stress, exhaustion, hyperventilation, the use of potentially dangerous equipment and prolonged isolation (American Academy of Pediatrics 1983; Cowart 1986).

Excluded Sports

Rope climbing, climbing on bars, trampolining, mountaineering, high-diving, flying, hang-gliding, javelin throwing, archery, pistol shooting, SCUBA diving and competitive underwater swimming are probably the only sports from which an epileptic should be excluded (American Academy of Pediatrics 1983; O'Donohoe 1983; Cowart 1986; Couch 1987). Such choices, however, depend on the individual, as some programmes include several of these activities as part of a confidence-enhancing exercise for children with epilepsy.

Showering in an enclosed glass or plastic stall is also unwise.

Most authors agree that swimming is safe if under constant supervision (American Academy of Pediatrics 1983; Cowart 1986). Swimming and activities which are associated with isolation, for example backpacking and cross-country skiing can be made safer for epileptics with a 'buddy' system. Contact sports are considered to be safe provided adequate protection is used. Boxing, however, is more controversial, with some advocating a total ban. The small number of epileptics who are pre-disposed to fits following a mild head injury should not take up boxing or other contact sports, such as the various codes of football. Those who have been unconscious because of a head injury should also try to avoid loss of consciousness.

Cycling may be a problem for children suffering from absence seizures because in traffic a momentary lapse of concentration may be dangerous, but well-controlled epileptics should have no problems away from traffic or on uncrowded cycle paths.

'Permitted' Sports

Most sports or activities are good for epileptics and should be encouraged and undertaken at a moderate level as long as there is good seizure control. Activities which require a moderate level of aerobic fitness and concentration or technical skill without high levels of stress are probably the most suitable for epileptics.

High-level competitive sport, however, is often associated with high stress levels and exhaustion and therefore may be unsuited to epileptics.

Driving and Epilepsy

The recommendations given by the Australian Association of Neurologists and modified by the Department of Transport and Communications (1988) are those currently used in Australia (Australian Association of Neurologists' Advisory Committee 1988).

The general guide-lines suggest that a specific diagnosis of the type of seizure should be made and investigation under strict neurological guide-lines be carried out. If there is no clear diagnosis, a fit-free period of 2 years is recommended before a licence application is approved and thereafter an annual follow-up is required for 5 years.

The suspension of a licence after a fit is based on other factors such as:

- Withdrawal (under medical supervision) of the anticonvulsant medication
- Other intercurrent problems (infections etc.)
- The cessation of medication without medical advice
- The use or abuse of alcohol

These may cause the suspension of a licence from 1 month to 2 years.

If it can be proved that seizures only occur during sleep there may be no restrictions imposed on the individual at all.

Sports People Who Become Epileptics

There are no clear guide-lines for sports people who develop epilepsy and until good control or cessation of the seizures occurs, full participation in sport may not be possible.

Dangerous and potentially dangerous sports or activities may require cessation altogether, but these may be reintroduced later if good control can be established.

Participation in sport may depend on the athletes' compliance with their medication and its efficacy; however, lapses in the compliance will make any sport more dangerous for the individual.

The biggest problem facing the athlete may be the requirement to modify or lower his or her aspirations in their chosen sport and this may be more of a problem for the governing bodies than the individual who has very well controlled epilepsy.

CONCLUSIONS

There are few restrictions that need to be placed on epileptics with regard to sports and activities and common sense must be used when suggesting a suitable type of activity or counselling. A full and frank discussion by everyone involved, including the athlete, partner, parents and coaches will be needed to make participation safe. With comprehensive medical management, good seizure control and proper supervision, there is little risk from most activities or sports.

Epileptics should be encouraged to lead a full life and become involved in physical activities to the best of their ability, as more psychological and social problems are caused by a severe restriction of activity than by its associated risks.

REFERENCES

American Academy of Pediatrics (1983) Sports and the child with epilepsy. *Pediatrics* 72, 884–885.

Australian Association of Neurologists' Advisory Committee (1988) *Driving and Epilepsy: Medical Guidelines Regarding Driving Licences.*

Couch J. M. (1987) Special medical problems of athletes. *Journal of Physical Education, Recreation and Dance* 58, 104–107.

Cowart V. S. (1986) Should epileptics exercise? *Physician and Sportsmedicine* 14, 183–191.

Department of Transport and Communications (Australia) (1988) *National Guidelines for Medical Practitioners in Determining Fitness to Drive a Motor Vehicle.* Australian Government Publishing Service, Canberra.

Harden C. L. (1994) New antiepileptic drugs. *Neurology* 44, 787–795.

Hutchinson D. O. & Frith R. W. (1989) Epilepsy: Choosing the most appropriate therapy. *Current Therapeutics* 30, 57–77.

O'Donohoe N. V. (1983) What should the child with epilepsy be allowed to do? *Archives of Disease in Childhood* 538, 934–937.

Van Linschoten R., Backx F. J. G., Mulder O. G. M. & Meinardi H. (1990) Epilepsy and sports. *Sports Medicine* 10, 9–19.

PART III

DIABETES MELLITUS

D. J. Chisholm

TYPES OF DIABETES

Diabetes mellitus is a syndrome, characterized by high blood glucose levels (hyperglycaemia), which has multiple causes (Kahn 1985). In a very small percentage of cases there is a recognizable clinical condition which causes the diabetes (e.g. haemochromatosis or iron storage disease); sometimes these conditions are reversible with a 'cure' of the diabetic state. However, the vast majority of people with diabetes fall into two major categories — insulin-dependent (Type I, juvenile onset) or non-insulin-dependent (Type II, maturity onset) diabetes. These two conditions are quite separate from the pathophysiological viewpoint, and there are important differences in relation to appropriate management of vigorous exercise or sport.

Insulin-dependent Diabetes

This accounts for about 10–15% of all cases of diabetes in most Caucasian populations and is due to destruction of the β cells of the pancreas by the body's immune system, causing relatively complete insulin deficiency. It usually has a sudden and dramatic onset in childhood or young adult life and insulin therapy is needed from the outset. Interruption or reduction of insulin therapy leads to excess production of ketones, which may lead to the life-threatening condition of ketoacidosis.

Non-insulin-dependent Diabetes

This type of diabetes accounts for about 85–90% of all cases; it has a more insidious onset in middle age or later life and mild hyperglycaemia may be present for some years prior to diagnosis. The cause is less well understood, but involves a strong genetic predisposition plus the environmental factors of a reduced level of physical activity, excess calories and obesity. There are three major metabolic abnormalities in non-insulin-dependent diabetes:

- Impaired insulin action (insulin resistance) in the insulin responsive tissues of the body, the most important of which is muscle
- Relatively delayed and impaired insulin secretion
- Excessive liver glucose output

Management by diet alone is possible in many cases but tablet therapy is often required with sulfonylureas or biguanides. Sulfonylureas have their predominant effect in increasing pancreatic insulin production, but may also improve insulin action. The mechanism of action of the biguanides is less well understood, but almost certainly involves delayed carbohydrate absorption from the gut and reduced liver glucose output. There is a tendency for a gradual progression of the metabolic disorder and insulin therapy is often needed as the patient ages. However, all patients with non-insulin-dependent diabetes maintain some endogenous insulin secretion, even when they do need insulin injections.

One of the practical differences between insulin-dependent and non-insulin-dependent diabetes in the management of exercise or sporting activity is that people with the former type of diabetes have much greater fluctuations in blood glucose levels. Thus avoidance of severe hypo- or hyperglycaemia is much more of a problem than with non-insulin-dependent diabetes. Nevertheless with modern diabetes management, including finger-prick blood glucose monitoring, it is possible for most people with diabetes, even of a relatively brittle insulin-dependent type, to engage in vigorous physical activity and a wide variety of sports. This is evidenced by the fact that there have been a number of athletes with insulin-dependent diabetes at the top international level, including American Davis Cup tennis players and an Australian cricket captain. However, to maintain satisfactory metabolic control, appropriate manipulations of diet and medication are important.

POTENTIAL BENEFITS OF PHYSICAL ACTIVITY IN PEOPLE WITH DIABETES

Most physicians who are expert in diabetes management consider that regular aerobic physical activity is a desirable component of therapy (NHMRC 1994). This is particularly true in non-insulin-dependent diabetes (Schneider & Ruderman 1990), where regular physical exercise of an aerobic or endurance nature has the capacity to improve insulin sensitivity (Fig. 28.5), thereby partially reversing one of the major metabolic defects of this condition (Bogardus et al. 1984; Simon 1984). Regarding this, it is notable that there is increasing epidemiological evidence that a physically active life-style reduces the prevalence of non-insulin-dependent diabetes and improves other cardiovascular risk factors in a number of racial groups, well demonstrated by Zimmet and colleagues, most recently in the population of Mauritius (Zimmet et al. 1991). On the other hand, demonstration of actual improvement in the diabetic state in established cases of non-

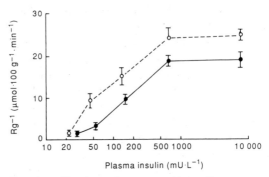

Fig. 28.5 Showing an improvement in insulin response in the red gastrocnemius muscle from exercise-trained animals (o) compared with sedentary animals (•). The data represent a dose–response curve for insulin action where Rg^{-1} is an index of glucose metabolism (James et al. 1985).

insulin-dependent diabetes has been somewhat equivocal (National Institutes of Health 1987; Berger et al. 1989). In both types of diabetes there is an increased risk of atheromatous arterial disease, which is the greatest cause of morbidity and mortality; as regular physical activity has been shown to have favourable effects on blood lipids, coagulation factors, platelets and blood pressure as well as 'cardiovascular fitness' (Simon 1984; Austin et al. 1994), it is reasonable to expect that it would reduce the cardiovascular risk and be of benefit in the long-term management of all diabetic patients.

Physiology and Pathophysiology of Carbohydrate Metabolism

During exercise in the non-diabetic person, muscular activity greatly increases glucose utilization. However, during exercise of moderate intensity, blood glucose levels remain remarkably stable for about 2 h, due to an increase in hepatic glucose output which precisely matches the glucose utilization. The mechanisms controlling the hepatic glucose output are not well understood. Insulin and the counter-regulatory hormones (especially catecholamines) undoubtedly play a part, but there are important regulatory processes which are independent of circulating levels of insulin and the counter-regulatory hormones (Jenkins 1986). Sympathetic neural stimulatory pathways and direct or indirect feedback effects of the blood glucose level itself on the liver are likely to be important.

In people with diabetes, the relationship between glucose utilization and hepatic glucose output is disturbed. Commonly, hepatic glucose output is quantitatively less than glucose utilization and the blood glucose level falls. However, there is considerable individual variation in the response, so that a rise in blood glucose is not uncommon, especially in children during vigorous physical activity. Moreover, when there is a state of relative insulin deficiency with a substantial elevation of blood glucose levels, exercise generally causes a further increase in hyperglycaemia and, in the insulin-dependent diabetic subject, may precipitate a degree of ketosis (Zinman 1989).

With regard to the longer-term effects of exercise, regular training improves insulin sensitivity and may lead to a reduced need for insulin or oral hypoglycaemic agents (National Institutes of Health 1987; Berger et al. 1989; Zinman 1989). However, the benefit is short-lived if the exercise training is interrupted. Importantly, a single bout of vigorous physical activity may increase insulin sensitivity for a period of up to 12–15 h. This may create a risk of a late hypoglycaemic reaction unless medication is reduced or carbohydrate intake increased during this period (MacDonald 1987).

PRINCIPLES OF MANAGEMENT

Some differences apply to the management of insulin-dependent or non-insulin-dependent diabetes, especially in regard to the metabolic responses (NHMRC 1994). Therefore the metabolic management will be discussed separately for each type, while other aspects of management common to both types of diabetes will be dealt with subsequently.

Insulin-dependent Diabetes (Wasserman & Zinman 1994)

The main consideration during vigorous physical activity in the person with insulin-dependent diabetes, is to avoid undue hypo- or hyperglycaemia. As there is commonly a fall in the blood glucose level during exercise, the routine approach is as follows:

- Increase carbohydrate intake. This is best done by taking complex carbohydrate prior to the activity if it is to last no more than about 70–80 min. A rough guide-line to carbohydrate intake would be 15 g of complex carbohydrate (e.g. one thick slice of bread) for each 20 min of moderately vigorous physical activity (say 60% $\dot{V}_{O_2max}$). Alternatively, simple sugar may be taken during the activity, for example 100 mL (half a can) of ordinary lemonade or other soft drink contains 12–15 g sugar. If carbohydrate is taken beforehand and the activity lasts more than about 70–80 min, it is wise to take a simple sugar, or a food that is easily digested containing a mixture of simple and complex carbohydrate, at intervals from 90 min onwards. Higher levels of physical activity would require proportionately more carbohydrate

- Reduce the dose of insulin operating at the time of the physical activity by 15–40% (e.g. a child playing a 0900 h game of football after taking his morning quick-acting (clear) and intermediate-acting (cloudy) insulin at 0700 h, might reduce the quick-acting insulin by 30%). For exercise of less than 30 min duration, it is usually not necessary to reduce the insulin dosage

It should be noted that neutral or regular insulin has an onset of action at about 30 min, peak effect at 2–3 h, and duration 6–7 h; for intermediate (Isophane or Lente) insulin onset is 1–2 h, peak 5–7 h and duration 12–14 h; for long-acting (Ultralente) insulin onset is 2–3 h, peak 8–14 h, duration 16–28 h. The shorter duration of action of different types of insulin compared to older estimates relates to a virtually complete shift to the use of human insulin formulations, which have shorter actions than pig and beef insulin.

It must be strongly emphasized that the above regimen represents a conventional approach to the average situation. In practice there is very considerable variation in the response of different individuals to the same activity, and of the same individual to different activities. Therefore the person with diabetes should be advised to follow the type of regimen suggested above, but it is important to check the finger-prick blood glucose level before and at the end of the period of physical activity to determine the response. When the exercise is prolonged, it may be helpful also to check the blood glucose during the activity if this is possible (e.g. between sets of a tennis game). If there is an elevation of blood glucose levels after the event, one would suggest a reduced carbohydrate intake or lesser reduction in the insulin dose on the next occasion. On the other hand, if blood glucose levels are unduly low, the reverse would apply. Once a response pattern is established for a particular person to a particular type and duration of exercise, it is likely that a similar response will occur on future occasions. Thus, when an appropriate adjustment of insulin and food intake is determined, this regimen can generally be repeated on future occasions with a satisfactory blood glucose response.

Two important issues with regard to insulin injections should be mentioned. First, although it may appear important to the diabetic subject to ensure avoidance of hypoglycaemia, it is unwise to make too large a reduction in the insulin injection prior to exercise, as excessive hyperglycaemia and ketosis may result (Zinman 1989). It is also wise to avoid giving the insulin injection prior to exercise into a limb that will be involved in the physical activity (Koivisto & Felig 1978) as the exercise will accelerate absorption of the insulin dose. Abdominal subcutaneous injection is generally the preferred site and injections in the thigh should be avoided if the subject is running.

The problem of late hypoglycaemia after exercise is of particular importance (MacDonald 1987). As mentioned above, a single bout of vigorous physical activity may increase insulin sensitivity for up to 15 h afterwards. Thus a person taking their usual dose of insulin may be at risk of hypoglycaemia during a period of 12–15 h after activity. For this reason it is often necessary to reduce the dose of insulin operating over that time period. For example, a child with a late afternoon football practice may need to have a small reduction in his evening dose

of quick and intermediate-acting insulin to avoid hypoglycaemia during the night. The occurrence of later hypoglycaemia after exercise seems to be unrelated to whether there was a rise or fall in blood glucose levels during the bout of exercise.

In a situation of moderately prolonged or very prolonged vigorous physical activity (Meinders et al. 1988; Sane et al. 1988), there is usually a need for a more substantial reduction of insulin dosage and the reduction is likely to involve the morning injection of both quick and intermediate-acting insulin. This would apply to situations such as an all-day cricket game, all-day skiing or an event such as a triathlon. Commonly, a reduction of 25–50% of the insulin dosage is required, but insulin has been omitted altogether without any adverse effects by some subjects involved in marathon running (Meinders et al. 1988). Once again, it is not possible to predict a response for each individual and blood glucose monitoring and urinary ketone measurements, during training sessions at the same time of day as the actual event, should be used as a guide in the manipulation of the insulin dosage and carbohydrate supplementation.

Non-insulin-dependent Diabetes (Schneider & Ruderman 1990)

In general, blood glucose levels are subject to much less fluctuation in non-insulin-dependent diabetes, so there is less risk of significant hypo- or hyperglycaemia. Nevertheless either problem can occur; so it is important to assess the individual response by a finger-prick using self-blood glucose monitoring, if this is possible. Two different types of oral hypoglycaemic agents are used in the management of non-insulin-dependent diabetes. Metformin, a biguanide, does not enhance insulin secretion and should not cause significant hypoglycaemia. Therefore, a patient taking Metformin only, should not be in danger of hypoglycaemia during exercise even if it is vigorous or prolonged. However, patients with diabetes controlled by Metformin alone usually only have mild hyperglycaemia; therefore, it would often be appropriate to omit the dose of Metformin on a day of vigorous physical activity, as the blood sugar is likely to be well controlled by exercise without additional medication. Sulfonylureas (e.g. tolbutamide, chlorpropamide, glibenclamide, gliclazide, glipizide, etc.) enhance insulin secretion and may cause hypoglycaemia. It is therefore appropriate to reduce the dosage in the same way as the insulin dosage is reduced in the case of insulin-dependent diabetes. An increase in carbohydrate intake is also advisable but, as hypoglycaemia is less likely, one might initially suggest half to two-thirds of the amount of carbohydrate suggested for the insulin-dependent subject. Some non-insulin-dependent subjects have progressed to insulin therapy, in which case their management is the same as for true insulin-dependent diabetes; however, they do not have the same potential problem of ketosis, nor are they liable to the same degree of blood glucose fluctuation.

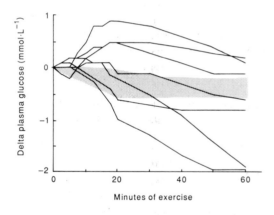

Fig. 28.6 Showing the individual variation in plasma glucose response to 60 min of exercise at 50% $\dot{V}_{O2max}$ in seven fasting subjects with non-insulin-dependent diabetes. Shaded area represents response in non-diabetic subjects (Jenkins *et al*. 1988).

Once again (Fig. 28.6) it is important to emphasize the variability of the blood glucose response (Jenkins *et al*. 1988) and the desirability of blood glucose monitoring, so that an appropriate adjustment of food intake or medication can be arranged on future occasions.

Considerations Applying to Both Insulin-dependent and Non-insulin-dependent Subjects

RECOGNITION AND TREATMENT OF HYPOGLYCAEMIA (NHMRC 1994)

Sweating and signs of increased sympathetic nervous activity usually provide the warning symptoms of hypoglycaemia, but are identical to sympathetic effects during exercise. Thus it may be difficult for the person with diabetes to distinguish between the symptoms of hypoglycaemia and the normal response to vigorous physical activity. If the sympathetic symptoms of hypoglycaemia are not recognized, more severe hypoglycaemia will result in poor co-ordination, mental confusion and mood change, possibly with aggression; the final stage is coma. It is therefore desirable for the person with diabetes, especially if on insulin, to engage in vigorous or prolonged physical activity in the company of a friend. The friend should know about the need to give a glucose drink or some other form of sugar should the diabetic become mentally confused due to hypoglycaemia. Ordinarily, early symptoms of hypoglycaemia can be treated with about 15 g of simple sugar such as seven jelly beans or half a can of lemonade. However, during vigorous exercise two to three times this amount of sugar may be necessary and should be followed by a continued intake of sugar in relation to the duration of exercise, as indicated earlier in this chapter. Should coma occur, intravenous administration of glucose or a subcutaneous (or intramuscular) injection of glucagon is required.

DISTURBED TEMPERATURE REGULATION

Hypoglycaemia can impair temperature regulation and could increase the risk of hypo- or hyperthermia should the subject be exercising under circumstances where there is a risk of these problems.

CARDIOVASCULAR RISK

People with diabetes have an approximately three-fold increased risk of coronary artery disease and, in the case of women, the risk of coronary artery disease prior to menopause becomes the same as for men of the same age. Thus the cardiovascular assessment for a person with diabetes contemplating a vigorous training programme is of considerable importance and a more detailed assessment is desirable at a younger age than for people without diabetes. Some authorities would suggest a stress electrocardiogram (ECG) prior to the commencement of an intensive exercise training programme in any patient with diabetes who is over the age of 31 years, or who is in the 20–30 age group and has had diabetes for more than 20 years (Vignati & Cunningham 1985). If the subject is over the age of 45 years, there is an even stronger reason for a formal cardiac assessment (see exercise testing in this chapter). While no one would question the desirability of a clinical cardiac assessment for such diabetic patients, the need for a stress ECG is debated by some. This is partly due to the lower predictive value of the stress ECG (especially false positives) in patients who do not have an established symptom of chest pain. Therefore, if the subject is prepared to embark on a very gradual increase in physical activity over a period of time, it may be reasonable to perform a clinical cardiac assessment and to advise the patient to report immediately if chest pain is experienced during exercise. In this case, a stress ECG could then be undertaken. In a patient with known coronary artery disease, an exercise ECG would normally be performed prior to undertaking or returning to an exercise programme.

FOOT PROBLEMS

People with diabetes commonly have a degree of peripheral neuropathy with some loss of sensation in the feet. In the middle-aged or older age groups, there is also a greatly increased risk of peripheral vascular disease. For this reason foot care is of enormous importance in subjects with diabetes. If such people have any degree of peripheral neuropathy or peripheral vascular disease, exercise involving high impact on the feet needs to be approached with great caution. There should be meticulous attention to footwear and appropriate preventive foot care and a podiatric consultation is usually desirable. It must also be remembered that ulcers and other lesions on the feet account for more than half of all hospitalization of people with diabetes.

RETINOPATHY

When patients with diabetes have retinopathy which is of the proliferative type, vigorous physical activity of any type, but especially anaerobic activity involving sudden stress, should be avoided, as the consequent rise in blood pressure could increase the chance of a vitreous haemorrhage. If the retinopathy becomes quiescent and the proliferative vessels regress after laser therapy, it may be safe to resume moderate aerobic activity.

REDUCTION IN HYPOGLYCAEMIC MEDICATION WITH REGULAR PHYSICAL ACTIVITY

When people with diabetes engage in regular physical activity there is often a significant improvement in insulin sensitivity so that the dose of insulin or sulfonylurea tablets needs to be reduced to avoid the risk of hypoglycaemia (National Institutes of Health 1987; Berger et al. 1989; Zinman 1989) If this is not anticipated by the patient or physician, the subject may experience some difficulty with repeated hypoglycaemic reactions.

Advice to Coaches

It is very important that coaches or instructors who have an athlete with diabetes in their squad take the trouble to become familiar with the requirements of each individual in regard to exercise. In particular, it is imperative that the athlete be allowed access to carbohydrate food or sugary fluids at all times. The coach/instructor should be aware of the possibility of hypoglycaemia causing a state of mental confusion and should ensure that sugary food or liquid is given immediately in such an eventuality. In the rare situation of coma, it is dangerous to administer fluid or food by mouth. Help should be sought immediately so that an intravenous injection of 30–50 mL of 50% glucose or a subcutaneous injection of 1 mg glucagon (a hormone which raises the blood sugar level) can be given without delay. Intravenous glucose is preferred to glucagon when hypoglycaemia occurs after prolonged exercise, as liver glycogen stores may be depleted; this could result in an inadequate blood glucose response to glucagon.

Sporting Activities which should be Avoided or Approached with Great Caution

Because of the risk of hypoglycaemia, people with diabetes who are receiving insulin injections (or who are on sulfonylurea medication which cannot be temporarily interrupted) should generally avoid activities where impairment of consciousness would pose a danger to life, or where circumstances might not allow glucose to be administered in the event of hypoglycaemia; for example, motor-car racing, hang-gliding, mountain climbing, solo yachting or SCUBA diving (where it may be necessary but dangerous to bring the person rapidly to the surface to administer glucose). Other activities which are potentially dangerous may be undertaken, with suitable precautions, where a 'buddy', who is familiar with the person's diabetes and knows how to deal with a hypoglycaemic reaction, is always in close proximity, for example surf-board riding, flying, long-distance running, triathlon, cross-country skiing, etc.

CONCLUSIONS

It is possible for most people with diabetes to engage in vigorous activity and to compete in most types of sport. Appropriate precautions must be taken to avoid high or low blood glucose levels during vigorous activity, and particular care must be taken in those subjects with insulin-dependent diabetes. Finger-prick blood glucose monitoring has greatly improved the ability to make appropriate adjustments in diet and medications to maintain good blood sugar control during and after exercise.

Preventive care of the feet is important when patients have neuropathy or peripheral vascular disease and caution should be exercised when there is known cardiovascular disease. Moreover, because of the increased risk of coronary artery disease, cardiovascular assessment is desirable at a younger age than in the non-diabetic population.

Not only should it be possible for people with diabetes to undertake most sporting activities; there is evidence that regular physical activity will improve the condition of non-insulin-dependent diabetes, by improving insulin sensitivity. Moreover, it is likely that people with either type of diabetes will derive some benefit from regular physical activity, which appears to reduce the likelihood of atheromatous cardiovascular disease.

REFERENCES

Austin A., Warty V., Janosky J. & Arslanian S. (1993) The relationship of physical fitness to lipid and lipoprotein (a) levels in adolescents with IDDM. *Diabetes Care* **16**, 421–425.

Berger M., Kemmer F. W. & Starke A. R. S. (1989) Exercise in non-insulin-dependent diabetes mellitus. In Larkins R., Zimmet P. & Chisholm D. J. (eds) *Diabetes 1988*, pp. 1217–1220. Elsevier, Amsterdam.

Bogardus C., Ravussin E., Robbins D. C., Wolfe R. R., Horton E. S. & Sims E. A. H. (1984) Effects of physical training and diet therapy on carbohydrate metabolism in patients with glucose intolerance and non-insulin-dependent diabetes mellitus. *Diabetes* **33**, 211–318.

James D. E., Kraegen E. W. & Chisholm D. J. (1985) Effects of exercise training on *in vivo* insulin action in individual tissues of the rat. *Journal of Clinical Investigation* **76**, 657–666.

Jenkins A. B., Chisholm D. J. & Kraegen E. W. (1986) Regulation of hepatic glucose output during exercise by circulating glucose and insulin in humans. *American Journal of Physiology* **250**, R411–417.

Jenkins A. B., Furler S. M., Bruce D. G. & Chisholm D. J. (1988) Regulation of hepatic glucose output during moderate exercise in non-insulin-dependent diabetes. *Metabolism* **37**, 966–972.

Kahn C. R. (1985) Pathophysiology of diabetes mellitus: An overview. In Marble A., Krall L., Bradley R., Christlieb A. & Soeldner J. (eds) *Joslin's Diabetes Mellitus*, pp. 43–50. Lea & Febiger, Philadelphia, PA.

Koivisto V. A. & Felig P. (1978) Effects of leg exercise on insulin absorption in diabetic patients. *New England Journal of Medicine* **298**, 79.

MacDonald M. J. (1987) Post-exercise late-onset hypoglycaemia in insulin-dependent diabetic patients. *Diabetes Care* **10**, 584–588.

Meinders A. E., Willekens F. L. A. & Heere L. P. (1988) Metabolic and hormonal changes in IDDM during a long-distance run. *Diabetes Care* **11**, 1–7.

National Health and Medical Research Council of Australia — Expert Panel on Diabetes (1994) *Diabetes and Exercise*, No. 4, *Diabetes Series*. Australian Government Publishing Service, Canberra.

National Institutes of Health (1987) Consensus development conference on diet and exercise in non-insulin dependent diabetes mellitus. *Diabetes Care* 10, 639–644.

Sane T., Helve E., Pelkonen R. & Koivisto V. A. (1988) The adjustment of diet and insulin dose during long-term endurance exercise in Type I (insulin-dependent) diabetic men. *Diabetologia* 31, 35–40.

Schneider S. H. & Ruderman N. B. (1990) (Technical Review). *Exercise and NIDDM Diabetes Care* 13, 785–789.

Simon H. B. (1984) Sports medicine. In Rubenstein E. & Federman D. (eds) *Current Topics in Medicine*, pp. 1–26. Scientific American Medicine, New York.

Vignati L. & Cunningham L. N. (1985) Exercise and diabetes. In Marble A., Krall L., Bradley R., Christlieb A. & Soeldner J. (eds) *Joslin's Diabetes Mellitus*, pp. 43–50. Lea & Febiger, Philadelphia, PA.

Wasserman D. H. & Zinman B. (1994) Exercise in individuals with IDDM. *Diabetes Care* 17, 924–937.

Zimmet P. Z., Collins V. R., Dowse G. K., Alberti K. G. M. M., Tuomiletito J., Gareeboo H. & Chitson P. (1991) The relation of physical activity to cardiovascular disease risk factors in Mauritians. *American Journal of Epidemiology* 134, 862–875.

Zinman B. (1989) Overview of exercise and insulin-dependent diabetes mellitus. In Larkins R., Zimmet P. & Chisholm D. (eds) *Diabetes 1988*, pp. 1213–1216. Elsevier, Amsterdam.

PART IV

PODIATRY

A. S. Watson

Podiatry includes the study of the normal and abnormal function of the foot, as it relates to the lower limb, as well as the clinical practice of management of pathological foot problems.

Modern podiatry is based on a biomechanical approach. James *et al.* (1978) identified anatomical or biomechanical factors as important in the susceptibility of athletes to overuse injury.

Root *et al.* (1977) define as 'abnormal' no motion, excessive motion or incorrect timing of motion within the gait cycle. Functional orthoses are designed to control not only the extent but the timing of joint motion in the foot. Podiatrists often prescribe, fabricate and fit functional orthotic devices in order to relieve pain, control foot posture and improve foot and lower limb function. Temporary or long-term podiatric orthoses may assist in providing protected function for the rehabilitation of acute lower limb injuries and allow more comfortable sports participation for those with permanent congenital or acquired foot deformity.

PODIATRIC BIOMECHANICS

The Gait Cycle

The major functions of gait, both during walking and running, are the propulsion of the body in a forward direction and single limb stability. The gait cycle has two phases: stance and swing.

The stance phase begins with footstrike and ends with toe off. It is normally divided into three components:

- The loading response or contact phase, where initial impact is absorbed and the bodyweight is progressively placed on the foot
- Mid-stance, during which the body progresses over a stationary foot with the foot flat on the surface
- Terminal stance or propulsion phase, during which the heel lifts and weight is shifted anteriorly over the metatarsal heads and toes

The swing phase is divided into three sections:

- Follow-through, during which the limb lifts from the surface with extension of the hip joint
- Forward swing to achieve toe clearance and forward propulsion, where the limb advances to maximum hip joint flexion and knee joint flexion
- Deceleration or foot descent phase, with continued tibial advancement towards knee extension to create step length. There is deceleration of the thigh and leg in this last subphase and stabilization of the foot to prepare for footstrike (James & Brubaker 1973)

Biomechanics and Pathomechanics of the Lower Limb Link Mechanism

FOOT SUPINATION AND PRONATION

Movement of the subtalar and mid-tarsal joints in the foot is a particularly important aspect of the biomechanics of gait. The foot becomes a mobile adaptor in the early stance phase to assist shock absorption and to provide a stable base for gait, by adapting to varying surface contours. The foot then converts to a rigid lever for efficient propulsion in the late stance phase (Sammarco 1980). This occurs with the normal movements of pronation (unlocking) and supination (relocking) of the sub-talar and mid-tarsal joints.

At the end of the swing phase, the foot is held in a supinated position (Fig. 28.7). As the lower limb adducts under the body, this further tilts the foot so that ground contact or footstrike occurs on the lateral border of the heel, mid-foot or forefoot. The rapid subtalar pronation (Fig. 28.8) that commences with heel strike is passive. This movement is restrained by the configuration of the joint itself, as well as by ligamentous restraints and the contraction of the supporting musculature, particularly the tibialis anterior and tibialis posterior.

Pronation in the subtalar joint involves slight dorsiflexion in the sagittal plane, eversion in the frontal plane and abduction in the transverse plane. As the foot becomes fixed on the ground, if frictional forces (traction) are high, abduction becomes impossible, thus the proximal limb of the joint must internally rotate. Pronation with the

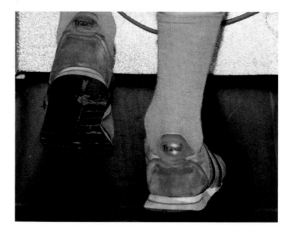

Fig. 28.8   The foot in early mid-stance undergoing rapid pronation.

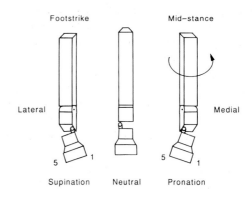

Fig. 28.9   Right foot closed chain motion (front view). A demonstration of the internal rotation of the leg which is associated with subtalar joint pronation if the foot is fixed on the ground (diagram of a model).

foot planted therefore causes internal tibial rotation (Fig. 28.9).

Pronation in the subtalar joint unlocks the mid-tarsal and other joints in the foot, lowering the medial longitudinal arch and allowing the foot to adapt to the running surface topography and absorb shock (Gross & Napoli 1993). This latter mechanism is ineffective if the foot lands in a maximally pronated position or is prevented from pronating sufficiently.

The motion of the subtalar joint during stance reduces the stresses on the ankle joint and restriction of the subtalar joint may cause increased rotational

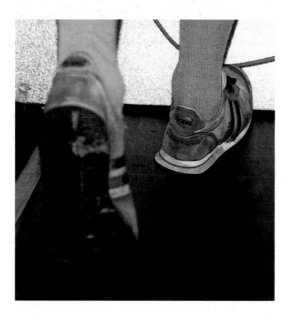

Fig. 28.7   The supinated position of the foot just prior to footstrike.

(a)　　　　　　　　　　(b)　　　　　　　　　　(c)

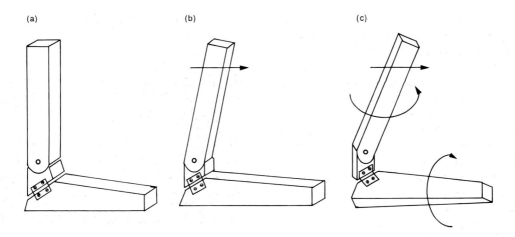

stress on the ankle. If pronation is very rapid and excessive, not only is shock absorption ineffective, but the internal rotation of the leg is excessive and prolonged. This may place additional rotational stress on the whole lower limb including the pelvis, hip, knee and patellofemoral joints.

Limitation of movement in one joint causes compensatory increased motion in the other joints in the link mechanism (Nicholas *et al.* 1977). As the body moves anteriorly over the planted foot in mid-stance, at least 10° of dorsiflexion are required of the ankle joint. If this movement is not possible due to joint abnormality or tight calf muscles, further dorsiflexion must be obtained from the subtalar and mid-tarsal joints. This dorsiflexion will only be obtained in conjunction with increased pronation at these joints (Fig. 28.10). This occurs at a time when the subtalar joint should be supinating (Sammarco 1980) and therefore restricts the ability of the foot to lock into a rigid lever required for efficient propulsion. If the arch is thus rendered structurally unstable in the propulsive phase, the dynamic stabilizers (especially the tibialis posterior) may be subject to overuse.

TRAINING SURFACES

The surfaces on which an athlete runs may also cause variations in biomechanical stress, as hard ones cause greater impact loading and require shoes with good shock absorption. Softer surfaces absorb more energy and require more force generation in the propulsive phase and uneven ones markedly

Fig. 28.10 Restriction of the ankle joint movement causing increased subtalar joint pronation and internal rotation of the leg. (a) A model of the right foot, subtalar joint, ankle joint and shank in the neutral position. (b) Dorsiflexion of the ankle blocked by joint stiffness. (c) Further dorsiflexion achieved by pronation at the subtalar joint.

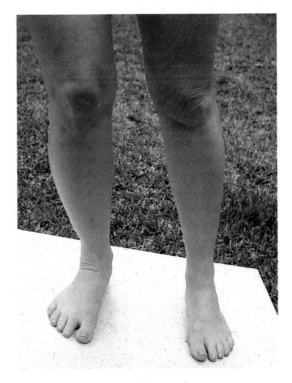

Fig. 28.11 Running or walking across a slope causes the uphill foot to pronate and the downhill foot to supinate.

increase the amount of subtalar motion causing increased rotational stress on the lower limb.

Surfaces sloped in a plane perpendicular to the line of progression cause supination of the downhill foot and pronation of the uphill foot (Fig. 28.11). The efficiency of shock absorption is reduced in the rigid supinated downhill foot, and there is greater and more prolonged internal tibial rotation with pronation of the uphill foot, or of the inside foot when running at high speed around an unbanked, curved running track. Running uphill may cause more dorsiflexion and thus more pronation at the subtalar and mid-tarsal joints and increased internal tibial rotation. This is more pronounced if the calf muscles are tight or if motion in the ankle joint is otherwise restricted.

PODIATRIC MANAGEMENT

Podiatric assessment should include the history of the condition, an evaluation of foot, lower limb, pelvis and back posture, static alignment, measurements, stance and subtalar neutral position, forefoot to rearfoot relationship, individual joint and muscle function and gait analysis (preferably on video).

Foot Types and Examples of Malalignment Syndromes

THE IDEAL FOOT

The term 'normal foot alignment' is not a statistical one. 'Normal' in this context means ideal. A large proportion of the population has less than ideal leg, heel and forefoot alignment.

The ideal foot has at least 10° of dorsiflexion available at the ankle. The calcaneus is in line with the lower one-third of the leg and perpendicular to the supporting surface in the normal relaxed stance when the subtalar joint is neutral. Furthermore, the plane of the forefoot is perpendicular to the calcaneal bisection and there are no forces on the foot from the leg above in any of the three body planes, which cause it to invert or evert, abduct or adduct, dorsiflex or plantar flex (Fig. 28.12).

MALALIGNMENT SYNDROMES

Deviation from the normal relationships between the leg, the rearfoot and the forefoot are termed malalignment syndromes and these may be described in the three cardinal body planes.

The site, severity and nature of secondary deformity or overuse injury caused by structural malalignment of the foot or lower limb is determined not by the primary problem itself but by the site and type of biomechanical compensation. It may be quite complex and may be congenital or acquired, such as that caused by malunion of a fracture or from soft tissue shortening following injury. Table 28.3 lists common malalignment syndromes.

Fig. 28.12 A diagrammatic representation of (a) ideal leg/heel/foot alignment, (b) subtalar varus and (c) forefoot varus as seen in the neutral position of the subtalar joint (non-weight-bearing).

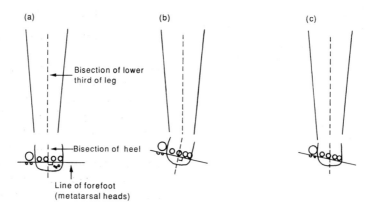

(a)   (b)   (c)

Bisection of lower third of leg

Bisection of heel

Line of forefoot (metatarsal heads)

Table 28.3 Common foot malalignment syndromes

Malalignment	Associated factors	Injury
Sagittal plane		
Talipes equinus	No subtalar motion	Plantar forefoot callosities
		Calcaneal apophysitis (Sever's disease)
	Mobile subtalar joint	Pathological flat foot
		Hallux valgus, hammer toes, plantar calcaneal periostitis, plantar fasciitis, plantar callosities
Frontal plane		
Subtalar varus	Excessive pronation	Metatarsalgia
	Hypermobile first (metatarsal) ray	Callus under second and third metatarsal heads
		Posterior tibial stress syndrome
		Stress fracture of the foot and leg
		Navicular apophysitis
		Posterior tibial tendinitis
		Patellofemoral joint pain
Subtalar valgus (rare)	Flat foot	Intolerance to arch supports
Forefoot varus (neutral subtalar joint)	Excessive and prolonged pronation	Medial tibial stress syndrome
		Posterior tibial tendinitis
	Eversion of rearfoot	Patellofemoral joint pain
Forefoot valgus, plantar flexed first (metatarsal) ray	Rapid reversal of pronation into supination	Navicular stress fracture
		Inversion injury of ankle, sesamoiditis
Leg length discrepancy	Pelvic tilt	Iliotibial band friction syndrome
	Postural scoliosis	Patellofemoral joint pain
		Back pain
Transverse plane		
Internal rotation tibia	Poor propulsion	
	Abnormal heel contact	Heel fat pad injury
Metatarsus adductus	'C-shaped' foot	Hallus valgus (bunion)
Metatarsus primus adductus	Broad forefoot	Footwear intolerance
External rotation tibia	Internal rotation knee	Patellofemoral joint pain

The frontal plane malalignments particularly of tibial, subtalar and forefoot varus, forefoot valgus and plantar flexed first metatarsal ray may be adequately treated using orthoses.

Orthotic Devices

Orthotic devices (orthoses) can be divided into three main categories:

• Palliative
• Functional
• Corrective

PALLIATIVE ORTHOSES

These are primarily for the purpose of alleviating foot symptoms, allowing more comfortable ambulation (Fig. 28.13). They range from simple flat innersoles with heel cushioning, to specific cushioning to redistribute pressure away from areas taking excessive weight. A moulded palliative orthotic device provides a more even distribution of weight-bearing and the bulk of material underneath the medial longitudinal arch is capable of blocking extremes of pronation and the associated symptoms, if pronation is excessive. Additions to the orthoses,

Fig. 28.13 Examples of palliative orthotic devices (orthoses).

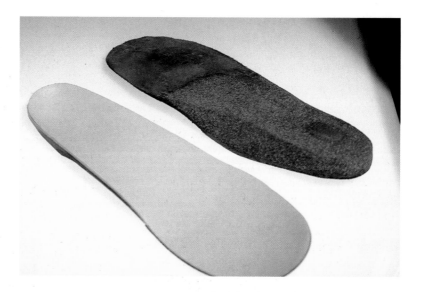

called wedges or postings, may be made to give an element of correction or some control. The material used depends on the age and weight of the patient and the sporting, occupational or recreational activity. 'Unifoam', 'Plastazote' or other thermo-moulding plastic foams may be used, and postings are often made from 'Corex' or other firmer

Fig. 28.14 Examples of the more rigid functional orthoses.

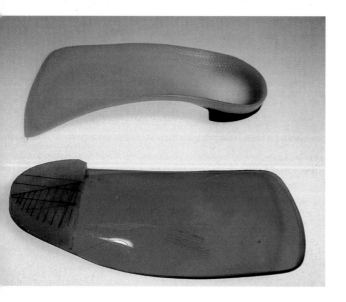

material. These orthoses are often very useful for sprinters or footballers, particularly as a first meas-ure, as they are relatively easy and cheap to fabricate and modify. Recent evidence suggests that softer orthotics made of these materials, if posted with glued-on rearfoot and forefoot wedges, may be effective in treating some overuse syndromes in runners, such as the patellofemoral syndrome (Eng & Pierrynowski 1993). This somewhat blurs the demarcation between palliative and functional orthoses. It appears that to be effective softer orthotics need to be accurately prescribed and well fabricated, in the manner of a functional orthosis rather than simply a heat-moulded insole.

FUNCTIONAL ORTHOSES

Functional orthoses require a thorough and precise assessment and an extremely accurate neutral cast. A negative mould is made using plaster splints laid around the foot, which is held with the subtalar joint in the neutral position and the mid-tarsal joint fully pronated. The orthotic shell is then vacuum-moulded over a balanced positive mould, which is made by pouring moulding plaster into the negative impression. Wedges or postings are then added as appropriate (Fig. 28.14). Functional orthotic devices allow the patient's feet to function as closely as possible to the neutral position. They should eliminate or decrease compensatory motion caused by extrinsic or intrinsic factors, as they control not only position but also foot motion and timing.

Orthotic devices of this type are not prescribed to eliminate pronation, but to reduce or control the extent and duration of pronation (McCulloch *et al.* 1993). A normal amount of pronation is required for the purpose of shock absorption and adaptation to the playing or training surface.

The materials used for the shell of the orthoses are normally thermoplastics. The stiffness and thickness of the acrylic or polypropylene material used depends on the sporting application. Such orthoses are particularly efficient in runners for reducing the symptoms of posterior tibial syndrome and symptomatic flat foot due to varus malalignment (D'Ambrosia 1985). They are also prescribed as part of the treatment of metatarsalgia, plantar fasciitis, iliotibial band friction syndrome, symptomatic cavus foot, patellofemoral pain syndrome, Achilles tendinitis and stress fractures of the foot or the leg related to abnormal biomechanics.

Recently, there has been evidence to support the use of functional orthoses to enhance efficiency and performance, particularly in sports such as ice skating and skiing (Greenberg *et al.* 1991) where edge control and balance are critical for elite performance.

CORRECTIVE ORTHOSES

These are made of material similar to functional orthotic devices, such as high-density polyethylene or the acrylic 'Polydur' or laminations of Kevlar and carbon fibres. They are usually made from a corrected cast and are only used when there is suitable joint mobility and an absence of any upper body postural malalignments. They are mainly used for paediatric problems.

FOOTWEAR FOR SPORT

Sporting footwear has three main overlapping functions: protection, comfort and modification of weight-bearing and locomotion forces. Those features relevant to comfort include fit, weight, flexibility, ventilation (heat exchange) and waterproofing while those related to force attenuation or modification include:

- Shock absorption
- Flexibility
- Foot motion control
- Traction
- Shoe fit

It is important that for each sporting application these considerations in shoe design should be optimized by modifications in the design and construction of the outer sole, the mid-sole, the inner sole and upper. Figure 28.15 illustrates the

Fig. 28.15 The components of sports shoe design.

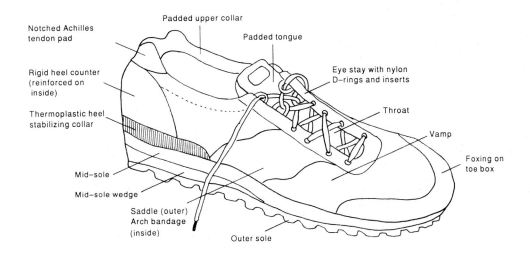

various parts and the design characteristics of a sports shoe.

Whereas it is accepted that modern running shoes may reduce the risk of certain injuries particularly when running on hard, man-made surfaces or rough, uneven, natural surfaces, some maintain that the sensory insulation inherent in modern running shoe design may be responsible for some overuse injuries associated with running. These injuries, such as plantar fasciitis and particularly stress fractures of the foot, have been termed 'pseudo-neuropathic' (Robbins & Hanna 1987). It appears that sensory feedback largely from the skin of the sole of the foot is important in developing adaptations which enhance the ability of the foot to provide impact absorption and protection against running-related injuries. This may be a significant factor in injuries caused by running in ill-fitting, over-padded or 'too soft' shoes. This may also provide a basis for the use of some barefoot training on ideal surfaces to reduce the incidence of some overuse running injuries by enhancing the natural protective functions of the foot.

Shock Absorption

Each foot strikes the ground approximately 900 times per kilometre. Eighty per cent of runners land on their heel, showing a typical bimodal pressure peak of between two and three times bodyweight under the heel on impact and under the ball of the foot on propulsion (Cavanagh 1980). Those with a rigid high arched pes cavus have a very high peak under the forefoot, and those runners with excessive pronation or pes planus have a very high impact peak under the heel. It is a good idea to attenuate the forces in the first peak as this relates to impact and may cause injury, but it is less desirable to attenuate the forces in the second peak, as this represents active propulsion and is required for efficient performance.

Flexibility

Running shoes need to flex through about 30° in a line just proximal to the metatarsal heads. If the shoe is too stiff in this area, the windlass action of the plantar fascia wrapping around the flexing toes is inhibited. The plantar fascia normally lifts and stabilizes the arch passively in this manner, aiding supination in propulsion and protecting the metatarsals from bending stress (Sammarco 1980; Fig. 28.16). The lever arm of the foot in propulsion is also effectively lengthened by an inflexible sole, thus placing greater stress on the plantar flexors and predisposing to injury such as Achilles tendinitis.

Weight

An increase in shoe weight of 100 g may add 1–2 min to a marathon time by increasing energy expenditure by about 1% (Frederick 1987). Decreased weight, however, may mean a decrease in foot control and shock absorption. The trend towards lightweight materials in shoe construction reduces the ability of shoes to resist compression, distortion and wear. This restricts the average life of a typical modern running shoe to no more than 1000 km. Although outwardly the shoe may appear to be in

Fig. 28.16 The function of the plantar fascia in the propulsive subphase of the stance during gait. The fascia acts as a windlass, wrapping around the metatarsophalangeal joints and lifting and supporting the longitudinal arch on heel lift.

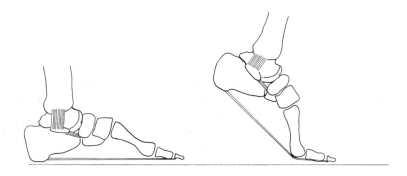

good repair, it may need replacing. Nothing will slow a runner more than injury and thus a well-designed, slightly heavier but more protective running shoe is more sensible for all but the most elite runners.

Foot Motion Control

Some pronation is desirable; however, excessive or prolonged pronation decreases the efficiency of shock absorption and propulsion and also increases rotational stress on the lower limb, which may cause overuse injury (James *et al.* 1978).

Shoes with a large lateral sole flare catch early on footstrike, increasing the speed and extent of pronation around the longer lever arm. Similarly, shoes with too soft a mid-sole collapse on the lateral edge, increasing the inverted attitude of the rearfoot at footstrike. A greater amount of pronation is thus required to achieve forefoot contact. Conversely, the soft mid-sole may collapse on the medial edge allowing a greater degree of, and prolonged, pronation.

Pronation is more effectively controlled if shoes have a straight last (i.e. less medial curve of the front part from the centre line of the shoe), a stiffer 'board last' construction, harder heel wedge material and a firm heel counter reinforced with a collar.

Excessive pronation may also be controlled if heel height is increased as this decreases dorsiflexion. However, this heel raise should only be integrated into the shoe structure, as the insertion of commercially available, firm, flat heel raises may result in significantly decreased control, increased shock and heel irritation.

Shoe Fit

For motion control and comfort it is important that shoes should fit well. The correct width, weight, last shape and mid-sole construction should be chosen for the individual, depending on bodyweight, foot shape and size, foot mechanics, sporting activity and running surfaces. If orthoses are to be worn, all standard shoe inserts should be removed to provide a firm base for the orthoses.

FOOT CARE

Blisters are collections of fluid or blood between the layers of the skin and are caused by shearing forces often related to ill-fitting shoes. They can be prevented by carefully wearing in new shoes and conditioning the feet to an increase in activity. Absorbent acrylic or cotton/acrylic blend socks made of crease-resistant material (tube socks), combined with the taping of vulnerable areas with adhesive, smooth-surfaced tape, may reduce friction. Once the skin has been damaged by blister formation, however, sterile shear-reducing gel under conforming adhesive tape may reduce pain and further injury.

Blisters should not be 'deroofed' unless infected. Drainage of fresh blisters through adjacent normal skin with a fine gauge sterile needle should be followed by careful protective taping with the gel dressing.

'Open' or deroofed blisters should be dressed by removing unwanted skin with sterile scissors and then applying an antibiotic preparation such as '*Betadine*' (once iodine allergy has been excluded). Covering with sterile, non-adhesive protective bandages and allowing the wound to heal is then appropriate.

Bunions result from hallux valgus deformity and the syndrome includes dorsomedial exostoses of the first metatarsal head and inflammation of the skin and deeper structures with or without bursa formation on the medial side of the first metatarsophalangeal (MTP) joint (Fig. 28.17). Bunions are often the result of an underlying biomechanical abnormality and exercises, orthoses, padding and splinting may be required.

Corns and calluses are thickenings of heavily keratinized skin related to abnormal weight-bearing or ill-fitting footwear, and these can be treated symptomatically by paring away the thick keratinized skin. The foot and lower limb should be biomechanically evaluated and functionally corrective orthoses with or without padding used to alleviate pressure on the affected part.

Warts are caused by a virus and are often mistaken for corns or calluses as they commonly occur over

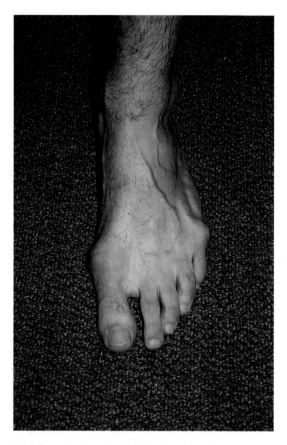

Fig. 28.17 Hallux valgus deformity with bunion formation.

pressure points, such as the heels and metatarsal heads. In these sites they can cause pain with weight bearing, which may be severe enough to affect the biomechanics and execution of sports manoeuvres (Ramsey 1992). Plantar warts penetrate deep under the skin and have a clearly defined border, the centre often being dark brown, black or rust coloured. Warts are more painful when side to side pinching pressure is applied rather than direct pressure. If not treated, they may resolve spontaneously with time, or spread and multiply and be transmitted to other persons. Salicylic acid paint or nightly applications of 5D-fluorouracil in saturated pyruvic acid, protective dressings and measures to prevent cross-infection are useful. Specialist attention should be sought if the above measures do not resolve the problem. Surgical excision of plantar warts does not represent a certain cure and the risk of a life-long painful scar is extremely high.

Fungal infections often present as burning or itching on the bottom and sides of the feet and the spaces between toes, particularly the third, fourth and fifth toes. The toenails may also be infected. Fungus infection between the toes causes the skin to become moist, white and fissured. Infected nails appear abnormally thickened and flaky with brown or yellow discoloration rendering the nail opaque. Care must be taken to prevent cross-infection and the feet should be kept as dry as possible, socks changed twice daily and footwear removed as often as possible. Topical treatment with antifungal creams, used regularly for some weeks, is usually effective. Treatment for fungal infections of the nails is not usually necessary in athletes unless the nail is painful. Occasionally, long-term systemic antifungal therapy with avulsion of the infected nail is required. The benefit of this treatment should be weighed up against the often significant side-effects of the medications.

Ingrown toenails are caused by the imbedding of the sides of the nails into the skin surrounding the nail plate. Small calluses form under the rolled nail edge, further increasing pressure. Swelling may occur with infection, and chronic granulation tissue may overhang the margin of the nail plate. Prevention involves careful fitting of shoes and cutting the nails straight across or in a slight V shape. Definitive treatment involves total removal of the offending border of the nail right down to the nail bed to prevent further spicules forming (Hlavac 1977).

Ingrown toenails, blood blisters under the nail, thickened nails, or repeated seasonal shedding or loss of the nail may have a biomechanical basis. Any varus malalignment which causes prolonging of pronation into the propulsive phase and instability of the forefoot contributes to such injuries of the nail of the big toe (Head 1994).

CONCLUSIONS

Some athletes experience difficulty with major or minor foot problems, which may affect gait and cause discomfort while competing. Appropriate podiatric treatment often alleviates foot and lower leg discomfort and these athletes should be referred to a podiatrist for assessment. Orthotic devices should not be used as a substitute for an overall management plan for injured running athletes. Comprehensive treatment includes modified rest, training modification, and change in the running surface or shoe. Proper conditioning, remedial and maintenance exercise programmes are also important for injury prevention and treatment of specific injuries. In many cases medical or physiotherapy evaluation and treatment may be necessary; however, surgical intervention is only rarely required.

REFERENCES

Cavanagh P. R. (1980) The biomechanics of running. *The Running Shoe Book*, pp. 78–96. Anderson World, Mountain View, CA.

D'Ambrosia R. D. (1985) Orthotic devices in running injuries. *Clinics in Sports Medicine* 4, 611–618.

Eng J. J. & Pierrynowski J. R. (1993) Evaluation of soft foot orthotics in the treatment of patellofemoral pain syndrome. *Physical Therapy* 73, 62–70.

Frederick E. C. (1987) The running shoe: Dilemmas and dichotomies in design. In Segesser B. & Pförringer W. (eds) *The Shoe in Sport*, pp. 26–35. Year Book/Wolfe, London.

Greenberg S. B., Sanderson D. J., Taunton J. E. & Macintyre J. G. (1991) Control of subtalar motion with the use of ski boot footbeds. *Clinical Journal of Sports Medicine* 1, 188–192.

Gross M. L. & Napoli R. C. (1993) Treatment of lower extremity injuries with orthotic shoe inserts — An overview. *Sports Medicine* 15, 66–70.

Head J. (1994) The biomechanics and treatment of hallux nail damage in athletes. *Sport Health* 12, 44–48.

Hlavac H. F. (1977) *The Foot Book*, pp. 164–186. World Publications, Mountain View, CA.

James S. L. & Brubaker C. E. (1973) Biomechanical and neuromuscular aspects of running. *Exercise and Sport Science Review* 1, 189.

James S. L., Bates B. & Osternig L. (1978) Injuries to runners. *American Journal of Sports Medicine* 6, 40–50.

McCulloch M. U., Brunt D. & Vander Linden D. (1993) The effect of foot orthotics and gait velocity on lower limb kinematics and temporal events of stance. *Journal of Sport Physical Therapy* 17, 2–9.

Nicholas J. A., Grossman R. B. & Hershman E. B. (1977) Simplified classifications of motion in sport. *Orthopedic Clinics of North America* 8, 499–532.

Ramsey M. L. (1992) Plantar warts, choosing treatment for active patients. *Physician and Sports Medicine* 20, 69–88.

Robbins S. E. & Hanna A. M. (1987) Running-related injury prevention through barefoot adaptations. *Medicine and Science in Sports and Exercise* 19, 148–156.

Root M., Orien W. & Weed J. (1977) *Normal and Abnormal Function of the Foot*, Vol. 2, pp. 8–22. Clinical Biomechanics Corp., Los Angeles, CA.

Sammarco G. J. (1980) Biomechanics of the foot. In Frankel V. H. & Nordin M. (eds) *Basic Biomechanics of the Skeletal System*, pp. 193–220. Lea & Febiger, Philadelphia, PA.

PART V

EXERCISE STRESS TESTING

B. E. F. Hockings

Exercise testing is used in the assessment of physical fitness and the training of athletes. It is also an important diagnostic and prognostic procedure in the assessment of patients with coronary artery disease. In clinical practice, continuous recording of the electrocardiogram (ECG), enables displacement of the ST segment to be measured, together with various non-ECG parameters including exercise tolerance, symptoms and changes in heart rate and blood pressure. These are used to estimate the likelihood and extent of coronary disease and determine functional capacity as well as assessing the effects of different therapies. Standard exercise protocols can be enhanced by combining them with radionuclide imaging or echocardiography for selected patients. Exercise testing also provides the basis for exercise prescription, which is used in the rehabilitation of patients with cardiovascular disease and to help prevent the development of this condition.

EXERCISE PHYSIOLOGY

The anticipation of exercise can itself result in an increase in resting cardiac output due to increased sympathetic activity and vagal withdrawal. The haemodynamic responses to physical activity also vary with body posture.

During light to moderate exercise in the upright position, cardiac output increases as a result of an increase in stroke volume as well as heart rate. With more intense physical activity further increases in cardiac output are primarily due to an increase in the heart rate. At the same time additional sympathetic activity and diminished parasympathetic stimulation result in vasoconstriction of most circulatory beds except for those of the exercising muscle groups and cerebral and coronary circulations. Further, sympathetic activity also enhances ventricular contractility.

With exercise skeletal muscle blood flow can increase by more than 20-fold (Guyton 1992) and oxygen extraction by muscle tissue from each millilitre of blood flowing through it, increases up to three-fold (Wilmore & Costill 1994). This means that the total oxygen uptake by muscle may increase by 40–60 fold (Evans 1994). As well, total peripheral resistance falls and systolic blood pressure, mean arterial pressure and pulse pressure increase. In normal individuals diastolic blood pressure may be unchanged or increase or decrease by approximately 10 mmHg, while cardiac output can increase four to six times. Maximum heart rate and maximum cardiac output decrease with age. The maximum heart rate can be estimated from the formula $220 - $ age (years) with a standard deviation of 10–12 beats$\cdot$min^{-1} (Froelicher & Marcondes 1989).

In the supine position the cardiac output and stroke volume are somewhat higher at rest than in the upright position and with exercise in this position the increase in cardiac output results almost entirely from an increase in heart rate with only a small contribution from an increased stroke volume. Most normal subjects achieve approximately 10% increases in exercise time, cardiac index, heart rate and rate pressure product (systolic blood pressure × heart rate) at peak exercise in the upright position compared with supine exercise. On the cessation of exercise haemodynamic parameters return to baseline within minutes.

The total oxygen uptake in excess of the resting oxygen uptake during the recovery period is the oxygen debt. Lactate begins to accumulate in the blood when a healthy untrained subject reaches 50–60% of maximal capacity for aerobic metabolism (Wilmore & Costill 1994). Lactate builds up as exercise continues and metabolic acidosis can occur. The gas exchange ventilatory threshold is the point at which minute ventilation increases disproportionately to respiratory oxygen uptake and work. Ventilatory threshold, under most conditions, coincides with the lactate threshold (American College of Sports Medicine 1991). Changes in the lactate or ventilatory threshold for an individual can be used to assess improved cardiovascular fitness with training as well as in patients, progression of disease and response to treatment.

The heart utilizes aerobic metabolism and oxygen extraction in the coronary circulation is nearly maximal at rest (Evans 1994). To allow increased myocardial oxygen consumption with exercise, there must be an increased blood flow to the heart and this is achieved by decreased resistance of the coronary arterioles coupled with an increased cardiac output. In patients with coronary artery disease obstructing the lumen of the epicardial arteries, an increase in coronary flow beyond the narrowing may not be possible and the patient may develop symptoms of angina pectoris, ECG changes and changes in cardiac function with localized impairment of cardiac contraction. Thus, for patients with coronary artery disease, physical activity not only imposes an increased myocardial oxygen demand but there may be also localized limitation of coronary flow reserve.

THE EXERCISE TEST

Purpose of the Test

The indications for exercise testing are listed in Table 28.4 and contraindications in Table 28.5. While peripheral vascular disease is not a contraindication to exercise testing, it may limit a subject's

Table 28.4 Indications for exercise stress testing

Clinical
  Patients with known or suspected heart disease
  To assist with diagnosis
  To assess prognosis
  Evaluation of possible re-stenosis following coronary angioplasty
  Assessment of exercise-induced arrhythmias or other symptoms
  To determine capacity for sustained work performance
  To aid in development of exercise prescription
  (Exercise stress testing is not indicated as a screening test for asymptomatic individuals because of the frequency of false positive results)
Exercise and sports training
  Assessment of functional capacity
  Assessment of the effect of exercise training

Table 28.5 Contra-indications for exercise stress testing

Major	Unstable angina
	Severe aortic stenosis
	Acute myocarditis
Relative	Uncontrolled hypertension
	Uncontrolled heart failure
	Recent myocardial infarction
	Musculoskeletal problems
Circumstances where ECG changes are unreliable	Left bundle branch block
	Wolff-Parkinson-White syndrome
	Pre-existing ST–T abnormalities

Table 28.6 Indications for stopping on exercise test

Major	A fall in systolic blood pressure ≥10 mmHg repeatable within 15 s
	Significant chest pain suggestive of angina associated with diagnostic ST segment depression or elevation
	Sustained ventricular arrhythmias
Relative	Diagnostic ECG changes
	Chest pain
	Lack of rise of blood pressure
	Dizziness or ataxia
	Excessive fatigue or dyspnoea

performance so that target heart rate is not achieved and the test is inconclusive. In clinical practice most stress tests are undertaken to assist with the diagnosis and to assess the prognosis of patients with suspected or established coronary artery disease. For this purpose a maximal or symptom-limited stress test is usually performed during which the subject is taken to the limit of their endurance unless a specific indication for stopping the test is evident (Table 28.6). After myocardial infarction, for patients making an uncomplicated recovery a submaximal stress test is frequently performed sometimes as early as 3–4 days post-infarction. During such a test the patient exercises to a heart rate which does not exceed 120 beats·min^{-1} unless symptoms or significant ECG changes occur at a lower work load.

Preparation

Subjects should be advised to wear comfortable clothes and shoes and not to eat a meal for at least 3 h before the test. The referring physician needs to advise whether medications (particularly beta-blocking agents and some calcium channel blocking drugs) should be discontinued (for up to 48 h) so that the patient's heart rate response will not be limited during the test. A brief history should be obtained by the physician conducting the test; if the patient has had recent chest pain and/or ECG changes then the test may be contraindicated. The test is explained to the patient and a brief demonstration of how to walk on the treadmill or pedal the bicycle is given. Written consent for the test is not considered necessary in Australia but is necessary in North America and some European countries. A standard 12 lead ECG is obtained immediately before the test for comparison with later recordings and the patient's blood pressure is recorded in the erect position. Meticulous skin preparation, good quality electrodes and appropriate support of the lead cables are all essential to obtain

Fig. 28.18 An exercise stress test in progress.

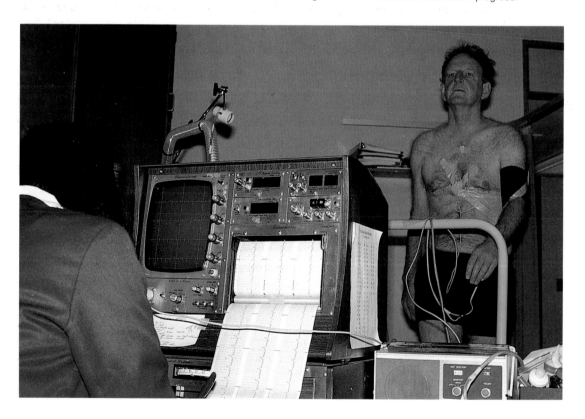

high quality artefact-free ECG tracings during exercise. Note the position of the limb lead electrodes to allow the subject to exercise unhindered (Fig. 28.18). Computerized signal averaging of the ECG recording is now standard to minimize motion and other artefacts, but it is important that the raw ECG data be reviewed and seen to be of good quality, otherwise the averaged signal may be distorted and not recognized as such. Computer programs are also available to measure and plot ST segment depression and other ECG parameters.

Regular determination of the rating of perceived extension (RPE) is a useful adjunct to recording heart rate, blood pressure. It is especially useful with patients on medication which restricts heart rate (American College of Sports Medicine 1991).

Safety

Complications of exercise testing are rare but can include death, myocardial infarction, serious cardiac arrhythmias and hypotension. The risk depends on the clinical circumstances, but even for patients who have had a recent myocardial infarction the mortality rate is $<0.03\%$ (Hamm *et al.* 1989). In an unselected patient population mortality is $<0.01\%$ (Stuart & Ellestad 1980). A defibrillator and a resuscitation trolley, including manual ventilation equipment and standard medications for dealing with cardiac arrest must be available in the room while exercise testing is in progress. Patients must have continuous ECG monitoring under supervision until any exercise-induced ECG changes have returned to baseline. The attending physician must remain in the room with the patient during the test and for at least 5 min after cessation of exercise. Two attendants must be present during the test and both must be competent in defibrillation and cardiopulmonary resuscitation.

Exercise Protocols

BICYCLE ERGOMETRY

Various standardized exercise protocols are available which provide a graduated increase in load over timed stages using either a mechanically braked bicycle or the more reliable but more expensive electronically braked equivalent. Bicycle exercise testing is quieter and there may be less motion artefact than with a treadmill as the subject's thorax is relatively stable and it is easier to determine blood pressure. Some patients are unable to use a bicycle ergometer satisfactorily whereas they can walk on a treadmill, while other patients with osteoarthritis of their weight-bearing joints will find bicycle ergometry easier than walking on a treadmill. Regardless of the mode of exercise, the equipment must be calibrated frequently to ensure correct speed and grade or watts.

TREADMILL STRESS TESTING

Standardized stepped protocols (Bruce, Naughton, etc., Table 28.7) are available which provide gradually increasing motorized treadmill speeds and gradients, which are maintained for timed stages. The subject may use the handrail for balance but not support themselves otherwise functional capacity can be significantly overestimated. The treadmill should slow down gradually for at least 45–60 s at the termination of the test to minimize the likelihood of syncopal episodes which occasionally follow abrupt cessation of exercise.

Symptoms

Chest discomfort induced by physical activity is suggestive of angina pectoris. Some patients with ischaemic heart disease will develop chest discomfort during the test without any associated ST segment changes and it is a matter of clinical judgement when to discontinue the test under such circumstances. If the symptoms are suggestive of angina and are becoming increasingly severe, then exercise should be discontinued.

Blood Pressure

In normal subjects systolic blood pressure increases progressively with exercise up to about 160–220 mmHg; with older subjects reaching the higher levels. Diastolic blood pressure usually only varies from resting values by ± 10 mmHg. If the systolic blood pressure does not rise >120 mmHg or there is a decrease of ≥ 10 mmHg confirmed within 15 s,

Table 28.7 A comparative analysis of commonly used maximal stress testing protocols indicating oxygen uptake, MET values and fitness classification

Functional class	Clinical status	O₂ cost mL·kg⁻¹·min⁻¹	METS	Bicycle ergometer (1 watt = 6 KPDS)	Bruce (3 min stages) mph	Bruce %GR	Cornell (2 min stages) mph	Cornell %GR	Balke-Ware (% Grad at 3.3 mph)	Naughton (2 min stages) %GR 3 mph	Naughton %GR 3.4 mph	Weber (2 min stages) mph	Weber %GR
				For 70 kg bodyweight	5.5	20							
Normal and I	Healthy Dependent on age, activity	55.0	16		5.0	18	5.0	18	26 / 25	32.5	26		
		52.5	15	KPDS					24 / 23	30	24		
		49.0	14	1500			4.6	17	22	27.5	22		
		45.5	13	1350	4.2	16	4.2	16	21 / 20 / 19	25	20		
		42.0	12	1200					18	22.5	18		
		38.5	11	1200			3.8	15	17 / 16	20	16	mph	%GR
	Sedentary Healthy	35.0	10	1050	3.4	14	3.4	14	15 / 14 / 13	17.5	14	3.4	14.0
		31.5	9	900					12 / 11 / 10	15	12	3.0	13.0
		28.0	8	750			3.0	13	9 / 8	12.5	10	3.0	12.5
		24.5	7	600	2.5	12	2.5	12	7 / 6	10	8	3.0	10.0
II	Limited Symptomatic	21.0	6	450			2.1	11	5 / 4	7.5	6	3.0	7.5
		17.5	5	300	1.7	10	1.7	10	3 / 2	5	4	2.0	10.5
III		14.0	4	300	1.7	5	1.7	5	1	2.5	2	2.0	7.0
		10.5	3	150						0		2.0	3.5
		7.0	2		1.7	0	1.7	0				1.5	0
IV		3.5	1									1.0	0

METS = multiple of resting metabolic rate (1 MET = 3.5 mL O₂·kg⁻¹·min⁻¹); m.p.h. = mile·h⁻¹. 1 m.p.h. = 1.61 km·h⁻¹; KPDS = kiloponds. Adapted from Chaitman (1992).

or a fall in systolic blood pressure below standing rest values then these are abnormal responses and the test should be terminated. These features correlate with the presence of three vessel or left main coronary disease (Ellestad 1986; Froelicher 1987). It is important to distinguish between a fall in blood pressure during exercise and post-exertional hypotension; the latter occurs occasionally, usually in younger subjects and although the patients may be symptomatic at the time, post-exertional hypotension does not correlate with the presence of coronary disease (Fleg & Lakatta 1986).

Maximal Work Capacity

This is an important variable in stratifying risk for patients with coronary disease. Poor exercise tolerance is associated with increased morbidity and mortality. Exercise testing is more accurate in predicting prognosis in patients with ischaemic heart disease than it is for making the diagnosis of coronary artery disease. Patients who exercise to a higher workload and, for example, can reach stage 4 of the Bruce protocol without significant symptoms or diagnostic ECG changes, have a low risk of cardiac events within the 12 months following the test irrespective of whether coronary artery disease is present or not. Normal standards for peak functional capacity are available against which an individual's performance can be compared.

Electrocardiographic Changes

- *ST segment depression.* The PQ segment is taken as the isoelectric line and the ST segment is usually measured relative to this 80 ms after the

J point. If the baseline is depressed >1 mm below the isoelectric line for three consecutive beats in at least two adjacent leads then it is considered an abnormal response (Fig. 28.19)

- *ST segment elevation.* >1 mm ST segment elevation above the PQ isoelectric line 80 ms after the J point for three consecutive beats in at least two adjacent leads is also considered an abnormal response and in a non-Q-wave lead, is usually associated with more severe coronary artery disease than is ST segment depression

- *T wave changes.* These are non-specific as the T-wave morphology is influenced by body position, respiration and hyperventilation

- *Bayesian theory.* There are problems with false positive and false negative stress test results particularly if ST segment changes are considered in isolation. Bayesian theory relates the pretest likelihood of disease being present to the sensitivity and specificity of the test in order to calculate the post-test probability of coronary disease. In other words, ST depression in an elderly male with multiple risk factors is more likely to be a true positive result than is ST depression in a young woman with no risk factors where there is a low probability of coronary artery disease being present. The theory explains why maximal exercise testing as a screening procedure is not useful because the test does not significantly alter the post-test risk of coronary disease being present, and also why it is important to include all the non-ECG variables in the final assessment of a patient and in the interpretation of the stress test; which should not be labelled simply 'positive', 'negative' or 'inconclusive'

The leads affected by ST segment depression do not necessarily indicate the site of myocardial ischaemia but ST segment elevation is more specific for the region of the affected myocardium (Mark *et*

Fig. 28.19 A signal-averaged ECG recording taken during a treadmill test. The ST segment depressions in leads V4, V5 and V6 were associated with typical exertional chest discomfort which increases the likelihood of significant coronary artery disease.

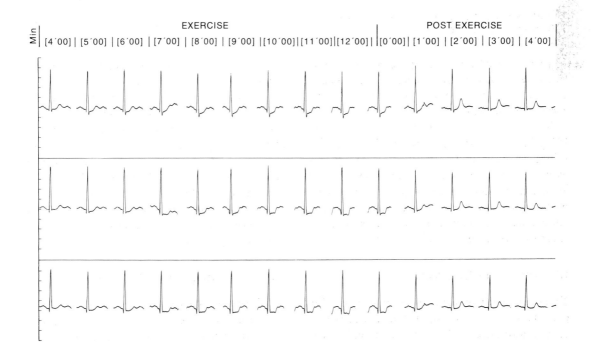

Min

EXERCISE   POST EXERCISE

[4´00] | [5´00] | [6´00] | [7´00] | [8´00] | [9´00] |[10´00]|[11´00]|[12´00] | [0´00] | [1´00] | [2´00] | [3´00] | [4´00]

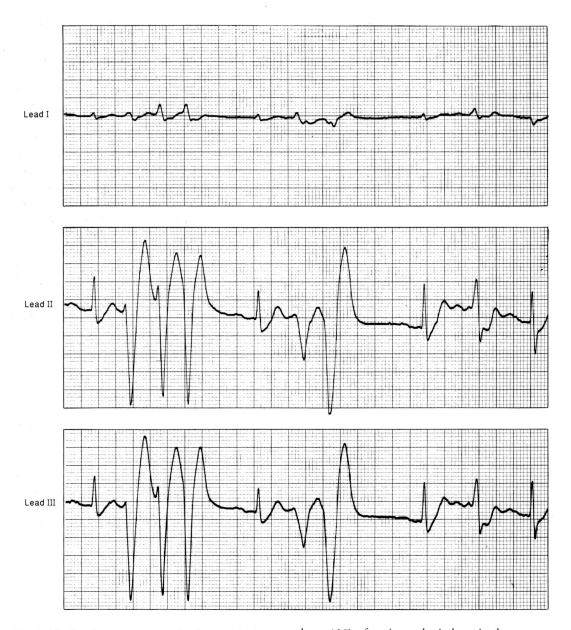

Fig. 28.20 Ventricular ectopic activity after exercise is present demonstrating single couplets and 'three in a row' ventricular ectopic beats.

al. 1987). ST segment depression due to myocardial ischaemia is usually progressive with increasing exertion and persists for up to 10 min in the recovery phase. Sometimes, however, the ischaemic ST response is seen only during exercise whereas in

about 10% of patients the ischaemic changes may only be present in the recovery phase.

Rhythm Disturbance

In normal subjects ventricular ectopic activity, when present, usually decreases with exercise. Ventricular ectopic activity increasing with physical activity and continuing to exceed 20% of the QRS com-

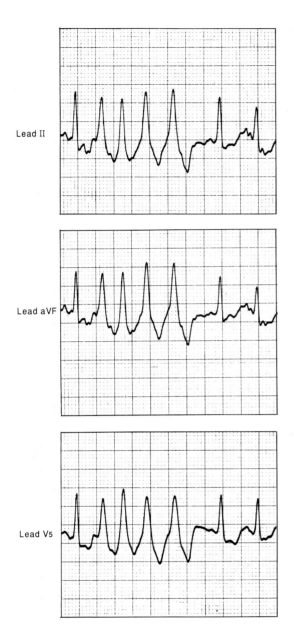

Lead II

Lead aVF

Lead V5

Fig. 28.21 Non-sustained ventricular tachycardia. Note the flat ST segments in the flanking normal beats which indicate a probable ischaemic basis for this rhythm disturbance.

plexes, frequent multiform ventricular ectopic beats (VEB), ventricular tachycardia or ventricular fibrillation are all abnormal responses.

SUBMAXIMAL EXERCISE TESTING

Submaximal exercise testing is a means of evaluating a person's functional aerobic capacity, which can be defined as the ability to sustain a whole body activity such as running, cycling or swimming over a considerable period of time. In selecting a test of aerobic endurance or physical work capacity the two most important considerations are reliability and validity. Maximal exercise testing usually performed in the laboratory and involving expired gas analysis is the most valid and reliable test; however, this form of testing is time consuming and requires sophisticated equipment and trained technicians. Furthermore, the American College of Sports Medicine (1991) recommends that a physician be present at all times when maximal exercise testing is being performed on males over 40 years and females over 50 years. Thus, on many occasions maximal exercise testing would be impractical and submaximal exercise testing, from which maximal capacity can be estimated, is a reasonable compromise.

The two most common submaximal exercise tests are the Physical Work Capacity 170 Test (PWC 170), and the Tri-Level Exercise test (Telford *et al.* 1987). The PWC 170 fitness test aims to estimate the workload that a given subject can complete at a heart rate of 170 beats·min^{-1} while working at a lower heart rate on a cycle ergometer. It is important to note that this heart rate value will change depending on the age of the subject. For this test the subject must ride a bicycle at a pedal rate of 60 revolutions·min^{-1}, over a series of three workloads. The first workload is estimated so that the subject's heart rate will be between 115 and 130 beats·min^{-1}, the second level increases the rate to 130–145 beats·min^{-1}, and the third should produce a heart rate between 145 and 165 beats·min^{-1}. These heart rate ranges will vary with the age of the subject. Workloads last for 4 min or until a steady-state heart rate is obtained. The subject's heart rate along with the workloads is graphed and a predicted work capacity for the subject can be determined.

The Tri-Level fitness test aims to estimate the workload that can be completed at a given subject's

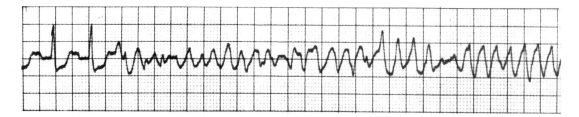

Fig. 28.22 Ventricular fibrillation occurring during exercise.

target heart rate (THR). THR is calculated using the following formula: THR = (220 − age) × 0.75. The Tri-Level exercise test also involves performing on a cycle ergometer. The subject begins cycling at the slow rate of 25 W·min⁻¹, and this workload is increased by 25 W·min⁻¹ at the end of each minute. Heart rates are monitored in the last 20 s of each minute and the subject keeps cycling until THR is reached or exceeded. The subject's aerobic capacity is estimated using an interpolation method to determine the workload at the subject's THR.

Both these submaximal exercise tests use heart rate as the measure of work intensity and the aim is for subjects to complete the test at a target heart rate of between 120 and 165 beats·min⁻¹ (age related). The maximum oxygen uptake ($\dot{V}_{O_2max}$) can be estimated using heart rate values obtained, based on the principle that a linear relationship exists between heart rate and oxygen consumption.

There are other forms of submaximal exercise tests such as step tests and field runs, which can be undertaken in a more natural environment. These may be more cost-efficient means of exercise testing, but the validity of such tests is open to question.

Except for special circumstances such as early after myocardial infarction, symptom-limited or clinical maximal exercise tests are preferred to submaximal testing for assessing the cardiovascular response of patients with coronary heart disease.

CONCLUSIONS

Exercise testing is a very useful procedure both in sports medicine and clinical practice. For the latter,

an understanding of the strengths and limitations of the test is required, particularly with regard to false positive and false negative results, if inappropriate patient management is to be avoided.

REFERENCES

American College of Sports Medicine (1991) *Guidelines for Exercise Testing and Prescription*, 4th edn. Lea & Febiger, Philadelphia, PA.

Chaitman B. (1992) Exercise stress testing. In Braunwald E. (ed.) *Heart Disease: A Textbook of Cardiovascular Medicine*, 4th edn. W. B. Saunders, Philadelphia, PA.

Ellestad M. H. (1986) *Stress Testing Principles and Practice*, 3rd edn. F. A. Davis, Philadelphia, PA.

Evans D. E. (1994) Exercise. In Case R. M. & Waterhouse J. M. (eds) *Human Physiology: Stress and Environment*. Oxford University Press, Oxford.

Fleg J. L. & Lakatta E. G. (1986) Prevalence and significance of post exercise hypotension in apparently healthy subjects. *American Journal of Cardiology* 57, 1380–1384.

Froelicher V. F. (1987) Exercise and the heart. *Clinical Concepts*, 2nd edn. Year Book Medical Publishers Inc., Chicago, IL.

Froelicher V. F. & Marcondes G. D. (1989) *Manual of Exercise Testing*. Year Book Medical Publishers Inc., Chicago, IL.

Guyton A. C. (1992) *Human Physiology and Mechanisms of Disease*, 5th edn. W. B. Saunders, Philadelphia, PA.

Hamm L. F., Crow R. S., Stall G. A. & Hannon P. (1989) Safety and characteristics of exercise testing early after acute myocardial infarction. *American Journal of Cardiology* 63, 1193–1197.

Mark D. B., Hlatky M. A., Lee K. L. et al. (1987) Localising coronary artery obstructions with the exercise treadmill test. *Annals of Internal Medicine* 106, 53–55.

Stuart R. J. & Ellestad M. H. (1980) National survey of exercise stress testing facilities. *Chest* 77, 94–97.

Telford R. D., Minikin B. R., Hooper L. A. et al. (1987) The tri-level fitness profile. *Excel* 4, 11–13.

Wilmore J. H. & Costill D. L. (1994) *Physiology of Sport & Exercise*. Human Kinetics Publishers, Champaign, IL.

PART VI

EATING DISORDERS

P. N. Gilchrist and L. Burke

Eating disorders can have a devastating effect on the lives of individuals and their families. Once established, an eating disorder may become chronic and in a small number of cases be fatal. The treatment is often prolonged and a successful outcome is not always assured. An eating disorder may develop after a period of conscious dieting by vulnerable individuals, such as young women. Or, it may be the result of a period of restricted food intake following facial or dental surgery, illness or stress, leading to an increasing preoccupation with issues of weight and food (Garfinkel & Garner 1982). Media publicity, with emphasis on the dietary component, has tended to trivialize these conditions and downplay the extent of the disruption they can cause. Athletes encouraged to follow rigid dietary programmes or to diet to reach a specific weight for competition and those engaged in sports or activities where physical appearance and/or low body fat levels are stressed (e.g. gymnastics and distance running), seem to be particularly at risk (Sundgot-Borgen 1994). In striving to improve performance, athletes may focus on weight/body fat and diet and develop beliefs which are increasingly idiosyncratic, or behaviours which are compulsive and not dissimilar to eating disordered patients. Such individuals should be carefully monitored.

There are two main eating disorders recognized, namely anorexia nervosa or the so-called 'slimmer's disease' and bulimia nervosa, which is a loss of control of appetite and binge eating/vomiting.

Diagnostic criteria for anorexia nervosa and bulimia nervosa proposed in the 'DSM-IV' or Diagnostic and Statistical Manual of Mental Disorders (American Psychiatric Association 1994) are summarized in Tables 28.8 and 28.9. These criteria represent the extreme manifestation of eating disorders. Many individuals, including athletes who suffer from eating disorders may not completely fulfil these criteria. In essence, both anorexia nervosa and bulimia nervosa are characterized by a body image disturbance, where a 'normal' weight/body fat level is viewed as unacceptable. The perception of themselves as overweight can better be under-

Table 28.8 Diagnostic criteria for anorexia nervosa

Refusal to maintain bodyweight at or above a minimally normal weight for age and height (e.g. weight loss leading to maintenance of bodyweight less than 85% of that expected; or failure to make expected weight gain during period of growth, leading to bodyweight less than 85% of that expected)

Intense fear of gaining weight or becoming fat, even though underweight

Disturbance in the way in which one's bodyweight or shape is experienced, undue influence of bodyweight or shape on self-evaluation, or denial of the seriousness of the current low bodyweight

In postmenarcheal females, amenorrhoea, i.e. the absence of at least three consecutive menstrual cycles. (A woman is considered to have amenorrhoea if her periods occur only following hormone treatment, e.g. oestrogen administration.)

Table 28.9 Diagnostic criteria for bulimia nervosa

Recurrent episodes of binge eating. An episode of binge eating is characterized by the following:

Eating, in a discrete period of time (e.g. within any 2 h period), an amount of food that is definitely larger than most people would consume

A sense of lack of control over eating during the episode (e.g. a feeling that one cannot stop eating or control what or how much one is eating)

Recurrent inappropriate compensatory behaviour in order to prevent weight gain, such as self-induced vomiting; misuse of laxatives, diuretics, enemas or other medications; fasting; or excessive exercise

The binge eating and inappropriate compensatory behaviours both occur, on the average, at least twice a week for 3 months

Self-evaluation is unduly influenced by body shape and weight

The disturbance does not occur exclusively during episodes of anorexia nervosa

Adapted from the American Psychiatric Association (1994).

stood if 'being fat' is seen as 'not being good enough', or even 'worthless'. The extent of self-loathing in eating-disordered patients is often extreme.

ANOREXIA NERVOSA

Anorexia nervosa is characterized by an intense pursuit of thinness, with marked weight loss and avoidance of fatty or carbohydrate foods. As well as abstaining from eating, individuals may use a variety of strategies to lose weight, such as compulsive purposeless exercise (in excess of their normal training load), vomiting, fluid restriction, self-administered diuretics, appetite suppressants or laxative abuse. Strategies employed by various individuals are limited only by their creativity in such matters or their degree of desperation.

There may be a change in eating habits to what might at first be considered a 'healthy diet' but with increasing restrictions, both in the type and quantity of food consumed. Self-description as a 'vegetarian' is often an early clue to restricted dietary practices, although the athlete does not actually follow a true (balanced) vegetarian diet with alternative dietary sources of protein and

minerals. As the anorexic condition develops, the individual may spend much time preparing food for others, but go to great lengths to avoid eating food personally. In addition they become expert at concealing such behaviour, preoccupied with the calorie content and/or fat content of food and frequently keep extensive records of the calorie content of meals as a means of controlling food intake.

Despite often radical changes in behaviour and dramatic weight loss, there is a strenuous denial at first that there is anything wrong, much to the frustration of family and friends. In a competitive environment, such as a training camp or sports institute, an athlete's excessive self-weighing or checking of skinfold thickness may be viewed by some as a wish to improve performance rather than an indication of compulsive behaviour and the beginnings of an anorexic condition.

BULIMIA NERVOSA

Bulimia nervosa, as a clinical entity, has only relatively recently been described in the literature (Russell 1979), although like anorexia nervosa it is not a new condition. It is characterized by a loss of control of appetite, the consumption of large quantities of readily digestible food and is followed by a variety of strategies aimed at avoiding a feared weight gain. The commonest techniques used to avoid this gain are self-induced vomiting or regurgitation.

The bulimic individual is often more difficult to identify, as he or she may appear to be of relatively normal weight, but this weight may fluctuate significantly. If there is no dramatic weight loss, no immediate suspicions may be raised and in the case of an athlete, his or her performance may initially not be affected.

In the absence of overtly disturbed eating patterns, an eating disorder may be suspected through complications of such behaviour. For example, unexplained electrolyte changes may be seen on routine blood biochemistry tests, especially decreased serum potassium or a metabolic alkalosis. There may be a deterioration in dental hygiene (a classical sign is the loss of enamel from the posterior surfaces of the lower teeth as a result of vomiting the acidic contents of the stomach) or swollen parotid glands. Occasionally, enlarged masseter muscles are found in individuals who excessively chew and then spit out their food. A haematemesis due to a Mallory-Weiss tear of the oesophagus may be the only presenting sign.

The secretive behaviour of the bulimic is carefully concealed and this in part is related to the bizarre behaviour which they wish to hide, as well as the fear of being discovered. These individuals are often caught out if there is a change in their routine, such as when expected to engage in group activity or share accommodation in a communal living situation (such as a training camp or a sports institute), where visits to the toilet or unusual eating habits may be more noticeable.

An unexpected increase in food requirements may be the first hint of a problem. Sufferers of bulimia nervosa often consume enormous quantities of readily digestible food as quickly as possible until they can eat no more and then induce vomiting. They may repeat this behaviour throughout the day or have periods of relative control, only to resume the behaviour during times of stress or when depressed and lonely. Others find that they are unable to induce vomiting or are repulsed by the idea and alternate between bingeing and fasting, or bingeing and abusing laxatives. Others, although far less commonly, binge and then spit out the food.

It is often difficult to appreciate the compulsive nature of the bulimic's behaviour, but the day can be taken up with planning and preparing to carry out the binge/vomiting behaviour. Such behaviour is difficult to understand until it is appreciated that the binge eating is pleasurable and perceived by the bulimic as a comfort and as a solution to a serious underlying emotional issue. What is unacceptable and not pleasurable is the idea of gaining weight as a result of the large amount of food consumed, which in turn leads to vomiting behaviour.

There is often an overlap between anorexia and bulimia in patients. Many bulimic patients have been anorexic previously and develop overeating and vomiting behaviour when they can no longer maintain an abstaining and underweight condition,

while others alternate between bulimia nervosa and anorexia nervosa.

ATYPICAL AND SUBCLINICAL DISORDERS

Some individuals who have had a previous episode of anorexia nervosa, regain weight without resolving the underlying psychological issues. These and other individuals who are obsessed about issues of weight, body image and food, but are within a normal weight range, have been more recently referred to as 'restrained eaters'. The latest edition of the DSM (American Psychiatric Association 1994) has included a classification of *Eating Disorder Not Otherwise Specified* to characterize disturbances in eating behaviour that do not fully meet their criteria for anorexia nervosa and bulimia nervosa. This could include overweight individuals who binge but do not purge, thus failing to meet the criteria for bulimia nervosa and individuals who appear to have anorexia but have regular menses or a normal/slightly below normal bodyweight.

Sundgot-Borgen (1994) and others have used the term anorexia athletica to describe athletes who exhibit fears of weight gain, restricted eating and other distorted eating behaviour, but whose symptoms and bodyweight loss do not meet DSM-IV criteria for anorexia nervosa or bulimia nervosa. The use of the term anorexia athletica should be discouraged, as these individuals do not fit any pattern which is different from the population of atypical eating disorders. However, it is important to increase the recognition of these atypical or 'subclinical' eating disorders in athletes as it is a concern that the severity of conditions which do not meet full DSM-IV criteria may be overlooked or the behaviour justified as being merely part of the individual's sports routine.

ARE ATHLETES AT GREATER RISK?

Recent publication of studies reporting eating disorders in groups of athletes and public announcements of eating disorders in famous athletes have prompted the inquiry 'does sport cause eating disorders?' It is apparent that in some cases, sport is not the cause but a camouflage for eating disorders. It has been suggested (Thompson & Sherman 1993; Sundgot-Bergen 1994) that some sports may attract individuals with pre-existing eating disorders, or who are at high risk to contrast eating disorders, because these individuals see exercise as an opportunity to expend extra kilojoules, or to justify their abnormal eating and dieting behaviour. These athletes seek and participate in sports that condone low bodyweight, excessive exercise and rigid eating, in an attempt to legitimize or hide their condition and to delay any intervention.

However, in most cases it appears that the eating disorder presents or develops after the individual has become involved in a sport. It is therefore reasonable to speculate whether sports participation predisposes them to a greater risk of eating disorders. However, well-conducted, longitudinal studies of large numbers of athletes and non-athletes have not yet been undertaken. Nevertheless, the following circumstantial evidence has led Brownell and Rodin (1992) and Sundgot-Borgen (1994) to suggest that:

- A higher than expected occurrence of eating-related problems occur in athletes when they are compared with the rates given for the general population
- More frequent problems occur in athletes than in controls or non-athletes
- Problems occur more frequently in sports in which low body fat levels and weight restrictions are important, than in sports in which weight is not so important

There are many cross-sectional studies which have attempted to measure or comment on the prevalence of eating disorders in athletes and detailed summaries of these studies have been made by Wilmore (1991) and Brownell and Rodin (1992). Most of these studies have used surveys or questionnaires to gather information about preoccupation with food, weight and body fat level, disturbed body image or the use of pathogenic weight control methods. Estimates of the prevalence of symptoms or the existence of eating disorders varies from less than 1% of athletic populations (Warren et al. 1990) to nearly 50% of the athletic group (Rucinski

1989). In some studies the prevalence of eating problems was reported to be greater among athletes than in control groups of non-athletes and higher than the rates of eating disorders estimated in the general population (Wilmore 1991; Brownell & Rodin 1992). Nevertheless, results are not always consistent between studies and there are errors inherent in some of the methods used.

Reasons for the wide variation in the results of these studies include the composition of the athletic population investigated, whether self-reports or clinical interviews were used and the methodological instrument used (Sundgot-Borgen 1994). Studies which use the DSM IV criteria to diagnose eating disorders would be expected to produce lower prevalence rates than studies which collect data on individual symptoms or behaviours of eating disorders, since many athletes who demonstrate eating problems will fail to meet these strict diagnostic criteria. Other studies have attempted to measure the prevalence of problem attitudes and behaviours using individually developed questionnaires or standardized instruments such as the Eating Disorder Inventory (EDI; Garner et al. 1984) and the Eating Attitude Test (EAT; Garner & Garfinkel 1979). While these methods are well-known and useful as diagnostic tools, they may not have been validated with athletes (Brownell & Rodin 1992).

Indeed there is evidence that these self-reporting instruments are inappropriate for athletes, or that individuals are not always truthful in their responses. Brownell and Rodin (1992) cite the following cases:

- Questionnaires were given to 110 elite female athletes representing seven different sports. Anonymity was guaranteed and coaches and athletic officials were not to see the results. Of 87 respondents, not one scored in the disordered eating range of the EAT and there were few indications of serious disorders in other parts of the questionnaire. However, within 2 years of the completion of the study, 18 of the athletes had received either inpatient or outpatient treatment for eating disorders
- The EDI was administered to nine amenorrhoeic and five eumenorrhoeic runners during a study of nationally ranked female distance runners.

Three subjects were identified as having 'possible' problems but not clear eating disorders. Subsequently, seven of the nine amenorrhoeic runners were diagnosed as having eating disorders. No problems developed in the eumenorrhoeic runners

Despite these methodological problems and conflict between individual surveys, the current literature of cross-sectional studies indicates that there is a greater risk of problems with eating behaviour and attitudes in sport, particularly among female athletes. Sports in which rigid bodyweight standards are enforced, or in which a low body fat level is seen as important, appear to be 'high-risk' sports (Brownell & Rodin 1992; Sundgot-Borgen 1994) and include distance running, ballet dancing, gymnastics, figure skating and light-weight rowing. It is uncertain from studies whether eating problems are more common in the most highly trained or elite competitors of these sports. One could speculate that elite performers might be more at risk from the pressures or factors that create risk. However, it might also be expected that athletes with eating disorders might have difficulty performing at an elite level and may discontinue their participation or that the sub-elite may be tempted to strive harder to improve performance to reach the elite level. Indeed one study of ballet dancers reported a greater prevalence of eating disorders among the lower level ballet schools, than among the more elite companies (Hamilton *et al.* 1988).

As most of the surveys have studied only women athletes, it is difficult to make definite statements on the prevalence of eating disorders in male athletes, relative either to the general male population or to female athletes. Nevertheless, it seems logical to conclude from population estimates that females make up 90–95% of cases of eating disorders (American Psychiatric Association 1994) and that male athletes are at less risk of developing eating disorders than are female athletes.

The second source of evidence to support the connection between eating disorders and sport is the recognition that many of the known risk factors for eating disorders exist in sport and indeed are sometimes self-selective for good sports performance. For example, a number of the psychological risk factors for eating disorders are common in athletes. These include perfectionist attitudes, competitiveness; the ability to be rigid and driven to complete tasks; and the ability to undertake a 'spartan' life-style of intense exercise, precise time management and food control. These attributes are some of the factors that may drive an individual to participate in sport in the first place and then assure them of success. Furthermore, the high pressure environment of sport and the close level of competition may create an intense external stress pushing athletes towards any behaviour or strategy that offers the promise of performance improvements. The athlete's own strong desires may be matched and in some cases overwhelmed, by the goals of parents, coaches and other pivotal people in their lives.

The focus on low body fat levels and competition weight restrictions in many sports may provide an unnatural view of weight control, dieting, body image and food intake. It is true that weight and body fat levels do influence sports performance in some events. Lower body fat levels are generally predictive of good performance in sports where a high power-to-weight ratio is important, particularly when events are endurance-based (e.g. distance running, road cycling, triathlons, jumps, gymnastics, cross-country skiing). Furthermore, it is undeniable that aesthetics play a part in performance in activities such as gymnastics, diving, ballet and figure skating and that the present culture in these sports prizes low body fat levels. In sports such as light-weight rowing, horse racing and combative events (wrestling, boxing, judo), an athlete is not eligible to compete unless a weight division has been reached. It is easy to see that athletes attempting to gain even the smallest advantage or competitive edge may undertake eating and dieting strategies that promote weight/fat loss rather than healthy nutritional status. The situation seems worse for female athletes, reflecting the dissatisfaction of females in the general population with their body image and the tendency for female athletes to have higher body fat levels despite undertaking the same training and eating less calories than their male counterparts.

In summary, sport and sports coaches do not 'cause' eating disorders in athletes. However, it is understandable that the combination of individuals with high-risk personalities and an environment that is highly pressured and focused on body-weight/fat levels and control of food and exercise can lead to the development of eating disorders.

SYMPTOMS OF EATING DISORDERS IN ATHLETES

If an athlete is known to have unusual eating behaviour, is abusing laxatives or diuretics, or is regarded as a compulsive exerciser (is exercising beyond the requirements of the sport or programme), then a coach or sports psychologist may need to check for other psychological problems. Even in groups where extreme demands on exercise time are made and dietary restrictions are present, it is usually obvious to other members of that group when any one individual has exceeded expected requirements. Peers may be reluctant to say anything for fear of being seen as disloyal or interfering with another's preparation, especially if dieting or exercise behaviour had initially been encouraged by their coach. Coaches, who have a special relationship with athletes under their control, can easily underestimate the influence they have on an individual and their role in the development of an eating disorder. Similarly, parents who have unrealistic expectations of their children may figure in the development of eating disorders.

On a practical level, a disorder may be recognized by the need to either continue to exercise excessively against advice or to the individual's physical detriment, together with the other behaviours mentioned above. In some sports, where it may be necessary to lose weight or to increase training requirements prior to a particular event in order to improve performance, it is the inability after the event to return to a less vigorous exercise requirement, or the wish to lose further weight, that may indicate an eating disorder.

An unexpected alteration in routine, such as a forced change to training due to injury, may expose an eating disorder. If an individual has been able to control an eating disorder by maintaining a rigid exercise programme and this strategy is no longer

Table 28.10 Warning signs for eating disorders in athletes

Warning signs for anorexia nervosa
  Dramatic loss in weight
  A preoccupation with food, calories and weight
  Wearing baggy or layered clothing
  Relentless, excessive exercise
  Mood swings
  Avoiding food-related social activities

Warning signs for bulimia nervosa
  Noticeable weight gain or loss
  Excessive concern about weight
  Bathroom visits after meals
  Depressive moods
  Strict dieting followed by eating binges
  Increasing criticism of one's body

National Collegiate Athletic Association, cited in Wilmore (1991).

possible, this can make an individual acknowledge that there is a problem and thereby confront the behaviour.

Warning signs, such as those publicized by the National Collegiate Athletic Association (Table 28.10) can be an indication of a developing or undetected eating disorder in athletes. It is important to recognize that the presence of these signs is not necessarily indicative of an eating disorder; the absolute diagnosis should be done by an appropriate health professional. Indeed the observation of other specific behaviours deemed to be predictive of eating disorders in non-athletes may, at times, simply be a part of the requirements for participation and good performance in sport. These might include the possession of a 'calorie counter'/food composition manual to constantly evaluate meals, rigid adherence to an intense exercise programme, compulsion to rise in the early morning and follow a strict daily timetable of activities. Such behaviours and activities cease being 'normal' when the athlete becomes obsessive about them, particularly when they are continued despite evidence that they are causing harm to health and performance.

FACTORS CONTRIBUTING TO EATING DISORDERS

Figure 28.23 is offered as a guide to the source of stressors that can contribute to the development

670

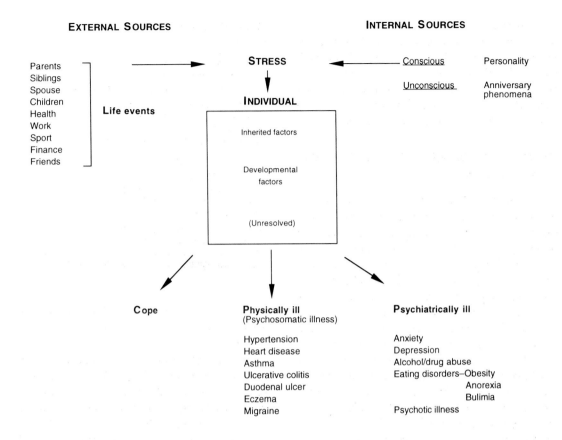

EXTERNAL SOURCES

INTERNAL SOURCES

Parents
Siblings
Spouse
Children
Health
Work
Sport
Finance
Friends

Life events

STRESS

INDIVIDUAL

Inherited factors

Developmental
factors

(Unresolved)

Conscious   Personality

Unconscious   Anniversary
phenomena

Cope

Physically ill
(Psychosomatic illness)

Hypertension
Heart disease
Asthma
Ulcerative colitis
Duodenal ulcer
Eczema
Migraine

Psychiatrically ill

Anxiety
Depression
Alcohol/drug abuse
Eating disorders–Obesity
                          Anorexia
                          Bulimia
Psychotic illness

Fig. 28.23 Factors which may lead to eating disorders.

and perpetuation of an eating disorder. When either anorexia nervosa or bulimia nervosa is seen as a powerful solution to an athlete's problems, the reluctance to give up such behaviour is understandable.

From Fig. 28.23 it can be seen that any individual is a product of inherited and developmental factors. We inherit biological bases to personality styles as well as to physical and psychiatric illness. The developmental factors relate to the life experiences that shape our attitudes and aspirations. There may be significant psychological issues in any one individual, depending on the circumstances of his or her birth, whether planned, illegitimate or complicated by illness in the mother. Similarly, an individual is shaped by parental personalities, childhood experiences and expectations in the parents, who may attempt to act out their own ambitions through their children. If there are unresolved major

conflicts, whether they be in relationship to parents, siblings or peers, they can continue to influence behaviour and sensitize the individual in later life.

The external sources of stress are self-explanatory and are regarded as life events, but may reactivate unresolved developmental issues, leading to an emotional over-reaction on the individual's part.

The internal sources of stress relate to both conscious factors and unconscious factors. On a conscious level some personalities will tolerate stress and competition better than others and what may be seen as insurmountable by one person could well be regarded as an exciting challenge by another. The unconscious sources of stress are more difficult to discern. An example of this sort of distress is the unresolved grief towards a loved one where, if not confronted, the emotional turmoil remains even though the death may have occurred many years earlier. If an athlete develops or already has an eating disorder, it is probable that such issues are contributing and will need to be explored. In some cases an individual's athletic activities may be an attempt to keep these issues under some sort of control.

Sundgot-Borgen (1994), from a series of studies of athletes with eating disorders, has identified a number of external sources of stress and triggers that may contribute to eating problems in vulnerable athletes. These are summarized in Table 28.11 and include traumatic events in the life of the athlete, interruption to sports participation and unsupervised advice or pressure to lose bodyweight/fat. In summary she suggests that it is not necessarily dieting *per se* that may be important in triggering an eating disorder, but whether the athlete received guidance and sensible advice to help achieve weight loss goals.

SHOULD AN ATHLETE WITH AN EATING DISORDER CEASE TO COMPETE?

There is no simple answer to this and factors such as the severity of the condition, the age of the individual, the risk of physical sequelae and the attitudes of the various sporting bodies need to be considered. If the perceived benefits of continuing the behaviour are high, then it is unlikely that reason will prevail. In the pursuit of excellence or in achieving goals, some athletes are prepared to place their physical health at risk and it is unlikely that the severity of an eating disorder will be acknowledged if it satisfies a short-term goal.

Whatever decision is made, it should be emphasized that the individual's disturbed eating is not simply a dietary or weight problem but is an indication of significant psychopathology. Often it is only when athletes are confronted with the fact that their weight or behaviour is obviously outside acceptable standards, or when they develop significant physical complications that they are prepared to acknowledge and explore the determining psychological factors.

TREATMENT OPTIONS

To hope that the eating disorder problem will just go away is wishful thinking. On the other hand, recent work has indicated that relatively simple education methods outlining basic dietary requirements may benefit some individuals.

However, the majority of cases require more intensive treatment, either by a therapist familiar with eating disorders or by referral to a specialist weight disorder unit (Kalucy *et al.* 1984). The principles of treatment include weight gain if underweight, control of disordered eating patterns and other weight controlling strategies, combined with the exploration and resolution where possible of psychological factors. A multidisciplinary team approach is often useful. Individual psychotherapy and at times, family therapy, may be required. Associated depressive symptoms and obsessive–compulsive behaviour often benefit from pharmacotherapy.

Table 28.11 Risk factors and triggers for eating disorders in vulnerable athletes

High risk	Low risk
Recommendation to lose weight without guidance	Recommendation to lose weight with guidance
Start of sport-specific training at an early age	Start of sport-specific training at a later age
Start of dieting at an early age	Start of dieting at a later age
Low acceptance of puberty by athlete (from a performance perspective)	High acceptance of puberty by athlete (from a performance perspective)
Sudden increase in training volume	
Injury	
Loss of coach	

Adapted from Sundgot-Borgen (1994).

CONCLUSIONS

Eating disorders are not uncommon in the general population and as such could be expected to occur in groups of athletes (Ben-Tovim 1988, 1990). Recurring themes in eating-disordered patients relate to issues of self-worth and control. If athletes are encouraged to lose weight as a means of improving performance and if this is linked with improving their own sense of self-worth and/or to impress significant others in their lives (such as their coach, family or peers), then they are at risk of developing an eating disorder. In an impressionable group of young athletes, any advice to diet should be made cautiously, with clear guide-lines of lower limits and should be seen as an adjunct to performance and not aligned with self-worth. Although eating disorders are more common in females, they should not be overlooked in males.

REFERENCES

American Psychiatric Association (1994) *Diagnostic and Statistical Manual of Mental Disorders (DSM-IV)*. American Psychiatric Association, Washington, DC.

Ben-Tovim D. I. (1988) Diagnosis and prevalence of bulimia in Australia. *American Journal of Psychiatry* 145, 1000–1002.

Ben-Tovim D. I. (1990) Epidemiology of anorexia nervosa in South Australia. *Australian & New Zealand Journal of Psychiatry* 24, 182–186.

Brownell K. D. & Rodin R. (1992) Prevalence of eating disorders in athletes. In Brownell K. D., Rodin R. & Wilmore J. H. (eds) *Eating, Body Weight and Performance in Athletes*. Lea & Febiger, Philadelphia, PA.

Garfinkel P. E. & Garner D. M. (1982) *Anorexia Nervosa: A Multidimensional Perspective*. Brunner/Mazel, New York.

Garner D. M. & Garfinkel P. E. (1979) An index of symptoms of anorexia nervosa. *Psychological Medicine* 9, 273–279.

Garner D. M., Olmsted M. P. & Polivy J. (1984) *Manual of Eating Disorder Inventory (EDI)*. Psychological Assessment Resources, Odessa.

Hamilton L. H., Brooks-Gunn J. & Warren M. P. (1988) The role of selectivity in the pathogenesis of eating problems in ballet dancers. *Medicine and Science in Sports and Exercise* 20, 560–565.

Kalucy R. S., Gilchrist P. N., McFarlane C. M. & McFarlane A. C. (1984) The evolution of a multitherapy orientation. In Garner D. M. & Garfinkel P. (eds) *Handbook of Psychotherapy for Anorexia Nervosa and Bulimia*. Guildford Press, New York.

Rucinski A. (1989) Relationship of body image and dietary intake of competitive ice skaters. *Journal of the American Dietetic Association* 89, 98–100.

Russell G. F. M. (1979) Bulimia nervosa: An ominous variant of anorexia nervosa. *Psychological Medicine* 9, 429–448.

Sundgot-Borgen J. (1994) Eating disorders in female athletes. *Sports Medicine* 17, 176–188.

Thompson R. A. & Sherman R. T. (1993) *Helping Athletes with Eating Disorders*. Human Kinetics Publishers, Champaign, IL.

Warren B. J., Stanton A. L. & Blessing D. L. (1990) Disordered eating patterns in competitive female athletes. *International Journal of Eating Disorders* 5, 565–569.

Wilmore J. H. (1991) Eating and weight disorders in female athletes. *International Journal of Sport Nutrition* 1, 104–117.

ORCHARD SPORTS INJURY CLASSIFICATION SYSTEM

J. Orchard

The Orchard Sports Injury Classification System (OSICS) is an injury classification system designed for use by practitioners who regularly see sports injuries. It is simple to use (with each diagnosis being made up of three characters only (but provides an extensive list of the diagnoses which are seen in sports medicine. The system can be expanded, so it is anticipated that regular updates will be published. Individual users and centres may create their own codes by varying the third character (to one other than the numbers 1–7, which are used in the list of common diagnoses).

Currently, this system is being used by the Australian Institute of Sport, the major football codes in Australia and several sports medicine centres. Copyright is owned by Dr John Orchard, but use of the system for research is free and encouraged by the author. Potential uses also include the compilation of an injury data base and statistics, archiving of files and comparison of injury profiles between groups.

EXPLANATION OF CODES:

FIRST CHARACTER
(Body area)

HEAD and NECK

H–   Head
N–   Neck

UPPER LIMB

S–   Shoulder
U–   Upper arm
E–   Elbow
R–   Forearm
W–   Wrist
P–   Hand

TRUNK

C–   Chest
O–   Abdomen
D–   Thoracic back
L–   Lumbar back

LOWER LIMB

B–   Buttock
G–   Groin/hip
T–   Thigh
Q–   Lower leg
A–   Ankle/heel
F–   Foot

GENERAL

X–   Multiple areas
M–   Medical problem
Z–   Area not specified

SECOND CHARACTER
(Type of pathology)

BONE
-F-   Fracture (*not* stress or avulsion)
-G-   Avulsion or chip fracture
-S-   Stress fracture
-Q-   Old fracture mal- or non-union

JOINT
-D-   Dislocation
-U-   Recurrent instability/subluxation
-C-   Articular/chondral damage
-J-   Minor joint trauma ± synovitis
-P-   Atraumatic arthritis/effusion/joint pain/
        chronic synovitis/gout/other rheumatological
        condition
-A-   Chronic degenerative arthritis (including
        avascular necrosis)
-L-   Ligament tear or sprain

SOFT TISSUE
-M-   Muscle tear or strain
-Y-   Muscle spasm/cramps/soreness/trigger
        points/myalgia/overuse
-T-   Tendinitis/bursitis/enthesopathy/
        apophysitis/periostitis
-R-   Complete rupture of tendon
-H-   Haematoma/bruising/cork
-K-   Laceration/skin condition

OTHER
-B-   Developmental anomaly
-I-   Infection
-E-   Tumours
-O-   Visceral damage/trauma/surgery
-N-   Neural condition/nerve damage
-V-   Vascular condition
-X-   Systemic disease process
-Z-   Undiagnosed

THIRD CHARACTER

−1 to −7   Common diagnoses (see attached list)
−8   Character to be used when making a
                diagnosis not included in common
                diagnosis list

−9   Character to be used when specific
                diagnosis is not known or supplied
−A to −Z   Special diagnoses used for individual
                centre research or expansion

Abbreviations used in the listing of codes

#	fracture	jt	joint
disl	dislocation	lig	ligament
spr	sprain	pts	points (as in
str	strain		trigger points)

HEAD (see also Medical section)

HF1	# Nose
HF2	# Skull
HF3	# Mandible
HF4	# Facial bone(s)
HG1	Avulsed/# tooth
HD1	Disl temporomandibular jt
HJ1	Spr temporomandibular jt
HY1	Facial muscle trigger pts
HH1	Head/facial haematoma
HK1	Scalp laceration
HK2	Facial laceration
HO1	Eye injury/trauma
HO2	Perforated ear drum
HN1	Concussion
HN2	Intracranial bleed
HN3	Chronic brain injury
HV1	Epistaxis
HI1	Otitis externa (otitis media — see Medical section MI1)
HI2	Cellulitis/skin infection, face
HZ1	Headache/pain undiagnosed

NECK

NF1	Stable cervical #
NF2	Unstable cervical #
NG1	Avulsion # cervical spine (e.g. spinous process)
NC1	Cervical disc prolapse
NC2	Cervical disc degeneration
NJ1	Whiplash/neck spr
NP1	Cervical facet jt pain
NA1	Cervical facet jt degenerative arthritis
NM1	Neck muscle str
NY1	Neck muscle trigger pts/spasm/torticollis

NH1   Neck haematoma
NK1   Neck laceration
NB1   Cervical developmental anomaly
NO1   Laryngeal trauma
NN1   Cervical nerve root compression/stretch
NN2   Neck spinal injury
NN3   Cervical spinal canal stenosis
NZ1   Neck pain undiagnosed

SHOULDER
SF1   # Clavicle
SF2   # Scapula
SF3   # Neck of humerus
SG1   Avulsion # shoulder
SS1   Stress # coracoid process
SD1   Disl shoulder
SD2   Acromioclavicular jt disl (Grade 3)
SU1   Shoulder subluxation/chronic instability
SJ1   Shoulder jt spr
SJ2   Acromioclavicular jt spr
SP1   Adhesive capsulitis or frozen or stiff
       shoulder
SA1   Shoulder jt degenerative arthritis
SA2   Acromioclavicular arthritis/distal clavicle
       osteolysis
SM1   Shoulder muscle str
SY1   Shoulder trigger pts/posterior muscle
       soreness
ST1   Rotator cuff tendinitis/subacromial
       bursitis
ST2   Biceps tendinitis
SR1   Rotator cuff tendon rupture/large tear
SR2   Rupture of long head of biceps tendon
SH1   Shoulder haematoma
SK1   Shoulder laceration
SB1   Cervical rib
SE1   Tumour, shoulder region
SN1   Brachial plexus traction injury/burner/
       stinger
SN2   Axillary nerve palsy
SN3   Non-traumatic brachial plexus lesion
       (including thoracic outlet impingement)
SN4   Suprascapular nerve entrapment or palsy
SV1   Axillary vessel thrombosis/insufficiency
SZ1   Shoulder pain undiagnosed

UPPER ARM
UF1   # Shaft of humerus

UM1   Upper arm muscle str
UY1   Upper arm muscle soreness/trigger pts
UR1   Pectoralis major tendon rupture
UH1   Upper arm haematoma
UK1   Upper arm laceration

ELBOW
EF1   Supracondylar # humerus
EF2   # Humerus condyle(s)
EF3   # Head of radius or olecranon
EG1   Elbow avulsion #
ED1   Disl elbow
ED2   Disl head of radius (including pulled
       elbow)
EU1   Elbow valgus instability
EC1   Osteochondritis elbow ($\pm$ loose bodies)
EJ1   Spr/jarred elbow
EP1   Elbow atraumatic synovitis
EA1   Elbow jt degenerative arthritis
EL1   Elbow medial collateral ligament str or
       tear
ET1   Lateral epicondylitis ('tennis elbow')
ET2   Medial epicondylitis ('golfer's elbow')
ET3   Olecranon bursitis/apophysitis/triceps
       tendinitis
EH1   Elbow haematoma
EK1   Elbow laceration
EI1   Elbow infection
EN1   Ulnar neuropathy, elbow
EN2   Posterior interosseus nerve entrapment
EZ1   Elbow pain undiagnosed

FOREARM
RF1   # Radius $\pm$ # ulna
RS1   Stress # radius or ulna
RM1   Forearm muscle str
RY1   Forearm muscle trigger pts
RY2   Forearm compartment syndrome
RT1   Extensor tenosynovitis/intersection
       syndrome (see also — Wrist WT1)
RH1   Forearm haematoma
RK1   Lacerated forearm
RK2   Forearm skin lesion

WRIST
WF1   # Scaphoid
WF2   # Other carpal bone
WF3   Intra-articular # radius

WS1	Radial epiphysis lesion or carpal stress fracture
WQ1	Non-union # scaphoid
WD1	Disl carpus
WU1	Carpal instability
WU2	Distal radio-ulnar jt instability
WC1	Wrist fibrocartilage tear
WJ1	Spr/jarred wrist jt
WP1	Wrist jt synovitis (including impingement syndromes)
WA1	Wrist osteoarthritis (including avascular necrosis of lunate or capitate)
WL1	Carpal ligament tear
WT1	Extensor tenosynovitis/de Quervain's disease (see also — Forearm RT1)
WT2	Wrist ganglion
WT3	Flexor tenosynovitis
WH1	Wrist haematoma
WK1	Wrist laceration
WN1	Wrist nerve compression (including carpal tunnel syndrome)
WV1	Aneurysm of vessel near wrist
WZ1	Wrist pain undiagnosed

HAND

PF1	Bennett's #/disl
PF2	# Metacarpal
PF3	# Phalanx
PG1	Avulsion # phalanx
PQ1	Malunion finger #
PD1	Disl metacarpophalangeal or interphalangeal jt
PU1	Chronic jt instability of finger or thumb
PJ1	Spr metacarpophalangeal or interphalangeal jt
PP1	Finger jt chronic synovitis
PP2	Hand Reflex Sympathetic Dystrophy
PA1	Finger degenerative arthritis
PL1	Spr ulnar collateral ligament (skier's) thumb
PL2	Other hand or finger ligament tear
PT1	Trigger finger
PT2	Hand tendinitis
PR1	Ruptured finger tendon (including mallet finger)
PH1	Hand haematoma
PH2	Subungual haematoma/fingernail problem

PK1	Hand/finger laceration
PK2	Hand/finger blisters/contact dermatitis/ callus
PK3	Hand wart or other skin lesion
PI1	Hand/finger infection

CHEST

CF1	# Rib(s)
CF2	# Sternum
CS1	Stress # rib(s)
CC1	Costal cartilage/costochondral jt injury
CJ1	Sternoclavicular jt injury
CM1	Chest muscle str
CY1	Chest muscle trigger pts
CH1	Bruised ribs/chest wall (excluding sternum)
CH2	Bruised sternum
CO1	Pneumothorax (see Medical section for other lung and heart diseases)
CZ1	Chest pain undiagnosed

ABDOMEN

OO1	Abdominal trauma to internal organs
OM1	Abdominal muscle str
OY1	Abdominal muscle trigger pts or spasm or winding
OT1	Rectus abdominus tendinitis
OH1	Abdominal haematoma
OZ1	Abdominal pain undiagnosed (see Medical section for internal organ diseases)

THORACIC BACK

DF1	# Thoracic vertebrae
DG1	# Thoracic transverse or spinous process
DC1	Thoracic disc prolapse
DJ1	Thoracic facet jt spr
DP1	Chronic thoracic facet jt pain/stiffness
DA1	Thoracic facet jt degenerative arthritis
DY1	Thoracic back trigger pts
DM1	Thoracic extensor muscle str
DT1	Scheuermann's disease
DH1	Thoracic back haematoma
DK2	Upper back skin lesion
DB1	Thoracic scoliosis
DE1	Tumour, thoracic spine
DZ1	Thoracic pain undiagnosed

LUMBAR BACK (see also Buttock section)

LF1   # Lumbar vertebrae
LG1   # Lumbar transverse or spinous process
LS1   Stress # pars interarticularis
LQ1   Non-union lumbar fracture
LC1   Disc prolapse
LC2   Disc degeneration
LJ1   Lumbar facet jt spr
LP1   Chronic lumbar facet jt pain
LA1   Lumbar facet jt degenerative arthritis
LL1   Lumbar region ligament injury
LM1   Lumbar muscle str
LY1   Lumbar trigger pts
LH1   Lumbar haematoma
LK1   Lumbar laceration
LB1   Spondylolisthesis/lysis
LB2   Lumbar scoliosis
LB3   Other lumbar anomaly (e.g. spina bifida occulta, 'extra' lumbar vertebra)
LE1   Tumour, lumbar spine
LN1   Lumbar spinal injury
LN2   Lumbosacral nerve root impingement
LN3   Lumbar spinal canal stenosis
LN4   Lumbosacral nerve stretch/traction injury
LZ1   Lumbar pain undiagnosed

BUTTOCK (see related sections of Lumbar back, Hip and Groin and Thigh)

BF1   Fractured sacrum/coccyx
BG1   Avulsion # ischial tuberosity
BP1   Sacro-iliac jt pain (including spondyloarthropathies)
BP2   Sacrococcygeal jt pain
BM1   Gluteal muscle str/tear
BY1   Gluteal muscle or piriformis trigger pts
BT1   Ischial bursitis
BT2   Gluteal tendinitis/enthesopathy
BH1   Buttock haematoma
BK1   Buttock laceration
BI1   Ischial abscess
BN1   Piriformis syndrome (with sciatic nerve impingement)
BZ1   Buttock pain undiagnosed

HIP and GROIN

GF1   # Neck of femur
GF2   # Pelvic ring
GF3   # Ilium
GG1   Pelvic avulsion # (iliac spines and pubic rami) (see also Buttock — BG1 for ischial tuberosity)
GS1   Osteitis pubis
GS2   Stress # neck of femur
GS3   Pelvic bone stress #
GD1   Disl hip jt
GC1   Hip chondral lesion
GJ1   Hip jt spr/jar
GP1   Hip jt synovitis
GA1   Hip jt osteoarthritis/avascular necrosis
GA2   Slipped capital femoral epiphysis
GA3   Perthes' syndrome
GM1   Hip flexor (including Psoas) muscle str/tear
GM8   Groin muscle str (unspecified)
GY1   Groin soreness or trigger points
GT1   Adductor tendinitis/tear
GT2   Hernia/inguinal canal/conjoint tendon tear
GT3   Iliopsoas tendinitis/bursitis
GT4   Trochanteric bursitis
GH1   Haematoma, hip region
GH2   Testicular haematoma (see Medical section for other testicular conditions, e.g. MO2 and ME1)
GK1   Groin laceration or abrasion
GB1   Congenital dislocation hip
GI1   Groin rash/fungal infection
GI2   Hip jt infection
GO1   Damage to pelvic organ
GN1   Lateral cutaneous nerve of thigh entrapment (meralgia paraesthetica)
GZ1   Groin pain undiagnosed

THIGH

TF1   # Shaft of femur
TS1   Stress # shaft of femur
TM1   Hamstring str/tear
TM2   Quadriceps str/tear
TM3   Adductor muscle str/tear
TY1   Hamstring spasm/cramps/trigger pts
TY2   Quadriceps spasm/cramps/trigger pts/ wasting
TY3   Posterior thigh compartment syndrome

TH1 Haematoma of thigh/hamstrings ± myositis
TK1 Thigh laceration
TE1 Tumour, thigh region
TZ1 Thigh pain undiagnosed

KNEE (see also Lower Leg)
KF1 # Patella
KF2 Knee # intra-articular
KS1 Stress # patella
KD1 Disl patella
KD2 Disl knee
KU1 Knee jt chronic instability
KU2 Patella instability
KC1 Knee articular cartilage damage
KC2 Medial meniscus tear
KC3 Lateral meniscus tear
KC4 Knee osteochondritis (± loose bodies)
KC8 Knee joint cartilage injury (unspecified)
KJ1 Knee jt str/jar
KP1 Patellofemoral jt pain
KP2 Knee jt rheumatological condition/ atraumatic effusion
KP3 Knee synovial plica
KA1 Knee jt degenerative arthritis
KL1 Anterior cruciate ligament str/tear/rupture
KL2 Posterior cruciate ligament str/tear/rupture
KL3 Knee medial collateral lig str/tear/rupture (± Pellegrini-Stieda syndrome)
KL4 Knee lateral collateral ligament str/tear/ rupture
KL5 Knee arcuate ligament complex strain/tear
KT1 Iliotibial band syndrome
KT2 Patellar tendinitis (or Siding-Larsen-Johansson syndrome or fat pad impingement)
KT3 Hamstring tendinitis/bursitis
KT4 Osgood-Schlatter syndrome/tibial tuberosity pathology
KT5 Popliteus tendinitis
KT6 Prepatellar bursitis
KT7 Quadriceps tendinitis or suprapatellar bursitis

KR1 Ruptured patellar tendon
KH1 Knee haematoma (extra-articular)
KH2 Infrapatellar fat pad haematoma +/− bursitis
KK1 Lacerated knee
KB1 Bipartite patella
KB2 Discoid meniscus
KI1 Infected knee jt
KE1 Tumour, knee region
KO1 Complication of knee jt surgery
KZ1 Knee pain undiagnosed
KZ2 Knee jt haemarthrosis caused by internal derangement not yet diagnosed

LOWER LEG
QF1 # Tibia ± fibula
QF2 # Fibula
QS1 Stress # tibia
QS2 Stress # fibula
QD1 Disl superior tibiofibular jt
QP1 Baker's cyst (± rupture)
QJ1 Spr superior tibiofibular jt
QM1 Calf muscle str
QY1 Calf muscle cramps/spasm/trigger pts
QY2 Compartment syndrome
QY3 Lower leg delayed onset muscle soreness
QT1 Medial tibial stress syndrome ('shin splints')
QH1 Bruised shin
QH2 Calf haematoma
QK1 Lacerated skin
QK2 Lacerated calf
QI1 Lower leg soft tissue infection
QE1 Tumour, lower leg
QN1 Common peroneal nerve palsy (foot drop)
QV1 Deep venous thrombosis
QV2 Calf/ankle oedema
QV3 Varicose veins
QV4 Popliteal artery entrapment or arterial insufficiency (including claudication)
QZ1 Lower leg pain undiagnosed

ANKLE and HEEL (see also Foot section)
AF1 Pott's #
AG1 Chip/avulsion # ankle
AS1 Stress # Calcaneus or Talus

AD1   Disl ankle
AU1   Ankle instability
AC1   Ankle osteochrondral lesion (inc. talar dome)
AJ1   Ankle anterior capsule spr
AJ2   Inferior tibiofibular syndesmosis spr
AP1   Ankle jt synovitis (including meniscoid lesion)
AP2   Ankle reflex sympathetic dystrophy
AP3   Sinus tarsi syndrome
AA1   Ankle jt degenerative arthritis
AF2   # Talus or # calcaneus
AL1   Spr lateral collateral ligament ankle
AL2   Spr medial collateral (deltoid) ligament ankle
AT1   Achilles tendinitis/retrocalcaneal bursitis
AT2   Sever's disease
AT3   Ankle posterior impingement
AT4   Ankle anterior impingement
AT5   Ankle extensor tendinitis (incl. Tibialis Anterior)
AT6   Peroneal tendinitis or subluxation or disl
AT7   Tibialis posterior or flexor hallucis tendinitis (ankle)
AR1   Achilles tendon rupture
AH1   Ankle haematoma
AK1   Ankle laceration
AI1   Ankle infection
AE1   Osteoid osteoma (ankle)
AN1   Tarsal tunnel syndrome
AN2   Medial calcaneal nerve entrapment
AZ1   Ankle pain undiagnosed

FOOT (see also Ankle and Heel section)
FF1   # Tarsal bone (other than talus or calcaneus)
FF2   # Metatarsal(s)
FF3   # Phalanx (foot)
FG1   Foot avulsion #
FS1   Stress # midtarsal bone (navicular, cunieforms, cuboid)
FS2   Stress # metatarsal
FQ1   Non- or mal-union foot fracture
FD1   Disl toe
FD2   Disl jt(s) of foot (incl. Lisfranc injury)
FC1   Foot osteochondrosis (including Kohler's and Frieberg's disease)

FJ1   Spr foot jt
FJ2   Spr toe/'turf toe'
FP1   Sesamoiditis/1st metatarsophalangeal jt pain
FP2   Tarsal jt pain/synovitis
FP3   Metatarsalgia
FP4   Gout (foot)
FP5   Foot Reflex Sympathetic Dystrophy
FA1   1st metatarsophalangeal jt degenerative arthritis
FA2   Other foot jt degenerative arthritis
FL1   Foot ligament spr (including 'spring' ligament)
FM1   Foot muscle str
FY1   Foot muscle spasm/cramps/trigger pts
FT1   Plantar fasciitis/strain calcaneal spur
FT2   Foot extensor tendinitis
FT6   Cuboid syndrome or foot peroneal tendinitis
FT7   Tibialis posterior insertion tendinitis
FR1   Ruptured tibialis posterior tendon
FH1   Foot haematoma
FH2   Toenail problem/haematoma
FH3   Heel fat pad bruise
FK1   Foot laceration
FK2   Foot blistering/callus
FK3   Plantar wart
FB1   Tarsal coalition
FB2   Symptomatic accessory bone of foot
FB3   Foot deformity (including claw, hammer toes, bunions, 'club' foot)
FI1   Athlete's foot (tinea)
FI2   Foot cellulitis/infected ulcer
FE1   Osteoid osteoma (foot)
FN1   Morton's neuroma or Joplin's neuritis
FZ1   Foot pain undiagnosed

MULTIPLE AREAS
XU1   Generalized jt hypermobility
XP1   Widespread rheumatological jt condition
XY1   Fibromyalgia/multiple trigger pts
XY2   Generalized muscle spasticity/jt hypomobility
XK1   Rash or other dermatological condition
XB1   Congenital disease affecting musculoskeletal system (e.g. Marfan's syndrome, dystrophies)

MEDICAL ILLNESSES (see also Multiple Areas or specific body part which condition affects)

MI1 Otorespiratory infection (includes tonsillitis, otitis media, bronchitis) (for otitis externa see Head section — HI1)

MI2 Gastrointestinal infection (including food poisoning)

MI4 Systemic non-specific virus

MI5 Virus proven by serology (e.g. Epstein-Barr, hepatitis B, HIV)

MI6 Genitourinary infection

MI8 Infection, other

ME1 Non-musculoskeletal tumour (e.g. lymphoma)

MO1 Appendicitis

MO2 Urological including haematuria, varicocoele

MO3 Dental, eye, ear, nose or throat disease (not including ear and throat infections — use MI1 or trauma, see Head section)

MO8 Other surgical diagnosis

MN1 Neurological including epilepsy, migraine, coma (excluding head trauma, see Head section)

MV1 Cardiovascular

MX1 Environmental condition (including hyperthermia, barotrauma)

MX2 Condition due to drug use, overdose, poisoning

MX3 Asthma/allergy/hay fever/respiratory

MX5 Gynaecological

MX6 Psychological/psychiatric

MX7 Nutritional or haematological or enterological or endocrinological or immunological

MX8 Other medical diagnosis

MZ1 Tired athlete undiagnosed

MZ2 Other medical symptoms or signs, non-specific

MISCELLANEOUS

ZZ1 Paperwork (certificate, referral, prescriptions, etc.)

ZZ2 Pre-participation screening or precompetition or insurance medical examination

ZZ3 Immunizations or preparation for overseas travel

ZZ4 Advice regarding equipment (e.g. suitable footwear)

INDEX

(*f* = figure, *t* = table)